Oxford Specialist Handbooks

Addiction Medicine

Second Edition

Edited by

John B. Saunders

Professor and Consultant Physician in
Internal Medicine and Addiction Medicine,
University of Queensland, University of
Sydney, and St. John of God Health Care,
Wesley Health Care, and South Pacific
Private Hospital, Sydney, Australia

Katherine M. Conigrave

Professor in Addiction Medicine and
Public Health, Sydney Medical School,
University of Sydney, and Addiction
Specialist Royal Prince Alfred Hospital,
Sydney, Australia

Noeline C. Latt

Addiction Medicine Specialist, Royal
North Shore Hospital, and Sydney Medical
School, University of Sydney, Australia

David J. Nutt

Professor of Psychopharmacology,
Division of Brain Science, Department
of Medicine, Hammersmith Hospital,
Imperial College London, UK, and
Founding Chair of DrugScience, UK

With a Foreword by **Karl Mann**

E. Jane Marshall

Consultant Psychiatrist, Alcohol Service,
South London and Maudsley National
Health Service Trust and the National
Addiction Centre, Institute of Psychiatry,
King's College London, UK

Walter Ling

Integrated Substance Abuse Program
(ISAP), School of Medicine, University
of California at Los Angeles (UCLA),
and formerly Commissioner for
Narcotics and Dangerous Drugs
Commission, Los Angeles, CA, USA

Susumu Higuchi

Director, National Hospital
Organization Kurihama Medical and
Addiction Center and Director of the
World Health Organization (WHO)
Collaborating Centre on Research and
Training of Alcohol-Related Problems,
Kanagawa, Japan

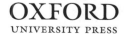

OXFORD
UNIVERSITY PRESS

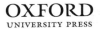

OXFORD
UNIVERSITY PRESS

Great Clarendon Street, Oxford, OX2 6DP,
United Kingdom

Oxford University Press is a department of the University of Oxford.
It furthers the University's objective of excellence in research, scholarship,
and education by publishing worldwide. Oxford is a registered trade mark of
Oxford University Press in the UK and in certain other countries

Published in the United States of America by Oxford University Press
198 Madison Avenue, New York, NY 10016, United States of America

British Library Cataloguing in Publication Data

Data available

Library of Congress Control Number: 2015955010

ISBN 978–0–19–871475–0

Printed and bound in China by
C&C Offset Printing Co. Ltd

Preface

Origin of this handbook

This Oxford Specialist Handbook *Addiction Medicine* is the result of many years, preparation by a group of colleagues who have been clinicians, teachers, and researchers in the addictive disorders field for many years. The present edition replaces the first edition, which was published in 2009. That had its origins in a series of lecture notes produced for the University of Sydney more than 30 years ago and clinical protocols developed separately and in collaboration by the authors and constantly updated over this time.

The scope of the second edition has been expanded in several ways. It now includes the behavioural addictions such as gambling and gaming and includes a broader range of psychoactive substances. It aims to be international in scope. The editors are drawn from the United Kingdom, Australia, United States of America, and Japan and there are contributing authors from 25 countries worldwide.

Our aim continues to be to offer a contemporary, broadly based, and clinically grounded text that summarizes the scientific basis and the practice of addiction medicine.

Evidence and practice

Evidence-based practice continues to increase in impact and there is an expectation that the approaches made in management of addictive disorders and the selection of medications, therapies, and overall strategy are based on scientific data from controlled clinical trials and other relevant studies. This applies in addiction medicine as much as it does in any other field of healthcare. We recognize, however, that as in other areas the scientific evidence base is not comprehensive, particularly when a person with an addictive disorder has different co-morbidities or when standard treatment approaches have been exhausted, or simply where the evidence base does not exist.

Our approach to the second edition has been to draw upon the following sources:

1. Current guidelines developed according to prevailing international standards for clinical guidelines and which include guidelines published by the World Health Organization, government departments of health and human services (e.g. from the US, UK, Australia, Japan, Germany, France, Sweden, and other Nordic countries) and those produced by relevant professional organizations, academies, and associations, which have been based on systematic reviews of the literature and undergone extensive processes of validation.
2. Publically accessible scientific evidence on the efficacy of treatment (with an emphasis on systematic reviews, meta-analyses, and

randomized controlled trials), supplemented by other scientifically valid clinical, psychometric, and epidemiological studies.

3. The clinical practice and experience of the authors, ensuring that the recommendations are appropriate to many clinical practice settings and, where there is an absence of evidence from scientific studies, that the material published here represents a distillation of practice which we consider to have international relevance and to be effective and safe.

It should be emphasized that in clinical practice, decisions need to be made often in the absence of scientific evidence. This may be simply because there is none or, very typically, the clinical situation develops beyond what scientific evidence exists or could ever realistically be expected to exist. In clinical practice, the focus is on the individual (or it may be on a couple, a family, or a group) and individuals and groups of individuals are infinitely variable. Scientific data will never exist to cover the multiple variations and eventualities in terms of comorbid disorders, previous treatment experience, lack of response to an approved treatment, individual patient or family preference, and some of the unknowns such as vital diagnostic or background information not being available at the time the clinical decision has to be made. These are the realities of the clinical life and in producing this handbook we recognize these as realities. Clinical practice is not merely the application of the evidence base to a particular person. Rather, the evidence base informs and guides clinical practice.

Who is this book for?

This handbook is intended as a concise and practical guide for students and practitioners of medicine, nursing, psychology, and other health professionals whose work brings them into contact with people with addictive disorders. In particular, it is designed for students and post-graduate trainees and fellows in addiction medicine, internal medicine, psychiatry, emergency medicine, pain management, gastroenterology, and general medical (family physician) practice. We believe it will be useful and relevant to nurses, particularly those working as specialists in addictive disorders, clinical psychologists, psychologists and counsellors, and social workers and for staff in specialist multidisciplinary agencies which provide help, support, and treatment for people with addictive disorders.

Why is this book important?

Alcohol and other substance use rank among the five top risk factors contributing to the global burden of disease. In recent years, there has been a rapid increase in non-substance forms of addiction such as gambling, internet gaming, and various other behavioural or 'process' addictions. In Asia and several other parts of the world, these latter disorders represent the biggest burden of ill health and social problems of any of the addictions. Substance use disorders can cause, mimic, underlie, or complicate a large number of medical and psychiatric conditions. All addictive disorders can cause immense personal suffering as well as harm and costs to families, communities, and society as a whole. Often this is not recognized. People with addictive disorders may be reticent about revealing their substance use and may not see its relevance. The fact that many patients use more than one substance, sometimes multiple substances and sometimes a substance used in combination with a behavioural addiction, further adds to the complexity. Making a correct diagnosis of an addictive disorder can greatly facilitate management, often avoid unnecessary tests and procedures, shorten hospital stays, and make both the clinician's and the patient's life easier. The ability to diagnose addictive disorders and initiate appropriate management is a responsibility for all health professionals. Historically, however, most have not been confident in their ability to diagnose and manage these disorders, as they have often been omitted from student and postgraduate courses. Recent years have seen the development of a comprehensive knowledge base and an understanding of the skill set and professional practice behaviour necessary for good professional practice in this field. Addiction medicine now has a range of approaches that compare in their effectiveness with those in other areas of medicine.

What is covered?

This handbook provides a practical guide to the management of people with addictive disorders. The first chapters provide important background information and summarize the overall principles of diagnosis and management. There follow several chapters on specific types or groups of psychoactive substance. The nature of the substances, their pharmacological properties, and the clinical syndromes that result are described, together with specific guidance on diagnosis and management which takes into account both their generic addictive properties and their specific pathophysiological ones. The latter part of the book is devoted to the management of specific groups of patients and people seen in specific settings, together with an account of relevant medicolegal and ethical issues. Following the main text, the final chapter comprises a series of practical tools, such as questionnaires, which assist in systematic clinical practice.

The handbook provides detailed guidelines on how to elicit a history of substance use and other addictive activities, together with ways of diagnosing the core clinical syndromes and the physical, psychiatric, and social disorders that may flow from them. It includes practical guides to brief intervention, management of intoxication, withdrawal management ('intoxication'), pharmacotherapies, and psychological therapies aimed at relapse prevention, together with an account of support approaches and the principles and practice of self-help.

Foreword

Addictions are highly prevalent. They cause harm to the afflicted and their families and are costly to society. While the clinical symptomatology in people suffering from addictions is similar around the world, treatment and prevention are not. Research in recent years has provided enormous progress in our understanding of these disorders resulting in a multitude of new evidence-based treatments. However, most conditions remain under-served and treatment approaches vary substantially around the world. All of these facts call for an up-to-date and universal appraisal of the current situation. A comprehensive overview on emerging strategies would be instrumental in this and could help to meet the actual challenges.

The *Oxford Specialist Handbook—Addiction Medicine* provides such a global perspective. The editors and authors are eminent researchers and clinicians in our field. They come from a large variety of areas such as Australia, Asia, Europe, and North America. While the first edition of the textbook in 2009 already provided a very broad view on addictions and ways of dealing with them, the revised version gives an update of current concepts and newly emanating strategies. Important extensions have been made providing several new chapters and incorporating new fields such as gambling and gaming as examples for behavioural addictions. The handbook now also includes evidence-based recommendations from the most recent clinical guidelines from around the world.

Prof. John Saunders of Sydney and Queensland Universities and his colleagues are to be congratulated for their enormous efforts. Their book *Addiction Medicine* gives the necessary detail to understand and respond to actual problems in an individual patient. The long standing teaching experience of most of its authors has resulted in a text which is well structured and easy to read and thus offers information not only to the professional but also to the patient and his or her family and to others in search of some quick and valid information on the troublesome but also fascinating field of addiction.

Karl Mann, MD
Emeritus Professor of Addiction Research
Central Institute of Mental Health
Medical Faculty Mannheim
University of Heidelberg
Germany

Contents

Acknowledgements *xi*
Editors and authors *xii*
Contributors *xv*
Symbols and abbreviations *xxiii*

1	The nature of addictive disorders	1
2	Epidemiology and prevention	7
3	Pharmacology and pathophysiology	31
4	The scope of intervention	55
5	Establishing the diagnosis	67
6	Acute care	85
7	Ongoing management of substance use disorders	103
8	Tobacco	119
9	Alcohol	151
10	Cannabis	235
11	Opioids	249
12	Pain and opioids	295
13	Benzodiazepines and the other sedative-hypnotics	307
14	Psychostimulants	327
15	Hallucinogens and dissociative drugs	355
16	Other drugs	363
17	Polysubstance use	391
18	Injecting drug use	407
19	Gambling	427
20	Gaming	441
21	Other addictive disorders	449
22	Psychiatric co-morbidity	461

23 Specific clinical situations	483
24 Special populations	493
25 Substance use and specific healthcare settings	545
26 Legal and ethical issues	563
27 Resources	589

Index 629

Acknowledgements

In presenting this handbook to our colleagues and students, we would in turn like to thank our own teachers. We wish to dedicate this handbook to those who helped influence and shape our own professional careers, including Griffith Edwards, Alex Paton, David Graham-Smith, Markku Linnoila, Boris Tabakoff, Harding Burns, Norman Sartorius, and Harold Kalant.

We would like to acknowledge the contribution of our colleagues in reviewing and helping finalize parts of this book, and in particular, Robert Batey, Glenys Dore, Anne Lingford Hughes, Martin Raw and Carina Walters.

We would particularly like to highlight and acknowledge the key role played by Corinne Lim, Editorial Officer, throughout the preparation of this book.

Editors and authors

Professor John B. Saunders MA, MB BChir, MD, FRCP, FRACP, FAChAM, FAFPHM is a Professor and Consultant Physician in Internal Medicine and Addiction Medicine, with appointments at the University of Queensland and University of Sydney in Australia, and with several private hospital groups. He graduated in pharmacology and then medicine from the University of Cambridge, and undertook specialist medical training in internal medicine, gastroenterology, and addiction medicine. His career as a clinician, service director, researcher, and academic in addictive disorders extends back over 40 years, and he has extensive clinical experience in hospital and community settings. He has been a member of many state and federal Australian government committees, including the Australian National Council on Drugs (2001–2007). He has worked with the World Health Organization since 1981 and was responsible for developing the AUDIT Questionnaire. He is a member of the WHO's Expert Advisory Panel on Substance Abuse and the ICD 11 Substance-Related and Addictive Disorders Workgroup. He has published four books and over 330 scientific papers, reviews, and book chapters. He is an ISI highly cited scientist.

Professor Katherine M. Conigrave MB BS (Hons), PhD, FAFPHM, FAChAM is Senior Staff Specialist in Addiction Medicine and Public Health Medicine at Royal Prince Alfred Hospital and Concord Hospital in Sydney, Australia, where she provides clinical care in out-patient, general hospital, and residential detoxification and rehabilitation settings. She has been involved for many years in training medical and other health professionals through Sydney Medical School, University of Sydney, and through training sessions for practising health professionals. Professor Conigrave's research has a focus on detection and early intervention for alcohol problems, and on improving implementation of evidence-based practice in prevention and treatment of substance use disorders. Over the past 15 years, Professor Conigrave has also worked in partnership with Aboriginal communities in urban, regional, and remote Australia. She has over 100 peer-reviewed academic publications, has received the Senior Scientist Award for the Australasian Professional Society for Alcohol and Other Drugs, and has acted as a consultant to the World Health Organization on alcohol screening and brief intervention. She is on the Editorial Advisory Boards of *Alcohol and Alcoholism*, and of *Addiction Science & Clinical Practice*.

Dr Noeline C. Latt MBBS, MPhil, MRCP, FAChAM is a Senior Staff Specialist in Addiction Medicine at Royal North Shore Hospital, Clinical Lecturer at the University of Sydney, and a Foundation Fellow of the Chapter of Addiction Medicine, Royal Australasian College of Physicians. She is a Physician and Addiction Medicine Specialist with extensive experience in clinical pharmacology and internal medicine. After a period as a medical director in the Pharmaceutical Industry, she became a Specialist in Addiction Medicine at Westmead Hospital and as Director of the Ryde and Hornsby Drug & Alcohol Service she developed a drug and alcohol unit offering consultation liaison services and teaching programmes in alcohol and substance use disorders. Her research interests have focused on platelet monoamine oxidase activity, and treatment of alcohol and substance use disorders, alcoholic liver disease and hepatitis C in injecting drug users, and substance-induced psychosis.

Professor David J. Nutt MA, MB BChir, DM, FRCP, FRCPsych, FMedSci is Consultant Psychiatrist and the Edmund J. Safra Professor of Neuropsychopharmacology in the Division of Brain Science, Department of Medicine, Hammersmith Hospital, Imperial College London. Here he uses a range of brain imaging techniques to explore the causes of addiction and other psychiatric disorders and to search for new treatments. He has published over 400 original research papers, a similar number of reviews and book chapters, eight government reports on drugs, and 28 books, including one for the general public, *Drugs: Without the Hot Air*, that won the Transmission Prize in 2014. He is currently the President of the European Brain Council and Founding Chair of DrugScience (formerly the Independent Scientific Committee on Drugs (ISCD)). Previously he has been president of the British Association of Psychopharmacology, the British Neuroscience Association, and the European College of Neuropsychopharmacology. He broadcasts widely to the general public both on radio and television. In 2010, *The Times Eureka* science magazine voted him one of the 100 most important figures in British science, and the only psychiatrist in the list. In 2013, he was awarded the John Maddox Prize from Nature/Sense about Science for standing up for science.

Dr E. Jane Marshall MB BCh BAO MRCP (Ireland) FRCPsych is a Consultant Psychiatrist in Alcohol Services at the South London and Maudsley NHS Foundation Trust and Senior Lecturer in the Addictions at the National Addiction Centre, Institute of Psychiatry, King's College London. She trained in Psychiatry at St Patrick's Hospital, Dublin, and St Bartholomew's and the Maudsley Hospitals in London. Her clinical work is currently focused on a specialist out-patient and in-patient alcohol service, and also a service for addicted healthcare professionals. She is lead clinician for the MSc programme in Addiction at the Institute of Psychiatry. Research interests include the evaluation of treatment for alcohol problems in specialist and generalist settings and, in particular, and treatment for addicted healthcare professionals. Dr Marshall acts as a medical supervisor and examiner for the General Medical Council and as a medical advisor for the General Dental Council. Within the Royal College of Psychiatrists she is Co-Director of Flexible Training, and a member of the executive committee of the Faculty of the Addictions and Psychiatrists' Support Service Committee. Dr Marshall has contributed to national guidelines, and has been a member of a number of Working Parties, including the Royal College of Physicians Working Party on Alcohol in the General Hospital (2001); an Alcohol Concern Research Forum (2002); and a Department of Health Working Group on Alcohol-related Brain Damage (2007).

Professor Walter Ling, MD, is Professor of Psychiatry and the Founding Director of the Integrated Substance Abuse Programs (ISAP) at UCLA, one of the foremost substance abuse research groups in the US. He is board certified in neurology and psychiatry, is active in research and clinical work, and has been listed in 'Best Doctors in America'. Dr Ling's research in opiate pharmacotherapy provided pivotal information for the approval of buprenorphine and naltrexone. His current focus of research includes abuse and dependence on methamphetamine, cocaine, heroin, and prescription opiates; opiate-induced hyperalgesia, treatment of pain in opiate-maintained patients, including those treated with buprenorphine, and the role of buprenorphine in the management of pain in these patients. Dr Ling is a fellow of the American Academy of Neurology; he has served as Commissioner for the Narcotics and Dangerous Drugs Commission, Los Angeles County, California; and a consultant on narcotics for the World Health Organization, the United Nations, and the U.S. Department of State. As Principal Investigator of NIDA's Clinical Trial Network's Pacific Region Node, Dr Ling has extended ISAP's research beyond the US to China, Southeast Asia and the Middle East.

Professor Susumu Higuchi, MD, PhD is Director of the National Hospital Organization Kurihama Medical and Addiction Center and Director of the World Health Organization (WHO) Collaborating Centre on Research and Training of Alcohol-Related Problems in Yokosuka, Japan. He has principally worked on genetics and clinical studies of alcohol use disorders, especially on the implications of genetic variations of alcohol-metabolizing enzymes on pharmacokinetic and pharmacodynamic effects, organ damage, and alcohol-use disorders. He has published more than 220 scientific papers in well-recognized international journals, and more than 400 papers in domestic journals. He is President of the International Society for Biomedical Research on Alcoholism (ISBRA), congress president in 2014, a director of the International Society of Addiction Medicine, and President of the Japanese Society of Alcohol-Related Problems. For the past decade, he has worked on alcohol policy and programmes, and has served as chair or a member of many committees of the Japanese government. He has contributed to WHO initiatives to reduce global alcohol-related harm as a member of the WHO Expert Advisory Panel and a delegate of the Japanese government to the World Health Assembly and other WHO meetings. Clinically, he has been the leading psychiatrist in the field of alcohol dependence and behavioural addiction, especially Internet addiction in Japan.

Contributors

Professor Peter Anderson
Professor, Substance Use
Policy and Practice, Institute of
Health and Society, Newcastle
University, UK
*Chapter 2: Epidemiology and
prevention*

**Associate Professor Sawitri
Assanangkornchai**
Associate Professor, Epidemiology
Unit, Faculty of Medicine, Prince
of Songkla University, Songkhla,
Thailand
*Chapter 4: The scope of intervention;
Chapter 24: Special populations*

**Associate Professor Tatiana
Balachova**
Associate Professor of Pediatrics,
University of Oklahoma Health
Sciences Center, Department
of Pediatrics and the Center
on Child Abuse and Neglect,
University of Oklahoma,
Oklahoma City, USA
Chapter 24: Special populations

Professor Robert Batey
Professor in Hepatology and
Addiction Medicine, University
of Sydney and Flinders University
South Australia; Consultant
Physician, Department of
Medicine, Alice Springs Hospital,
Australia
*Chapter 9: Alcohol;
Chapter 11: Opioids;
Chapter 18: Injecting drug use*

Dr Jenny Bearn
Consultant in Addiction Psychiatry,
Maudsley Hospital, South London
and Maudsley NHS Foundation
Trust, UK
Chapter 16: Other drugs

Dr James Bell
Consultant Physician, Addictions
Clinical Academic Group, Kings
Health Partners, London, UK
Chapter 12: Pain and opioids

**Associate Professor Renee
Bittoun**
Associate Professor, Sydney
Medical School, Faculty of
Medicine, University of Sydney;
Director, Smoking Cessation
Unit, and Smokers Clinics, Brain
and Mind Research Institute,
Camperdown, NSW, Australia
Chapter 8: Tobacco

**Associate Professor
Yvonne Bonomo**
Associate Professor and Consultant
Physician in Addiction Medicine,
St Vincent's Hospital Melbourne,
and Departments of Medicine
and Paediatrics, University of
Melbourne, VC, Australia
Chapter 24: Special populations

Dr Henrietta Bowden-Jones
Consultant Psychiatrist, Director
and Lead Clinician, National
Problem Gambling Clinic and
Honorary Senior Lecturer, Division
of Brain Science, Imperial College,
London, UK
Chapter 19: Gambling

Dr Jonathan Brett
Consultant in Clinical
Pharmacology, Toxicology and
Addiction Medicine, Royal Prince
Alfred Hospital and Clinical
Lecturer, University of Sydney;
Sydney, NSW, Australia
*Chapter 16: Other drugs;
Chapter 25: Substance use and spe-
cific healthcare settings*

Dr Adam Brodie

Consultant Addiction Psychiatrist, Clinical Director Addictions (NHS Lanarkshire), Coathill House, Coatbridge, UK
Chapter 16: Other drugs

Professor Katherine M. Conigrave

Professor in Addiction Medicine and Public Health, Sydney Medical School, University of Sydney, and Addiction Medicine Specialist, Royal Prince Alfred Hospital, Sydney, Australia
Chapter 2: Epidemiology and prevention; Chapter 8: Tobacco; Chapter 9: Alcohol; Chapter 11: Opioids; Chapter 16: Other drugs; Chapter 18: Injecting drug use; Chapter 24: Special populations; Chapter 26: Legal and ethical issues

Professor Jason P. Connor

Professor of Clinical Psychology, Discipline of Psychiatry and Centre for Youth Substance Abuse Research, The University of Queensland, Royal Brisbane and Women's Hospital, QLD, Australia
Chapter 17: Polysubstance use

Professor Ilana B. Crome

Emeritus Professor of Addiction Psychiatry, Keele University, UK; Honorary Consultant Psychiatrist, South Staffordshire and Shropshire Healthcare NHS Foundation Trust, Staffordshire, UK; Honorary Professor, Queen Mary University, London, UK; Senior Research Fellow, Imperial College London, UK
Chapter 24: Special populations

Professor H. Valerie Curran

Professor of Psychopharmacology, Clinical Psychopharmacology Unit, Brain Sciences, University College London, UK
Chapter 10: Cannabis

Professor Louisa Degenhardt

NHMRC Principal Research Fellow and Professor, National Drug and Alcohol Research Centre, University of New South Wales, Sydney, NSW, Australia
Chapter 2: Epidemiology and prevention

Associate Professor Glenys Dore

Clinical Director and Senior Staff Specialist Psychiatrist, Northern Sydney Drug & Alcohol Service, and Clinical Associate Professor, University of Sydney, Sydney Medical School - Northern; Royal North Shore Hospital, Sydney, NSW, Australia
Chapter 5: Establishing the diagnosis; Chapter 6: Acute care; Chapter 14: Psychostimulants; Chapter 22: Psychiatric co-morbidity; Chapter 24: Special populations; Chapter 26: Legal and ethical issues

Professor Colin Drummond

Professor of Addiction Psychiatry, Addictions Department, National Addiction Centre, Institute of Psychiatry, Psychology and Neuroscience, King's College London, South London and Maudsley NHS Foundation Trust, UK
Chapter 9: Alcohol

Associate Professor Gerald F. X. Feeney

Consultant Physician and Medical Director, Alcohol and Drug Assessment Unit, Princess Alexandra Hospital and the Centre for Youth Substance Use Research, The University of Queensland, Brisbane, QLD, Australia
Chapter 17: Polysubstance use

Dr Emily Finch

Clinical Director and Consultant Addiction Psychiatrist, South London and Maudsley NHS Foundation Trust, and Addictions Clinical Academic Group, London, UK
Chapter 26: Legal and ethical issues

Mr Bradley Freeburn

Drug and Alcohol and Mental Health Unit, Aboriginal Medical Service, Redfern, NSW, Australia
Chapter 24: Special populations

Dr Sanju George

Consultant in Addiction Psychiatry, Birmingham and Solihull Mental Health NHS Foundation Trust, Birmingham, UK; and now Senior Consultant in Psychiatry, Rajagiri Hospital, Aluva, Kerala, India
Chapter 19: Gambling

Professor Paul Haber

Clinical Director, Drug Health Services, Sydney Local Health District; Professor and Head, Discipline of Addiction Medicine, Sydney Medical School, University of Sydney, Camperdown, NSW, Australia
Chapter 18: Injecting drug use

Professor Wayne Hall

Director, University of Queensland Centre for Youth Substance Abuse Research and the University of Queensland Centre Clinical Research, The University of Queensland, Brisbane, QLD, Australia; and National Addiction Centre, King's College London, UK
Chapter 2: Epidemiology and prevention

Associate Professor Takayuki Harada

Associate Professor, Department of Psychology, Faculty of Human Sciences, Mejiro University, Tokyo, Japan
Chapter 21: Other addictive Disorders

Professor Susumu Higuchi

Director, National Hospital Organization Kurihama Medical and Addiction Center and Director of the World Health Organization (WHO) Collaborating Centre on Research and Training of Alcohol-Related Problems, Kanagawa, Japan
Chapter 19: Gambling
Chapter 20: Gaming
Chapter 21: Other addictive disorders

Dr Ralph Hingson

Director, Division of Epidemiology and Prevention Research, National Institute on Alcohol Abuse and Alcoholism, National Institutes of Health, Bethesda, MD, USA
Chapter 26: Legal and ethical issues

Professor Kazutaka Ikeda

Professor, Addictive Substance Project, Tokyo Metropolitan Institute of Medical Science, Tokyo, Japan
Chapter 3: Pharmacology and pathophysiology

Dr Marianne Jauncey

Medical Director, Sydney Medically Supervised Injecting Centre, NSW, Australia
Chapter 24: Special populations

Associate Professor Stephen Jurd

Consultant Psychiatrist and Associate Professor, Discipline of Psychological Medicine, Sydney Medical School, University of Sydney, and Director of Training in Psychiatry, Macquarie Hospital, North Ryde, NSW, Australia
Chapter 7: Ongoing management of substance use disorders

Ms Shivani R. Khan

Pre-doctoral Fellow, Department of Epidemiology, College of Public Health and Health Professions & College of Medicine, University of Florida, Gainesville, FL, USA
Chapter 16: Other drugs

Dr Yasunobu Komoto

Chief of Psychiatry, National Hospital Organization, Kurihama Medical and Addiction Center, Yokosuka City, Japan
Chapter 19: Gambling

Dr Noeline C. Latt

Addiction Medicine Specialist, Royal North Shore Hospital and Sydney Medical School, University of Sydney, NSW, Australia
Chapter 5: Establishing the diagnosis; Chapter 6: Acute care; Chapter 9: Alcohol; Chapter 11 Opioids; Chapter 13: Benzodiazepines and the other sedative-hypnotics; Chapter 23: Specific clinical situations; Chapter 26: Legal and ethical issues

Professor Michael Levy

Professor, Medical School, College of Medicine, Biology and Environment, Australian National University, Acton, ACT, Australia
Chapter 24: Special populations

Ms Corinne Lim

Editorial Officer, 'Addiction Medicine'; formerly The Australian Financial Review, Fairfax Media Limited, Australia
Chapter 24: Special populations

Professor Walter Ling

Integrated Substance Abuse Program (ISAP), School of Medicine, University of California at Los Angeles (UCLA), and formerly Commissioner for Narcotics and Dangerous Drugs Commission, Los Angeles, CA, USA
Chapter 14: Psychostimulants

Professor Anne Lingford-Hughes

Professor of Addiction Biology, Centre for Neuropsycho-pharmacology, Division of Brain Sciences, Department of Medicine, Imperial College London, UK
Chapter 22: Psychiatric co-morbidity

Dr E. Jane Marshall

Consultant Psychiatrist, Alcohol Studies Services, South London and Maudsley National Health Service Trust and the National Addiction Centre, Institute of Psychiatry, King's College London, UK
Chapter 6: Acute care; Chapter 9: Alcohol

Professor Ross McCormick
Consultant in Addiction Medicine, and Associate Dean (Postgraduate Studies), Faculty of Medical and Health Sciences, University of Auckland, New Zealand
Chapter 24: Special populations

Ms Satoko Mihara
Chief, Department of Clinical Psychology, National Hospital Organization Kurihama Medical and Addiction Center, Kanagawa, Japan
Chapter 21: Other addictive disorders

Professor Hisatsugu Miyata
Professor, Department of Psychiatry, Jikei University School of Medicine, Tokyo, Japan
Chapter 8: Tobacco

Dr Hideki Nakayama
Chief of Psychiatry, National Hospital Organization Kurihama Medical and Addiction Center, Yokosuka, Japan
Chapter 20: Gaming

Dr Tim Neumann
Senior Specialist, Department of Anaesthesiology and Intensive Care Medicine, Charité-Universitätsmedizin Berlin, Germany
Chapter 25: Substance use and specific healthcare settings

Dr Daisuke Nishizawa
Addictive Substance Project, Tokyo Metropolitan Institute of Medical Science, Tokyo, Japan
Chapter 3: Pharmacology and pathophysiology

Professor David J. Nutt
Professor of Psychopharmacology, Division of Brain Science, Department of Medicine, Hammersmith Hospital, Imperial College London, UK, and Founding Chair of DrugScience (formerly the Independent Scientific Committee on Drugs), UK
Chapter 3: Pharmacology and pathophysiology; Chapter 9: Alcohol; Chapter 10: Cannabis; Chapter 11: Opioids; Chapter 13: Benzodiazepines and the other sedative-hypnotics; Chapter 14: Psychostimulants; Chapter 15: Hallucinogens and dissociative drugs; Chapter 19: Gambling

Dr Sally Porter
Regional Clinical Director, Turning Point Substance Misuse Services, Croydon, UK
Chapter 26: Legal and ethical issues

Professor Richard Saitz
Chair, Professor of Community Health Sciences and Medicine, Department of Community Health Sciences, Boston University Schools of Public Health and Medicine, Boston, MA, USA
Chapter 9: Alcohol; Chapter 25: Substance use and specific healthcare settings

Dr Hiroshi Sakuma
Chief of Psychiatry, National Hospital Organization Kurihama Medical and Addiction Center, Kanagawa, Japan
Chapter 20: Gaming

Dr Taku Sato
Psychiatrist, National Hospital Organization Kurihama Medical and Addiction Center, Treatment of Pathological Gambling and Research Section, Kanagawa, Japan
Chapter 19: Gambling

Professor John B. Saunders

Professor and Consultant Physician in Internal Medicine and Addiction Medicine, University of Queensland, University of Sydney, and St. John of God Health Care, Wesley Health Care, and South Pacific Private Hospital, Sydney, NSW, Australia
Preface; Chapter 1: The nature of addictive disorders; Chapter 3: Pharmacology and pathophysiology; Chapter 4: The scope of intervention; Chapter 5: Establishing the diagnosis; Chapter 6: Acute care; Chapter 7: Ongoing management of substance use disorders; Chapter 9: Alcohol; Chapter 10: Cannabis; Chapter 11: Opioids; Chapter 13: Benzodiazepines and the other sedative-hypnotics; Chapter 21: Other addictive disorders; Chapter 22: Psychiatric co-morbidity; Chapter 23: Specific clinical situations; Chapter 25: Substance use and specific healthcare settings; Chapter 26: Legal and ethical issues

Professor Andrew J. Saxon

Professor, Department of Psychiatry & Behavioural Sciences; Director, Addiction Psychiatry Residency Program, University of Washington; WA, USA; Director, Center of Excellence in Substance Abuse Treatment and Education (CESATE), VA Puget Sound Health Care System, Seattle, WA, USA
Chapter 11: Opioids

Professor Janie Sheridan

Professor, School of Pharmacy and Centre for Addiction Research, Faculty of Medical and Health Sciences, The University of Auckland, New Zealand
Chapter 16: Other drugs

Dr Iain Smith

Consultant in Addiction Psychiatry, Kershaw Unit, Gartnavel Royal Hospital, Glasgow, UK
Chapter 16: Other drugs

Professor Claudia Spies

Professor, Department of Anaesthesiology and Intensive Care Medicine, Charité-Universitätsmedizin Berlin, Germany
Chapter 25: Substance use and specific healthcare settings

Professor Tim Stockwell

Director, Centre for Addictions Research of BC and Professor, Department of Psychology, University of Victoria, BC, Canada
Chapter 2: Epidemiology and prevention

Professor John Strang

Professor of Addiction Psychiatry and Head of Department, National Addiction Centre, Institute of Psychiatry, King's College London, UK
Chapter 18: Injecting drug use

Dr Pierluigi Struzzo

General Practitioner, Head of the Research and Innovation Area of the Regional Centre for the Training in Primary Care, Department of Life Sciences, University of Trieste, Italy
Chapter 25: Substance use and specific healthcare settings

Assistant Professor Catherine Woodstock Striley

Assistant Professor, Department of Epidemiology, College of Public Health and Health Professions, College of Medicine, University of Florida, Gainesville, FL, USA
Chapter 16: Other drugs

Professor David Taylor

Director of Pharmacy and Pathology, South London and Maudsley NHS Foundation Trust, Pharmacy Department, Maudsley Hospital, London, UK
Chapter 16: Other drugs

Associate Professor Peter Thompson

Senior Staff Specialist, Emergency Medicine, and Associate Professor, Rural Clinical School, Rockhampton, QLD, Australia
Chapter 6: Acute care

Dr Sue Wilson

Senior Research Fellow, Centre for Neuropsychopharmacology, Division of Brain Sciences, Imperial College London, UK
Chapter 23: Specific clinical situations

Dr Adam R. Winstock

Consultant Psychiatrist and Addiction Medicine Specialist, South London and Maudsley NHS Trust; Senior Lecturer, King's College London, UK
Chapter 15: Hallucinogens and dissociative drugs;
Chapter 16: Other drugs

Professor Kim Wolff

Professor in Addiction Science, King's College London, Institute of Pharmaceutical Science, London, UK
Chapter 24: Special populations

Professor George Woody

Professor, Department of Psychiatry, University of Pennsylvania and Treatment Research Institute, Philadelphia, PA, USA
Chapter 11: Opioids

Professor Nicholas Zwar

Professor of General Practice, School of Public Health and Community Medicine, University of New South Wales, Sydney, NSW, Australia
Chapter 8: Tobacco

Symbols and abbreviations

5HIAA	5-hydroxyindoleacetic acid
5HT	5-hydroxytryptamine (serotonin)
AA	Alcoholics Anonymous
Ab	antibody
ACE	angiotensin-converting enzyme
ADH	antidiuretic hormone
ADHD	attention deficit hyperactivity disorder
ADIS	Alcohol and Drug Information Service, Australia
AFP	alpha-fetoprotein
Ag	antigen
AIDS	acquired immune deficiency syndrome
ALP	alkaline phosphatase
ALT	alanine aminotransferase
Anti-HBc	anti-hepatitis B core antibody
Anti-HBe	anti-hepatitis B e antibody
Anti-HBs	anti-hepatitis B surface antibody
Anti-HCV	hepatitis C antibody
APTT	activated partial thromboplastin time
ARND	alcohol-related neurodevelopment disorder
ASI	Addiction Severity Index
ASPD	antisocial personality disorder
ASSIST	Alcohol, Smoking and Substance Involvement Screening Test
AST	aspartate aminotransferase
ATS	amphetamine-type stimulants
AUD	alcohol use disorder
AUDIT	Alcohol Use Disorders Identification Test
AWS	Alcohol Withdrawal Scale
BAC	blood alcohol concentration
BAP	British Association of Psychopharmacology
BBV	blood-borne virus
BP	blood pressure

BWS	Benzodiazepine Withdrawal Scale
CAGE	acronym for four alcoholism screening questions
CAL	chronic airways limitation (also known as COPD)
CB_1	cannabinoid receptor type 1
CB_2	cannabinoid receptor type 2
CBD	cannabidiol
CBT	cognitive behavioural therapy
CCF	congestive cardiac failure
CDT	carbohydrate deficient transferrin
CIDI	Composite International Diagnostic Interview
CIWA-Ar	Clinical Institute Withdrawal Assessment for Alcohol-revised
CIWA-B	Clinical Institute Withdrawal Assessment for Benzodiazepines
CK-MB	creatine kinase isoenzyme
C-L	consultation-liaison
CNS	central nervous system
CO	carbon monoxide
COMT	catechol-O-methyltransferase
COPD	chronic obstructive pulmonary disease
CPK	creatine phosphokinase
CRP	C-reactive protein
CT	computed tomography
CVS	cardiovascular system
CXR	chest X-ray
DA	dopamine
DALY	disability-adjusted life year
DD	differential diagnosis
DDS	Delirium Detection Scale
DIS	Diagnostic Interview Schedule
DNA	deoxyribonucleic acid
DSM-IV	*Diagnostic and Statistical Manual*, 4th edition
DSM-5	*Diagnostic and Statistical Manual*, 5th edition
DTs	delirium tremens
DVLA	Driver and Vehicle Licensing Agency (UK)
ECG	electrocardiogram

ECHO	echocardiogram
ED	emergency department
EDOU	emergency department observation unit
EEG	electroencephalogram
EMR	Eastern Mediterranean region
ERCP	endoscopic retrograde cholangiopancreatography
ESR	erythrocyte sedimentation rate
EU	European Union
EUC	electrolytes, urea, and creatinine
FAE	fetal alcohol effects
FAS	fetal alcohol syndrome
FASD	fetal alcohol spectrum disorder
FBC	full blood count
FCTC	World Health Organization Framework Convention on Tobacco Control
FLAGS	Feedback, Listen, Advice, Goals, Strategies (acronym for core elements of brief intervention)
fMRI	functional magnetic resonance imaging
FTQ	Fagerström tolerance questionnaire
GABA	gamma aminobutyric acid
GAD	generalized anxiety disorder
GCS	Glasgow coma scale
GDP	gross domestic product
GGT	gamma-glutamyl transferase
GHB	gamma hydroxybutyrate
GI	gastrointestinal
GIT	gastrointestinal tract
GP	general practitioner
HADS	Hospital Anxiety and Depression Scale
Hb	haemoglobin
HBcAb	hepatitis B core antibody
HBeAg	hepatitis B e antigen
HBsAg	hepatitis B surface antigen
HBV	hepatitis B virus
Hct	haematocrit
HCV	hepatitis C virus

HCV Ab	anti-hepatitis C antibody
HDL	high-density lipoprotein
HDV	hepatitis D virus
HIV	human immunodeficiency virus
HoNOS	Health of the Nation Outcome Scales
h	hour(s)
ICD 10	International Classification of Diseases, 10th revision
IDU	injecting drug user
IgG	immunoglobulin G
IgM	immunoglobulin M
IM	intramuscular
INR	international normalized ratio
IV	intravenous
IU	international units
IUGR	intra-uterine growth retardation
K, Special K	ketamine
kg	kilogram(s)
L	litre(s)
LDL	low-density lipoprotein
LFT	liver function test
LSD	lysergic acid
MAOI	monoamine oxidase inhibitor
mcg	microgram(s)
MCV	mean corpuscular volume
MDMA	methylenedioxymethamphetamine
MEOS	microsomal ethanol oxidizing system
min	minute(s)
mL	millilitre(s)
mmHg	millimetres of mercury
MRI	magnetic resonance imaging
MRSA	meticillin-resistant *Staphylococcus aureus*
MSE	Mental State Examination
NA	Narcotics Anonymous
NAD	nicotinamide adenine dinucleotide (oxidized form)

NADH	nicotinamide adenine dinucleotide (reduced form)
NARS	Nicotine Assisted Reduction to Stop
NaSSA	noradrenaline and specific serotonergic agent
ng	nanograms(s)
NMDA	N-methyl-D-aspartate
NMS	neuroleptic malignant syndrome
nocte	at night
NRT	nicotine replacement therapy
NSAID	non-steroidal anti-inflammatory drug
OCD	obsessive–compulsive disorder
OST	opioid substitution treatment
OTC	over-the-counter
PAT	Paddington alcohol test
PAE	prenatal alcohol exposure
PCP	phencyclidine
PCR	polymerase chain reaction
PET	positron emission tomography
PFC	prefrontal cortex
PMA	para-methoxyamphetamine
PO	per oral (orally)
PPP	purchasing power parity
PRN	pro re nata (as required)
PTSD	post-traumatic stress disorder
RASS	Richmond Agitation-Sedation Scale
RIMA	reversible inhibitor of monoamine oxidase A
RNA	ribonucleic acid
RTA	road traffic accidents
SAD	social anxiety disorder
SADQ	Severity of Alcohol Dependence Questionnaire
SAM	substance abuse module
SC	subcutaneous
SCAN	Schedules for Clinical Assessment in Neuropsychiatry
SDS	Severity of Dependence Scale
sec	second(s)

SF14, SF36, SF96	quality of life questionnaires
SIDS	sudden infant death syndrome
SE	side effects
SL	sublingual
SNRI	serotonin and noradrenaline reuptake inhibitor
SNS	social networking service
SODQ	Severity of Opiate Dependence Questionnaire
SSRI	selective serotonin reuptake inhibitor
STI	sexually transmitted infection
$t_{1/2}$	half-life
TB	tuberculosis
TCA	tricyclic antidepressant
TFT	thyroid function test
THC	tetrahydrocannabinol
TIA	transient ischaemic attacks
TSH	thyroid-stimulating hormone
TTFC	time to first cigarette
TWEAK	Tolerance, Worried, Eye-opener, Amnesia, K/ Cut-down
UN	United Nations
UNODC	United Nations Office on Drugs and Crime
VDRL	venereal diseases research laboratory test for syphilis
VSM	volatile solvent misuse
VTA	ventral tegmental area
WBC	white blood cell count
WE	Wernicke's encephalopathy
WHO	World Health Organization
WPR	Western Pacific Region

Chapter 1

The nature of addictive disorders

What are addictive disorders? 2

What are addictive disorders?

The nature of addictive disorders

'Addictive disorders' is the term applied to disorders and conditions that occur as a result of the single or repeated use of a psychoactive substance which has dependence-inducing or 'addictive' properties. It includes acute intoxication from an addictive substance, even though there may be no features of dependence or addiction present. More broadly, it encompasses disorders which have arisen as a result of repetitive use of a dependence-inducing substance or an addictive activity.

Included in the latter are various forms of gambling and gaming. Many behavioural addictions have developed with advances in technologies that encourage highly repetitive actions by the participant. These technologies may be applied to gambling, gaming, social communication, and the use of sexual images (pornography).

There is debate about the extent to which normal, unremarkable, and generally healthy human activities such as exercise, work, and the consumption of food can develop into an addiction.

Addictive disorders can potentially occur in any human being. Studies on human volunteers show that there are common responses seen in all individuals. However, there are also individual differences in susceptibility, which may reflect genetic and other familial factors, experience of adverse events in early life (such as child abuse) and trauma at any stage, the presence of underlying psychiatric disorders, and less commonly, underlying physical disorders. Some of the predisposing factors have a small percentage effect on susceptibility; others such as genetic influences and abuse in childhood appear as strong influences.

Any predisposing factors need to be identified when information about addictive disorders is being elicited, and there is an increasing expectation that clinicians and agencies practising in the field of addictive disorders will have a keen understanding of the relevance of abusive and traumatic experiences in the genesis of these disorders.

Characteristics of addictive substances

The pharmacological properties of substances that have dependence potential may be summarized as follows:

- They have pleasurable effects, which the individual finds cause euphoria and excitement, and also may relieve dysphoric states.
- The effects are rapid in onset and therefore particularly reinforcing.
- With repeated exposure, tolerance occurs as a neuroadaptive response. More of the substance is required to produce the desired effect.
- The reward system is profoundly re-set such that normal human pleasures and rewards become ineffective; this is referred to as the 'hijacking' of the reward circuitry by the psychoactive substance. The person affected descends into a state of low mood, low motivation, and inactivity.

- Other neuroadaptive changes result in hyperactivity of excitatory circuits, which typically results in exaggerated responses to triggers for psychoactive substance use and also a general increase in anxiety, with the development of agitation and irritability.
- In many cases, withdrawal symptoms occur on cessation or reduction in the use of the psychoactive substance, and this can lead to strong cravings and therefore a return to further substance use.

Predisposing factors

Although substance use and addictive disorders can develop in any human (being subject only to repeated exposure to a psychoactive substance with dependence or abuse properties or a repetitive behaviour with addictive characteristics), some people are more susceptible to develop these disorders than others.

In addition, there are certain environments which predispose to the development of repetitive patterns of substance use or addictive behaviours.

The development of an addictive disorder reflects the complex interplay between the person and his/her individual characteristics, the setting (and the broader social and environmental influences), and the addictive characteristics of the particular substance or behaviour.

Individual predisposing factors

Among individual predisposing factors that are recognized as increasing the risk of having an addictive disorder are the following:

- Genetic (inherited) predisposing factors—although there are many areas of the human genome which appear to influence susceptibility to substance disorders, gene variations associated with a greater likelihood of such a disorder than average include (i) those involved in neurotransmission including opioids, dopamine, serotonin (5-HT), and gamma aminobutyric acid (GABA); (ii) genes coding for response to substances including taste and the extent of the effect; (iii) those coding for cell microstructure; and (iv) those coding for signal transduction within neurons. Some genetic variants reduce susceptibility, notably gene variants coding for aldehyde dehydrogenase, which results in an unpleasant and adverse reaction to alcohol in many Asian populations.
- Adverse experiences in childhood including:
  - physical abuse
  - sexual abuse
  - severe emotional abuse (e.g. abandonment in early life).
- Trauma in youth or adult life, which may include:
  - combat trauma in the armed forces
  - traumatic experiences occurring in the civilian forces such as the Police, Fire Brigade, Ambulance, and Rescue Services
  - severe domestic and interpersonal violence.

- Underlying psychiatric disorders:
  - Several psychiatric disorders are associated with predisposition to substance use and addictive disorders—but not all.
  - The strongest associations are with bipolar disorder, schizophrenia, and post-traumatic stress disorder, and there are weaker associations with various types of depression and anxiety disorder. These latter disorders, being numerically more common, are operational for a higher proportion of people who have substance disorders than bipolar disorder and schizophrenia which are rarer conditions.
  - Some mental health disorders have not historically been associated with predisposition to substance use and addictive disorders. These include obsessive–compulsive disorder, anorexia nervosa, and autistic spectrum disorder; however, over the past generation, disorders such as these which seemed not to be predisposing conditions are now more evident in this capacity.
  - Several personality disorders, especially those in Cluster B are associated with substance dependence.
- Several *physical disorders* predispose to substance dependence, especially when repeated or chronic pain is prominent or, rather less commonly, when the person experiences persistent disability or chronic ill health.

Social influences and mechanisms

Substance use occurs in a context and there are many environmental influences which increase the likelihood of unhealthy substance use developing and substance use disorders emerging. These include broad environmental factors such as the following:

- Cultural characteristics, especially in relation to social sanctions to drink alcohol, smoke cigarettes, engage in psychoactive substance use, and gambling.
- Characteristics of the subculture, be it a sports group, youth group, and musical interests.
- The physical availability of the substance in terms of outlets, e.g. licensed outlets for purchase of alcohol, tobacconist shops or supermarkets, nightclubs, and the extent of the illicit drug market.
- Economic availability of psychoactive substances such as the cost of a substance in relation to disposable income, and the extent of taxation.
- The legal status of a substance—in general when a substance is illicit there is a reduction in its availability, with fewer people taking up its use; however, there may be opposite forces at play including making use of an illicit substance attractive and seductive to potential users and also the impact of criminalizing people who are simply in possession of an illicit substance for personal consumption.

More restricted environmental factors include the following:

- Peer pressure—from elder siblings, friends, and members of certain social groups and sporting clubs.
- Advertising of products (especially alcohol and tobacco) but including broader promotional activities to keep the particular substance (most commonly alcohol and tobacco) in public view.

Psychological mechanisms

Psychoactive substance use and repetitive behaviours such as gaming perform a function for the individual in many ways and several psychological mechanisms are operative. These include the following:

- Classical (Pavlovian) conditioning, where an association is established between a situation or experience which acts as a trigger or 'cue'. A conditioned association is established between the cue and the response, which results in urges and craving occurring even when the substance itself is unavailable.
- Operant conditioning, where the response such as the effect of substance use acts as a reinforcer (or alternatively a deterrent), and thus influences subsequent use of that substance.
- Social learning influences, which emphasize the importance of the social environment as well as interior milieu in the response to a psychoactive substance and the subsequent appetite for that substance.

Neurobiological mechanisms

In the last two decades, much information has been gained into the mechanisms by which a pattern of repetitive use of a psychoactive substance or an addictive activity becomes progressively stereotyped. Psychoactive substances with addictive properties interact with several neurocircuits in the extended amygdala located in the midbrain and lower forebrain and subserve the following mechanisms:

- Reward mechanisms, including the sensation of pleasure and reinforcement of substance use because of this.
- Alertness, which is subserved by a balance between the excitatory and sedating neural mechanisms involving principally glutamate and GABA respectively.
- Salience, which reflects the priorities in a person's life ranging from essential survival responses through to optional activities; these also influence the extent of the incentive of a particular substance or activity and the consequent motivation to respond by either substance use or another activity.
- The behavioural control pathways which seek to dampen more primitive responses (as listed earlier), through pathways which course from the prefrontal gyrus of the frontal lobe to the lower forebrain and midbrain nuclei, dampening down the more primitive responses (listed earlier) through a degree of cognitive control. Substance dependence diminishes the activity in these behavioural control pathways to result in a resetting of activity which is persistent.

The outcome of these physiological changes is that a persistent internal driving force to use and continue use of the substance or engage in the repetitive behaviour is established. This is little influenced by external circumstances and activities, instead becoming more determined by a persistent physiological need to continue substance use. At a certain point when substance use is discontinued, the person may develop a withdrawal state consisting of unpleasant physical and psychological symptoms, the relief of which requires continued use of that substance.

Neuroplasticity phenomena occur—in large measure induced by excessive amounts of released dopamine—and cause the 'rewiring' of these brain circuits such that the drive to use the substance becomes enduring, typically lasting for some years, and maybe the lifetime of the individual.

Some conclusions

Substance use and addictive disorders may start out as elaborations of unremarkable, repetitive human behaviour. However, with the passage of time, profound neurobiological changes to key neurocircuits develop and have the effect of perpetuating substance use through an internal drive that the person may experience (as craving) or continue that behaviour or activity in a way which is fairly unthinking and may be subconscious.

Fig. 1.1 illustrates in a simplistic way how substance dependence and addictions come about and also identifies the individual and social influences on the development of repetitive use, the addictive process itself, and the multiple complications which may arise, affecting the person's physical health, brain functioning, psychological status, and social condition.

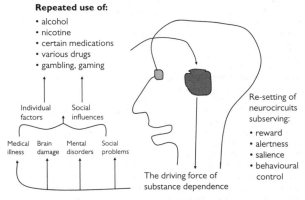

Fig. 1.1 A schematic representation of substance dependence and addiction.

Epidemiology and prevention

Epidemiology of substance use 8
Reducing harmful substance use through
  policy and prevention 26

Epidemiology of substance use

Alcohol

Burden of alcohol

Alcohol is the world's fifth leading risk factor for ill health and premature death. In 2010, it was responsible for the loss of 97 million years of healthy life lost (97 million disability-adjusted life years (DALYs)).

- Alcohol can cause harms both to the drinker and to those around them. The DALYs estimate includes some harms to people other than the drinker (e.g. injuries), but not all harms (e.g. the impact of alcohol during pregnancy). At present, it is not possible to fully quantify the magnitude of harms to others.
- *Gender*: men experience 3.5 times more alcohol-attributable loss of functional life than women.
- *Age*: the burden of death and disability from alcohol use is greatest in those 50 years of age and older; however, in relative terms, alcohol contributes the greatest percentage of all healthy life years lost in those aged 35–64 years.
- *Wealth*: in general, people living with lower income experience more harm per litre of alcohol consumed than people living with higher income.
- The greatest burden of alcohol use globally is in Eastern Europe and Central Asia (Fig. 2.1). The lowest burden is in the Eastern Mediterranean region, due to high rates of abstinence.

Trends since 1990

After correcting for population structure, the burden of disease and death from alcohol use worldwide has fallen between 1990 and 2010 (from 1636 to 1444 DALYs per 100,000 people) (Table 2.1). This decrease has been observed among both men and women. However, over the same period the percentage of all years of healthy life lost (as DALYs) that are attributable to alcohol use has increased from 2.9% to 3.9% (an increase of 32.5% in DALYs). This increase can be explained by an increase in alcohol consumption among low-income countries. Alcohol use is strongly correlated, up to a certain level, with the gross domestic product of a country (adjusted for purchase power parity) and there has been a shift in the deaths and burden of disability from infectious diseases to non-communicable diseases among low-income countries.

Table 2.1 Healthy life years lost from all causes that are attributable to alcohol or tobacco (expressed as DALYs/100,000 people)

	Total	Female	Male
Alcohol	1444	653	2234
Tobacco	2385	1195	3683

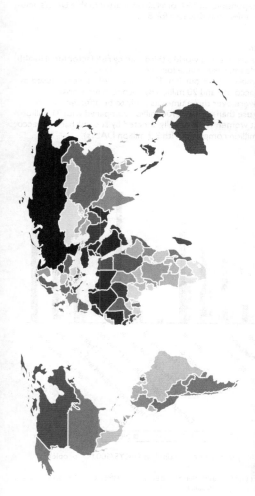

Fig. 2.1 (See also Colour plate 1.) Healthy life years lost because of alcohol use globally in 2010 (as age-adjusted DALYs per 100,000 people attributed to alcohol).

Reproduced with permission from Institute for Health Metrics and Evaluation (IHME), GBD Compare. Copyright (2013), with permission from the University of Washington. Available from http://vizhub.healthdata.org/gbd-compare (Accessed 1 February 2014.)

Impacts on health

Alcohol use exerts its adverse health effects on the drinker most often through mental and behavioural disorders (18% of all alcohol-attributable DALYs), and then next through cardiovascular and circulatory diseases (15%), and then cirrhosis of the liver (15%) (Fig. 2.2). Non-communicable diseases were responsible for 59% of all alcohol-attributable DALYs, injuries for 33%, and infectious diseases for 8%.

Tobacco

Burden of tobacco

In 2010, tobacco use was the world's third leading risk factor for ill health and premature death, responsible for 157 million DALYs.
- *Second-hand smoke*: of this burden, 137 million DALYs were caused by first-hand tobacco use and 20 million by second-hand smoke.
- *Gender*: men were over three times as likely to be affected by first-hand tobacco use than women (106 million compared with 31 million DALYs), whilst women were equally affected by second-hand tobacco smoke (10.0 million compared with 9.9 million DALYs).

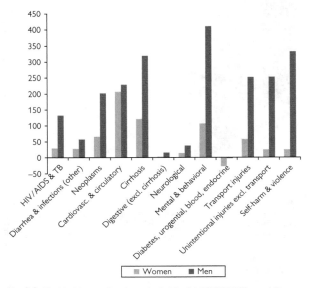

Fig. 2.2 Healthy life years lost from alcohol (as DALYS/100,000 people) by disorder.
Source data from Institute for Health Metrics and Evaluation (IHME). GBD Compare. Copyright (2013), University of Washington.

- *Age*: the DALYs attributable to tobacco were highest for infants aged 0–27 days, followed by those aged 70–79 years. However, as a percentage of all healthy years of life lost, tobacco had the largest impact on those aged 60–69 years.
- *Region*: the greatest burden of tobacco use globally was in Eastern Europe and Central Asia (Fig. 2.3). Western, Eastern, and Central sub-Saharan Africa experienced the least harms caused by tobacco smoking, with this region having a comparatively lower prevalence of smoking when compared to other regions.

Trends since 1990

After correcting for population structure, the burden of tobacco use decreased between 1990 and 2010 (from 3379 to 2385 DALYs per 100,000 people) (Table 2.1), and this decrease was observed among both men and women. However, while the absolute burden of disease decreased, the percentage of all DALYs attributable to tobacco use increased from 6.1% to 6.3% (an increase of 4%); this increase was only observed for men and not for women.

Impacts on health

Tobacco use exerted its adverse health effects most often through cardiac and circulatory diseases (42% of all tobacco-attributable DALYs), then through chronic respiratory diseases or neoplasms (each representing 20% of tobacco-attributable DALYs), lower respiratory infections and other common infectious diseases (7%), diabetes (2%), and tuberculosis (1.3%; Fig. 2.4).

Illicit drug use

'Illicit drug use' refers to the non-medical use of a variety of drugs (see Table 2.2) including:

- cannabis
- various psychostimulants, including amphetamine-type stimulants (e.g. methamphetamine, amphetamine, and MDMA)
- cocaine
- opioids (including heroin and prescribed opioid pain killers)
- miscellaneous drugs which are used for their psychoactive effects, such as gamma-hydroxybyrate (GHB), ketamine, and d-lysergic acid (LSD).

Some of the miscellaneous drugs are used by comparatively fewer persons and/or in a limited number of countries, and both the nature and extent of harm is less well documented. Accordingly this section focuses upon the four major drug classes.

Worldwide, between 167 and 315 million adults use illicit drugs each year.

How common is illicit drug use?

The illegality of illicit drug use makes it difficult to quantify the levels of use. Illicit drug users are 'hidden' and thus difficult to identify, and even when they can be located and interviewed, they may conceal their drug use. The United Nations Office on Drugs and Crime (UNODC) publishes estimates of the prevalence of past-year illicit drug use, but the

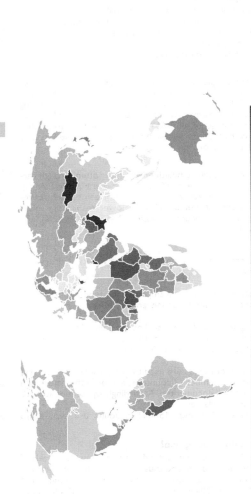

Fig. 2.3 (See also Colour plate 2.) Healthy life years lost because of tobacco use globally in 2010 (as age-adjusted DALYs lost attributable to tobacco per 100,000 people).

Reproduced with permission from Institute for Health Metrics and Evaluation (IHME). GBD Compare. Copyright (2013), with permission from the University of Washington. Available from http://vizhub.healthdata.org/gbd-compare. (Accessed 1 February 2014.)

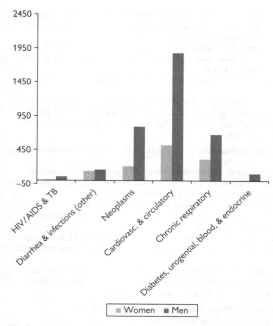

Fig. 2.4 Healthy life years lost from tobacco (as DALYS/100,000 people) by disorder.

Table 2.2 Some major drug classes	
Cannabis	A generic term for psychoactive preparations (e.g. marijuana, hashish, and hash oil) derived from the *Cannabis sativa* plant
Amphetamines	A class of sympathomimetic amines with powerful stimulant action on the central nervous system (CNS)
Cocaine	An alkaloid CNS stimulant that is derived from the coca plant
Opioids	Derivatives of the opium poppy (such as heroin and morphine), their synthetic analogues, and endogenous compounds which act upon the opioid receptors in the brain. They relieve pain and produce a sense of euphoria, as well as cause stupor, coma, and respiratory depression

quality of the data used varies dramatically from country to country. However, it remains the only source of estimates for some countries.
  Cannabis is the most widely used illicit drug.

- In 2011, around 180 million adults (range 129–230 million; 3.9% of the global population aged 15–64 years) were thought to have used cannabis in the past year.
- Europe generally has lower rates of use than Australia, Canada, and the US.
- Limited data from low- and middle-income countries suggest that with exceptions (e.g. South Africa), rates of cannabis use are much lower in Africa, Asia, and South America than in Europe and English-speaking countries.

The term 'amphetamine type stimulants' (ATS) refers to a range of drugs related to amphetamine.

- Methamphetamine and amphetamine are the major ATS available worldwide, followed by 3,4- methylenedioxymethamphetamine (MDMA, or 'Ecstasy' as it is commonly known).
- The diversion of prescription stimulant drugs such as dexamphetamine has been reported, but this is less of a problem than illicitly produced ATS.
- Use appears to be increasing in many parts of the world, but many countries have scant or no data on the prevalence, routes, and forms of use.
- Problematic use of amphetamines appears more prevalent in East and South East Asia, North America, South Africa, New Zealand, Australia, and a number of European countries.

Cocaine is reportedly the least widely used of the illicit drugs:

- Around 17 million adults were thought to have used cocaine in 2011 (range 14–21 million), with use heavily concentrated in North America, Latin America, and some European countries.
- The reported prevalence of cocaine use in other high-income countries is typically much lower than that in the US.

Illicit opioids are the third most common form of illicit drug use.

- Globally, illicit opioids—including pharmaceutical opioids—were estimated to have been used by around 32 million people in 2011 (range 28–36 million).
- Opiates, such as heroin and opium, were estimated to have been used by around 16 million (range 13–20 million).
- Most research on the epidemiology and natural history of opioid use is with dependent users. The distinction between 'use' and 'dependence' is an important one that is briefly discussed in the following section.

Use versus problematic use

Not all drug use causes harm to users. Efforts have been made on an international level to classify the behaviours or symptoms associated with use that does cause problems to the user. This problematic use is the target for most interventions.

The International Classification of Diseases (ICD) distinguishes between 'harmful drug use' and 'drug dependence'.

- Harmful drug use is defined by clear evidence that the substance use is responsible for physical (e.g. organ damage) and psychological harm (e.g. drug-induced psychosis).
- In ICD 10, drug dependence requires the presence of three or more of the following: a strong desire to take the substance; impaired control over the use; a withdrawal syndrome on ceasing or reducing use; tolerance to the effects of the drug; requiring larger doses to achieve the desired psychological effect; a disproportionate amount of the user's time is spent obtaining, using, and recovering from drug use; and the user continuing to take the drug(s) despite associated problems (see p. 68).

It is difficult to estimate the number of people who make up the 'hidden population' of dependent or problematic drug users, the group who probably suffer the bulk of problems related to their drug use and who are in most need of treatment. The preferred strategy is to look for convergence in estimates produced by a variety of different methods. These approaches are of two broad types, *direct* and *indirect*.

- Direct methods attempt to estimate the number of illicit drug users in representative samples of the population.
- Indirect estimation methods attempt to use information from known populations of illicit drug users (such as those who have received treatment, or died of overdoses) to estimate the size of the hidden population of illicit drug users.

In the 2010 Global Burden of Disease (GBD 2010) study, mathematical modelling was used to estimate country, region, and global prevalence of drug dependence, taking into account data gaps and uncertainties.

- Opioid and amphetamine dependence were the two most common forms of illicit drug dependence globally (15.4 million and 17.2 million estimated cases, respectively; Fig. 2.5).
- There were 13.1 million cannabis-dependent and 6.9 million cocaine-dependent persons.
- Males formed the majority of cases (64% each for cannabis and amphetamines, and 70% each for opioids and cocaine).

Geographical variation

The geographic distribution of cases of dependence reflects variations in prevalence and country populations (Fig. 2.5).

- An estimated 57.8% of amphetamine-dependence cases were found across the Asian regions (9.3 million cases), but the highest prevalence estimates were for Southeast Asia (0.42%) and Australasia (0.41%).
- North America High-Income (NA-HI) was estimated to contain 13.4% of cannabis-dependent people, with a high prevalence (0.6%).
- The highest levels of cocaine dependence were estimated in NA-HI (0.53%) and Latin America.
- Australasia had among the highest levels of opioid dependence (0.46%) although the largest populations were in East and South Asia.
- Estimated levels of illicit drug dependence were generally lower in African and Asian regions.

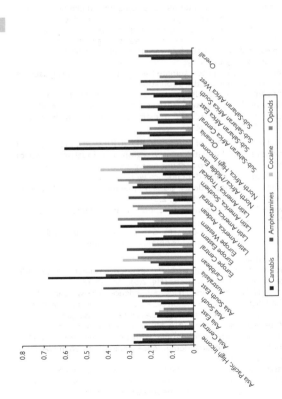

Fig. 2.5 Age- and sex-standardized prevalence of cannabis, amphetamine, cocaine, and opioid dependence in 2010 (% by GBD region).

The harms related to drug use

The adverse health effects of illicit drug use can be considered under four headings:

- *Acute toxic effects*, including overdose
- *Acute effects of intoxication*, such as injuries and violence
- *Dependence* on the drug
- *Adverse health effects* of sustained regular use, such as chronic physical disease (e.g. cardiovascular disease and cirrhosis), blood-borne infections, and mental disorders.

Measuring the impact of disease: DALYs

Measuring the impact of disease was revolutionized in 1993, when the World Bank provided estimates of causes of global disease burden using the DALY. For each disease or injury, DALYs are calculated as the sum of years lost due to premature mortality and the years of lost health due to disability. One DALY represents the loss of one healthy year of life. The DALY is a standard metric that allows the mortality and morbidity of different diseases to be compared.

GBD 2010 evaluated the nature and quality of evidence for illicit drug use as a risk factor for many health outcomes. In order for risk-outcomes to be included in the comparative risk assessment component, a number of eligibility criteria needed to be met to justify a causal inference between drug use and the harm, namely, evidence: of an association, that drug use preceded the outcome, and that excluded reverse causation and confounding.

Unfortunately, very few putative consequences of illicit drug use have the quality or quantity of data to be eligible for inclusion. Many studies report associations, but it has been difficult to determine if these are *causal* relationships.

Available literature suggests that:

- the risks of cannabis use are much more modest than those of other illicit drugs, largely because cannabis does not produce fatal overdoses and it cannot easily be injected
- the quality of evidence varies widely across drug type and health outcomes: there are more data on cannabis use from prospective population-based cohorts, and for the drugs, more data from selected treatment cohorts
- the magnitude of the effect is often poorly quantified.

Globally, greatest burden was due to opioids, and least to cannabis. Fig. 2.6 shows geographic variation in the burden of disease attributed to specific drug types.

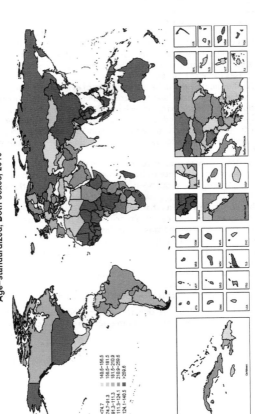

Opioid use disorders DALYs per 100,000 people,
Age-standardized, Both sexes, 2010

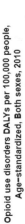

Fig. 2.6 (See also Colour plate 3.) a) Opioid-dependence DALYs per 100,000 persons. b) Amphetamine-dependence DALYs per 100,000 persons.
c) Cocaine-dependence DALYs per 100,000 persons. d) Cannabis-dependence DALYs per 100,000 persons.
Reproduced from *The Lancet*, 382(9904), Degenhardt L, Whiteford H, Ferrari AJ, Baxter A, Charlson F, Hall W, et al., The global burden of disease attributable to illicit
drug use and dependence: Results from the GBD 2010 study, pp. 1564–74, Copyright (2013), with permission from Elsevier.

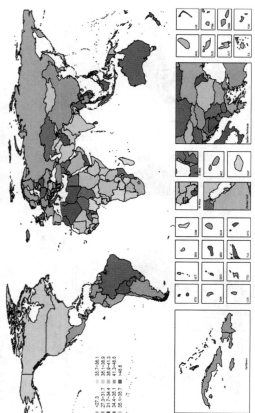

Amphetamine use disorders DALYs per 100,000 people,
Age-standardized, Both sexes, 2010

Fig. 2.6 (Contd.)

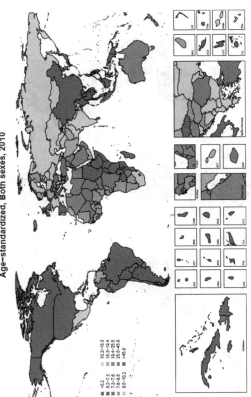

Cocaine use disorders DALYs per 100,000 people,
Age-standardized, Both sexes, 2010

Fig. 2.6 (Contd.)

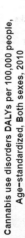

Cannabis use disorders DALYs per 100,000 people,
Age–standardized, Both sexes, 2010

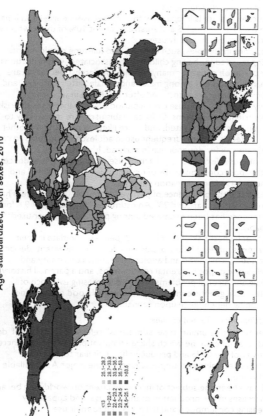

<13
13–22.4
23.2–24.5
24.5–25.1
25.1–28.7
28.7–33.9
33.3–35.7
35.7–53.5
>53.5

Fig. 2.6 (Contd.)

The natural history of illicit drug use

Cannabis

The best data on the prevalence of cannabis use and its correlates come from the US, Canada, and Australia, where the levels of use appear to have been the highest. Generally, rates of use have been higher among young people in high-income countries, but rates of recreational use may be increasing among young people in low- and middle-income countries. Studies suggest the following:

- Cannabis use typically begins in the mid to late teens, and is most prevalent in early adulthood.
- Most cannabis use is irregular, with very few users engaging in long-term daily use. In the US and Australia, about 10% of those who ever use cannabis become daily users.
- Transitions in life roles, such as entry into full-time employment, getting married, or having children, are associated with reductions in or cessation of use for many people. The largest decreases are seen in cannabis use among males and females after marriage, and especially during pregnancy and after childbirth in women.
- Heavy (daily) cannabis use over a period of years increases the risks of experiencing problems. Daily cannabis users are more likely to be male, less well educated, and more likely to regularly use other drugs. Weekly or more frequent use in adolescence appears to carry significant risk for dependence in early adulthood.
- Cannabis use disorders (e.g. harmful use or abuse or dependence) are the most common forms of drug problems after alcohol and tobacco, based on population surveys.
- In Australia, the prevalence of past-year cannabis use disorders has been estimated at around 2%. An estimated lifetime risk of 9% for dependence has been estimated among persons who ever used cannabis.
- Those at highest risk of developing dependence initiate in their early teens, have a history of poor academic achievement, deviant behaviour in childhood and adolescence, non-conformity and rebelliousness, poor parental relationships, and a parental history of drug and alcohol problems. There is increasing evidence of a substantial genetic contribution to the likelihood of using and developing dependence upon cannabis.

Psychostimulants: ATS and cocaine

The term 'amphetamine type stimulants' refers to a range of drugs related to amphetamine which share stimulant properties that increase the activity of the CNS and produce effects similar to adrenalin.

- Methamphetamine and amphetamine are the major ATS available worldwide.
- ATS have been the subject of increased attention worldwide because of increases in the production of these drugs, and apparently increasing consumption and harm related to their use.

- Cocaine use has typically been more concentrated in regions where the coca plant is grown or those regions nearby.
  - The US has had by far the greatest problem with cocaine (and 'crack' cocaine) worldwide, particularly in the late 1980s and early 1990s.
  - More recently, there have been increases in the availability and use of cocaine in Western Europe.
  - The use of cocaine is much less common in Asia, Oceania, and African countries.

Psychostimulants are most commonly taken orally, intranasally, the vapours inhaled (smoking), or injected.

Dependence has been associated with mental health, physical, occupational, relationship, financial, and legal problems.

- It is likely that most of the harm related to psychostimulant use occurs among those who have developed dependence on the drug.
- Users with a history of other drug and mental health problems may be at greater risk of developing dependence.
- There has been concern about associations between psychostimulant use and HIV risk via risky sexual behaviour.

Both route of administration and forms used are important factors affecting the nature and extent of associated harms.

- The increase in use of the crystalline form of methamphetamine, for example, has been associated with increased problems related to dependent and binge patterns of use.
- Smoking and injecting have also been associated with a higher risk of dependent or problematic use than swallowing or snorting of the drug.
  - There is evidence that 'smoking' crystal methamphetamine and 'crack' cocaine also carries harms related to the inhalation of possibly toxic chemicals, and possibly blood-borne virus transmission through the sharing of smoking implements.

Few studies have documented the natural history of psychostimulant use. Our current understanding derives largely from cross-sectional studies. US prospective studies have suggested that relapse following treatment is common. The concentration of such research in samples from treatment and prison populations makes it difficult to draw inferences about amphetamine use in the general population, since most users never come into contact with either treatment or law enforcement agencies. As a result, little is known about the aetiology and consequences of psychostimulant use that does not come to the attention of police or treatment services.

Opioids

Cohort studies indicate that dependent opioid users may continue to use opioids for decades, with periods of use interrupted by time spent in treatment, prison, and, for some, extended periods of abstinence. These studies have largely been conducted in high-income countries (particularly North America and Western Europe), though there are increasing studies in Asia. Nonetheless, the evidence available suggests that opioid-dependent persons may have difficulty controlling their use for significant portions of their lives. Data from the US have suggested that one in four people who use opioids illicitly may develop dependence upon them.

Although opioids are used by far fewer people than cannabis, opioid *dependence* may be more common globally than cannabis dependence, and carries a significantly greater mortality risk. Multiple reasons exist for this including:

- drug overdose risk, suicide, accidents, and trauma
- the consequences of blood-borne viral infections such as HIV and hepatitis C virus (HCV), and generally poorer physical health contribute to shorter life expectancy and poorer quality of life for this group.

Although in the past heroin has typically been the primary form of opioid dependence, in many countries (particularly in the US, South Asia, and Eastern Europe) dependence upon pharmaceutical opioids is an increasing problem.

Summary and implications

Although we have some data on the scope of the problem, there is much that we do not understand about the extent, context, and natural history of illicit drugs, particularly in low- and middle-income countries where drug use may be increasing. We still have much to learn about the extent of drug use and the nature and magnitude of harms that may result.

Despite these gaps, several things are clear:

- There is considerable and possibly increasing demand for illicit drugs in the general population
- Demand for and consumption of drugs is dynamic
- Drug supply may both respond to and drive demand for drugs
- Responses to drug use must reflect these drivers.

Benzodiazepines and other sedative-hypnotics

Benzodiazepine use is common in many countries around the world. Iatrogenic dependence is relatively common, and deliberate misuse is regularly reported, with associated overdoses, injuries, and crime.

In the developed world, benzodiazepines usually require a prescription for supply, whereas in some developing countries they are available over the counter in pharmacies. The rise of Internet drug sales has also led to increased avenues for access to non-prescribed benzodiazepines.

The data on prevalence of self-reported benzodiazepine use worldwide is limited, and monitoring is challenging given the wide range of anxiolytic and sedative hypnotic medications available. Large quantities of benzodiazepines are legally produced and global consumption of anxiolytics was estimated at around 21 billion defined daily doses in 2009 (S-DDD: defined daily dose for statistical purposes). In Europe, anxiolytic use was estimated to be 42 S-DDD per 1000 inhabitants per day in 2007–2009, and for sedatives it was 22 S-DDD in 2006–2008.

Use of benzodiazepines without a prescription is relatively common, and these medications are both sold on the 'black market' or shared. Among 15- to 16-year-old students in EU member states or Norway, 2–15% had at some stage used 'tranquillizers or sedatives' without a doctor's prescription in 2011.

The prescription rate for benzodiazepines across Medicaid has grown steadily in the US, from 8.0 million in 1991 to 17.1 million in 2009. In Manitoba province, Canada, 6.1% of the respondents to a population-based survey reported benzodiazepine use in 2011–2012. Rates of prescription and use in other countries, such as Australia, have fluctuated, and the pattern of use may mirror both the reinforcing properties of the medications available, and the regulatory mechanisms controlling availability.

Inhalants

A wide range of inhalants are misused, ranging from household products to petrol (fuel) and nitrous oxide. Only limited data are available on their levels of use or misuse. However, we know that inhalant misuse is more common in the young (under 30 years), and in subpopulations experiencing disadvantage. Up to 12% of UK adults report inhalant misuse at some point in their life, and 1–2% of 13–15-year-olds report it. Nitrous oxide has become a popular inhalant of misuse in the UK with 6% of 16–24-year-olds reporting use.

While females are as likely to use inhalants, males are more likely to die as a result of their use. Increased prevalence of inhalant misuse has been reported in rural and remote regions (e.g. in the US or Australia).

Further reading

Center on Addiction and Substance Abuse (2007). *You've Got Drugs! V: Prescription Drug Pushers on the Internet*. A CASA White Paper, National Center on Addiction and Substance Abuse (CASA). New York, NY: Columbia University. Available at: http://www.casacolumbia.org/addiction-research/reports/youve-got-drugs-perscription-drug-pushers-internet-2008

Degenhardt L, Whiteford H, Ferrari AJ, et al. (2013). The global burden of disease attributable to illicit drug use and dependence: results from the GBD 2010 study. *Lancet* 382:1564–74.

European Monitoring Centre for Drugs and Drug Addiction (EMCDDA). *Benzodiazepines Drug Profile*. Available at: http://www.emcdda.europa.eu/publications/drug-profiles/benzodiazepine

Hall W, Degenhardt L. (2007). Prevalence and correlates of cannabis use in developed and developing countries. *Curr Opin Psychiatry* 20:393–7.

Lim SS, Vos T, Flaxman AD, et al. (2012). A comparative risk assessment of burden of disease and injury attributable to 67 risk factors and risk factor clusters in 21 regions, 1990–2010: a systematic analysis for the Global Burden of Disease Study 2010. *Lancet* 380:2224–60.

Macleod J, Oakes R, Copello A, et al. (2004). Psychological and social sequelae of cannabis and other illicit drug use by young people: a systematic review of longitudinal, general population studies. *Lancet* 363: 1579–88.

Shield D, Rehm J. (2015). The effects of addictive substances and addictive behaviours on physical and mental health. In: Anderson P, Rehm J, Room, RR (eds) *The Impact of Addictive Substances and Behaviours on Individual and Societal Well-Being*, pp. 77–118. Oxford: Oxford University Press.

Shield KD, Rehm M, Patra J, et al. (2011). Global and country specific adult per capita consumption of alcohol, 2008. *J Addiction Res Pract* 57:99–117.

Volkow ND, Lellan TA. (2011). Curtailing diversion and abuse of opioid analgesics without jeopardizing pain treatment. *JAMA* 305:1346–47.

Reducing harmful substance use through policy and prevention

Government policies play a critical role in defining the context of substance use and the extent to which associated harms are experienced by both users and other community members. Government policy in relation to any particular substance can be usefully classified according to a 'continuum of control' illustrated in Table 2.3, ranging from total prohibition with criminal penalties to a laissez-faire free-market approach. An historical perspective is given here followed by some implications for levels of substance use and related harms in a population that flow from particular policy approaches.

Historical context

Substance use can be traced back to Neolithic times and attempts to formally limit related harms have been documented in many societies down the millennia. The policy context has become far more complex over the past century as a multiplicity of both natural and manufactured psychoactive substances have become more available, more widely distributed, and readily stored for longer periods. In earlier times, alcohol and other substances made simply from plants and seeds would typically be available for use only in specific places and for limited times. One of the first types of formal regulatory response to psychoactive substance use was the licensing of approved individuals to sell alcohol and tobacco products. The main motivation for licensing systems was undoubtedly the higher collection of taxes though there is also evidence of concerns about public order and extreme harms, e.g. death from alcohol overdose.

Making psychoactive substances available only on prescription can be understood as a form of licensing their distribution for exclusively therapeutic purposes. There is, however, a strong connection between illicit supply and medical practice. Many drugs now available through illicit markets were initially developed purely for therapeutic purposes, e.g. heroin was developed as a powerful, injectable pain reliever. Echoes of this phenomenon include the flooding of illicit drug markets in the UK in the 1960s with pharmaceutical heroin due to overprescribing by 'approved' private practitioners. More recently, prescribed injectable strong opioid drugs like OxyContin® (oxycodone) have flooded illicit drug markets in Canada and the US and once again with a relatively small number of practitioners contributing to the great bulk of overprescribing.

Worldwide, the phenomena of illicit drug use and illicit drug markets have flourished especially since the 1960s. In response, the UN has facilitated a series of international treaties designed to control both trade and personal use of 'narcotic drugs'. Different member states have pursued 'drug wars' and prohibition with criminal sanctions with different degrees of enthusiasm. In the US, the war on drugs ushered in during the Reagan administration has been credited with an astonishing rise in rates of imprisonment, especially of ethnic minority groups.

The last 50 years has seen opposite trends in relation to policy-making for the two most common legally available drugs: alcohol and tobacco.

Table 2.3 Alternative models of substance use control and consequences

	Prohibition	Decriminalization	Prescription	Regulation	Free market
Controls	Criminal sanctions	Civil sanctions, i.e. fines	Medical certification	Government authority	Profitability
Supply	Illicit drug dealers	Dealers or home grown	Approved doctors	Licensed sellers	Internet sales
Examples of substances	Heroin, UN members	Cannabis, parts of EU, Argentina	Opioids, OECD	Tobacco, OECD	Designer drugs
Alternatives examples	Alcohol in some Islamic countries	Use of tobacco in public spaces in many OECD countries	'Medical marijuana' in Canada and parts of US	Swedish government alcohol monopoly	Highly caffeinated drinks, most countries
Impacts on use and harm	Concentrates use to high risk settings and users	Limited impact on level of use, reduces harm from criminalization	Depends on effectiveness of controls on suppliers	Powerful levers for controlling use and harm	Maximizes levels of use and related harm

EU, European Union; OECD, Organization for Economic Cooperation and Development; UN, United Nations.

International efforts to create free-trade zones such as the EU and the North American Treaty countries have mostly contributed to fewer restrictions on the price and availability of alcohol. The only countervailing policy direction has involved increased restrictions on alcohol-impaired driving. By contrast, tobacco sale and promotion has been heavily regulated with spectacular reductions in use and associated serious diseases. International efforts at tobacco control have also been supported by international conventions. By contrast, international efforts to limit alcohol-related harms are represented by a much weaker resolution by the World Health Assembly to reduce alcohol misuse and report regularly on progress.

New challenges for policymakers are ever present. At the time of writing, health departments and governments are scrambling to make policy in relation to e-cigarettes which can deliver nicotine, the addictive ingredient in tobacco, into the bloodstream with apparently negligible health consequences. An increasing number of jurisdictions are flouting the UN convention on narcotic drugs by legalizing the use of cannabis. Increasing evidence that harm reduction initiatives can successfully limit the spread of blood-borne viruses and keep illicit drug users alive (e.g. prescribed heroin, needle exchange, and self-administered opioid antagonist programmes) also pose challenges to jurisdictions bent on enforcing laws to prohibit any use of illicit drugs.

Implications of policy measures for levels of use and related harm

Government policies have major implications for the types of health problems which clinicians will be presented with and also for the range of interventions at their disposal. This is a very large subject area and some key references are provided for more in-depth reading. Two general observations will be noted based here.

1. Prohibition with criminal sanctions can limit overall use but may amplify problems experienced by those who continue to use

Many of the health and social problems experienced by illicit drug users are driven by the fact that the markets supplying these drugs rarely offer any quality control so that supplies may be contaminated, be of uncertain purity, administered with infected equipment and in unhygienic settings, encouraging hurried use. Police crackdowns on illicit drug markets are known to disrupt supplies of clean drug-using paraphernalia, discourage safe drug-use behaviours, and disconnect users with harm reduction services. Undoubtedly, however, making presently illegal substances legally available will increase the number of users in a community—these will include both heavy users at risk of dependence and other problems as well as more occasional, recreational users. Legal markets in a free enterprise system can usually deliver cheaper drugs and, as with almost any traded commodity, lower prices mean greater use.

2. Regulatory systems provide opportunities to discourage hazardous patterns of use and reduce harms

Evidence from policy experiments around the world shows that regulatory systems can be developed which favour lower-risk forms of psychoactive substances by making these more affordable and available. Prices which reflect the amount of harmful ingredients in substances (e.g. ethanol) and, in particular, target the cheapest brands favoured by heavy users can reduce harm. Restrictions on sales to high-risk individuals (e.g. imposing a purchase age) and on high-risk times (e.g. restrictions on bar and club trading hours) have also been shown to reduce levels harm. The success of such policies owes a lot to their degree of enforcement and also levels of community support. The therapeutic supply of lower-risk substances is another variation on this approach usually specifically for those who have developed a serious substance use disorder. Examples include prescribed heroin administered in safe consumption sites for those who have failed abstinence treatment; the provision of regulated doses of beverage alcohol to severely dependent drinkers with a preference for more dangerous non-beverage alcohol; and nicotine patches, sprays, and e-cigarettes as a safer alternative to regular cigarettes.

Conclusions

It is important that clinicians are fully aware of the policy context in which they treat their patients, many of whom will present with conditions which are caused by or influenced by their substance use. Opportunities to implement harm reduction interventions or to advocate for these will be partly determined by this context. Health practitioners as a group can provide a critical counterbalance to commercial vested-interest groups who invariably espouse a free market over regulatory systems which could benefit public health and safety. They can also advocate for compassionate responses to individuals suffering the serious consequences of that substance use and who have failed with abstinence. Arguably, the ultimate goal of reduced harms from substance use is best served by a greater involvement of experienced and compassionate clinicians in the business of making government policy.

Health practitioners need to be actively engaged in shaping policies concerning the appropriate legal status, availability, affordability, and treatment options for psychoactive substance use and users.

Further reading

Babor T, Caetano R, Casswell S, et al. (2010). *Alcohol: No Ordinary Commodity – Research and Public Policy* (2nd ed). Oxford: Oxford University Press.

Babor T, Caulkins J, Edwards G, et al. (2010). *Drug Policy and the Public Good*. Oxford: Oxford University Press.

Stockwell T, Gruenewald P, Toumbourou J, et al. (2005). *Preventing Harmful Substance Use: The Evidence Base for Policy and Practice*. Chichester: John Wiley and Sons.

Pharmacology and pathophysiology

Pharmacology *32*
Pharmacology of individual substances *35*
The neurobiology of substance use disorders *48*
The genetics of substance use disorders *52*

Pharmacology

Many thousands of psychoactive substances exist and many have abuse and dependence potential. Different drugs can be classified in various ways, e.g. according to their chemical structure, their pharmacological actions, their legal status, and their place in different societies. A pharmacological approach is taken in the present text, on the basis that this most clearly illustrates what effects they have, why people use them, and what problems may emerge as a consequence of their actions.

A conventional pharmacological classification is provided in Table 3.1.

Table 3.1 Commonly self-administered psychoactive drugs (street names in brackets)

CNS depressants	CNS stimulants	Hallucinogens	Others or mixed
Alcohol	Amphetamine-type	Hallucinogens	Solvents
Sedative-hypnotics	substances	LSD (acid)	Petrol, paint
Benzodiazepines	Amphetamine	Mescaline	Inhalants
(benzos, pills)	(speed; uppers, goey,	Psilocybin	Amyl nitrite,
Barbiturates	whiz, velocity)	(magic	nitrous oxide
z-drugs:	Methamphetamine	mushrooms)	MDMA—a
zopiclone, zolpidem	(ice, shabu, crystal,		stimulant and
Opioids	yaba, crystal meth)		empathogen
Heroin (H, horse,	**Cocaine** (coke;		(e, Ecstasy, XTC,
hammer, smack)	crack; snow, charlie)		eckies)
Prescribed	**Caffeine**		**Anabolic**
Analgesics	**Nicotine**		**steroids**
Morphine			
Pethidine			
Methadone			
Buprenorphine			
Oxycodone			
Pentazocine			
Dextromoramide			
Fentanyl			
Pharmacy or			
over-the-counter			
analgesics			
Codeine			
Cannabis (dope;			
ganga; yandi; grass;			
weed; hashish)			
GHB (fantasy, liquid			
ecstasy, grievous			
bodily harm)			
Ketamine			
(Special K)			

A more informative approach, however, is to consider psychoactive substances as being located on two axes.

Their *primary* effects fall along a dimension of *sedation–stimulation*.

A *second* axis reflects alterations of *perceptions and feelings*.

For example, MDMA as well as being a moderate stimulant is also an empathogen (empathy-enhancing) substance. Magic mushrooms and LSD alter consciousness to cause novel phenomena such as hallucinations and a disordered sense of time and being (hallucinogens or psychedelics).

Characteristics of addictive substances

Addictive substances have certain characteristics in common, despite their pharmacological dissimilarities. However, it must be recognized that dependence on (or addiction to) a psychoactive substance develops on the basis of a complex interaction between:

- the pharmacological properties of the drug
- individual vulnerability
- the influence of the environment.

Within this overall understanding, the characteristics of addictive drugs may be summarized as follows:

1. They generally have a biphasic mode of action.
2. The initial effects are typically pleasurable and perceived as rewarding.
3. These pleasurable effects are rapid in onset and may result in positive reinforcement effects.
4. In the second ('restorative') phase the feelings experienced may be less pleasant or somewhat aversive (e.g. 'hangover' symptoms).
5. More of the substance may be consumed in order to relive the unpleasant experiences (i.e. the substance is taken for its 'medicinal' effects).
6. Repeated exposure induces tolerance as a neuroadaptive response: more of the drug is required to produce the same effect.
7. As a consequence of this neuroadaptation, withdrawal symptoms may occur on cessation or reduction of substance use.
8. Such negative reinforcement of abstinence, is associated with strong craving, and so encourages return to substance use.

Primary targets and CNS effects

Table 3.2 shows the primary targets and CNS effects of various drugs.

Table 3.2 Primary targets and CNS effects of various drugs

Drug	Primary (proximal) target	Brain effects
Alcohol	Agonist at GABA and antagonist at glutamate receptors	Increases GABA function Blocks NMDA glutamate receptors
Benzodiazepines	Agonist at benzodiazepine site on $GABA_A$ receptor	Increases GABA function
GHB	GHB and $GABA_B$ receptor agonist	Mimics GABA Switches off dopamine
Ketamine	NMDA glutamate receptor antagonist	Blocks glutamate
Caffeine	Antagonist at adenosine A_{2A} receptor	Reduces sedation Increases noradrenaline
Heroin and other opioids	Agonist at endorphin receptors	Produce euphoria, reduce pain
Khat	Releases ephedrine, a dopamine releaser	Mild increase in noradrenaline and dopamine
Cannabis	Cannabis CB_1 receptor agonist	Stimulate endocannabinoid signalling → change cortical and memory functions
Cocaine	Blocks dopamine reuptake site	Large increase in dopamine
Amphetamines	Release dopamine and block reuptake	Large increases in dopamine and noradrenaline
Nicotine	Agonist at (nicotinic) acetylcholine receptors	Small increase in dopamine
MDMA	Blocks serotonin and dopamine reuptake	Increases serotonin and dopamine
Mephedrone	Releases dopamine and blocks reuptake	Increases dopamine, and possibly serotonin too
Psychedelics	Agonist at serotonin $5HT_{2A}$ receptors	Change across-cortex signalling

Further reading

Nutt DJ. (2012). *Drugs: Without the Hot Air*. Cambridge: UIT Cambridge.
Nutt DJ, Lingford-Hughes A (2008). Addiction: the clinical interface. *Br J Pharmacol* 154:397–40.

Pharmacology of individual substances

What follows is a summary of the pharmacology of the main groups of psychoactive substances that cause human disorders and problems. This is designed to allow comparison between the main substance types, and complements and introduces the material on pharmacology found in each of the substance-specific chapters. Both pharmacokinetic and pharmacodynamic properties are included.

Tobacco

- Nicotine is the principal addictive constituent of tobacco.
- Nicotine levels are detectable within 30 seconds of smoking a cigarette and peak at 5–10 mins. It has a short duration of action (half-life of 20–40 minutes).
- Smoking tobacco is the most effective means of delivering nicotine to the reward centres of the brain.
- Nicotine receptor sites occur throughout the brain. Neuronal nicotinic receptors have acetylcholine as their natural ligand on the $\alpha_4\beta_2$ subunit. Nicotine is a potent agonist at these subunit sites (and possibly others).
- After interacting with these receptors, nicotine facilitates neurotransmission involving multiple neurotransmitters and local hormones such as dopamine, serotonin, β-endorphin, noradrenaline, vasopressin, acetylcholine, and many others. When this occurs at sites such as the hippocampus and nucleus accumbens, mood, memory, and cognitive ability may be enhanced.
- Nicotine has effects on many neurotransmitter systems, which tend to have positive psychological effects in people.
- In general, smokers report relaxation and stimulation, as well as anxiolytic effects.
- Dependence on nicotine develops rapidly; the average number of cigarettes required to induce dependence is four.
- The plasma nicotine level is the principal determinant of whether a dependent smoker feels psychologically 'normal' or in a withdrawal state (craving for a cigarette).
- With as little as one inhalation from a cigarette, dependent smokers immediately feel less anxious, less moody, less distressed, less hungry, and less aggressive, are able to concentrate more effectively, and are relieved of strong urges to smoke.
- These withdrawal treating effects are powerfully reinforcing, and so ensure that smoking is self-perpetuating; they are the basis for nicotine dependence.
- Nicotine has effects on the cardiovascular system, causing mild increases in blood pressure and pulse, particularly in naïve smokers.
- There are complex metabolic interactions between nicotine and many substances that people use.

Alcohol

- Alcohol (more accurately termed ethyl alcohol or ethanol) is a highly water-soluble, small-molecular-weight molecule.
- After oral ingestion, alcohol is readily absorbed from the upper small intestine (80%) and to a lesser extent (20%) from the stomach.
- Peak blood alcohol concentrations are reached after 30–60 minutes.
- Absorption is delayed by food or drugs which delay gastric emptying.
- Alcohol is widely distributed throughout the body, with a volume of distribution roughly equivalent to total body water.
- As women have a lower proportion of body water and a higher proportion of fat, blood alcohol concentrations are higher in women than in men after ingestion of equivalent amounts of alcohol.
- Metabolism is mainly in the liver, but a smaller amount of ethanol is also metabolized in the stomach wall (gastric first-pass metabolism).
- Alcohol is primarily broken down by the enzyme alcohol dehydrogenase (ADH) to acetaldehyde. This step is rate limiting. Women have 20% lower gastric alcohol dehydrogenase activity than men.
- A healthy 70 kg person metabolizes approximately 10 grams alcohol (one standard drink in many countries) per hour, which equates to an alcohol elimination rate of ~0.015 g% (or 15 mg %) (BAC) per hour.
- Acetaldehyde is, in turn, metabolized by aldehyde dehydrogenase (ALDH) to acetate which enters the Krebs cycle, and is ultimately oxidized to carbon dioxide and water (Fig. 3.1).
- A small percentage (2–3%) of alcohol is excreted unchanged in the urine, expired air, and sweat. This can be detected in breath, urine, or by transdermal alcohol assays.
- Some people, especially those of Japanese and Chinese origin, have an inactive form of ALDH, which results in their experiencing higher levels of acetaldehyde and aversive effects (as seen with the disulfiram reaction), including flushing, headaches, and nausea.
- A cytochrome P450 (CYP2E1) system metabolizes a smaller amount of ethanol (3–5%) in healthy subjects.
- From alcohol oxidation, hydrogen equivalents are generated, which lead to the production of lactic acid, ketone bodies, and neutral fats.

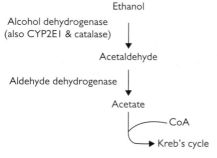

Fig. 3.1 Metabolism of alcohol (ethanol).

Cannabis

- Cannabis is a generic term for a group of approximately 100 cannabinoids derived from the marijuana plant *Cannabis sativa* and also *Cannabis indica* species of Indian hemp. Many of these cannabinoids are biologically active and have psychotropic properties.
- The principal active ingredient is delta 9-tetrahydrocannabinol (THC) which produces many of the desired psychological effects of cannabis smoking, through stimulation of brain cannabis CB_1 receptors.
- The next most common constituent is cannabidiol (CBD), which has effects different from, and in some ways opposite to, those of THC.
- New preparations of cannabis (e.g. 'skunk') can have more deleterious mental effects due to higher THC and lower CBD content, with the result that the actions of THC are not attenuated.
- After smoking, cannabis is rapidly absorbed from the alveolar membrane of the lung, and plasma levels are detected within 5 minutes.
- Peak levels are reached in 20–30 minutes and the effect lasts 2–4 hours or more, depending on the dose.
- Plasma levels show a biphasic elimination profile: the first [redistribution phase lasts about half an hour, and reflects the distribution of (highly fat-soluble) THC into fatty organs such as the brain and fat.
- The second elimination phase last 20–80 hours or more and reflects the clearance of cannabis and its metabolites via the liver and kidneys.
- THC is metabolized in the liver to 11-nor-THC-9-carboxylic acid.
- THC metabolites may be detected in the urine weeks after a single joint or up to 8 weeks after repeated daily use because of the residual amounts of drug and metabolites leaching out of fat stores.
- The very enduring presence of inactive cannabis metabolites is very easy to detect in urine screens so individuals may be found 'drug positive' weeks after the effects of cannabis have worn off (these generally disappear within a day).
- There are two types of cannabis receptors, CB_1 and CB_2, which have quite different functions and locations, with CB_2 receptors being predominantly located in the immune and gastrointestinal systems.
- Endogenous cannabinoids, such as anandamide, act as natural ligands for cannabinoid receptors.
- Endogenous cannabinoids are synthesized from brain membrane phospholipids usually as a result of neuronal depolarization.
- Endogenous cannabinoids interact with CB_1 receptors in the brain; they influence second messenger processes involved in mood, learning, and memory.
- Other effects of smoked cannabis preparations, especially effects on the gastrointestinal tract, are mediated by the less prevalent CB_2 receptors.

Opioids

- The opioids are a group of drugs, some of which occur naturally and some are chemically synthesized.
- They include morphine, diacetylmorphine (heroin), methadone, dextropropoxyphene, fentanyl, pentazocine, oxycodone, pethidine, codeine, and buprenorphine.
- Opioids act on opioid receptors in the brain to produce analgesia and varying amounts of euphoria and sedation. These receptors are of three main types:
    - μ *(mu) receptors*: euphoria, sedation, analgesia, miosis, reduced gastrointestinal motility, respiratory depression and physical dependence.
    - κ *(kappa) receptors*: located principally in the spinal cord, basal ganglia, and temporal lobes result in drowsiness and dysphoria.
    - δ *(delta) receptors*: mediate analgesia and also have cardiovascular effects (hypotension, bradycardia).
- Stimulation of mu (and possibly delta) opioid receptors is involved in 'reward' systems (see 'Neurobiology of dependence', pp. 48–51). In mice that have the mu receptor 'knocked out' the rewarding effects of opioids are abolished, and those of alcohol and cocaine attenuated, but the analgesic effect of delta receptor agonists is retained.

Heroin, morphine, and codeine

- Heroin (diamorphine) is highly lipid-soluble, and crosses the blood–brain barrier more rapidly than morphine or other opioids. Within a minute or two after intravenous heroin there is a characteristic 'rush' associated with warm flushing of the skin.
- Heroin is metabolized in the brain and in the liver to active metabolites 6-monoacetyl morphine and then to morphine, which is then conjugated with glucuronic acid—hence, heroin is a pro-drug of morphine (Fig. 3.2).
- Codeine is also a prodrug of morphine—being converted to it by CYP2D6—it is misused for this reason. Persons with low functioning 2D6 (e.g. from drugs such as paroxetine), will get less effect from codeine. Conversely, rapid metabolizers will get greater effects.
- With repeated administration, tolerance develops to most opioid effects, except miosis and constipation, and withdrawal may occur on cessation of use. Cross-tolerance is the norm among the opioids as they share a common target receptor.
- Oral morphine has a high first-pass effect and for a therapeutic effect, the oral dose is higher than the parenteral dose. Morphine is metabolized by conjugation in the liver, but one of the major metabolites, morphine-6-glucuronide, is also a mu receptor agonist and is used as an analgesic.

Methadone

- Methadone is a synthetic opioid mu receptor agonist with properties similar to morphine, but is much longer-acting.
- It is available as syrup or in the form of tablets. Methadone tablets are used for the relief of pain, while methadone syrup is indicated for

Brain effects

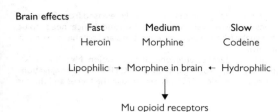

Fig. 3.2 Heroin and codeine are 'prodrugs' of morphine.

the treatment of opioid dependence, as its administration is easier to supervise. On single dose testing, 30 mg of methadone is equivalent to 15 mg of morphine.

- Methadone is well absorbed after oral administration, and reaches a peak at about 4 h, and readily crosses the blood–brain barrier. 90% is bound to plasma proteins.
- Methadone has a much longer plasma half-life than morphine (mean 22 hours, range 15–32, versus 2 hours for morphine), enabling once-daily administration.
- It is extensively metabolized by n-demethylation and cyclization in the liver, and excreted in the urine and bile. Some of the details of methadone's neuropharmacology and metabolism remain poorly defined.
- Rifampicin and phenytoin accelerate the metabolism of methadone by inducing cytochrome P450 enzymes and may precipitate withdrawal symptoms. In contrast, fluvoxamine decreases the metabolism of methadone and may result in symptoms of opioid intoxication.

Buprenorphine
- Buprenorphine is a long-acting mu receptor partial agonist and kappa receptor antagonist; it has a high affinity for both receptors.
- Buprenorphine competes with and displaces heroin or methadone from the mu receptor sites and is sometimes referred to as a mixed agonist-antagonist. Because of its low intrinsic activity and 'ceiling effects', it has a much lower risk of respiratory depression and, thus, is considerably safer than either heroin or methadone (Fig. 3.3).
- Buprenorphine is more potent than either heroin or methadone (Table 3.3). The smallest sublingual dose of buprenorphine (0.4 mg) is equivalent to 10 mg morphine (intramuscular injection), and 2 mg of sublingual buprenorphine is equivalent to 30 mg oral methadone.
- Onset of action occurs within 30–60 minutes. Peak plasma levels are reached in 1–2 hours and the half-life is approximately 20–70 hours (average 35 hours), Steady state levels are achieved in 3–7 days. Duration of action is dose dependent and ranges from 4 to 12 hours for low doses to 48–72 hours for high doses.

- Buprenorphine is highly lipophilic and slowly released from fat stores. It undergoes extensive first-pass metabolism and, hence, needs to be given sublingually (though depot preparations and patches are under development).
- Buprenorphine undergoes enterohepatic circulation. Metabolism is by hepatic enzymes, involving cytochrome CYP3A4 and conjugation with glucuronic acid. Most (70%) is excreted in the faeces and the rest in the urine.

Characteristics of buprenorphine
- More potent than morphine or methadone per mg (up to 30×)
- Good sublingual absorption (60%+) in most patients
- Poor gastric absorption and high first-pass metabolism (only 10% of dose enters systemic circulation)
- Partial agonist at the mu opioid receptor
- High affinity means it blocks access of other opioids to the mu receptor so reduces 'on-top' use.
- Half-life (including active metabolite) from one to several days as dose increases
- If there has been recent use of other opioids, buprenorphine can displace these off opioid receptors, precipitating a withdrawal reaction in dependent users (because of its high affinity and lower agonist activity at the opioid receptor).

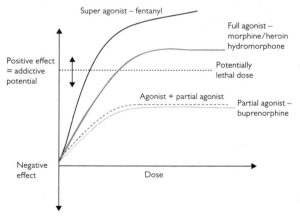

Fig. 3.3 Mu partial agonists—safety and antagonist action.

Table 3.3 Comparison of the pharmacology of three opioids

	Heroin	Methadone	Buprenorphine
Receptor	Mu agonist	Mu agonist	Partial mu agonist Kappa antagonist
Administration	IV	Oral usually. May be given in reduced dose, IM or subcutaneously when a person is nil by mouth	Sublingual
Peak plasma levels	1–2 min	2–4 h	1–2 h
Plasma half-life	2 h	22 h	Approx. 36 h (20–72 h, increases with dose)
Onset of effect	Minutes	30–60 min	30–60 min
Peak effect	1–2 min	3–6 h	1–4 h
Duration of effect	4–5 h	16–30 h dose dependent	12 h, low dose 72 h, high dose
Liver metabolism	Hydrolysis	MEOS CYP3A4	MEOS CYP3A4 Conjugation
High first-pass metabolism	Yes	No	Yes
Drug interactions	MAOIs Sedatives	MAOIs Sedatives Protease inhibitors	MAOIs Sedatives Protease inhibitors
		CYP3A4 inducers: Phenytoin Rifampicin Carbamazepine Methadone has complex effects on 3A4, induces and blocks	Antimycotics Ca channel blockers Macrolide antibiotics
		CYP3A4 inhibitors Fluvoxamine	

Sedative-hypnotics

The principal sedative-hypnotics are drugs of the benzodiazepine class. In addition, there are the barbiturates, z-drugs, and miscellaneous sedatives.

- Benzodiazepines have sedative/hypnotic, anxiolytic, anticonvulsant, and muscle relaxant properties.
- They increase GABA inhibition by acting as indirect modulators on the $GABA_A$ receptor, which has specific binding sites for these drugs—the so-called benzodiazepine receptor.
- Benzodiazepines are well absorbed after oral use. A number of long-acting benzodiazepines (e.g. diazepam) are metabolized in the liver to active metabolites (e.g. nordiazepam) and excreted in the urine.
- The duration of action of benzodiazepines depends on the half-life of the parent drug and its active metabolite (see Table 3.4). Because of long half-lives, urine drug screens of long-acting benzodiazepines may test positive for up to several weeks after use.

Table 3.4 Benzodiazepine and 'Z' drugs half-life and conversion table

Form of benzodiazepine	The dose of that benzodiazepine which is approxi-mately equivalent to diazepam (5 mg)	Approximate $t_{1/2}$ (hours)
Ultra-short acting benzodiazepines ($t_{1/2}$ < 4 h)		
Triazolam	0.25 mg	1–3
Midazolam	15 mg	1–3
Short- to intermediate-acting benzodiazepines		
Oxazepam	15 mg	4–15
Lorazepam	1 mg	12–16
Temazepam	10 mg	5–15 (10)
Bromazepam	3 mg	20
Alprazolam	0.5 mg	6–25
Flunitrazepam	1 mg	20–30
Clobazam	10 mg	17–49
Nitrazepam	5 mg	16–48
Long-acting benzodiazepines includes effects of active metabolites:		
Clonazepam	0.5 mg	22–54
Diazepam	5 mg	20–80
Chlordiazepoxide	10 mg	>50
Flurazepam	15 mg	>50
Clorazepate	10 mg	>50
'Z' drugs:		
Zolpidem	10 mg	2.4
Zopiclone	7.5 mg	5.2
Zaleplon	10 mg	1.5

- Short half-life drugs have a higher risk of withdrawal problems with inter-dose and early morning anxiety. Long half-life preparations have more residual day time drowsiness and cognitive impairment.
- There are several different subtypes of the GABA-A receptor that are thought to mediate the various actions of benzodiazepines.
- Alpha 1-GABA$_A$ receptors mediate sedation/ataxia, some anterograde amnesia and some seizure protection; alpha 2- and 3-GABA$_A$ subunits mediates anxiolysis, and some anticonvulsant and skeletal muscle relaxation; alpha 5 units are highly localized in hippocampus and contribute to the amnestic actions.
- In a setting of illicit drug use, oral benzodiazepines may be crushed or otherwise prepared for injecting. Very lipophilic benzodiazepines, such as flunitrazepam, are sometimes crushed and snorted.

Psychostimulants

All stimulants cause CNS arousal, excitation and have sympathomimetic effects similar to noradrenaline. Their pharmacological properties are summarized here and in Table 3.5.

Amphetamine and amphetamine-type stimulants (ATS)

- The primary action of amphetamines is to activate the release of the monoamines dopamine, noradrenaline, and serotonin from central storage sites in presynaptic nerve terminals, and to a lesser extent to inhibit their reuptake. Amphetamines act as substrates for transporters of these biogenic amines and increase central synaptic concentrations of dopamine, noradrenaline, and serotonin. Noradrenaline release contributes to the sympathomimetic effects, dopamine to central stimulant and rewarding effects, and serotonin to the mood effects.

Table 3.5 Half-life and approximate time course of pharmacological action of various stimulants

Psychostimulant	Approximate $t_{1/2}$	Onset of action	Duration of effect
Amphetamines (ATS)	7–12 h (up to 36 h)	Rapid after IV use through to 20 min after oral use	8–36 h
Metham-phetamine	7–12 h	Within minutes after smoking	At least as long as for amphetamines
MDMA	7–9 h	30–60 min	8–9 h
Cocaine	Variable and dose dependent: 18 min	5–10 s (inhalation)	Up to 20 min
		½–2 min (IV)	Up to 90 min
		1–3 min (intranasal)	Up to 90 min (metabolite benzoylecgonine can be detected in urine 48 h later)

Note that the time course differs with the route of administration.

- Methamphetamine has similar effects to amphetamine though is rather longer-acting.
- Higher brain levels are reached for the same dose and smoking of crystal methamphetamine ('ice', 'crystal meth') produces a very rapid brain entry, and so a greater euphoria.
- Amphetamines and ATS can be smoked, snorted, injected, or taken orally, including rubbing on gums. Occasionally, they are taken anally ('shelving').
- Onset of effect is rapid and depends on the mode of administration, occurring within minutes after intranasal administration and even faster after inhalation or intravenous administration.
- Most amphetamine users take the drug for the 'rush' or 'high' associated with use, but some use amphetamines to stay awake longer (students and truck drivers), to give more energy and attenuate the sedative effects of alcohol (e.g. at parties), to lose weight (young women), or for increased sexual desire or performance.
- Amphetamines are metabolized in the liver by isoenzymes of cytochrome P450 to active metabolites. Methamphetamine is partly converted to amphetamine and amphetamine to 4-hydroxyamphetamine.
- Depending on the pH of the urine, a significant proportion is excreted unchanged by the kidneys. As renal excretion is increased in acidic urine, overdose can be treated by acidifying the urine. Urine drug screen remains positive for 2–4 days.

3,4-Methylenedioxymethamphetamine (MDMA, Ecstasy)

- MDMA, a synthetic derivative of the amphetamines, possesses both CNS stimulant and empathetic (entactogenic) effects. It is popular at dance parties and 'raves', and is generally taken for its empathetic and stimulant effects, and for generating feelings of closeness with others (it is sometimes called the 'hug drug').
- MDMA was previously used as an appetite suppressant and psychotherapeutic aid; it is now being used as an adjunct in treatment for PTSD.
- Like the amphetamines, MDMA releases central monoamines particularly serotonin but probably also dopamine and noradrenaline by reversing the action of their transporters. MDMA also may inhibit tryptophan hydroxylase, the rate limiting enzyme in serotonin synthesis, and so may reduce central serotonin levels.
- Recent neuroimaging studies have revealed MDMA suppresses brain activity in limbic regions such as amygdala.
- MDMA is usually taken orally but can be injected or inserted anally. Typically, it is taken as 1–2 tablets at weekly to monthly intervals, but occasionally a number of tablets are taken consecutively ('stacking'), and uncommonly dependence may occur. Onset of effect occurs within 30–60 minutes and peaks at 90 minutes. The duration of effect is approximately 8 hours.
- MDMA is metabolized in the liver to an active metabolite MDA.

Cocaine

- Cocaine is an alkaloid present in the leaves of *Erythroxylum coca*. Cocaine hydrochloride is a crystalline white water-soluble compound which is readily absorbed following either intranasal administration ('snorting', 'sniffing') and intravenous administration. The cocaine free base (crack), formed when cocaine is heated in an alkaline solution, is more volatile so can be smoked or inhaled (snorted). It is more rapidly absorbed and, thus, has greater addictive potential.
- Cocaine is similar in function to amphetamine sulphate, but is significantly more rewarding due to faster onset of effects and the magnitude of the increase in dopamine concentrations in the nucleus accumbens.
- Cocaine inhibits the reuptake of dopamine, noradrenaline, and serotonin from the synaptic cleft by blocking the transporters of these biogenic amines. The block of the noradrenaline transporter produces the sympathomimetic effects sometimes leading to cardiotoxicity.
- Cocaine's vasoconstrictor and local anaesthetic actions have led to its use as a topical anaesthetic when a blood-free field is necessary, e.g. in eye surgery.
- Onset of effect of euphoric effect of cocaine is rapid, occurring within minutes, and within seconds when smoked as the free base.
- Duration of effect is short, approximately 30–90 minutes depending on the mode of administration.
- Because of its short duration of intense euphoria, cocaine is at times used repeatedly, in a binge pattern over several hours, which places the user at increased risk of toxicity and transmission of sexually transmitted infections and HIV/AIDS.
- Cocaine is metabolized, mainly in the liver, by choline esterase to an inactive demethylated metabolite benzoylecgonine and ecgonine methyl ester. A small proportion (1–2%) is excreted unchanged in the urine. Metabolites can be detected in blood or urine for 36 hours and in the hair for weeks to months after use.
- When cocaine is used with alcohol a longer-acting metabolite cocaethylene is formed that can have more prolonged stimulant and cardiotoxic actions.
- Cocaine is sometimes taken together with heroin ('speedballing').
- Many of the acute complications of cocaine tend to result from overstimulation of the CNS sympathomimetic effects and/or vasospasm.

Hallucinogens and dissociative drugs

- These include:
  - lysergic acid diethylamide (LSD)
  - psilocybin (magic mushrooms)
  - ibogaine
  - ayahuasca.
- These drugs probably act through altering brain 5HT function especially in the cortical and hippocampal regions. They have high affinity for $5HT_{2A}$ receptors and act as agonists or partial agonists at these.

- Recent studies suggest that the psychedelic 5HT agonists produce different actions on intracellular second messengers or subpopulations of cortical pyramidal cells than do other non-psychedelic $5HT_2$ acting drugs, which probably explains their effects.
- Ayahuasca is a herbal drink made from two separate plants. One is a source of the active ingredient dimethyltryptamine (DMT). This is a potent $5HT_{2A}$ receptor agonist but is not orally active due to its metabolism by MAO in gut and liver. The other plant provides a source of MAO inhibition that allows the DMT to work. Ayahuasca is used by certain churches at subpsychedelic doses to produce a sense of well-being and group harmony.
- Recent human imaging studies have revealed that the psychedelic state produced by these drugs reduces activity (and thus the function) of cortical connector hubs that integrate brain function and enhance aspects of hippocampal memory function.

GHB (gamma hydroxybutyrate) and analogues

Also known as Fantasy, Liquid Ecstasy, G, or Grievous Bodily Harm.

- GHB is an endogenous short-chain fatty acid found in the CNS. It is a putative neurotransmitter. In some countries it is used to treat narcolepsy (in the form sodium oxybate).
- Two closely related drugs are GBL (often found in cleaning fluids) and butanediol, both of which are converted to GHB in the body.
- GHB use leads to a transient decrease followed by increase in dopamine levels possibly with an increase in endogenous opioid release.
- Often prepared in crude home laboratories, there is inconsistent composition and purity that, when added to marked variation in individual tolerance, makes titration difficult.
- The effects of GHB appear rapidly, commencing within 15–30 minutes, peaking at between 30–60 minutes after use, with duration of effect of 2–4 hours (the effects of the pro-drugs may be slower and may be delayed further when mixed with alcohol). Intoxication may resemble alcohol intoxication with slurring of speech and sedation.
- GHB has a half-life of 27 minutes and is excreted as CO_2 and H_2O. It is not routinely detected on urine drug screens.
- Deaths are well recognized particularly when GHB is used with alcohol.

Ketamine

- Ketamine is an anaesthetic agent, which is widely used in developing countries and in veterinary practice.
- It is now being evaluated as a rapidly acting antidepressant.
- It is a non-competitive NMDA antagonist, like phencyclidine (PCP), though it has a shorter half-life and is associated with less problematic emergence phenomena.
- It has actions at many receptor sites on many neurotransmitter systems, most significantly glutaminergic and monoaminergic neurotransmission, responsible for its sympathomimetic effects.

- The majority of the parent drug is eliminated within 24 hours though extended effects due the presence of active metabolites can be seen.
- Ketamine has a short half-life (17 minutes). Following intranasal or intravenous use it has a rapid onset of action with duration of effect of 1–2 hours. Repeated dosing over the course of a using session is common, often in association with other drugs.
- Because ketamine, like GHB, can impair memory, it may become difficult to remember the total number of doses consumed and other drug consumption over a period of time, leading to additional complications.
- Long-term effects include cognition impairment and bladder damage.

The neurobiology of substance use disorders

Neurobiology of the dependence syndrome

There have been remarkable advances in the neuroscience of drug and alcohol dependence in the past two decades. The target sites of action of most misused substances have been identified at the molecular and cellular level, and the brain circuits that underpin drug reward (pleasure) have been identified. Furthermore, the higher-level control systems that regulate behaviours, such as planning, wanting, and resisting drug use, are becoming understood in humans through the use of techniques such as positron emission tomography (PET) and functional magnetic resonance imaging (fMRI) scanning.

Animal studies, mostly in rodents, although with some key confirmatory ones in primates, have revealed a brain circuit that appears to be common to the rewarding effects of most if not all drugs, as well as other reinforcing behaviours, such as eating, thirst, and sexual drives. This brain circuit comprises a dopamine pathway that runs from the ventral tegmental area into the ventral part of the striatum (the nucleus accumbens) and into the prefrontal cortex (Fig. 3.4). Activation in this pathway is believed to lead to the learning of associations between behaviours and the relevance that they have for the individual. The landmark discovery here was that the self-administration of cocaine to rats is associated with a great release of dopamine in the nucleus accumbens. Subsequently, most other drugs that are misused have been found to do this (the main exception being the benzodiazepines).

From this developed the dopamine theory of addiction—addictive substances release dopamine—this is pleasurable so the behaviour is repeated (reinforced). However, as drugs stimulate greater dopamine release than natural reinforcing activities, such as food, water, and sex, they 'hijack' the system, thus directing motivation and behaviour to drug use, rather than other activities. For instance, rats allowed to electrically stimulate this brain circuit do so relentlessly, not stopping to eat or drink, to the point where they may die unless the electricity is turned off; a phenomenon that has striking parallels with some human binge drug use. In Fig. 3.4 the pathway is shown along with the sites at which drugs act. Some, e.g. cocaine, work at the level of the dopamine terminals to cause dopamine release; others, e.g. the opioids and cannabis, act to switch off an inhibitory GABA neuron that normally gates the firing of the dopamine neurons, so indirectly lead to dopamine release.

More recently, it has been discovered that the state of dopamine neurotransmission may itself influence vulnerability to repeated drug use. A landmark human imaging study by Volkow and colleagues revealed that human volunteers with a lower density of dopamine D_2 receptors in the striatum gained more pleasure from intravenous stimulant administration than those with a higher level. Attempts were made to back-translate this to animal models with remarkable results. It has now been shown both in monkeys and rats that the baseline density of D_2 receptors predicts the

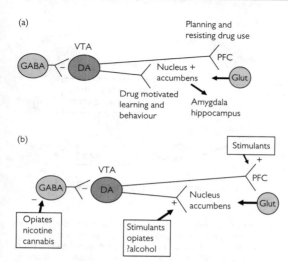

VTA = ventral tegmentalar; PFC = prefrontal cortex; DA = dopamine glutamate

Fig. 3.4 (a) The dopamine reinforcement pathway. (b) The dopamine reinforcement pathway: sites of drug action.

extent of cocaine use when access is allowed—low levels of receptors before exposure to drug leads to greater regular use of cocaine. In mice, low levels of these receptors are associated with alcohol intake and if the level is changed, e.g. by transfecting a virus that adds receptors to the nucleus accumbens, then preference declines. Moreover, repeated use of some drugs, especially stimulants and perhaps alcohol, leads to a reduction in the number of dopamine D_2 receptors so a vicious cycle of use and repeated use can be predicted (see Fig. 3.5). Very recent human studies have confirmed the view that a functioning dopamine system is critical in resisting compulsive drug use as treatment-resistant addicts and groups with high familial risk of addiction show lower dopamine function than relevant controls.

One powerful aspect of this dopamine receptor theory is that it can help explain other factors that are known to relate to drug use, e.g. stress and social deprivation, as each of these in animals has been shown to lead to reduced D_2 receptor number or function. It also leads to testable predictions about the role of dopamine receptor mutations that may alter neurotransmitter function as vulnerability markers. Also the basal ganglia dopamine systems are critical in the process whereby recreational drug use becomes compulsive addiction.

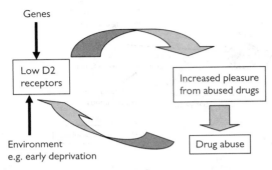

Fig. 3.5 Dopamine can help explain social aspects of addiction also.

It is too simplistic to believe that, in the human, all drug reinforcement can be explained simply in terms of changes in the dopamine system. For instance, not all drugs have been shown to release dopamine in humans, examples being opioids and benzodiazepines. Also, dopamine blocking drugs, e.g. neuroleptics, have little impact on human drug-taking so it is likely that other neurotransmitter systems play a part in human addiction. There is a good body of evidence to support an involvement of the brain endogenous opioid system—the endorphins—in addiction also. These peptides provide natural reinforcement, as well as regulating pain behaviour and may be released in parallel with, or in place of, dopamine to provide reward (e.g. from alcohol), and recent work finds stimulants release endorphins in humans. There is good and growing imaging evidence that brain opioid receptors are abnormally elevated in some addictions and that this may be associated with craving and relapse, as well as being a possible vulnerability factor to dependence. The involvement of endogenous opioids in addiction probably explains why opioid antagonists, such as naltrexone and nalmefene have utility in the treatment of alcohol, as well as heroin addiction.

Another critical aspect of drug misuse is the role of high-level cortical processing in behaviour. It has been known for a long time that people who misuse drugs, especially when addicted, have numerous deficits in mental functions, such as attention, memory planning, and impulse regulation. The use of new imaging techniques has revealed that these processes reside in subregions of the frontal cortex, particularly the orbitofrontal cortex and its limbic projection regions, especially the amygdala, and clear abnormalities of these brain regions have now been observed in many different addictions. The idea that addiction represents a fundamental remodelling of these pathways leading to long-term consequences for self-regulation has been put forward by Volkow and colleagues. A diagrammatic representation is provided in Fig. 3.6.

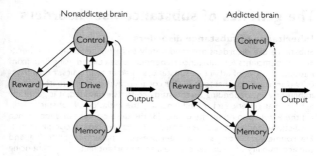

Fig. 3.6 Changed reciprocal brain control relationships in addiction.

Reproduced from *Neuropharmacology*, 56(Suppl. 1), Volkow ND, Fowler JS, Wang GJ, Baler R, Telang F., Imaging dopamine's role in drug abuse and addiction, pp. 3–8, Copyright (2009), with permission from Elsevier.

The extent to which these reflect predisposing factors or are a consequence of drug-induced damage is still under investigation, and both are likely to be relevant to differing extents in different people. Also there may well be particular aspects of dysfunction that explain a particular person's problems, e.g. in one person impulsivity may be the major problem, whereas in others compulsion to use may predominate. This offers a new approach to targeting treatments at the major risk factor in a person and also the prospect of new pharmacological approaches such as cognition enhancers.

Following repeated drug use, pathways of reward drive and memory become over-established and detached from higher-level control centres, so perpetuating drug use.

Further reading

Nutt DJ, Lingford-Hughes A, Erritzoe D, Stokes P (2015). Dopamine and addiction: 40 years of highs and lows. *Nature Reviews Neuroscience* 16:305–312.

Volkow ND, Fowler JS, Wang GJ, *et al.* (2009). Imaging dopamine's role in drug abuse and addiction. *Neuropharmacology* 56:3–8.

The genetics of substance use disorders

Inheritance of substance disorders

Substance use disorders are moderately to highly heritable. The heritability coefficients for substance dependence, calculated using data from national surveys of addictive substances in adult twin pairs, range from 0.39 (for hallucinogens) to 0.72 (for cocaine). Although estimates of heritabilities vary, depending on the study cohorts examined, it is generally agreed that genetic factors influence (1) the initiation of substance use, (2) the extent and regularity of use, (3) the development of dependence (addiction), and (4) the development of certain physical complications. Environmental factors, such as peer pressure, parental monitoring, and the accessibility of a substance, are also important factors in influencing the development of substance use disorders, as is the interplay between genetic and environmental factors.

The genetics of substance use disorders are not easily understood because the hereditary pattern is not simple like that of Mendelian disorders, in which a single mutation in the structure of DNA causes a single basic defect with pathological consequences. Rather, the influences are polygenic and sometimes with complex interactions. Many genetic variations can be involved in combination and heterogeneously in the development of substance use disorders or endophenotypic components. Although the heritabilities of substance use disorders are substantial, a single genetic variation can explain only a small portion of the total heritability. The remaining 'missing heritabilities' are expected to be uncovered in future studies.

Candidate genes for substance disorders

Candidate gene, genome-wide, and linkage analyses have been conducted to identify genetic variations associated with the vulnerability to substance use disorders in human studies. Some are common to several substances, others are specific to a certain substance such as alcohol. Leading candidates are described here and in Table 3.6.

Nicotine (tobacco)

The most striking evidence of an association with nicotine dependence/ smoking behaviour reported to date from genome-wide association studies (GWASs) is for a locus at 15q25 among subjects of European or African ancestry. This locus is represented by a synonymous rs1051730 single-nucleotide polymorphism (SNP) or non-synonymous rs16969968 SNP in the region of *CHRNA5–CHRNA3–CHRNB4*. These encode neuronal nicotinic acetylcholine receptor subunits.

Alcohol

The well-known functional SNPs for alcohol are East Asian-specific polymorphisms, Glu487Lys and His47Arg, in the aldehyde dehydrogenase 2 family (*ALDH2*) and alcohol dehydrogenase 1B (*ADH1B*) genes, respectively. The variant type 487Lys results in an inactive form of mitochondrial ALDH. The 47His variant is associated with a highly active form of ADH (1B) compared with the wildtype. Both these variants facilitate

Table 3.6 Genetic polymorphisms associated with substance use disorders in humans

Substance	Gene	Polymorphism
Nicotine	CHRNA5–CHRNA3–CHRNB4	rs16969968, rs1051730
	CYP2A6	rs1801272, rs4105144
	DAT1	3'UTR VNTR
	TTC12–ANKK1–DRD2	Taq1A (rs1800497)
	SLC6A4	5-HTTLPR
Alcohol	ALDH2	Glu487Lys (rs671)
	ADH1B	His47Arg (rs1229984)
	GABRA2	rs567926
	SLC6A4	5-HTTLPR
	TTC12–ANKK1–DRD2	Taq1A (rs1800497)
	IL10	−592C>A (rs1800872)
	HTR1B	−161A>T (rs130058)
Cocaine	CNR1	rs6454674
	HTR1B	−161A>T (rs130058)
	OPRD1	rs678849
Heroin	OPRM1	A118G (rs1799971)
	HTR1B	−161A>T (rs130058)
	BDNF	Val/Met (rs6265)
Metham-phetamine	BDNF	Val/Met (rs6265)
	AKT1	rs3730358
	GABRG2	315C>T, 1128+99C>A
Mixed substances	BDNF	Val/Met (rs6265)

UTR, untranslated region; VNTR, variable number of tandem repeat

accumulation of acetaldehyde, which is toxic and leads to an aversive experience with alcohol. Hence, these variants are protective against the development of alcohol dependence.

Heroin (opioids), cocaine, and methamphetamine
Although genetic variations with large effect sizes, as exemplified earlier in this topic, have not been reported for these drugs, several genetic polymorphisms in genes with neurobiological relevance have been associated with opioid and psychostimulant use disorders—and confirmed in meta-analyses (Table 3.6).

Further reading

Ducci F, Goldman D. (2012). The genetic basis of addictive disorders. *Psychiatr Clin North Am* 35:495–519.
Li MD, Burmeister M. (2009). New insights into the genetics of addiction. *Nat Rev Genet* 10:225–31.

The scope of intervention

Principles and scope of intervention 56
Treatment 59
Harm reduction 63

Principles and scope of intervention

The term 'intervention' applies to any approach that seeks to prevent a problem, offer early identification and treatment, or provide treatment for a disorder which has become established. The main body of this handbook is concerned with practical ways in which medical and other healthcare professionals can diagnose substance use and addictive disorders and provide practical assistance to those affected with a view to promoting recovery or reducing the risk of subsequent harm.

Although this handbook is aimed at practical aspects of intervention for clinicians, it is important to note the spectrum of approaches broadly designed to minimize harm from substance use and addictive disorders in the community as a whole. The most effective approach to reduce harm from these disorders at a population level derives from broad preventative approaches such as public policy focused on promotion of health, control of availability of substances and other addictive activities, supported by educational approaches such that the importance of such a policy and legislation is understood and accepted.

Many countries have established concerted programmes to reduce the harm caused by unhealthy substance use at a population level. These have taken different forms in different countries and range from punishment-based approaches to educational ones. In English-speaking Western countries, there have been well-publicized campaigns to limit harmful substance use. These include the 'war on drugs' which was initiated in the US in the early 1970s, the National Campaign against Drug Abuse in Australia which began in 1985, and the UK's 10-year drug strategy. Some of these strategies have been groundbreaking in their approaches and benefits; some have been abject failures.

The following sections summarize the four main components of health interventions.

Prevention (primary intervention)

The preventative approach aims to discourage unhealthy substance use and other addictive activities in the community as a whole. Examples include the following:

- Supply reduction: includes controls on availability of psychoactive substances and public policy and legislation to support this.
- Demand reduction: includes the provision of information and advice to the population as whole or specific subgroups, and includes mass media campaigns and school- and college-based education.
- Addressing underlying risk factors such as social disadvantage.
- Enhancing protective factors such as supporting and strengthening families and providing supportive environments within the community.

Although primary prevention is mainly channelled through government policy and programmes, there is a substantial contribution in many countries from voluntary and non-governmental organizations. Individual clinicians also help preventative efforts by providing information and advice to parents and other members of the community in a way that helps family members or galvanizes a community into prevention initiatives.

Early intervention (secondary intervention)

Early intervention proactively seeks to identify hazardous patterns of substance use or other addictive behaviours before these become established and dependence, addiction, or serious consequences have arisen.

All healthcare professionals can have a major role in early intervention including general practitioners, hospital doctors, nurses, psychologists and other therapists, social workers, and health educators.

- The emphasis of early intervention is on simple and effective identification (sometimes using screening questionnaires) and the provision of advice and (or) brief therapy at the point of first contact.
- The screening or early detection component may form part of a systematic activity in a medical practice, hospital or clinic for all new patients or for all patients attending (e.g. every 2 years).

Treatment (tertiary intervention)

Treatment and care aim to provide one or a combination of therapies, medications, or other approaches designed to improve the health and well-being of a person who has been diagnosed with a substance use or other addictive disorder.

- The aim is to help that person establish health and stability, typically based on cessation of use of the substance or addictive activity in the long term.
- This goal reflects the knowledge that when a dependence/addiction has developed (see Fig. 4.1), it is very difficult and may be essentially impossible for that person to maintain moderate levels of use of the substance because of the ever-present likelihood of substance use

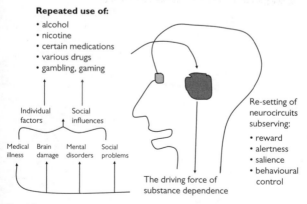

Fig. 4.1 A schematic representation of substance dependence and addiction.

escalating due to the internal persistent drive that is characteristic of addictive disorders.
- Alternative goals, but still with improvements in health and well-being as the overarching aim, include maintenance on a steady dose of a psychoactive substance. This is best developed in the area of opioid agonist maintenance for patients with injecting or other illicit or inappropriate opioid use; methadone and buprenorphine are the two principal opioid agonist agents.
- Psychostimulant and cannabinoid maintenance are also feasible approaches for many patients but are less well developed or publically accepted.

Harm reduction

Harm reduction is variably defined and this has caused considerable difficulties at various times and in various cultures in its acceptance as a legitimate approach to substance use disorders.
- A narrow understanding is that it involves a range of approaches to minimize the experience of harm in individuals (and in populations such as injecting drug users) while recognizing that such individuals may not be interested or able to engage in treatment based on a fundamental change in harmful substance use. A broader conceptualization of harm reduction is set out in a later section (see pp. 63–5).
- Essentially, harm reduction approaches aim to relieve symptoms and assist in everyday functioning and independence to the greatest possible extent.
- It may be a transitional phase through which people journey, with recovery and rehabilitation based on abstinence from the substance being a goal that may be attainable subsequently.

Treatment

Key components of treatment

The key components of treatment can be summarized as the following ten items (Box 4.1). These exist in somewhat of a chronological order but it should not be assumed that there is an invariable progression from one item to the next. The exact sequence will depend on how the individual has been recognized to have a substance use or addictive disorder and the access to the various forms of treatment and support that exist in their environment. There are many uncertainties in a person journeying out of an addiction into a life of stability and restoration of health, well-being, and social functioning.

1. Information and understanding

A principle of modern healthcare is that the patient is a key partner in his/her treatment. Accordingly it is vital for each individual to be provided with information about his/her disorder so that they develop an understanding of its nature and the relevance and importance of treatment. Just as diabetes education has contributed to improved blood sugar control and reduction in the physical complications of diabetes, so developing an understanding helps the person with a substance use or addictive disorder engage more effectively in treatment. A helpful approach is to provide visual material so that the person understands the essence of addictive disorders 'at a glance'. Fig. 4.1 is an example of a visual depiction of addictive disorders.

Box 4.1 The ten key components of treatment

1. Information and understanding
2. Acceptance and engagement
3. Initiating treatment: diagnosis and detoxification
4. Pharmacotherapies
5. Psychological therapies
6. Identification and treatment of underlying and complicating disorders
7. Family and social support
8. Self-help fellowships
9. Aftercare
10. Lifestyle and environmental change

2. Acceptance and engagement

A key requirement for making progress in treatment is that the person affected accepts a level of personal responsibility for making efforts to recover from the disorder.

- No form of treatment for a substance use or addictive disorder can help if the person is unwilling to engage in treatment—unless there are provisions in the country or state for compulsory treatment or if the person has a mental health disorder for which compulsory treatment under mental health legislation is appropriate.
- Accepting the situations the patient needs to engage with, an understanding that recovery is a priority for them and that commitment and effort on their part is vital. Whenever a therapist is working harder on a patient's recovery than the patient is, something is badly wrong.
- Acceptance and engagement tends to be a process which occurs over time; sometimes it occurs rapidly when the person has experienced a life-changing problem (known by many as 'rock bottom'). Sometimes there is a degree of encouragement, pressure, and coercion by family members on the individual.
- In other situations, the individual may have reality thrust upon them through being charged by the police for an offence or experiencing some other form of personal or psychological crisis.

3. Initiating treatment: diagnosis and detoxification

Although some people with substance and addictive disorders gain recovery without having treatment or being involved with self-help fellowship, the outlook is better with treatment than without it. For patients with established substance dependence it is highly likely that detoxification will be required initially, as most forms of treatment and therapy will be negated by continuing substance use.

- Detoxification is an entry point to treatment by ensuring that the person ceases substance use in a supervised way such that any withdrawal symptoms are prevented or minimized and the person is sufficiently physically and psychologically stable to gain from further intervention. At this point, the diagnosis will be clarified.
- Typically it may not be possible to make firm diagnoses of all the relevant substance use, psychiatric, and physical disorders at the time of presentation. Many symptoms are directly due to the effects of substance use or a withdrawal syndrome.
- A definitive diagnosis is more easily made after detoxification when the immediate substance-related features have settled. At this point, the opportunity should be taken by the patient to develop a personal plan for recovery, at least covering the next few weeks ahead.

4. Pharmacotherapies

The term 'pharmacotherapy' is applied to the range of medications that may be prescribed following detoxification and which aim to enhance the likelihood of the patient achieving recovery. Broadly the pharmacotherapies affect the neurobiological mechanisms which are implicated in the development and perpetuation of substance dependence.

- Several pharmacotherapies are known to exert their effects on the reward circuitry and CNS excitatory systems.
- Some medications have aversive effects, an example being disulfiram (Antabuse (R)) which results in an unpleasant reaction within a few minutes of alcohol being consumed.
- Other drugs are pharmacological agonists of the substance that has resulted in the dependence; the best known are methadone and buprenorphine.
- Others are pharmacological antagonists and these include opioid, benzodiazepine, and cannabinoid antagonists.
- A related approach is the use of vaccines for prevention or treatment but these are not available for routine clinical practice as yet.

5. Psychological therapies

The term 'psychological therapies' is applied to the range of individual and group-based therapies which are aimed at prevention of relapse and typically employ a range of cognitive, behavioural, and sometimes systems approaches to facilitate recovery.

- The aim of psychological therapy may be based on attainment of abstinence from the substance or addictive activity; in some cases where the person does not have an established dependence, goals such as moderated use may be appropriate.
- There is a large number of psychological approaches, many of which have evidence-based effectiveness in the treatment of addictive disorders. They range in intensity and frequency but typically the sessions occur at weekly intervals.

6. Identification and treatment of underlying and complicating disorders

Substance use and addictive disorders are comorbid in a high proportion of patients with mental health disorders, such as depression, anxiety disorders, bipolar disorder, and trauma-related disorders.

- Effective diagnosis and treatment of these comorbid disorders is vital to the health of the individual and to support continuing work on relapse prevention.
- These approaches encompass pharmacological ones (antidepressants, mood stabilizers, antipsychotic agents), psychological therapies directed specifically at the mental health disorder, and occasionally procedures such as electroconvulsive therapy, and anaesthetic and other pain management procedures. Treatment for the range of physical sequelae is also included here.

7. Family and social support

Human beings are described as social animals and for the great majority of people with substance use or addictive disorders, engagement or re-engagement with family or friends provides vital support for recovery, particularly maintaining recovery which is rewarding. Support from partners and family cannot be guaranteed as often a climate of mistrust and disengagement has developed due to the effects of the addiction. Support from family is more readily gained and is more effective when the individual with the addictive disorder has demonstrated some form of personal responsibility and commitment to move forward in life.

8. Self-help fellowships

By far the most available forms of support for recovery from an addictive disorder are the self-help fellowships. In the Western world these are typically founded on the 'Twelve Steps' recovery programme of Alcoholics Anonymous (AA). Numerous AA-aligned fellowships exist for those who have become dependent on opioids, psychostimulants, cannabis (marijuana), and sedative-hypnotics, and also various behavioural and electronic addictions. In many countries, such groups represent the most accessible form of support for recovery and are often available in areas which are poorly provided with formal treatments.

9. Aftercare

Substance use and addictive disorders have usually developed over an extended time and have resulted in often profound changes in the individual's sense of priorities (e.g. substance use versus family obligations, personal care, and moral code). Recovery from an addictive disorder typically involves a personal journey over time. The formal approaches involving detoxification, pharmacotherapy, and psychological therapies are valuable to initiate the recovery process.

- However, addictive disorders tend to have a relapsing course and continued support and appropriate treatment is important for many patients in the longer term.
- Many authorities consider that recovery from an established substance use or addictive disorder can take 2–5 years and the initial course may be characterized by periodic relapses.
- Persistent treatment (i.e. aftercare), is designed to reduce the risk and frequency of any relapses.
- The nature of the aftercare varies from person to person and may include periodic consultation, medical advice, pharmacotherapies, and some form of continued psychological therapy (often directed at recovery from the effects of trauma or managing depression, anger, or social anxiety).
- It is not possible to identify in advance exactly what form aftercare should take, but the principle of aftercare should be introduced to patients at the earliest possible opportunity.

10. Lifestyle and environmental change

Recovery from an addictive disorder is based partly on correct diagnosis of the addictive and other disorders, engagement in appropriate treatment, involvement with a self-help fellowship, and support from various family members. However, there are, importantly, many changes to a person's lifestyle and environment which are vital for continuing and rewarding recovery.

- These include healthy relationships with an intimate partner, key family members, and friends.
- Opportunity should be taken to review the person's work (source of income) and in particular identify unhealthy work environments or schedules.
- Recovery is difficult in areas which represent substance use or addictive 'hotspots' and the opportunity should be taken to consider whether a move to another area is preferable, recognizing that problems can be transferred geographically and not always left behind.
- Lifestyle also means establishing a healthy daily routine.

Harm reduction

Definition

Harm reduction refers to public policies or interventions that aim to reduce harm associated with substance use among people who do not want to cease using a harmful substance or are unable to do so.

Harm reduction has a population-wide goal and an individual one. In an individual sense it is analogous to palliation, which refers to the relief or alleviation of symptoms of a disorder, without effecting a cure, or in the case of addictive disorders, seeking or achieving recovery.

Goals and principles of harm reduction

- The goal of harm reduction is to minimize the harm associated with substance use.
- In the case of injecting drug use, the two priority goals are to minimize the risk of contracting infectious diseases (e.g. HIV/AIDS and hepatitis B and C viruses (HBV and HCV)) and of overdosing.
- Other goals of harm reduction include reduced violence, injury, crime, psychiatric disorder, nutritional deficiency, and improved healthcare.
- Harm reduction interventions are based on pragmatism and humanistic principles, which accept that some use of a psychoactive drug is a part of human experience and that a user's decision to use the drug is accepted as fact and no moralistic judgement is made about it.
- Harm reduction emphasizes an immediate and realistic goal, which is the reduction of drug-related harm rather than focusing on long-term abstinence.
- Harm reduction not only aims to reduce risk to individual drug users, but also harm to their families and the broader society.
- The latter goal is achieved through protecting the wider population through reduced transmission of blood-borne viruses in the injecting drug-using community (through needle-syringe availability programmes and education about safe sex practices), reduced public nuisance and crime, and reduced traffic deaths and injuries (e.g. through drink-driving prevention programmes).

General harm reduction strategies include education, which aims to provide accurate information about the consequences and risks of drug use, intervention to change high-risk behaviours, provision of a safe environment to minimize the risks of negative consequences to health or quality of life, and promoting social and community support.

The evidence base

Injecting drug use

Evidence-based harm reduction strategies for injecting drug users include:

- HIV/HCV counselling and testing
- needle-syringe availability/exchange programmes (NSPs)

- substitution therapy with opioid agonists for opioid dependence— examples include methadone maintenance treatment (MMT), and buprenorphine maintenance
- heroin prescribing for heroin-dependent persons not responding to other treatments
- supervised injecting and drug consumption facilities
- overdose intervention and prevention (e.g. through the use of naloxone)
- prevention of sexually-transmitted infections (STIs) through promotion of condom use
- ready access to treatment for STIs
- HBV vaccination.

Alcohol

Alcohol harm reduction policies and strategies include:

- campaigns against drinking and driving
- sobering-up shelters for heavily intoxicated individuals or homeless drinkers
- server training and risk assessments in bars
- serving alcohol in shatter-proof glass to prevent injuries
- brief interventions and advice for problematic drinkers, pregnant women, or young people
- drinking-in-moderation treatment goals
- thiamine supplements to reduce brain damage.

Tobacco

Examples of tobacco harm reduction interventions include:

- reduced-exposure products
- reducing consumption
- long-term nicotine replacement therapy, including e-cigarettes
- smokeless tobacco products
- using replacement products for temporary abstinence.

The role of clinicians

Although harm reduction is usually seen as a public health approach and deals with policy intervention, clinicians seeing individuals who use drugs should be familiar with the principles and interventions based on this approach.

Clinicians may be involved in the identification of specific harms, their causes, and decisions about appropriate interventions that require proper assessment of the problem and the actions needed. With increasing evidence of effectiveness and cost-effectiveness of harm reduction strategies, clinicians should be open and up to date with the harm reduction interventions existed in their community.

Clinicians may also help promote the interventions through partnerships with law enforcement, public health and government officials, researchers, and injecting drug users. However, this should be done safely within professional standards of confidentiality and other professional ethics. This is particularly important for those countries whose standards in this aspect leave much to be desired.

Clinicians may help in dissemination of information and materials about harm reduction, and development of scientific and the regulatory frameworks needed to deliver harm reduction interventions.

Principles of harm reduction practice for clinicians

Effective principles for clinicians working on harm reduction strategies include:

- accepting people who use drugs as they are and avoiding being judgemental
- being familiar with potential harms attributable to various types of drug use
- assessing individuals' risks based on knowing the type of drug used, method of administration, and pattern of use
- setting short-term pragmatic goals to meet users' current needs (e.g. wound care and vein maintenance in case of injection site infection), encouraging their ability to care for themselves, and acknowledge any positive change made (e.g. decreasing the number of injections or better cleaning of the paraphernalia)
- using a collaborative approach with the users to address as many suitable harm reduction interventions as possible and involving them in planning and the decision-making process
- providing simple, accurate, peer-based, factual information about the consequences of drug use and promoting behaviours that reduce the risks
- focusing on individuals' own risk behaviours and providing different options to reduce risk, e.g. advising non-injecting instead of injecting routes of administration
- supporting users to access the information, services, and other interventions in their community that can help keep them healthy and safe, and encouraging them to enrol into a treatment programme
- being cautious about promoting abstinence in individuals who are ambivalent about abruptly abstaining
- tailoring interventions to individuals' risks and harm while taking into account other specific factors that render them vulnerable, such as age, gender, comorbidity, or imprisonment
- working with teams of allied professionals in planning and implementing harm reduction programmes.

Further reading

Hunt N, Ashton M, Lenton S, et al. (n.d.). *A Review of the Evidence-Base for Harm Reduction Approaches to Drug Use.* [Online] Available at: http://www.forward-thinking-on-drugs.org/review2-print.html

Nutt DJ, Lingford-Hughes A, Chick J (2012). Through a glass darkly: can we improve clarity about mechanisms and aims of medications in drug and alcohol treatments? *J Psychopharmacology* 26:199–204.

Establishing the diagnosis

Presentations and diagnoses 68
History and antecedent conditions 69
Clinical examination 71
Mental state examination 73
Laboratory and other tests 77
Seeking the truth 78
Common presentations 79
Screening instruments and questionnaires 82
Formulation and diagnosis 83

Presentations and diagnoses

Patients may present with:

- Medical complications of substance use or issues such as insomnia, injuries, drug-seeking, repeated requests for medical certificates
- Psychiatric complications or psychiatric co-morbidity, e.g. anxiety, depression, suicidality, psychosis
- Social complications: family conflict, relationship breakdown, absenteeism from work, financial difficulties
- Legal or forensic complications, e.g. drink driving offence, aggression, violence, assault.

Substance use disorders should be diagnosed according to accepted diagnostic criteria. See pp. 590–9 for details of these.

Acute intoxication/overdose (ICD 10; DSM-5)

The features are related to the pharmacological effects of the substance when it is taken in excessive amounts.

Non-dependent substance use

- *Unhealthy use:* refers to the spectrum of use that can result in harmful consequences and as such includes hazardous (risky) use, harmful use, substance abuse, substance use disorder, and dependence.
- *Hazardous (risky) use:* repetitive use of alcohol or another substance which confers the risk of harmful consequences. Most commonly applied to alcohol: see Chapter 9 for national safe drinking guidelines.
- *Harmful use (ICD 10):* repetitive use of alcohol and other substances that results in actual harm (physical or mental harm) but does not fulfil the criteria for dependence.
- *Substance abuse (DSM-IV):* repetitive use of a substance essentially causing social or legal problems.
- *Substance use disorder (DSM-5):* an umbrella diagnosis which includes dependent and non-dependent substance use. Mild substance use disorder is generally non-dependent use.

Substance dependence (ICD 10)

This is defined as a psychobiological syndrome that reflects an internal driving force to use the substance. It comprises impaired control over alcohol or substance use, compulsion or craving, tolerance and withdrawal symptoms, and continued use despite harmful consequences.

Substance use disorder (DSM-5)

As mentioned earlier, this is an umbrella term which encompasses a wide range of disorders. Moderate or severe substance use disorder generally denotes dependence on (or addiction to) the substance.

Substance withdrawal syndrome (ICD 10; DSM-5)

This is defined as a cluster of symptoms and signs which occur on cessation or a marked reduction in substance use when that use has previously been excessive. Most commonly, the person fulfils the criteria for dependence but this is not a prerequisite.

History and antecedent conditions

A high level of awareness of the possibility of an alcohol or other substance use disorder is required. Insomnia, anxiety, depression, or other psychiatric symptoms are common clues to substance misuse; similarly physical or social problems can be reminders of the need for a more detailed substance use history.

Good interview and history-taking skills

To establish good rapport and develop a therapeutic relationship with the patient:

- Show an empathic and non-judgemental approach and sensitivity to the patient's current life situation and cultural background.
- Use an appropriate questioning style and content.
- Introduce alcohol consumption or other substance use as an unremarkable occurrence or as any other health risk factor.
- It can be helpful to place onus of denial on the patient when substance use is suspected (*When did you last …?*).
- Be alert to diversionary tactics and persevere —politely; do not abandon appropriate enquiry into substance use.
- It can be helpful to suggest a high level of consumption to the patient (*30 drinks in an evening …?*) when you suspect a more severe substance disorder.

History taking should also include use of:
- sedative-hypnotics (especially benzodiazepines)
- cannabis (marijuana) and synthetic cannabinoids
- heroin and other illicit opioids
- prescription and pharmacy-purchased (over-the-counter) opioids
- psychostimulants (amphetamines, cocaine)
- 'party drugs' such as MDMA (Ecstasy), GHB.

Note that many patients use more than one drug.

Record for each psychoactive substance:
- Quantity used (per day or session)
- Frequency of use:
- Pattern of use (daily or near-daily vs episodic use at weekends or at festivals)
- Duration of the major phases of use
- Time and date of last use
- Route of use
- Periods of abstinence
- Precipitants for relapse.

Past medical and psychiatric history

Include history of previous detoxification attempts, drug overdoses, suicide attempts, withdrawal syndrome, seizures, attendance at AA, NA, SMART recovery, rehabilitation.

Family history

- Alcohol and other substance misuse
- Major medical or psychiatric illnesses
- Childhood physical or sexual abuse, trauma.

Forensic history

Robbery, violence, assault, criminal activity, incarceration.

Social history

- Social deprivation
- Living arrangements: alone or with partner, friends, relatives, child under care
- Nutritional intake, available support systems (family, friends, community services, 'meals on wheels').

Medications

Prescribed medications: in addition to other prescribed medication, specifically inquire about use of:

- benzodiazepines and other sedative/hypnotics
- opioid analgesics—particularly patients with a history of chronic pain or previous heroin use
- antidepressants
- antipsychotics
- non-steroidal anti-inflammatory drugs (risk of gastric erosions in alcohol use disorders)
- over-the-counter preparations (codeine, paracetamol, antihistamines, etc.), which may be misused deliberately or unconsciously (see pp. 383–7 on pharmacy drugs).
- Internet-purchased medications

Antecedents

Enquire specifically about the predisposing factors or common underlying conditions listed in Box 5.1.

> **Box 5.1 Antecedent factors for alcohol and other substance misuse**
>
> - Genetic factors
> - Personality traits—impulsivity, risk-taking, rebelliousness
> - Family history of alcohol and other substance use disorders
> - Family history of psychiatric problems
> - Childhood abuse, trauma, and social deprivation.

Clinical examination

General appearance

In many patients with mild alcohol or drug use disorder (DSM-5) or non-dependent hazardous drinking or drug use (ICD 10), physical examination may be normal.

When the alcohol or other drug use disorder becomes more severe (DSM-5) or when harmful drinking or alcohol or drug dependence (ICD 10) sets in, the patient's appearance may provide more clues to the diagnosis.

Look for:

- Signs of poor self-care, malnourishment, vitamin deficiency
- Smell of alcohol on the breath and other signs of intoxication
- Facial flushing, telangiectasia, periorbital oedema, parotid swelling (alcohol misuse)
- Nicotine stains on the fingers (cigarette smoking)
- Needle track marks; If present, are they fresh or old? (injecting drug use; see Fig. 5.1)
- Signs of skin infections—thrombophlebitis, skin abscesses (Fig. 5.1)
- Pallor, fever, flushing
- Tremors (alcohol or benzodiazepine withdrawal)
- Sweating (benzodiazepine or alcohol withdrawal, also in-patients on methadone maintenance treatment)
- Conjunctival injection, i.e. red eyes (alcohol, cannabis)
- Pupil size—dilated in opioid withdrawal, constricted in opioid use (intoxication), unequal in head injury
- Jaundice (alcoholic liver disease, hepatitis C)
- Bruises of different ages (alcohol in particular)
- Excoriations (stimulants, liver disease)
- Dentition: bleeding gums, caries (opioids), tooth grinding (stimulants)
- Signs of injury or other trauma.

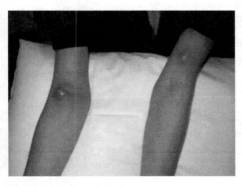

Fig. 5.1 Abscesses at injecting site.

Systematic examination of body systems

Respiratory system
- Chronic airways limitation in smokers
- Pneumonia or other respiratory infections
- Tuberculosis (poor self-care, poor living conditions, or suppressed immunity)
- Pulmonary oedema.

Cardiovascular
- Hypotension (opioid overdose) or hypertension (stimulant use, chronic alcohol excess, withdrawal states)
- Tachycardia (stimulant use, withdrawal states)
- Tachyarrhythmias, atrial fibrillation (alcoholic cardiomyopathy, alcohol-induced atrial fibrillation, stimulant use)
- Cardiac failure
- Heart murmurs (bacterial endocarditis, cardiomyopathy).

Gastroenterological
- Hepatomegaly (signs of hepatitis, fatty liver, or chronic liver disease)
- Splenomegaly, portal hypertension, signs of hepatic decompensation.

Musculoskeletal system
- Injury, scars, fractures (recent and/or old)
- Muscle weakness or wasting (alcoholic myopathy, chronic liver disease).

Neurological
- Is the patient intoxicated or in a withdrawal state?
- Is the patient drowsy, confused, or agitated?
- Speech (slurred with alcohol or benzodiazepines; may be slow with opioid or cannabis intoxication, or rapid or pressured with stimulant intoxication)
- Gait (ataxia with alcohol or benzodiazepine intoxication or Wernicke's encephalopathy or alcoholic cerebellar damage).
- Cerebellar signs in alcohol dependence
- Diplopia/lateral gaze palsies/nystagmus, Wernicke's encephalopathy
- Peripheral neuropathy (pain, diminished sensation, absent reflexes).

Mental state examination

The mental state examination (MSE) is a systematic assessment of the features of the patient's presentation, behaviour, and psychological experiences at the time of the interview.

Key areas to explore

Appearance and behaviour

General description of the patient, general reaction to the interview (e.g. friendly, cooperative, withdrawn, uncommunicative, hostile, guarded), physical appearance (level of self-care, unkempt, well dressed), abnormal motor activity (sweating, tics, tremor, restlessness, physical agitation, psychomotor retardation).

Rapport

The level of relatedness or connection between the patient and the health professional during the interview.

- Difficulties in establishing rapport may provide clues about difficulties the patient is having in establishing relationships with others, e.g. through mistrust, hostility, irritability, lack of warmth.
- The interviewer's reaction often reflects the nature of the patient's mental state. An elevated manic patient may provoke laughter; a depressed patient sadness; a hostile, threatening patient may provoke fear. Where patients are psychotic and thought disordered, the interviewer may be left feeling confused.

Speech and language (thought form)

- *Speech*: assess the rate (e.g. slow, hesitant, pressured), prosody (rhythm and intonation), volume (e.g. loud, soft, inaudible), quantity (e.g. poverty of speech). Note any abnormal articulation, e.g. stuttering or slurred speech.
- *Language*: assess amount and rate of thoughts (vague, poverty of ideas, slow, hesitant, flight of ideas), order of thoughts (logical, distractible, loosening of associations, tangential, circumstantial); disturbance of language (incoherent), repetitive language (perseveration).

Mood and affect

- *Mood*: the patient's subjective experience of their emotional state (depressed, angry, anxious, sad, fearful, elated).
- *Affect—objective*: what you observe of the person's emotional state by noting their appearance, level of movement, posture and general behaviour (normal, restricted, flat, anxious, elevated).

Thought content

- Preoccupations; anxious and obsessional thoughts; depressive thought content (hopelessness, helplessness, guilt, worthlessness).
- Delusional beliefs: false beliefs which are not amenable to reason or modifiable by experience, are not shared by a similar culture, religion, or background, are held with great conviction and experienced by the patient as part of their reality.

- Risk of harm to self: see section on suicide risk assessment (pp. 75–6).
- Risk of harm to others: ascertain whether the patient has any current thoughts, plans or intention to harm others pp. 553–4.

Perception

Look for abnormal experiences such as:

- illusions (distortions of real external stimuli) and misinterpretations (true perceptions, the meaning of which is misinterpreted), and hallucinations (the person hears, sees or smells something, but there is nothing there).
- hallucinations—may be auditory, visual, tactile, gustatory, olfactory or somatic. Formication is a form of tactile hallucination commonly experienced with excessive use of methamphetamine or cocaine. If hallucinations evident, consider drug-induced psychosis (psychostimulants, heavy cannabis use), co-morbid schizophrenia; alcohol withdrawal (withdrawal hallucinosis, delirium tremens), sedative withdrawal.

Cognitive state

- *Level of conscious awareness:* is the patient alert, drowsy, showing fluctuating level of consciousness, confused or delirious? (Rule out substance intoxication/withdrawal and other organic causes if confusion present.)
- *Orientation:* is the patient orientated in time, place, and person?
- *Attention and concentration:*
  - general behaviour during interview
  - simple arithmetic (addition, subtraction)
  - serial 7s (subtract 7 from 100 and from each subsequent answer)
  - months of year backwards or days of week backwards if serial 7s too hard.
- *Memory:*
  - immediate and short-term memory: give them three paired objects to remember; ask them to repeat immediately and 2–5 minutes later (e.g. white car, purple dress, 7 George Street)
  - recent memory: e.g. what they had for breakfast, what they did yesterday
  - long-term memory: relevant events from their past.
- *Intelligence:* this can be assessed by the patient's performance in the interview, their educational and occupational level, and their general knowledge. Specific tests can include name of the current prime minister, capital of their country, name of the US president.

More detailed bedside testing for suspected organic brain impairment

Consider use of:

- *Verbal fluency/executive function/visuospatial:*
  - draw a clockface and draw in the time 10 past 2
  - name as many words in 1 minute that begin with the letter 'F' but not the names of people or places (should get > 15; name as many animals as possible in 1 minute (should get >15)

- alternating trail making: on a page write the numbers 1–5 and capital letters A–E. Instruct the patient *'to draw a line, going from a number to a letter in ascending order. Begin here [point to (1)] and draw a line from 1 to A then to 2 and so on. End here [point to (E)].'*
- Mini mental state examination (MMSE).
- Montreal Cognitive Assessment (MOCA). This is a rapid screening test which takes around 10 minutes to administer and is more sensitive than the MMSE for mild cognitive dysfunction.
- Addenbrooke's Cognitive Evaluation (ACE)—see Chapter 27.

Insight and judgement

Insight refers to the patient's awareness of their psychological state; the impact of their behaviour on others; their understanding of their illness, and its likely causes, consequences, and treatment. Assessing the patient's judgement provides information about their ability for rational problem-solving and decision-making.

Specific tests: 'What would you do if you saw a fire in the rubbish bin?' 'What would you do if you found a wallet on the street?'

Suicide risk assessment

The overall assessment of suicide risk should take into account *risk factors* as well as *protective factors*.

Significant risk factors for suicide

- History of repeated suicide attempts
- Recent suicide attempt
- A clear plan and intention to suicide; access to lethal means
- Concurrent substance use
- Concurrent depression and/or hopelessness
- Concurrent untreated/poorly treated psychosis
- Significant recent losses and/or stressors
- Intercurrent medical illness, e.g. chronic pain, terminal illness
- Close friend or family member has attempted or completed suicide
- Recent discharge from hospital or a trusted practitioner.

Common protective factors

- Strong perceived social supports (family, friends, networks)
- Good coping and problem-solving skills
- Ability to seek help and engage with treating practitioners
- Positive values and beliefs e.g. religious beliefs, commitment to family
- Stable lifestyle (e.g. housing, work, absence of substance use disorder)

The General Screen and Risk Assessment section of the *PsyCheck Screening Tool* can be used to provide an overview of the patient's risk profile—for reference see p. 94.

Low-risk patients: have none or some thoughts of suicide but no specific plan, intention or means; minimal risk factors; evidence of protective factors (e.g. positive social supports).

Medium-risk patients: have some risk factors including suicidal thoughts and a plan with some specific detail; means are available with intention to act in the near future (but not immediately); some protective factors.

High-risk patients: often have previous suicide attempts and other risk factors; have suicidal thoughts with a clear and detailed plan, intent to act in near future, means are available (and potentially lethal); few protective factors.

Another contemporary suicide risk assessment tool is provided in Chapter 27.

Laboratory and other tests

Routine investigations
- Full blood count
- Liver function tests (LFTs)—(especially GGT, AST, ALT)
- Coagulation tests (INR/APTT)
- EUC—focusing on sodium, potassium and urea levels
- Magnesium (for alcohol dependence)
- Glucose—increased or decreased with heavy drinking; DD of delirium or coma.
- Viral serology: in injecting drug users screening for hepatitis B, hepatitis C, and HIV is important (p. 414).

Other laboratory tests depending on clinical presentation
- ESR/CRP
- Serum vitamin B_{12} and folate, if MCV elevated, or malnutrition is suspected
- Thyroid function tests (TFTs)
- Creatine phosphokinase (CPK, rhabdomyolysis from psychostimulant use or in patients who may have had a long period of coma)
- Cardiac enzymes (cocaine-induced myocardial infarction)
- Blood cultures (septicaemia, bacterial endocarditis)
- STI screen, e.g. including syphilis serology, chlamydia PCR, VDRL.

Specific tests for psychoactive substances
- Breath or blood alcohol concentrations
- COHb and cotinine
- Urine drug screens may provide useful information even though results may not be available for more than 24 hours. Results may help confirm suspected substance use, and/or use of more than one drug—which is common
- Carbohydrate-deficient transferrin (CDT)
- Ethyl glucuronide (EtG).

Other investigations
- Oximeter readings or blood gases (asthma/CAL/hypoxia)
- Chest X-ray (aspiration and other pneumonias)
- ECG (atrial fibrillation from acute heavy alcohol use or alcoholic cardiomyopathy, psychostimulant-induced arrhythmias)
- Abdominal fibroscan: cirrhosis of the liver
- ECHO—cardiac (alcoholic cardiomyopathy), abdomen (liver or gall bladder disease, pancreatitis, carcinoma of bowel)
- Brain CT/MRI (head injury, subdural haematoma, first seizure; Wernicke's encephalopathy).

Seeking the truth

Collateral and corroborative information

Some patients with alcohol and other substance use disorders are reluctant to divulge information about their substance misuse for fear of prejudice, or develop defence mechanisms to explain, understate, or rationalize their use to themselves and others. In many cases, the clinician will be faced with inconsistencies in the patient's history or the patient's report is at odds with the clinical signs or laboratory test results. In such cases, obtaining collateral or other corroborative information is important. These days one would seek the patient's consent to approach relatives or their GPs within the ethical framework for obtaining information. Other corroborative information comes from previous medical records/case notes, letters, and information from social service agencies, ambulance officers, and police.

In some emergency situations (e.g. acute overdose, acute psychosis, delirium), seeking the patient's consent is not possible. It is important that the ethics and implications of potentially revealing previously undisclosed information about the patient's substance use be carefully kept in mind.

Assessment as a continuing process

Diagnosis in alcohol and substance use disorders is not typically a spot diagnosis. In some cases, in the initial consultation a definitive diagnosis cannot be made, and the diagnosis is reviewed at follow-up interviews.

Always be open to new information. Repeated and incremental assessment is necessary to receive, process, and appraise new information, particularly if there is concern that the patient is understating or minimizing use and the impact it is having on him or her.

Be alert that patients commonly use more than one substance and consider whether there has been:

- missed or incorrect diagnosis of alcohol or substance use disorders, and inappropriate management
- missed or incorrect diagnosis of medical, psychiatric, and social complications of alcohol and other substance misuse, or co-morbidity, and inappropriate management
- lack of appropriate medical, psychiatric, or psychological treatment and follow-up services
- psychological factors—boredom, low self-esteem, stress
- environmental factors: lack of family or social support, peers/partners who drink excessively, or misuse substances.

Common presentations

See Table 5.1 for some common presentation of alcohol and other substance use disorders.

Table 5.1 Some common presentations of alcohol and other substance use disorders

Clinical problem	Presumptive diagnosis	Alcohol and other substance use-related diagnosis
GI system		
Dyspepsia, heartburn	Peptic ulcer; hiatus hernia	Alcohol-induced gastritis, oesophagitis
Vomiting, diarrhoea	Gastroenteritis	Alcohol withdrawal Opioid withdrawal
Upper GI bleeding	Oesophagitis Gastritis Peptic ulcer Carcinoma	Alcohol-induced: – Gastritis/oesophagitis – Mallory Weiss syndrome – Oesophageal varices NSAIDs ± alcohol
Lower GI bleeding	Diverticular disease, polyps Carcinoma Inflammatory bowel disease	Cocaine intoxication (bowel ischaemia from vasoconstriction)
Abdominal pain ± jaundice	Viral hepatitis Cholecystitis Pancreatitis	Alcoholic hepatitis/cirrhosis Viral hepatitis (hepatitis C, B secondary to IDU) Alcoholic pancreatitis
Cardiovascular system		
Palpitations, SOB, ankle swelling	Ischaemic heart disease, Tachyarrhythmias; AF Congestive cardiac failure (CCF)	Stimulant intoxication Alcoholic cardiomyopathy
High blood pressure	Essential hypertension	Alcohol-induced hypertension Stimulant-induced hypertension
Chest pain	Myocardial infarction, ischaemic heart disease	Cocaine-induced ischaemia/ myocardial infarction

(Continued)

Table 5.1 (Contd.)

Clinical problem	Presumptive diagnosis	Alcohol and other substance use-related diagnosis
Neuropsychiatric		
Anxiety, tremor, sweating, insomnia	Anxiety disorder	Alcohol (and/or sedative) withdrawal Stimulant intoxication
Depression	Major depressive illness	Stimulant 'crash' or withdrawal
Blackouts	Vasovagal or cardiac syncope Concussion—head injury	Alcohol intoxication
Seizures	Hypoglycaemia Epilepsy Cerebral neoplasms Head trauma Cerebral infections Hyponatraemia, hypomagnesaemia, Hypocalcaemia	Alcohol withdrawal seizures Benzodiazepine withdrawal seizures Stimulant-induced seizures
Confusion	Hypo- or hyperglycaemia Infections, etc. (As below for delirium)	Alcohol intoxication Alcohol withdrawal (mild to moderate) Benzodiazepine withdrawal Wernicke's encephalopathy
Delirium	Infections Hypoxia Trauma—head injury, subdural haematoma Post-ictal Hypo- or hyperglycaemia Hypo- or hyperthyroidism Electrolyte disturbances Cardiac failure Cerebrovascular accidents Hepatic encephalopathy Uraemia Cerebral neoplasm HIV/AIDS	Severe alcohol withdrawal/delirium tremens Severe benzodiazepine withdrawal Wernicke's encephalopathy

(continued)

Table 5.1 (*Contd.*)

Clinical problem	Presumptive diagnosis	Alcohol and other substance use-related diagnosis
Cognitive impairment	Dementia Alzheimer's disease Chronic subdural haematoma Syphilis HIV/AIDs Cerebral neoplasm Cerebrovascular disease Thiamine or B12 deficiency	Alcohol related brain damage Wernicke–Korsakoff syndrome
Coma	Trauma—subdural haematoma, head injury Hypo- or hyperglycaemia Cerebrovascular accident Cerebral and other infections Epilepsy Cerebral neoplasm	Alcohol intoxication. Opioid overdose Benzodiazepine overdose Ketamine overdose GHB overdose
Paranoid delusions and hallucinations	Schizophrenia	Alcoholic hallucinosis Delirium tremens Stimulant-induced psychosis Cannabis-induced psychosis

Screening instruments and questionnaires

Screening instruments

Screening and brief assessment instruments and questionnaires can often help the practitioner extract the salient points in the history (e.g. AUDIT variants and CAGE for alcohol problems; ASSIST is a combined screen for drug and alcohol misuse developed by WHO). These typically include ten items or fewer and are suitable for self-completion while in the waiting room or hospital clinic. These instruments are presented in Chapter 27. The Hospital Anxiety and Depression Scale (HADS) is also a useful brief screening tool for patients with underlying anxiety or depression.

Assessment instruments

More detailed assessment instruments such as SADQ (Severity of Alcohol Dependence Questionnaire), ASI (Addiction Severity Index), SDS (Severity of Dependence Scale), SODQ (Severity of Opiate Dependence Questionnaire), and quality of life questionnaires (SF14, SF36, SF96) are also sometimes used in specialist practices. See Chapter 27 for more information.

Diagnostic schedules

Complex interview-based schedules, such as CIDI (Composite International Diagnostic Interview), SAM (Substance Abuse Module), HoNOS (Health of the Nation Outcome Scales), SCAN (WHO Schedules for Clinical Assessment in Neuropsychiatry, DIS (Diagnostic Interview Schedule, National Institutes of Mental Health) cover a range of alcohol and substance use disorders from which validated diagnosis can be made. These are used by trained researchers for research purposes and are rarely used in clinical practice.

Formulation and diagnosis

With the assessment having been performed, information needs to be synthesized for a clear provisional diagnosis for each substance or group of substances, and for medical, psychiatric, and social complications and co-morbid conditions

In general, the clinician seeks the most parsimonious diagnosis. Alcohol and other substance use can explain a range of seemingly unrelated problems or conditions

Establishing a final diagnosis

Definitive diagnosis requires evaluation and a decision made on the presence or absence of the following (Fig. 5.2):

- Alcohol or other substance intoxication/overdose
- Non-dependent hazardous or harmful alcohol and/or other substance use (ICD 10) or mild to moderate alcohol and/or other substance use disorder
- Alcohol dependence or substance dependence (ICD 10) or moderate to severe alcohol use disorder or substance use disorder (DSM-5)
- Alcohol and/or other substance withdrawal syndrome
- Medical complications of alcohol or other substance use
- Psychiatric complications of alcohol or other substance use
- Primary or underlying mental health disorders, e.g. anxiety, depression, psychosis leading to alcohol and or substance use.
- Co-morbidity—usually taken to indicate a psychiatric disorder together with a substance use disorder
- Social complications of alcohol or other substance use
- Environmental factors: peers/partners who drink excessively or use substances
- Perpetuating factors for alcohol and substance misuse
- Polysubstance use prioritizing the different substance used.
- In addition the following information can be noted:
  - Are there major psychosocial stressors which are likely to impact on the treatment plan?

Once a diagnosis is made (Fig. 5.2), a treatment plan should be negotiated with, and agreed to by the patient. Early intervention measures will suffice for those with non-dependent hazardous/harmful use or mild alcohol or substance use disorders; for those with alcohol or substance dependence or severe alcohol or substance use disorders, the ideal goal is abstinence although this may not always be achievable.

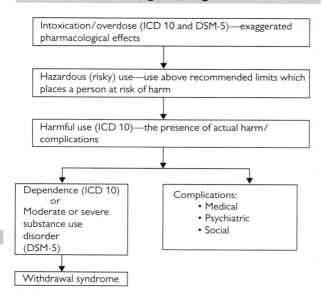

Fig. 5.2 Diagnosis of alcohol and substance use disorders.

Further reading

American Psychiatric Association (2000). *Diagnostic and Statistical Manual of Mental Disorders* (4th ed.). Washington, DC: American Psychiatric Association.

American Psychiatric Association (2013). *Diagnostic and Statistical Manual of Mental Disorders* (5th ed.). Washington, DC: American Psychiatric Association.

Babor TF, Higgins-Biddle JC, Saunders JB, et al. (2001). *The Alcohol Use Disorders Identification Test (AUDIT): Guidelines for Use in Primary Care* (2nd ed). Geneva: World Health Organization. Available at: http://apps.who.int/iris/bitstream/10665/67205/1/WHO_MSD_MSB_01.6a.pdf

Bradley KA, DeBenedetti AF, Volk RJ, et al. (2007). AUDIT-C as a brief screen for alcohol misuse in primary care. *Alcohol Clin Exp Res* 31:1208–17.

Saitz R, Saxon AJ, Hermann R. *Screening for Unhealthy Use of Alcohol and Other Drugs.* UpToDate®. [Online] Available at: http://www.uptodate.com/contents/screening-for-unhealthy-use-of-alcohol-and-other-drugs-in-primary-care

World Health Organization (1992). *The ICD 10 Classification of Mental and Behavioural Disorders. Clinical Descriptions and Diagnostic Guidelines.* Geneva: World Health Organization.

Acute care

Management of acute intoxication and overdose 86
Management of acute withdrawal syndromes 90
The suicidal patient 94
Confusion and delirium 95
Management of acute psychosis 98

Management of acute intoxication and overdose

Introduction and overview

Acute intoxication and overdose are challenging and dynamic events that cover a wide spectrum of presentations involving deliberate self-poisoning, and intoxication from alcohol, illicit and prescribed drugs.
- Both basic and advanced life support (BLS and ALS) techniques may be required together with ongoing intensive care support.
- Early identification and initiation of such supportive and restorative processes can result in good clinical outcomes.
- A myriad of complications can occur—a key imperative to clinical management is a simple hierarchical risk stratification and risk minimization approach.

Risk assessment

This is an essential step involving information from all sources, and should focus on:
- the individual:
  - the specific medical history (diabetes, asthma, chronic airways disease, cardiovascular and liver disease, epilepsy, mental health problems)
  - drug history (alcohol, benzodiazepines, opioids and other substances, injecting drug use)
  - risk factors (overdose, suicide attempt, trauma)
- the agent taken or potentially taken
- consideration of both the likely and the 'worst-case' scenario so that the necessary interventions can be put in place to avoid this. (See Box 6.1.)

This approach supports the clinician to deal with potentially time-critical management priorities in an appropriate order. The medical concerns when faced with a patient who has an altered level of consciousness or is at risk of becoming altered is whether they are able to protect their airway, ventilate well, and remain vitally stable with normal pulse rate and BP.

Box 6.1 Assessing acute intoxication/overdose
- What does the patient say?
- What information do the ambulance crew and paramedics have?
- What is the drug? How much has been taken?
- When was it taken? How long has it been?
- What does the Poison Centre advise?
- Where are the family, friends? What do they know?
- Why has this happened? Has this happened in the past?
- What else do we know of the patient?
- What is the expected clinical course?
- Document the initial management plan.

Resuscitation (ABCDE)

A. *Airway:* at risk with reduced consciousness: ensure it is patent.

B. *Breathing:* hypoventilation requiring assistance with bag valve mask.

C. *Circulation:* tachycardia or hypotension requiring intravenous bolus.

D. *Disability and neurological stabilization:* for altered mental state:
- Intravenous thiamine 200–500 mg three times per day (slowly—and before glucose)
- If BSL <4.0 mmol/L, correct hypoglycaemia with intravenous dextrose
- Intravenous naloxone in known or suspected opioid toxicity to reverse respiratory depression (see 'Assessment and management of opioid overdose', pp. 264–6 and pp. 408–11)
- Intravenous benzodiazepines (e.g. diazepam 10 mg and repeated every 10 minutes as necessary) for seizures /refractory seizures
- Note that flumazenil is not recommended even in suspected benzodiazepine overdose because of the risk of seizures.

E. *Exposure and elimination:*
- Remove clothing and external contaminants.
- Look for trauma, concealed weapons, or drugs.
- Look for needle tracts marks, abscesses; malnourishment, jaundice, bruises.
- Elimination:
  - multiple dose charcoal
  - urinary alkalinization
  - haemofiltration and haemodialysis
  - charcoal haemoperfusion.
- Decontamination needs to be balanced against risk of aspiration, obstruction, and perforation. Consider induced emesis, gastric lavage, activated charcoal, whole-bowel irrigation but usually these are not indicated.

Rapid systematic examination

- General appearance: malnourished, cachetic (malignancy; HIV)
- Body temperature:
  - correct hyperthermia:
    - — psychostimulant, hallucinogen, synthetic cannabinoid use
    - — drug withdrawal states
    - — serotonin syndrome
    - — neuroleptic malignant syndrome (NMS)
  - or correct hypothermia:
    - — use of opioids, sedative-hypnotics, alcohol or antipsychotics
- Blood pressure and pulse rate:
  - hypertension with tachycardia: use of psychostimulants, hallucinogens, nicotine, or anticholinergics, or withdrawal states from alcohol and other substances
  - hypertension with bradycardia: use of cholinergics; steroids

- hypotension with bradycardia: use of opioids, barbiturates, benzodiazepines
- tachyarrhythmias—psychostimulant use
- atrial fibrillation: alcoholic cardiomyopathy, caffeine, ischaemic or valvular heart disease.
- Heart murmurs: bacterial endocarditis (IDUs) in addition to other causes such as valvular heart disease.
- Respiration:
  - tachypnoea and hyperventilation: use of psychostimulants, hallucinogens, or methanol; alcohol and drug withdrawal states; alcoholic ketoacidosis
  - bradycardia and hypoventilation: use of opioids, alcohols, sedative hypnotics, antidepressants, antipsychotics, cholinergics, volatile solvents, muscle relaxants.
- Gastrointestinal tract:
  - stigmata of chronic and/or decompensated liver disease (alcohol with or without coexisting hepatitis B, C, D)
  - bleeding PR (bowel ischaemia—cocaine; inflammatory bowel disease, malignancy).
- Central nervous system:
  - level of consciousness
  - pupil size: mydriasis due to opioid withdrawal, anticholinergics, psychostimulants, hallucinogens, or serotonin syndrome; or miosis due to opioid toxicity, cholinergics, sedative-hypnotics, alcohols
  - unequal pupils: head injury, CVA
  - CNS depression: use of sedative hypnotics, opioids; alcohols, volatile inhalants, antidepressants, or GHB
  - CNS stimulation: use of psychostimulants or hallucinogens; drug withdrawal states;
  - neck stiffness: CVA, cerebral haemorrhage from psychostimulant use; meningitis
  - seizures: alcohol or benzodiazepine withdrawal states; psychostimulant use; epilepsy.

NB: patients often ingest more than one substance and this may cloud the clinical picture.

Investigations

- Standard investigations: FBC, EUC, LFTs, CRP, ESR; coagulation, CPK, TFTs, serum B_{12}/folate/magnesium; lactate
- Toxicology screen (blood /urine): serum paracetamol, salicylate levels, BAC; urine drug screen (UDS)
- Blood gases
- Screening: 12-lead ECG monitor.

Other investigations as indicated by clinical condition e.g.:
- Rhabdomyolysis—CK (creatine kinase): prolonged ischaemia/ immobilization, uncontrolled seizures, alcohol, psychostimulants, opioids, hallucinogens; NMS; serotonin syndrome—consider dialysis
- Head injury/subdural haemorrhage or cerebrovascular events from psychostimulants: brain CT; brain MRI

- SBE: blood culture (IDU)
- Blood-borne viral infections: serology (IDU)
- MSU
- Chest X-ray: non-cardiogenic pulmonary oedema (opioid toxicity, pulmonary irritants)
- Pregnancy test in women of child bearing age
- CSF.

Supportive care and monitoring

- *Stabilize in the ED*: if improved, then period of observation within suitable clinical environment able to deal with deterioration.
- *Admit to ED observation*: should be undertaken if monitoring required, deterioration not expected, and patient stable and compliant or sedated for care.
- *Criteria for ICD admission*:
  - airway control: $PaCO_2$ >45 mmHg
  - ventilation: emergency intubation
  - prolonged or invasive haemodynamic monitoring
  - haemodialysis
  - systolic BP <80 mmHg
  - QRS >0.12 seconds; AV block
  - unresponsive to verbal stimuli
  - post-ingestion seizures.

There is now an opportunity to reflect upon earlier decisions and consider if antidote is indicated or available.

Care plan

- Safe disposition and review has to be documented.
- This key step requires clarity of an ongoing plan.
- This may require retrieval to specialist unit in/outside the hospital.
- A proactive care plan will engage with the multidisciplinary team and ensure that all clinical and psychosocial components are addressed with an adequate clinical and mental health review in place.

Prevention

Acute intoxication often represents a severe exacerbation of a more chronic psychosocial disorder. Gaining insights into the history, and speaking with the family and community or specialist mental health workers who know the patient and their environment help in a rapid stabilization of not only the clinical situation but also the underlying crisis. Caring for such vulnerable patients can be exhausting within the context of a busy ED. Ensuring that a suitable strategy is in place for the patient and family to cope with a similar crisis in the future will also reduce recurrence and limit repeat presentations.

Further reading

Burns M. (2015). *General Approach to Drug Poisoning in Adults*. UpToDate®. [Online] Available at: http://www.uptodate.com/contents/general-approach-to-drug-poisoning-in-adults

Sivilotti MLA (2015). *Initial Management of the Critically Ill Adult with an Unknown Overdose*. UpToDate®. [Online] Available at: http://www.uptodate.com/contents/initial-management-of-the-critically-ill-adult-with-an-unknown-overdose

Management of acute withdrawal syndromes

Introduction and overview

In this section, we provide general guidance to the management of alcohol and drug withdrawal states. This section is intended to introduce the principles of withdrawal management and particularly in the acute care setting. Details and specific protocols, together with coverage of elective withdrawal management (often termed 'detoxification') are included in the chapters on specific substances.

Although elective detoxification can be carried out at home or on an ambulatory basis, in a hospital, clinic, or specialist detoxification unit, management of an acute withdrawal state is typically a role for the ED, acute general hospital ward, acute psychiatric unit, or some addiction specialist units.

Management of withdrawal in hospital is recommended for patients:
• who present in an acute withdrawal state
• who have severe alcohol or drug use disorders
• where confusion or delirium are present
• who have severe vomiting or diarrhoea, or are debilitated or malnourished
• who have a previous history of epilepsy or withdrawal seizures
• who have a history of DTs or complicated withdrawal syndromes
• who have acute psychiatric disorders and/or at risk of harm to self and to others
• who have severe concurrent medical illness
• in some cases who are living alone or in an unsupportive environment.

Sometimes, patients who have been admitted to hospital for treatment of medical, surgical, or psychiatric illnesses may circumstantially develop withdrawal symptoms from undiagnosed alcohol and other substance use disorders.

Assessment

Be alert for the possibility of a withdrawal syndrome and conduct a thorough assessment, in particular:
• full history of alcohol and other substance use
• systematic physical examination: monitor temperature, tremor, sweating, piloerection, pulse rate, BP, oximeter readings, pupil size, stigmata of liver disease, mental state examination, neurological observations
• use appropriate screening instruments (e.g. AUDIT)
• organize routine FBC, EUC, LFTs, BSL, magnesium levels, and other laboratory tests as indicated

- blood or breath alcohol levels and urine drug screen as required
- if clinically indicated, CPK, serum B_{12}, folate levels, TFTs, CXR, brain CT/MRI, ECG, arterial blood gases
- as IDUs are at risk of bacterial, fungal, and viral infections: serological investigations for hepatitis B, C, and HIV, blood cultures as well as CK-MB.

An alcohol withdrawal syndrome may occur concurrently with other withdrawal syndromes, e.g. benzodiazepines, barbiturates, baclofen, opioids, cannabis, and psychostimulants.

A range of medical and psychiatric disorders may mimic, or coexist with, the withdrawal syndrome, in particular:

- Wernicke's encephalopathy (alcohol), infections, hypoxia, hepatic encephalopathy, head injury, subdural haematoma and metabolic disturbances and other causes of delirium; if withdrawal seizures occur, be alert for DTs
- psychiatric illnesses either independent disorders (such as anxiety, depression, suicidality, psychosis) or related to alcohol and/or other drug use.

These, and other concurrent medical, psychiatric and social disorders need to be identified, and appropriately treated concurrently.

Management (4S's)

Management involves:

- Sedation
- Support and monitoring
- Supplements
- Standard (existing) treatments.

Sedation

- For acute alcohol and sedative drug withdrawal states, the predominant need is to control the withdrawal state by an appropriate sedative regimen, most commonly using a benzodiazepine.
- If the withdrawal syndrome is not speedily controlled, it may progress to a more severe disorder with complications such as seizures and delirium, acute dehydration, and (occasionally) renal failure.
- On the other hand, care must be taken to ensure that the sedative regimen does not compromise the patient's respiratory and cardiovascular status.
- Particular caution needs to be taken in patients with respiratory disease (especially respiratory failure), obstructive sleep apnoea, severe heart disease (especially heart failure), cirrhosis and other chronic liver disease (especially if there is portosystemic encephalopathy or other signs of hepatic decompensation) and in patients with head injury.

Support and monitoring
- Nurse patient in quiet, dimly lit room, provide constant reassurance and reorientation.
- Monitor withdrawal scores regularly at 2–4-hourly intervals with appropriate withdrawal scales, e.g. AWS, CIWA-AR (for alcohol, see pp. 606–16), benzodiazepine withdrawal scale (pp. 612–13), opioid withdrawal scale (p. 614, p. 615); cannabis withdrawal scale (p. 616).

Supplements
- Maintain hydration and fluid balance.
- Ensure normal electrolyte levels, especially potassium, and also magnesium levels.

Standard (existing) treatments
Although it may seem trite to mention it, the patient's existing medications and other treatments should be reviewed to ensure that essential medication is continued, but also that medication which may be contraindicated in a withdrawal state is identified and where necessary ceased.

Comments on management of specific withdrawal states

Alcohol withdrawal syndrome
- Sedate with benzodiazepines, generally the longer-acting diazepam or chlordiazepoxide. Use with caution in patients whose respiratory system is compromised or in those with head injury or decompensated liver disease.
- Vitamin supplementation: parenteral thiamine for patients with suspected or diagnosed Wernicke's syndrome, plus oral multivitamins.
- Antipsychotic medication may be necessary in addition if the patient remains agitated or has hallucinations—haloperidol 5 mg orally three to four times a day, or alternatively olanzapine 2.5–5 mg orally three to four times a day.
- Pharmacotherapy: following the withdrawal phase, treatment may be commenced with a medication such as naltrexone, acamprosate, or disulfiram in conjunction with a comprehensive relapse prevention programme.

Benzodiazepine withdrawal syndrome
- Generally, a pre-planned programme with a long-acting benzodiazepine-reducing regimen titrated according to response.
- Follow-up on discharge with further gradual dose reductions supervised by the addiction specialist or GP over a period of time, in conjunction with psychosocial counselling and support.

Heroin and other opioid withdrawal syndrome
- The preference is to manage withdrawal symptoms and signs using buprenorphine or methadone, which gives superior completion rates to non-opioid-based regimens.
- The alternative is to employ clonidine or lofexidine, together with symptomatic treatment with diazepam, loperamide, hyoscine, and (sometimes) quinine (the latter for muscle cramps).

Cannabis withdrawal syndrome
- Sedate with diazepam, where necessary and guided by a suitable withdrawal scale.
- Some authorities recommend the use of quetiapine, olanzapine, or mirtazapine (latter: 15–30 mg at night).

Psychostimulant withdrawal syndrome
- During the acute phase of stimulant use/intoxication, stimulant-induced psychosis may occur (p. 340).
- Following this, there is an initial withdrawal phase (the 'crash) which is characterized by dysphoria, fatigue, insomnia or hypersomnia, increased appetite, depression, and psychomotor agitation.
- Depressive symptoms and anxiety with increased risk of suicidality are features of the withdrawal syndrome.
- Therefore it is important to monitor for depression and suicidality and adopt suicide precautions and treatment where necessary.

Further reading

World Health Organization (2011). *mhGAP Intervention Guide for Mental, Neurological and Substance Use Disorders in Non-Specialized Health Settings*. Geneva: WHO. Available at: http://www.who.int/mental_health/publications/mhGAP_intervention_guide/en/

The suicidal patient

The patient and carer(s) should always be involved in the development of the management plan, including the treatment setting and any strategies to minimize the risk of suicide. Nominate a key worker/clinician to coordinate the care plan.

Determine the level of intervention required

Consider the following:
- Degree of insight and impulsivity
- Diagnosis and severity of illness
- Safety and security of current environment
- Ability to engage meaningfully with treating team
- Level of protective factors (e.g. social supports).

Enhance protective factors

- Instil hope
- Ensure family and social supports are in place
- Minimize substance use and intoxication
- Provide practical assistance with accommodation and food
- Provide psychological interventions to reduce distress and increase coping skills (e.g. problem-solving, anxiety management)
- Provide advice on sleep, exercise, and diet
- Treat underlying mental illness.

Determine the appropriate treatment setting

- Remove any objects in the immediate environment that pose a risk (e.g. razor blades, sharp knives)
- Consider referral for further assessment by mental health services
- Call ambulance and/or police if transfer to ED required
- Consider use of Mental Health Act and hospitalization if suicide risk escalates beyond ability of the health team and supports to manage.

Develop a contingency plan

- Establish clear directions for what to do when suicidality increases; written instructions may be helpful
- Generate a number of alternatives to suicide and self-harm: behavioural alternatives (e.g. mindfulness, exercise, journaling, call a friend); medication alternatives; urgent review
- Include support numbers for within and outside working hours (crisis team, ambulance, key support person, key clinician).

Clearly document your management plan including frequency of ongoing monitoring, and plan for rapid reassessment if symptoms or distress worsen.

Further reading

Lee N, Jenner L. *PsyCheck Screening Tool*. Available at: http://www.psycheck.org.au
NSW Department of Health (2004). *Framework for Suicide Risk Assessment and Management for NSW Staff*. North Sydney: NSW Department of Health. Available at: http://www.health.nsw.gov.au/mhdao/programs/mh/Publications/framework-suicide-risk-assess.pdf

Confusion and delirium

Introduction and overview

Confusion is the inability to think as clearly or quickly as usual for that person. It is typically associated with disorientation—in time, place, and/or person. It is a lay term, although one commonly used in medical and healthcare settings.

Delirium is a medical diagnostic term. It is an acute confusional state which is characterized by some or all of the following features:

- Disturbed consciousness ('clouding')
- Reduced concentration
- Reduced attention span
- Perceptual abnormalities: visual or auditory hallucinations, with an acute onset (hours to days) and fluctuating course, often worse in the evening
- Disorientation: in time, place, and/or person
- Disturbance in cognitive functions
- Lability of affect.

In alcohol and benzodiazepine withdrawal states, delirium is associated with agitation, tremulousness, and autonomic hyperactivity. Delirium can also present in a hypoactive way with drowsiness or lethargy.

If not diagnosed and treated early, delirium is likely to progress to stupor, coma, seizures, and death. Mortality in the untreated or poorly treated case may be as high as 40%

The prevalence of delirium in patients on medical wards is between 15% and 30%. The incidence of delirium (per patient, per hospitalization) in a general hospital is 5–50%, depending on the age of the individual, and 70–85% in intensive care patients.

Causes of delirium

For causes of delirium see Table 6.1.

It is often difficult to differentiate delirium from dementia particularly in the elderly and in those with pre-existing neurocognitive defects.

Management of delirium

1. Supportive care by trained nurses in an ICU or through 1:1 nursing in an acute medical or psychiatric unit.
2. Manage in a dimly lit, quiet room, constantly reassuring and reorientating the patient, facilitating visits from family and friends.
3. Identify, exclude, and treat the known underlying causes of delirium. See Table 6.1
4. Regular hourly to 4-hourly monitoring of BP, PR, respiration, oxygen saturation, neurological observations, AWS or CIWA-Ar or CIWA-B scores.
5. Ensure adequate fluid intake, and maintain nutrition.
6. Ensure appropriate fluid and electrolyte balance, and ensure that sodium, potassium, and magnesium levels are normal.

Table 6.1 Differential diagnosis of delirium in patients with substance use disorders

Condition	Differentiating factors
Wernicke's encephalopathy	Clinical features, low serum thiamine levels, low erythrocyte transketolase. Time is of the essence: give parenteral thiamine immediately if Wernicke Syndrome diagnosed or suspected.
Alcohol and drug intoxication delirium	Clinical features, BAC
Substance withdrawal delirium: Alcohol withdrawal delirium (DTs) Benzodiazepine withdrawal delirium Baclofen withdrawal Barbiturate withdrawal	Likely AWS >10; CIWA Ar >15 CIWA B >41
Infections (including HIV/AIDS, sepsis encephalitis, meningitis, brain abscess)	Clinical features, fever, blood cultures, CSF, antiGQ1b antibodies, full viral screen including HIV Ab, VDRL, MRI
Head injury/subdural haematoma	History of fall/assault/seizures, CT brain, brain MRI
Hypoxia	History of chronic heavy tobacco smoking; clinical features of respiratory insufficiency, blood gases, CXR
Hepatic encephalopathy	History of excess alcohol/IDU, clinical features of hepatic decompensation, LFTs, coags, AFP, hepatitis B , C serology
Uraemic encephalopathy	History, clinical features of renal failure, serum ammonia
Toxic encephalopathies/toxins (ethylene glycol, methanol, CO, cyanide)	History, urine drug screen; toxicology heavy metal screen
Cerebrovascular accidents	History, clinical features, CT brain, brain MRI
Cerebral neoplasms	History, clinical features, CT brain, brain MRI
Hypomagnesaemia	Serum magnesium levels
Hypo- or hypercalcaemia	Serum calcium, PO_4
Hypo- or hyperglycaemia	BSL
Hypo- or hyperthyroidism	Clinical features, TFTs
Fluid and electrolyte imbalances (from severe diarrhoea/vomiting/perspiration, diuretics)	Clinical features, EUC

Table 6.1 (Contd.)

Condition	Differentiating factors
Hypokalaemia or hyponatraemia	History of vomiting, diarrhoea, EUC, ECG
Acute psychotic illness Drug-induced psychosis (cannabis, psychostimulants, hallucinogens antipsychotics, antihistamines)	History, clinical features, UDS
Schizophrenia	History, psychiatric assessment
Vitamin deficiency states (B_1, B_{12}, possibly folate and niacin deficiency)	History, clinical features, serum B_{12}, folate levels
Serotonin syndrome	Drug interactions e.g. psychostimulant + SSRI, clinical features, blood tests

7. Have a high index of suspicion of a Wernicke syndrome in patients with alcohol use disorders and treat with parenteral thiamine. Always give thiamine before glucose and add multivitamins.
8. Sedate with benzodiazepines (diazepam, lorazepam, chlordiazepoxide) if patient is agitated, particularly if the patient is withdrawing from alcohol or benzodiazepines. Note that benzodiazepines may paradoxically worsen delirium in some patients.
9. Antipsychotic agents such as haloperidol (2.5–5.0 mg orally or IM every 4–6 hours) or olanzapine (2.5–5.0 mg every 6–8 hours).

Further reading

BMJ Best Practice (2014). *Assessment of Delirium.* [Online] Available at: http://bestpractice.bmj.com/best-practice/monograph/241.html

Francis J, Young GB (2014). *Delirium and Confusional States: Prevention, Treatment, and Prognosis.* UpToDate®. [Online] Available at: http://www.uptodate.com/contents/diagnosis-of-delirium-and-confusional-states

National Institute for Health and Care Excellence (2010, reviewed 2015). *Delirium: Diagnosis, Prevention and Management.* Clinical Guideline 103. London: NICE. Available at: https://www.nice.org.uk/guidance/cg103

Management of acute psychosis

Introduction and overview

Psychosis is a disorder of thinking and perception characterized by hallucinations, delusions, and thought disorder. Overarousal and hostility typically reflect positive psychotic symptoms. Irritability may indicate elevated mood. There may be disorganization, agitation, or aggression (see Table 6.2).

Assessment

The diagnosis is clinical:
- Undertake a medical and psychiatric history
- Conduct a mental state examination
- Seek collateral history
- Check for suicidality
- Investigations: FBC, EUC, thyroid function tests, LFTs, syphilis serology, BSL, CPK, BAC, urine drug screen, HIV testing where indicated, CT brain scan, MRI brain scan.

Management of acute psychosis

1. Ensure safety of patient, staff, and surrounding personnel. This is of paramount importance.
2. Physical restraint if there is danger to patient or others.
3. De-escalation techniques: approach patient in calm manner to defuse disturbed and disruptive behaviour.
4. Seclusion.
5. Nurse in a quiet, dimly lit room.
6. Observations: regular monitoring of temperature, BP, pulse rate, and respiratory rate, monitor oxygen saturation (pulse oximetry), neurological observations, Glasgow Coma Scale (GCS) score, ECG monitoring as required.
7. If hyperthermic, promote cooling.
8. Rapid tranquillization: follow local protocols.

Summary guidelines for rapid tranquillization

1. Offer oral drug treatment. If the patient is extremely agitated:
   - Lorazepam 1–2 mg or
   - Promethazine 25–50 mg or
   - Buccal midazolam 10–20 mg.
2. Consider an antipsychotic if not already taking one regularly:
   - Olanzapine 10 mg or
   - Risperidone 1–2 mg or
   - Haloperidol 5 mg (last resort: pre-treatment ECG needed).
3. Repeat lorazepam after 45–60 minutes.
4. Combine sedatives and antipsychotics as necessary.
5. Consider IM treatment if two oral doses fail or patient still very disturbed:
   - Lorazepam 1–2 mg
   - Promethazine 25–50 mg or

Table 6.2 Common causes of acute psychosis

Substance-induced psychosis:
a) Intoxication and overdose
	Psychostimulants (p. 337):
	  Amphetamines
	  Cocaine
	  MDMA
	Cannabis (p. 243)
	Hallucinogens (p. 359, pp. 359–60, p. 360)
	  LSD
	Phencyclidine
	Dextromethorphan
	Ketamine

b) Withdrawal states	Alcohol/DTs (p. 188, p. 189)
	Sedative hypnotics:
	  Benzodiazepines (p. 315)
	  Barbiturates (p. 323)

Mental health disorders	Schizophrenia Bipolar affective disorder Schizoaffective disorder Brief psychotic disorder Severe depressive episode in major depression
Medical illnesses	CNS: head trauma, CVA, epilepsy, infection, haemorrhage, neoplasms, delirium Infections: syphilis, HIV/AIDS Endocrine dysfunction: thyrotoxicosis Metabolic causes: hypoxia, hypoglycaemia, fluid and electrolyte abnormalities Dementia Severe hepatic and renal disorders Postpartum psychosis

- Olanzapine 10 mg or
- Aripiprazole 9.75 mg or
- Haloperidol 5 mg (high incidence of acute dystonia so be ready to give IM procyclidine).
6. Repeat after 30–60 minutes if needed.
7. If repeat IM treatment ineffective after 30–60 minutes try IV treatment. Diazepam 10 mg over at least 5 minutes (flumazenil should be available). Repeat after 5–10 minutes if insufficient effect (up to three times).

If this does not work seek expert advice.

Tranquillization using a benzodiazepine

An alternative to the previous protocol is to use repeated high doses of a benzodiazepine.

- Give diazepam 10–20 mg orally and repeat after 2 hours until the patient is calm and mildly sedated; typical dose of 60–100 mg in the first 24 hours.
- If the patient is extremely agitated or violent, it may be necessary to give IV diazepam (10 mg slowly over at least 5 minutes), titrating dose according to response. This may be repeated after 30 minutes if necessary. Then switch to oral diazepam as above.
- An alternative is midazolam 2.5–10 mg (IM or IV), repeated as necessary after 10 minutes, and with further doses given according to response up to a maximum of 20 mg.
- Some centres prefer lorazepam 0.5–2 mg three times per day orally or IM. Maximum oral dose 20 mg/day.
- Flumazenil should be available when using high doses of benzodiazepines.
- Patients requiring parenteral benzodiazepines should be nursed in an intensive care unit because of the risk of respiratory depression, aspiration, airway obstruction, or hypotension.

Antipsychotic agents

- When using antipsychotic agents, prescribe an oral preparation as first-line treatment.
- Give IM only when unable to take oral medication.
- Use only one antipsychotic drug, at the lowest effective dose.
- Give a second generation antipsychotic drug e.g. olanzapine 5–10 mg (maximum oral dose: 20 mg/day, less in lactating mothers) or quetiapine 50–100mg (maximum 200 mg/day in the first instance).
- Alternatively, use a first generation antipsychotic drug e.g. haloperidol 2.5–10 mg (maximum oral dose: 30 mg/day).
- Taper off and discontinue treatment with antipsychotic agents when symptoms resolve.

Acute dystonia

- For acute dystonia give procyclidine 5–10 mg IM/IV and repeat after 20 minutes if necessary; maximum 20 mg daily (or equivalent IM dose of benztropine).

Extrapyramidal side effects

- Treat side effects from first-generation antipsychotic agents with benztropine 1–2 mg orally three times per day.
- Alternatively give a second-generation antipsychotic, such as olanzapine 5–10 mg (maximum oral dose: 20 mg/day, less in lactating mothers), or quetiapine 25–100 mg.
- Do not give phenothiazines which lower seizure threshold.

Suicide risk assessment

- In psychotic disorders, the prevalence of suicide is high (in acute psychotic disorder it is approximately 35%).
- Suicidal risk assessment must be undertaken.

Psychosocial treatment

- Offer psychological counselling, psychotherapy, and family support.
- Continue to assess safety.

Continuing management

- In substance-induced psychosis, psychotic symptoms may persist for weeks or months after the substance has been eliminated from the body.
- Once psychotic symptoms have resolved, patients should be reviewed at monthly intervals.
- If symptoms recur, exclude continued substance use, review history, collateral history, and mental state.
- Consider differential diagnosis, including whether the patient might have schizophrenia or bipolar disorder.
- Note that substance-induced psychosis may precede, co-occur with, or develop subsequently to an independent or persistent mental health disorder.
- Psychosis may also coexist with medical illnesses or as part of a delirium, particularly in the elderly, and so causes of delirium should be excluded.

Further reading

BMJ Best Practice (2015). *Brief Psychotic Disorder.* [Online] Available at: http://bestpractice.bmj.com/best-practice/monograph/1118/diagnosis.html

National Institute for Health and Care Excellence (2015). *Violence and Aggression: Short-Term Management in Mental Health, Health and Community Settings.* NICE Guidelines 10. London: NICE. Available at: http://www.nice.org.uk/guidance/ng10

Rao H, Yeung WL, Jayaram M (2012). De-escalation techniques for psychosis induced aggression or agitation. (Protocol). *Cochrane Database Syst Rev* 7:CD009922.

Taylor D, Paton C, Kapur S. (2015). *The Maudsley Prescribing Guidelines in Psychiatry* (12th ed). Chichester: Wiley-Blackwell.

Ongoing management of substance use disorders

Natural history of substance disorders 104
Foundations of management 105
The ten key components of management 107
Mutual help and related groups 113
Other key considerations in treatment 116

Natural history of substance disorders

Natural history

The natural history of substance use disorders is difficult to summarize because of the huge spectrum of use and misuse of the various psycho-active substances. Longitudinal studies have been undertaken for many forms of substance use disorder but their duration varies considerably, being 40 or more years for alcohol use disorders, 10 years for opioid use disorders, but only 2–3 years for cannabis and psychostimulant use disorders. However there are some conclusions we can reach from the aggregate of natural history studies:

- The pathway to substance use disorders typically starts with experimental use. This may move on to repeated but occasional use, more regular use, use with harmful consequences, and then substance dependence and its various physical, mental, and social complications.
- In general, the higher the level of use, the greater frequency of use and the longer duration of use, the greater likelihood of development both of dependence and the harmful consequences of use.
- Population level studies show very different (and usually more favourable) outcomes to those of the clinical populations, reflecting differences in severity and the presence of comorbid disorders.
- Substance dependence (addiction) as seen in clinical populations tends to be a relapsing–remitting–relapsing disorder. Prevention of relapse is a key aim of treatment.
- Certain complications of substance use have particularly severe consequences for health and life. Examples include cirrhosis of the liver, where the decompensated form can result in death within weeks or months. Traumatic injuries may result in sudden death and disability. Substance use is a substantial risk factor for suicide and homicide.

Outcome after treatment

- Overall, treatment modifies the natural history of substance disorders.
- In general, the milder the form of substance use disorder, the greater the degree of scope for reduction in substance use and avoidance of harmful consequences.
- Numerous treatment outcome studies and randomized controlled trials provide evidence of the benefits of treatment and the comparative effectiveness of different forms of treatment respectively.
- Approximately 60% of patients achieve their stated goals after treatment for a substance use disorder.
- Cost–benefit studies demonstrate a return on investment of between 2:1 and 7:1, depending on the nature of the substance disorder and the type of intervention.
- Intervention is justified if the outcome for the individual is better than the expected natural history of the untreated disorder.

Foundations of management

Diagnosis as the basis of management

- The tradition of medicine and the clinical professions is for management to be based on determining the diagnosis for that person.
- Diagnoses are made on the basis of the information provided by the patient at interview, combined with observations made by the clinician, physical examination findings, and sometimes results of laboratory investigations and imaging and other procedures.
- The totality of this information is then compared by the clinician who judges how it conforms to the central features and boundaries of known substance use disorders.
- Often, in the substance use field, it is not possible to reach a definitive diagnosis during the first assessment of the patient; more likely a provisional diagnosis or set of differential diagnoses is reached.

In reaching the diagnosis the clinician should be particularly aware of the following:

- Symptoms of substance use disorders are often similar to those of common mental health disorders and a particular challenge is to distinguish the features of these two sets of disorders.
- Detoxification is typically necessary to achieve clarity of diagnosis by allowing transient symptoms and the masking effect of substance use to disappear, thus allowing a firmer and more confident diagnosis.
- Multiple diagnoses are to be expected in patients with substance use disorders, reflecting the core clinical syndrome of substance use, comorbid psychiatric disorders, and the physical sequelae.

Managing multiple disorders

Given that substance using patients often have multiple and interconnecting disorders, it is necessary to adopt a systematic approach to their delineation and treatment.

- In general, if the person has symptoms suggestive of a mental health disorder and their substance use is at the lower end of the spectrum, the mental health disorder is likely to be the primary condition.
- By contrast, where a person has severe substance dependence, it is more likely that the mental symptoms are a consequence of that, rather than a separate mental health disorder.
- Whenever there is uncertainty as to the presence and nature of substance use and mental health disorders, cessation of substance use should be an early goal to assist with the differential diagnosis and identification of the appropriate treatment.
- Rarely is treatment of a mental disorder successful when the substance dependence remains untreated and substance use uncontrolled.

Multidisciplinary understanding

Our knowledge of substance use disorders has been generated by multiple professional and scientific disciplines. There is no overarching 'model' of substance use disorders.

- Substance use is typically initiated and continued in a social setting. These include groups of friends, parties, after some sporting events, to celebrate birthdays and festive occasions, and in the evenings after study or work. Often the initial use is experimental and leads to no further involvement with that substance. Social influences are therefore of vital importance in sanctioning, facilitating, and indeed discouraging the uptake of use of various substances by young people. The nature of the peer group is highly important and in each generation this varies from the highly socially conservative to the impulsive and reckless. Certain peer groups are strongly linked to certain patterns of substance use and the latter may in effect be required to be accepted into a particular peer group. In addition broad environmental influences such as the availability, cost and legal status of particular substances influence its uptake and ongoing use.

- Behavioural psychology has contributed to our understanding of how patterns of repetitive substance use can develop and how they can become reinforcing through positive and negative contingencies and through principles of social learning.

- Physiological changes through key neurocircuits develop as an adaptive response to repetitive substance use and these changes cause a re-setting of neurocircuits involved with reward, alertness, salience (prioritization), and behavioural control. These are described in detail in Chapter 3 and in sections on pathophysiology in the chapters describing specific substance use disorders.

- There are, correspondingly, many and varied forms of intervention encompassing social approaches, psychological therapies, pharmacological treatments, environmental change, and self-support fellowships. No one profession offers a complete approach to management of substance use disorders. Instead, key elements from different disciplines are drawn upon and the patient encouraged to be engaged in a multidisciplinary programmatic approach.

Figure 4.1 (p. 57) presents an 'at a glance' depiction of the pathways to substance use, the development of dependence/addiction, and the complications that may arise, in a way that is readily understood by a wide spectrum of persons with substance use disorders.

The ten key components of management

The management of substance use disorders can be conveniently sub-divided into ten key components. These components are presented in some degree of chronological order but it must be emphasized that the actual sequence of these interventions varies considerably from patient to patient, and in the same patient, in different episodes of their substance use disorder.

1. Information and understanding

Given the many different perspectives on substance use, it is essential that accurate information is provided to the patient about the overall nature of their substance use disorder. It is convenient to explain this diagrammatically as is seen in Fig. 1.1/4.1. Substance use disorders, apart from acute intoxication, arise because of a repetitive pattern of use. The social, psychological, and neurobiological processes that occur can and should be simply explained to the patient. In this way, the patient and his (or her) family can develop a deeper understanding of the nature of their disorder, its likely natural history, the place of treatment, and why individual components of treatment will be recommended to them.

2. Acceptance and engagement

Seeking help typically represents a very significant step for the person with substance use disorder. Sometimes the person will realize the impact of their substance use and sense that life is becoming out of control. In many cases, however, the impact of the person's substance use is more apparent to others than to the individual. Sometimes a realization that a substance use disorder exists occurs because of a health or personal crisis.

Sources of advice and help range from the informal to professionally delivered treatments. They include the following:

- Informal advice and suggestions from family members, friends, and workmates
- Information from telephone lines and internet-based portals
- Advice from generic health and welfare staff
- Alcohol and drug counsellors
- General medical practitioners (family physicians)
- Specialist addiction psychologists
- Addiction medicine specialists
- Psychiatrists and internal medicine physicians with an addiction specialization
- Mobile phone applications
- Interactive websites.

The range of opportunities for advice and help is considerable in many countries, although minimal in others. See Chapter 27 for a list of overall resources that may be available.

3. Initiating treatment: diagnosis and detoxification

- When the person sees a qualified professional, the first essential is for a diagnosis to be made, both to provide clarity as to what the patient is experiencing and to ensure that the most appropriate intervention is offered.
- The initial intervention is often a form of detoxification.
- Detoxification is a supervised process by which someone with a substance use disorder ceases the use of that substance in a way that is safe and effective and minimizes the risk or severity of withdrawal symptoms.
- Following detoxification, the person's mental and physical status is reviewed. An initial provisional diagnosis can often be firmed up into a likely or even definitive diagnosis.
- There are various forms of detoxification, reflecting in the main the different pharmacological effects of the major substance groups and also the pattern of treatment services that is available in a particular area. Typically, detoxification is accompanied by a recommendation to cease the use of a particular substance (or substances) in the longer term.

4. Pharmacotherapies

Given the importance of neurobiological changes, pharmacological treatments are a logical approach to address substance dependence and they may have a role in lesser forms of substance use disorder. Broadly there are four pharmacotherapeutic approaches:

- Medications to suppress addictive processes
- Antagonist medications (often sharing the characteristics of the first group)
- Agonist maintenance medications (e.g. methadone and buprenorphine)
- Aversive medications of which the primary one is disulfiram (Antabuse (R)).

5. Psychological therapies

Here the focus is on:

- helping the patient to understand how substance using behaviours have developed in them
- providing a menu of options but also guidance as to which may be more likely to succeed for that individual
- consideration of the format of therapy, be it individual 1:1 therapy or group therapy typically comprising six to ten patients and with agreed group rules
- there are many types of therapy adapted from different disciplines but all aiming at minimizing the risk of relapse into heavy or dependent-type substance use; examples include:
  - cognitive-behaviour therapy
  - motivational enhancement therapy
  - therapy aimed at controlled substance use
  - couple and family therapy
  - network therapy

- contingency management approaches
- ongoing therapies may include anxiety management programmes, dialectical behaviour therapy (DBT)
- therapy for comorbid psychiatric disorders
- therapy for comorbid mental health disorders.

A key requirement is for the person to claim ownership of their sub-stance use disorder and to engage in treatment and therefore to be an important part of the solution to their disorder. But therapies which are by their nature passive (e.g. psychoanalysis and hypnosis) have no general role in the management of patients with substance use disorders.

6. Identification and treatment of comorbid disorders

Comorbid mental and physical disorders have an important influence on the patient's symptoms, prognosis, and treatment needs. Effective diag-nosis and management of a comorbid mental health disorder, particularly if it is an underlying one, contributes considerably to the patient's well-being and prognosis. Following detoxification, the opportunity should be taken to review the patient's mental state and identify what symptoms and features are still present. The opportunity should be taken to reach a firmer diagnosis given the transient mental features directly due to the substance dependence will have lessened or resolved, thus allowing any underlying psychiatric disorders to be better clarified. These disorders can then be treated as appropriate (see Chapter 22).

7. Family and social support

- People with substance use disorders often feel alone. They may take a view that they are the only person who has experienced what they feel, and many spiral downwards to a state of great isolation. It is important for the patient to recognize that recovery from a substance use disorder typically involves seeking and benefitting from help from others. These others may be family members or close friends, or members of a self-help fellowship (see point 8).
- In turn, family members and friends will need some understanding of the nature of substance use disorders and the particular type of disorder the person has developed. But typically, family members and friends misunderstand the nature of substance disorders, thinking that they are primarily self-inflicted conditions and/or that the solution is for the patient to simply cease the use of the substance. The concept of the psychobiological driving force of substance dependence is a key one for family members and friends to understand. Little progress will be made if this understanding is not achieved, when typically family and friends may make inadvertent and thus unhelpful comments. It may simply not be possible for the person to have any degree of control over a particular substance.
- Family members often respond by trying to control the person's substance use for them or impose arbitrary rules, which they may think will be helpful but often are not.

- Family members may also 'clear up the mess' as a result of the person's substance use, or explain it away for them, which negates the personal responsibility that the substance user needs to accept for their own behaviours; this is often termed 'enabling'.
- In other ways, family members can facilitate or 'enable' the person's continuing substance use and consequent problems.

8. Self-help fellowships

Uniquely prominent in the long term management of substance use and addictive disorders are mutual-(often called self-) help groups based on the 12 steps of recovery. For many patients and many healthcare practitioners, the patient's involvement in an appropriate self-help group would be seen as central to that person's management plan and recovery prospects. The original 12-step fellowship is Alcoholics Anonymous (AA), which was founded in the US in the mid 1930s. Since that time many such fellowships have arisen which seek to support recovery from many other psychoactive substances and addictive behaviours. Thus, self-help groups exist for those seeking recovery from illicit drugs (Narcotics Anonymous (NA), Marijuana Anonymous, Cocaine Anonymous, Crystal Meth Anonymous) and prescribed and pharmacy medications (Pills Anonymous) and addictive behaviours (Gamblers Anonymous, Sex and Love Addicts Anonymous).

For the healthcare professional, the self-help groups offer a valuable resource, but it is important to recognize that there is no direct link with the healthcare system. Self-help groups are independent and autonomous and exist only to support the recovery of their members. Many professional treatment programmes are based on the principles of the 12-step fellowships and abide by the corresponding 12 traditions, and some treatment and rehabilitation programmes are often described as 'institutionalized AA'. In addition, professional therapies such as '12-step facilitation' seek to inform patients about the 12-step fellowships and encourage their active involvement.

AA and similar 12-step fellowships are widely prevalent throughout Western countries and exist in many other countries in Asia and Africa. Sometimes these groups are predominantly for expatriate Western communities but increasingly 12-step fellowships have been established for local populations, often with suitable cultural adaptations.

Despite the widespread availability of 12-step fellowships there is relatively little research evidence attesting to their effectiveness. Indeed, it has been a principle of these fellowships not to engage in outcome research or specifically support it. This has had the effect of causing many health professionals to doubt the value of self-help fellowships on the basis that they do not represent an 'evidence-based' approach. It has to be acknowledged that the number of randomized controlled trials of 12-step-based approaches compared with no treatment or standard treatment is limited, but such evidence as exists indicates effectiveness comparable and on some criteria superior to conventional approaches. In addition there is evidence that patients who actively engage in 12-step fellowships are more likely to attend for medical and addiction specialist follow-up and to be engaged in aftercare therapy programmes. Many practitioners and treatment programmes encourage the involvement with 12-step fellowships to complement the medication and psychological therapy they provide.

Although the 12-step fellowships are numerically the largest of the self-help organizations, in other counties and cultures self-help groups of a different philosophy exist. These include Hudolin groups and Danshukai groups, which are discussed later in this section.

9. Aftercare

- It is recognized that substance use disorders respond to consistent and persistent care, especially if they are at the more severe end of the spectrum such as dependence. Intensive forms of treatment such as hospital-based treatment programmes typically of 3–4 weeks' duration should be regarded as providing an opportunity to undergo detoxification, to commence a programme of treatment and to be encouraged that personal change is feasible for the individual. However, aftercare is crucial to reinforce the initial programme of therapy and to ensure that the patient practises what he (or she) has learnt previously, at a time when they are living at home or at least in a relatively uncontrolled environment.

- Aftercare programmes exist in a variety of forms. A common form is a day or half-day programme which takes place once per week for 6–15 weeks. These typically comprise an initial 'check-in' meeting where those present review their progress or otherwise in the previous week. Following this, there are skills development or special topics meetings, often attendance at a 12-step fellowship, sometimes a didactic component, and then a final session to plan the week ahead. A cognitive behavioural framework is the most common one for a day programme.

- Individual CBT-based therapy sessions may be offered but the advantage of a group format is a sense of fellowship and common goals and also the opportunity for misconceptions to be addressed by other group members.

- A medical follow-up is very appropriate for many patients and for some, is the sole aftercare modality. Monitoring of relevant biochemical markers such as alcohol biomarkers or urine drug screening is a common approach undertaken by medical practitioners.

- A proportion of patients benefit from more long-lasting therapy programmes. These are typically based in residential facilities and run on therapeutic community principles. Here, the person with a substance use disorder moves through various levels of increasing personal and collective responsibility. Some residential programmes are specially designed for illicit drug dependent people, others for people with combined substance use and mental health disorders.

10. Lifestyle and environmental change

Natural history studies have shown that there are many informal changes in a person's life that facilitate recovery. Some of these may be assisted by the therapeutic process; others are outside the realm of formal treatment.

These changes include the following:

- Committing to a daily routine, personal care, meals, domestic responsibilities, work responsibilities, leisure time activities.
- Good nutrition, preferably with healthier alternatives to previous dietary habits.
- Regular physical exercise, which is known to enhance both physical and mental well-being.
- Development of the person's spiritual understanding, whether this be a belief in the Christian or another god, or another interpretation of a 'higher power' or humanistic sense of order in the world or amongst peoples.
- Achievement of a worthwhile role in life, be this paid work, voluntary work, membership of a fellowship group, family responsibilities.
- Review of their living arrangements in terms of location (easy avoidance of areas of high risk for drug use).
- Connectedness with others; in the longer term the establishment of a supportive personal relationship is known to be strongly associated with rewarding long-term recovery. Initially, however, avoidance of intimate relationships is helpful for the early months of recovery.

Mutual help and related groups

The original 12-step fellowship is Alcoholics Anonymous (AA), which commenced in 1935 from the chance meeting of a 5-month sober, unemployed stock analyst from New York with a still-drunken surgeon from Akron, Ohio. AA has grown organically to more than 2 million members, in over 150 countries.

The 12 steps may be summarized into six concepts:

- Admission of defeat
- Submission to a Higher Power
- Moral inventory
- Confession
- Restitution
- Helping others.

The invocation of a deity rankles with many clinicians. It is important to recognize that while spiritual, AA and NA fall far short of the piety one usually associates with belief in God. Commonly used shorthand for newcomers is to say that if they can't believe in God, then maybe they can believe in a Group Of Drunks, in Good Orderly Direction or more paradoxically, to suggest that they pray for the Gift Of Desperation.

Philosophy and approach

The philosophy of AA and sister fellowships borrows from the perseverance of the ancient Stoics and of fundamentalist Christians giving witness of their conversion, but the early fellowship specifically used both the pragmatist writings of William James as well as biblical writings, and acknowledged its debt to Jung.

- Given that AA is specific in its intention that each group is allowed autonomy, your patients may encounter a wide variety of experiences at AA, from those well-known meetings where members tell their story to a silent circle of bowed heads to lively topic meetings where readings are dissected and debated with some jocularity.
- Typically a meeting will reflect the local demography, so that wealthy suburbs have meetings with well-dressed members and inner city lunch time meetings have a mix of the unemployed and workers eager for a lunch time dose of recovery.
- Special purpose meetings exist in most large cities, for women or men only, for gays or lesbians, for doctors or health professionals.
- The 'mechanism of action' of the fellowships is likely to be the bonding that allows social contagion to occur, perhaps mediated by the oxytocin spike elicited in social engagement.

Sponsors

The favoured way of those successfully referring to AA is to identify a sponsor and introduce them to your patient, while the patient is still in your office. This overtly identifies your endorsement of engaging with the fellowship and confers some authority on this sponsor, who should arrange a specific meeting place at this first opportunity.

- The sponsor relationship is often crucial, so clinicians should take time to engage with likely sponsors who attend local meetings.
- Attempting to pair a patient to an appropriate sponsor seems sensible.
- Otherwise, a call to the local AA office may prove fruitful. A simple invocation to attend the meeting is rarely honoured by adherence.

The 12 traditions of AA and NA

- 12-step groups are a practical way to access all of the four non-treatment factors aiding recovery:
  - new relationships
  - new habits
  - new beliefs
  - external control.
- It is the 12 traditions which uniquely define AA and NA. Anyone can join and no one can be expelled (Tradition 3). No one gets rich through AA, not even AA (Tradition 6). No funding is sought from non-members (Tradition 7). No members are paid for helping other alcoholics and no payment is sought for AA services, but offices may need paid staff and literature costs money to produce (Traditions 8). Despite its size and influence on so many lives, AA remains poor, owning little property. AA does not seek to influence public policy, embracing a 'singleness of purpose' philosophy, the sole focus being 'helping the alcoholic who still suffers'.
- The fellowships represent a substantial repository of personal experience. Although no AA member speaks for AA, many freely share their opinions, not always in accordance with the latest professional wisdom.
- Patients may gain help from AA even though they may have previously rejected it. Treatment outcome studies have shown improved outcomes in those who engaged with AA in addition to clinic attendance.
- Despite some assertions to the contrary, AA does not have an opinion on the prescription of medications for patients. There is a useful pamphlet approved by AA's World Service Conference detailing how some people really need to stay on their medication (say for bipolar disorder) but others may be on medication which needs to be reduced or ceased once they get sober.

Japan's Danshukai

The Japanese Temperance Union was founded in the early 20th century. It introduced AA into Japan and the first meeting was held in Tokyo. A version of AA more culturally appropriate to Japan was desired. This was developed and established as 'Danshukai'. It shares the same principles as AA of staying sober and helping others to achieve and maintain sobriety. It teaches fundamental principles of attending meetings: 'Pursue your abstinence with your feet, not with your head'.

Danshukai is, however, not an anonymous organization. There is a list of members and costs are covered by membership fees and not by donations as with AA. There is little literature and Danshukai groups rarely use books. There is no equivalent to the AA 'Big Book'. Members learn the 'vows' in order to stay sober.

For many years Danshukai was the only self-help organization in Japan apart from a few AA groups for the expatriate community. In recent years, AA has grown among the Japanese culture and it appears to be more popular among younger alcohol dependent people, in part because of the principle of anonymity.

Other key considerations in treatment

The clinician's responsibilities

For a person with a substance use or addictive disorder, to move on from their present condition requires an understanding and acceptance of the need for change. That individual cannot be a passive recipient of treatment. There is no known method of recovering from a substance use or an addictive disorder without the patient putting in personal effort. Having said that, personal effort typically needs to be complemented by effective professional diagnosis and treatment and the support and involvement of others in that person's life. At any one time only about 25% of people with substance use or addictive disorders are in any form of treatment. This varies though from 10% of alcohol-dependent people up to 80% of heroin-addicted individuals, at least in certain countries.

The clinician has a vital role in steering and facilitating a person's recovery or in many cases adopting a harm minimization approach to try to minimize the risk of harm if the person is not of a mind to fundamentally change their substance use or other addictive behaviour. The clinician should provide a listening ear, empathy, and understanding of the patient's experience of their addictive disorder; a high level of awareness of the possibility of substance or other addictive behaviours; a diagnostic capacity to identify and characterize the disorders and their complications; and to provide or facilitate a range of treatments, therapies, and support appropriate to the individual.

The clinician should avoid the pitfall of trying to run the patient's life for him- or herself. There is a natural tendency for clinicians, particularly those trained in non-addiction speciality disciplines, to try to take on responsibilities for the patient's recovery which are typically the responsibility (and prerogative) of the patient. If the clinician finds that he or she is working harder than the patient is at recovery, something is fundamentally wrong.

Good prescribing practices

The history of medicine is littered with examples of medications and other treatments which have shown considerable promise, seemed relatively free of side effects, and have good patient acceptability and yet as time goes by have been shown to have serious limitations or complications.

A classic example of this is the benzodiazepine group of sedative-hypnotics. When they were introduced in the early 1960s they were welcomed as much safer medications than their predecessors (such as the barbiturates). In terms of acute toxicity they were a considerable improvement on their forerunners. The therapeutic ratio of benzodiazepines is far higher than that of barbiturates and they are associated with a much lower morbidity and mortality from overdose, either taken singly or in combination with other drugs or with alcohol.

Initially benzodiazepines were regarded as non-addictive and when case studies of addictive behaviours and withdrawal features were first described, the conclusion was that these were rare and essentially confined to people with existing mental health disorders.

Systematic studies have shown that benzodiazepines have predictable dose-dependent and duration-dependent addictive properties. Even with standard medically prescribed doses, addiction to benzodiazepines (e.g. as manifested by drug-seeking behaviour, tolerance, and withdrawal) occur in the majority of patients after prolonged administration.

For medically qualified practitioners and nurses and other practitioners who have prescribing rights, there is a very special responsibility to be cautious about prescribing benzodiazepines, other sedative-hypnotics, opioid analgesics, and psychostimulants. It is incumbent on the practitioner to make a firm, defensible diagnosis and to prescribe such medications only for such time as is clearly clinically indicated. International conventions and national and state legislation constrains the prescribing of these medications, typically by classifying them into categories or schedules, which require certain qualifications or levels of authorization to prescribe. It is incumbent on the practitioner to be aware of relevant national and local legislation. Penalties for neglecting such responsibilities can be severe, such as professional deregistration and criminal and civil legal proceedings.

Around the world, many medical registration authorities and professional associations provide rules and guidelines for responsible prescribing of psychotropic drugs. Some of these are listed here:

Referral options

Most people with substance use and addictive disorders are seen in primary care settings—in general (medical) practice, family physician rooms, community mental healthcare facilities, polyclinics, social welfare organizations, and in developing countries by generic health practitioners.

Complementing primary care in many countries are the specialist alcohol and drug (addiction) services. These exist in a variety of forms and include:

- medical specialists in addiction practice
- addiction psychologists and therapists and counsellors
- voluntary, charitable, and non-governmental organizations
- family support groups
- residential programmes and residential communities
- private hospital programmes.

For the practitioner working in a primary care facility, it is useful to be able to access colleagues and specialist facilities who can assist or take on the management of patients with substance use and addictive disorders. This is particularly the case when patients have significant psychiatric or physical co-morbidities or complex social situations. It is not possible here to give an outline of referral options for individual countries. Many countries, regions, states, and localities produce lists of referral options within the public health, private health, and voluntary/non-government sectors. These may be obtained in printed form through relevant websites via the Internet, in some cases via smartphone apps.

In some countries, conjoint care between primary healthcare practitioners and healthcare agencies and addiction specialists is facilitated through government-funded care programmes or through private health insurance schemes.

Social and welfare assistance

Many individuals with substance use and addictive disorders have experienced a major decline in their engagement with family, friends, and work under the impact of their disorder. Many are in great financial difficulties, particularly when they have been using illicit drugs or gambling, and this is often compounded by recent loss of employment or business. Furthermore, illicit drug dependence may have been supported by illicit activities such as drug dealing and property crime, and typically such a person wants to remove themselves not only from personal substance use but also from the activities, such as crime or prostitution, that have provided the wherewithal for their use.

Patients may or may not bring their social or financial situation to the attention of the health practitioner but it is often a major difficulty for them. Referral options for social and welfare assistance can include the following:

- Social welfare organizations
- A social worker or welfare officer in a community clinic or hospital
- Charitable and benevolent organizations
- Welfare facilities offered by professional and trade organizations
- Legal aid services (free of charge in some areas)
- Family groups.

Further reading

Johnson BA. (2011). *Addiction Medicine: Science and Practice*. New York: Springer.
Marshall EJ, Humphreys KM, Ball DM. (2010). *The Treatment of Drinking Problems: A Guide for the Helping Professions* (5th ed). New York: Cambridge University Press.
National Institute for Health and Care Excellence (2011, reviewed 2015). *Alcohol Use Disorders: Diagnosis, Assessment and Management of Harmful Drinking and Alcohol Dependence*. Clinical Guidelines No. 115. London: NICE.

Tobacco

Epidemiology *120*
Pharmacology *122*
Pathophysiology *124*
Clinical syndromes *126*
Natural history *128*
Complications *130*
Screening and brief intervention *131*
Clinical assessment and diagnosis *132*
Physical examination *133*
Laboratory tests and other investigations *134*
Screening or diagnostic instruments for nicotine
    dependence *136*
Management *137*
Harm reduction/palliation *150*
Prevention *150*

Epidemiology

Prevalence of smoking

- Over a third of men (36%) and one in 14 (7%) women worldwide currently smoke tobacco, with others using tobacco in other forms.
- Smoking cigarettes is the commonest method of use worldwide, but in many cultures smoking a pipe or a (water-cooled) hookah or shisha is usual. Tobacco may also be chewed or taken in the form of snuff.
- Smoking reached epidemic proportions in the Western world following the invention of the automated cigarette rolling machine in 1880, which allowed mass production of cigarettes.
- Cigarette smoking peaked in these countries in the 1940s and 1950s, when 75% of men and 30% of women smoked cigarettes. It has since declined greatly after concerted public health campaigns and legislation; in Australia, New Zealand, and some Nordic countries the prevalence among both sexes is now 16–20%.
- Elsewhere in Europe the prevalence of cigarette smoking is up to 50%.
- In South-East Asia and East Asia, the prevalence has risen hugely over the past two to three decades, with over 50% of men in Asia smoking cigarettes.
- One in every three cigarettes is smoked in China, where there are said to be 1000 cigarette brands.
- Disadvantaged, isolated, or indigenous communities can have smoking rates often greatly in excess of the general population (e.g. in remote Aboriginal communities in Australia, prevalence is up to 80%).

Impact of smoking

Smoking is the third most important cause of the global burden of disease. It is a well-recognized risk factor for:

- Acute disease:
  - respiratory infections
  - fire and burns
  - acute cardiovascular events.
- Chronic disease:
  - cardiovascular and respiratory disease
  - metabolic, endocrine, and renal disease
  - duodenal and gastric ulcers
  - lung cancer and a range of other cancers
  - perinatal and neonatal mortality.

In addition, tobacco addiction can contribute to financial hardship.

Disease from second-hand smoke

- In adults, second-hand smoke (passive smoking) is associated with increased risk of cancers and cardiovascular disease
- Maternal smoking in pregnancy increases the risk of miscarriage, and of babies being born prematurely or small-for-date
- Babies experience increased risk of respiratory infections, asthma and otitis media, and of Sudden Infant Death Syndrome (SIDS).

Risk factors for smoking

Smoking prevalence varies between and within countries:
- Globally, men are more likely to smoke than women.
- Within a population, lower socioeconomic status is the major risk factor for continued smoking in developed countries.
- Developing countries generally have less strict controls on advertising and sale of smoking, and some areas are seeing rises in smoking prevalence, and in smoking among children.

Initiation into smoking may be influenced by:
- prevailing social norms
- adolescent peer pressure, bravado, or rebellion
- curiosity, boredom
- desire for weight control.

In subgroups with high levels of stress (e.g. in mental illness, social disadvantage) smoking may be used for symptom relief.

Individual predisposing factors

Biological predisposition to a pleasant response to nicotine in the brain may explain the greater likelihood of uptake of tobacco smoking by some people. This is likely to lead to strong psycho-physiological rewards from smoking, and a predisposition to repeated use, which may initiate a lifelong 'relationship' with smoking.

In others, there may be greater ability to metabolize nicotine in the liver. Faster metabolizers are reported to smoke more and find quitting harder than slower metabolizers. Racial origin can also impact on nicotine metabolism.
- The reaction to the very first cigarettes smoked may be a clue as to whether a person will go on to smoke continuously.
- Identical twins separated from their parents and each other at birth are both more likely to be dependent smokers if their biological parents were dependent smokers, irrespective of personal histories of exposure or non-exposure, or environmental and cultural circumstances.
- Many smokers have discovered nicotine is anxiolytic and that it may have an antidepressant effect. They may 'self-medicate' with smoking tobacco to counteract anxiety or a depressed mood.

Pharmacology

Absorption, distribution, metabolism, and elimination

Absorption of nicotine across biological membranes depends on pH. Compared with absorption through mucous membranes (e.g. chewing tobacco, snuff, or nicotine gum), nicotine is rapidly absorbed from cigarette smoke through the lungs, presumably because of the huge surface area of the alveoli and small airways, and the pH (7.4) of cigarette smoke particulate matter.

- After a puff, high levels of nicotine reach the brain in 10–20 seconds, producing rapid behavioural reinforcement.
- Smokers can control nicotine intake by altering their puff volume, the number of puffs they take from a cigarette, the intensity of puffing, and the depth to which they inhale.

Nicotine is extensively metabolized, primarily in the liver and to a lesser extent in the lung and in the brain.

- In humans, about 70–80% of nicotine is converted to cotinine, with a smaller fraction metabolized to nicotine N'-oxide (4–7%) and nicotine glucuronide (3–5%).
- Cotinine is further metabolized to six primary metabolites: 3'-hydroxycotinine, 5'-hydroxycotinine, cotinine N-oxide, cotinine methonium ion, cotinine glucuronide, and nor-cotinine.
- CYP2A6 is primarily responsible for both the C-oxidation of nicotine to cotinine and for the oxidation of cotinine to trans 3' hydroxyl-cotinine.
- Recent findings show that slower metabolizers are at lower risk to develop nicotine dependence and may have lower risk for certain cancers.

Renal clearance accounts for about 10% (range 2–35%) of total nicotine clearance. Clearance of nicotine is influenced by various factors; nicotine clearance is increased:

- after a meal
- in women than in men
- in pregnancy
- in kidney failure.

In contrast, nicotine clearance is decreased in the elderly, and during sleep.

Pharmacologic actions on CNS nicotinic acetylcholine receptors

Nicotinic acetylcholine (ACh) receptors are encoded by nine alpha (α_1–α_{10}) and three beta (β_2–β_4) subunit genes, which are expressed in the nervous system and in several non-neuronal tissues.

Neuronal nicotinic receptors:

- are principally located at presynaptic or preterminal sites (where they modulate neurotransmitter release)
- are sometimes found on cell bodies or dendrites (where they mediate postsynaptic effects).

In the CNS, ACh-mediated innervation, acting through nicotinic receptors, regulates processes such as transmitter release, cell excitability, and neuronal integration. These processes are crucial for network operations and influence physiological functions such as arousal, sleep, fatigue, anxiety, the central processing of pain, food intake, and several cognitive functions.

Nicotinic receptors also have roles in neuronal development and plasticity. Because of this, nicotinic regulatory, plasticity, and developmental influences may be important in the aetiology of disease during development, adulthood, and ageing.

Cellular mechanism of nicotine dependence

Initially, the nicotinic receptors (mainly $\alpha_4\beta_2$ receptors) in the resting state are activated (depolarized) when nicotine first arrives in the brain. By the time the cigarette is finished, these receptors become desensitized, so that they cannot function by reacting to either nicotine or ACh.

This desensitization of nicotinic receptors is involved in acute tolerance:

- As an individual smokes several times during the course of a day, the background level of nicotine slowly increases.
- Therefore, nicotinic receptors become more desensitized by long-term nicotine exposure, eventually leading to an overall increase in the number of receptors as a homeostatic mechanism.
- During the length of time that smokers take between cigarettes, nicotine levels drop and some of the excess nicotinic receptors recover from desensitization. This results in an excess excitability of the nicotinic cholinergic systems of smokers.
- This hyperexcitability of nicotinic receptors could contribute to the unstable condition where smokers feel motivation for their next cigarette. That is, resensitization of the receptors initiates craving, due to the agitation arising in part, from the excess nicotinic receptors during abstinence.

Nicotine-associated learning

Nicotine-associated learning and memory appears to maintain nicotine use during periods of receptor desensitization, that is, when there is a loss or decrease in the biologic response to nicotine.

- Over months or years of smoking, long-term synaptic changes result in learned associations, including associations with the events, people, and context in which smoking takes place.
- Because environment is reinforced by repeated variable reinforcements from cigarettes, conditioned cues play a critically important role in the reinstatement or relapse to smoking in abstinent smokers.

Pathophysiology

Tobacco smoke is composed of:
- volatile phase substances (nitrogen, carbon monoxide (CO), carbon dioxide, ammonia, hydrogen cyanide, benzene, etc.)
- particulate phase substances (alkaloids nor-nicotine, anabasine, anatabine, myosmene, nicotyrine, nicotine, tar, etc.).

Inhalation of these gases and this particulate matter, including the estimated 3000 constituents of tobacco smoke, is associated with a wide range of morbidity and with mortality.

While nicotine is the component of tobacco that causes dependence, it is one of the least harmful components in terms of complications:
- Pure nicotine delivered slowly and in low doses (unlike from a cigarette, which is in high dose, bolus form) is associated with few medical consequences.
- In high-dose, bolus form (as with smoking), nicotine can cause vasoconstriction, tachycardia, nausea, and headaches in those naive to nicotine.

Respiratory disorders

Smoking impairs the cough reflex, ciliary function, and immune response, and these factors predispose to acute bronchitis.

Repeated episodes of acute bronchitis may be followed by chronic bronchitis and chronic obstructive pulmonary disease (COPD) including emphysema.

While structural destruction in emphysema is irreversible, smoking cessation leads to improved oxygen transfer capacity and improved ciliary function with improved clearance of particulate matter from the airways. These positive responses begin to occur within days of reduced exposure to the particulate matter and gases inhaled from smoking.

Cardiovascular disorders

The cardiovascular effects from smoking are due both to the acute effects of nicotine boluses, and the chronic effects of inhalation of CO and other toxins.
- Acutely, smoking impairs endothelium-dependent vasodilatation in both macro- and microvascular beds, and enhances platelet aggregation.
  These effects may in part be due to impaired nitric oxide formation.
- Chronically, smoking causes endothelial inflammation and promotes atheroma formation.
- The lipid profile is also altered in smokers with higher serum cholesterol, triglyceride, and low-density lipoprotein (LDL) levels, but lower high-density lipoprotein (HDL) levels than in non-smokers

These effects lead to increased risk of disease throughout the vascular system in both active and passive smokers, including myocardial infarction, cerebrovascular accidents, and peripheral ischaemia.

Many of the effects of smoking on the vascular system are reversible. Reversal begins within days of reduced exposure to the inhaled CO and other toxins, and with nicotine delivered in a less bolus-like manner.

Cancers

Risks of cancers, particularly lung cancer, are very high in smokers and continue to occur many years after quitting smoking. The risk of lung cancer in men who smoke is 22 times higher than for non-smokers. The cause of these cancers is likely to be multifactorial, and more than 20 carcinogens have been documented in tobacco smoke.

Other

Several other mechanisms are responsible for disease in the smoker or those affected by second-hand smoke. These include:

- activation of growth factors (angiotensin II, endothelin-1, and TGF-β1)
- renal tubulotoxic effects
- oxidative stress
- increased platelet aggregation
- impaired lipoprotein and glycosaminoglycan metabolism
- modulation of immune mechanisms
- vasopressin-mediated antidiuresis
- insulin resistance.

Clinical syndromes

Intoxication

As described previously in this chapter, nicotine use results in relaxation, anxiolysis, and improved concentration. In the novice smoker, nicotine may lead to light-headedness and nausea.

Nicotine dependence

Nicotine is a highly addictive substance, which provides reward and rein-forcement to the smoker.

- Nicotine dependence develops with repeated self-administration of nicotine which leads to tolerance to the adverse effects of smoking, withdrawal, and compulsive use of nicotine.
- Nicotine dependence typically involves daily use of nicotine for at least several weeks.
- Individuals with nicotine dependence smoke both for the positive rewards of nicotine and the relief of withdrawals.
- Dependent smokers adjust or titrate their nicotine blood levels by inhaling deeper or longer to bring about a higher nicotine level or inhaling more lightly and puffing more quickly to lower levels.

Development of tolerance: unlike most drugs of dependence, smokers do not require noticeably increasing nicotine plasma levels to achieve the effects desired. This is possibly due to the very short half-life of nicotine and that tolerance reduces even after overnight abstinence. Smokers do, however, develop tolerance to the adverse effects of smoking; e.g. deep inhalations cause initial light-headedness in novice smokers, but not in experienced smokers. There is also increased tolerance to nicotine across the course of each day.

Nicotine withdrawal

Nicotine withdrawal is defined as occurring where abrupt cessation of nico-tine use, or reduction in the amount of nicotine used, is followed within 24 hours by four or more of the following symptoms or signs:

Features of nicotine withdrawal
- Dysphoria (depressed mood)
- Insomnia
- Irritability, frustration or anger
- Anxiety
- Difficulty concentrating
- Restlessness
- Decreased heart rate
- Increased appetite or weight gain.

These symptoms cause clinically significant distress or impairment in social, occupational, or other important areas of function, and are not due to a general medical condition or another mental disorder.

Most regular smokers show at least some symptoms of nicotine with-drawal. This comprises a combination of anxiety, distress, aggressiveness, urges to smoke, inability to concentrate, increase in appetite, and general moodiness. These acute symptoms occur in some smokers even between cigarettes as nicotine blood levels quickly fall. On stopping smoking, withdrawals can persist for days or weeks.

- Longer-term symptoms of withdrawal can include depression and infrequent, but irritating, urges to smoke, linked to situations of psychological distress and other strong, often negative, triggers. Smokers have learned that these events can be 'cured' by smoking.
- Other physical symptoms of withdrawal that may occur within weeks of quitting include mouth ulcers and cough, which may appear for the first time or increase after quitting smoking.
- Relief from the acute symptoms of withdrawal usually occurs within the first few puffs of a cigarette. The learning of the 'relief' provided by smoking becomes an insidious factor encouraging further smoking.

Natural history

Smoking, as with any dependence on a psychoactive substance, can be viewed as a chronic illness. This can help understand why some smokers may not be receptive to messages about quitting or find it difficult to quit. Like any chronic illness, some smokers have:

- a long history—they may have been smoking for many decades
- remissions—they may have been able to occasionally cease smoking
- relapses—they typically have gone back to smoking many times
- poor spontaneous recovery—for dependent smokers, just stopping smoking without any effort is unusual
- limited treatment outcomes—at best, 50% of treatment-seeking smokers are able to quit for good.

Smoking shows convincing evidence of being an addictive behaviour, viz:
- 96% of smokers smoke daily
- Few smoke less than five cigarettes per day
- 50% smoke within 30 minutes of waking
- 48% have not abstained for more than 1 week in the past 5 years
- 67% say they wish to quit; and heavier smokers wish to quit equally
- 80% have tried to quit, 58% more than once
- 75% of self-quitting attempts fail in the first week
- Smokers who attempt to quit many times still want to quit.

Smokers have also 'learned' the pleasurable psycho-physiological effects of smoking in combination with other substances, such as alcohol, caffeine, and cannabis:
- Potent, cue-conditioned responses resulting in strong urges to smoke may accompany the use of those substances.
- Smokers are known to consume at least twice the amount of alcohol and caffeine as non-smokers, and may have lower tolerance to alcohol or caffeine toxicity on quitting smoking.

Some smokers have few symptoms of withdrawal when nicotine deprived; many spontaneously cease smoking without aid and do not relapse, while others self-report formidable and overwhelming withdrawal symptoms on cessation, and though persistently attempt to quit, always relapse.

The experienced relief provided by nicotine for negative symptoms, such as anxiety, means that smoking is used to relieve all types of anxiety states, or negative situations and events, as well as in withdrawal.

There is substantial evidence that most smokers want to quit:
- Relapse is endemic in smokers who make an unaided quit attempt, with 50–75% relapsing within 1 week of a concerted quit attempt, and more than 62% within the first 2 weeks, with an ever reducing likelihood of relapsing after 3 months.
- At best, about 5–15% of smokers committed to quitting on their own are still not smoking 1 year later.

Hence, the first 2 weeks, then the first 3 months are important target dates for interventions in helping smokers quit.

It is estimated that one in two smokers dies prematurely from smoking-related diseases. It is unclear why certain individuals are more susceptible to the adverse effects of smoking than others.

Smoking cessation has clear benefits for smokers:
- Among former smokers, the reduced risk of death compared with continuing smokers begins shortly after quitting and continues for at least 10–15 years.
- After 10–15 years' abstinence, the risk of all-cause mortality returns nearly to that of persons who never smoked.

Complications

Tobacco-related physical diseases include the following:

Cardiovascular disease
- Hypertension
- Cardiac arrhythmias
- Angina pectoris
- Myocardial infarction
- Cerebral infarction
- Peripheral vascular disease.

Pulmonary disease
- COPD
- Bronchial asthma
- Pneumonia
- Pulmonary tuberculosis
- Spontaneous pneumothorax.

Gastrointestinal disease
Peptic ulcers.

Metabolic disease
- Type 2 diabetes mellitus
- Dyslipidaemia with an increase in free fatty acid and LDL cholesterol, and a decrease in HDL cholesterol.

Endocrine disease
- Earlier menopause
- Impaired penile erection
- Osteoporosis.

Cancers
Smoking increases the risk of various kinds of cancer, including of the mouth, larynx, oesophagus, lung, stomach, pancreas, kidney, urinary bladder, and uterine cervix, as well as leukaemia.

Other diseases in the smoker
- Periodontal disease
- Cataract
- Adverse postoperative events
- Delayed bone and wound healing
- Renal disease
- Fire and burns.

Pregnancy and the neonatal period
Smoking during pregnancy nearly doubles the relative risk of having a low birthweight infant; the relative risks of spontaneous abortion and perinatal mortality are increased by one-third.

The relative risk of neonatal mortality is increased by a third.

Screening and brief intervention

Primary care has a major role to play in identifying tobacco use and offering smoking cessation support.
- The majority of the population sees a primary care health professional at least once a year and smokers attend more frequently.
- Brief advice from a general practitioner increases cessation rates by about two-thirds compared to no advice and is highly cost-effective.
- Practice nurses, pharmacists, allied health professionals, psychologists, and dentists also have an important role in providing this support.

The 5As approach

The 5As provide primary care clinicians with a framework for identifying tobacco use and for structuring smoking cessation support. The key features are as follows:
- *Ask:* regularly ask all patients if they smoke and record the information in the medical record. Tobacco use is a vital health issue and having a systematic approach to identification leads to more offers of cessation support.
- *Advise:* advise all smokers to quit in a clear, unambiguous way such as 'the best thing you can do for your health is to stop smoking'.
- *Assess:* assessment of interest in quitting helps to tailor advice to each smoker's needs and stage of change. Nicotine dependence should also be assessed and helps to guide treatment. Assessment of other relevant problems such as mental health conditions, other drug dependencies, and comorbidities is necessary to develop a comprehensive treatment plan.
- *Assist:* all smokers should be offered help to quit.
- *Arrange:* follow-up visits have been shown to increase the likelihood of long-term abstinence and are especially useful in the first few weeks after quitting.

When time is short, and referral options are available, the approach of 'very brief advice' is an alternative. The steps for this are as follows:
- *Ask:* establish smoking status.
- *Advise:* advise that the best way of quitting is with a combination of behavioural support and drug treatment.
- *Refer:* provide a referral to a specialized service.

In many countries, an option for referral is quit line telephone services. Internet-based services are another option. In some countries, specialized tobacco treatment services are available in government-funded or private practice settings.

Further reading

The website http://www.treatobacco.net provides information on treatment of tobacco dependence from the Society for Research on Nicotine and Tobacco and the Society for the Study of Addiction. The website has links to clinical practice guidelines for cessation from around the world.

UK National Centre for Smoking Cessation and Training (http://www.ncsct.co.uk/) provides online access to the Very Brief Advice Training Module.

Clinical assessment and diagnosis

Nicotine dependence or tobacco dependence

Considerable evidence indicates that nicotine is a primary active pharmacological ingredient, and has dependence potential. However, the non-pharmacological aspects of tobacco smoking may be more important as a conditioned reinforcer for establishing dependence than for other drugs of abuse. These non-pharmacological reinforcers include:

- the 'taste' of the tobacco smoke
- sensory responses in the throat and upper airway
- manipulation of the tobacco itself
- the smoke it produces
- the social aspects of tobacco smoking.

Diagnostic features of nicotine dependence

The diagnostic features of nicotine dependence, used in ICD 10 are:

- craving
- tolerance
- withdrawal
- impaired control
- social impairment
- risky use.

Tolerance to tobacco is exemplified by the disappearance of nausea and dizziness after repeated intake and with a more intense effect of tobacco the first time it is used during the day.

The most commonly endorsed tobacco withdrawal symptoms are irritability, anxiety, restlessness, and difficulty concentrating, followed by depression and insomnia.

- Physical aspects of tobacco withdrawal are increased appetite, in particular craving for sweet or sugary foods, and increased weight.
- Tobacco withdrawal usually begins within 24 hours of stopping or cutting down on tobacco use, peaks at 2–3 days after abstinence, and lasts 2–3 weeks.
- Withdrawal symptoms impair the ability to stop tobacco use, that is, smokers use tobacco to relieve or to avoid withdrawal symptoms. The large majority report craving when they do not smoke for several hours.

Compared to other drugs of abuse, use of tobacco rarely results in failure to fulfil major role obligations (e.g. interference with work, interference with home obligations), but persistent social or interpersonal problems (e.g. having arguments with others about tobacco use, avoiding social situations because of others' disapproval of tobacco use) or use that is physically hazardous (e.g. smoking in bed, smoking around flammable chemicals) occur at an intermediate prevalence. Although these criteria are less often endorsed by tobacco users, if endorsed, they can indicate a more severe disorder.

Physical examination

Given the wide range of physical disorders produced by smoking tobacco or by exposure to second-hand smoke, a careful physical examination is indicated, with an emphasis on respiratory and cardiovascular systems.

Laboratory tests and other investigations

Relevant investigations will vary according to the individual's history and examination, but may include:

- blood tests (e.g. EUC, blood sugar, lipids)
- spirometry
- ECG
- imaging:
  - chest X-ray examination
  - CT or MRI scan
- other investigations to confirm smoking status as indicated (see following subsections).

Carbon monoxide (expired air)

Breath measurements of expired air that contain 10–30 parts per million (ppm) CO usually indicate 20 cigarettes smoked within the past 8–12 hours. The CO meter is easy to use and can be a useful motivational tool. But the problem of exhaled CO as a biomarker is a lack of specificity. Elevated CO levels in the absence of smoking may be the result of exposure to environmental pollutants, such as faulty gas boilers, car exhausts, and smog, or heavy exposure to second-hand tobacco smoke.

Cotinine (plasma and saliva)

Cotinine can be measured if objective confirmation of recent smoking status is required. Cotinine has been most commonly used as a biomarker of daily nicotine intake both in cigarette smokers and in those exposed to second-hand tobacco smoke. The 16-hour half-life of cotinine makes it useful as a marker of nicotine intake. There is a high correlation among cotinine concentrations measured in plasma, saliva, and urine.

- Because of individual variability in the fractional conversion of nicotine to cotinine and in the rate of elimination of cotinine itself, plasma cotinine levels are not perfect quantitative markers of nicotine intake in individual smokers.
- However, the ratio of cotinine to its first metabolite 3-hydroxycotinine is a useful assay and can be done in urine. Fast metabolizers have a higher ratio. Fast metabolizers smoke more cigarettes per day and do not do well on one form of NRT alone. Generally, women are faster metabolizers than men.
- Another limitation to the use of cotinine is that levels reflect relatively short-term exposure to tobacco (over the past 3–4 days) due to its half-life.
- The cotinine level produced by a single cigarette is 8–10 ng/mL.
- A cotinine value >14 ng/mL typically is taken to indicate smoking.

Nicotine and cotinine in hair and nails

Hair or toenail measurements of nicotine or cotinine are promising bio-markers of tobacco exposure over several months. The average rate of growth of hair and toenail is 1 cm and 0.1 cm per month respectively.

Potential problems with the use of hair include:

* a strong influence of hair pigmentation on nicotine and cotinine binding and uptake. This makes comparison across individuals difficult
* nicotine and cotinine concentrations in hair may be influenced by the same substances contained in sweat (e.g. after recent smoking) and by tobacco smoke in the environment.

Other measures

A range of other tobacco-specific biomarkers have been used, but are not routinely available. These include anatabine (urine) and NNAL or NNAL-glucuronides (blood, urine). Other non-specific biomarkers of tobacco exposure are carboxyhaemoglobin (blood), 1-hydroxypyrene and other polycyclic aromatic hydrocarbon metabolites (urine), mercapturic acid metabolites (urine), acetonitrile (urine, blood, exhaled air), S-phenyl-mercapturic acid (urine), and thiocyanate (serum, saliva, urine). These biomarkers are influenced by non-tobacco factors including combustion products, diet, and vehicular traffic.

Further reading

Dani JA, Kosten TR, Benowitz NL. (2009). The pharmacology of nicotine and tobacco. In Ries RK, Fiellin DA, Miller SC, et al. (eds) *Principles of Addiction Medicine*, pp. 179–91. Philadelphia, PA: Lippincott Williams & Wilkins.

Henningfield JE, London ED, Pogun S. (2009). *Nicotine Psychopharmacology: Handbook of Experimental Pharmacology 192*. Berlin: Springer-Verlag.

Schmitz JM, Stotts AL. (2011). Nicotine. In Ruiz P, Strain E (eds) *Lowinson and Ruiz's Substance Abuse: A Comprehensive Textbook* (5th ed), pp. 319–34. Philadelphia, PA: Lippincott Williams & Wilkins.

Screening or diagnostic instruments for nicotine dependence

The best known screening instrument to identify smokers and their nicotine dependence severity is the Fagerstrom Test for Nicotine Dependence (FTND; see Chapter 27).

- The FTND is a standardized questionnaire for assessing level of physical dependence on nicotine.
- FTND scores may assist in tailoring treatment, e.g. higher scores suggest need for more intensive treatment compared with lower scores.
- FTND scores can be used to track progress over time.

Management

The main approaches to therapy for smoking cessation are brief intervention and more intensive interventions (see Table 8.1). These are not mutually exclusive.

There are two components to smoking cessation treatment:
• acutely arresting the activity of smoking, and then
• the maintenance of long-term abstinence.

Relapse to smoking is so endemic that the period within the first 2 weeks of a quit attempt should be the main focus of attention in the first instance when helping a smoker to quit.

• Some smokers in developed countries, who have been exposed to a strong antismoking climate, may be 'harder targets' who require intensive help, pharmacological interventions, and relapse prevention advice. They are often smokers who have medical repercussions from smoking but persist and, by definition, show high dependence.

• These smokers respond well to frequent counselling and medications. Interventions and time taken in consultations are related to successful permanent quitting. This level of intensity is reported to be at least as cost-effective in this group of smokers as any other medical intervention might be for any other illness.

• At best, with any single pharmacotherapy, about 30% of treatment-seeking smokers will remain abstinent from cigarettes 1 year after treatment. Increasing therapy (combining therapies and increasing doses, e.g. of NRT) and intensive counselling can improve permanent abstinence rates to around 50%. There typically is a close relationship between pharmacotherapy and frequency of counselling, as dependence on cigarettes is not solely a pharmacological process, but is also a psychosocial phenomenon.

Commonly used methods to quit smoking are described here:

'Cold turkey'

Simply stopping smoking without any medication is the commonest form of a quit attempt (80%). However, most smokers (92%) who attempt 'cold turkey' relapse and multiple attempts over many years are necessary to achieve permanent abstinence. A recent US study reports that it may take as many as 14 formal attempts to finally stop smoking.

Table 8.1 1-year success rates by intensity of intervention (across all settings)

No action	1%
Brief advice in primary care	5–8%
Brief advice plus NRT in primary care	10%
Intensive professional counselling alone	15–20%
Intensive professional counselling plus NRT	30–40%

Pharmacotherapies to assist in smoking cessation

Nicotine replacement therapies

One of the most effective and commonly available pharmacotherapies for treating nicotine dependence is NRT.

- Some researchers prefer the term 'nicotine reduction therapy' as the peak arterial blood levels these therapies deliver are often only one-fifth of the nicotine derived from cigarettes.
- Replacement therapies double the chance of achieving stable remission from smoking compared to an unmedicated quit attempt.

Nicotine gum

Nicotine is absorbed through the oral mucosa quite readily, as tobacco chewers and cigar smokers are aware, and considerable blood levels of nicotine can be obtained through the use of nicotine gum. Nicotine gum shows increased long-term success compared with placebo in all controlled trials to date.

- As the doses or combination of nicotine products increase, so do the positive outcomes, with validated abstinence rates of up to 40% or more at 12 months.
- If a smoker smokes within the first 20 minutes after waking and smokes more than 20 cigarettes per day, excluding medical contra-indications, they would be appropriate for 4 mg nicotine gum.
- Others should start with 2 mg gum and increase the frequency or dose if needed.

The nicotine patch

Slow-release, low-dose nicotine from the transdermal patch delivers nicotine, but the dose is not in a bolus form and, therefore, is less reinforcing than cigarette smoke or nicotine gum.

- Craving is the symptom most likely to abate with the use of a nicotine patch. Anxiety, irritability, low mood, and concentration all are also known to improve with patch use.
- Smokers who are highly dependent or who smoke a large number of cigarettes per day may find one patch is not sufficient and may need to add short-acting NRT (e.g. oral or inhaled) or in some cases, a further patch (Fig. 8.1).
- There is no evidence that weaning to lower doses of nicotine patch enhances long-term efficacy. The US Surgeon General's Clinical Practice Guidelines for Smoking Cessation reiterates that there is no need to wean off NRT.

Recommendations for nicotine patch use

- In most cases initiate patch at night prior to sleep—change every night
- Sleep disturbances—particularly vivid dreaming—are common, but rarely affect abstinence rates. If serious, transfer to 16-hour patch, applied every morning.
- Rotate patch around upper part of the body. Not on the waistline. Avoid fatty/hairy areas.
- Up to 10% of patch wearers can have severe skin irritation. This can be due to either patch adhesive or local high-dose nicotine on skin. Site rotation often prevents this. If not, hydrocortisone cream may provide relief.

Other forms of short-acting NRT

These are less widely available, but have shown excellent results:

- *Nicotine nasal spray:* trials have shown high long-term abstinence rates using nicotine nasal spray. Smokers with higher levels of nicotine dependence were more successful with this than on other types of therapy. However nasal bleeding is common. Nicotine nasal spray is available on prescription in many countries.
- *Nicotine lozenge and sublingual tablet:* these have varying availability. Smokers commonly under-use these pharmacotherapies. If sufficiently used, however, they show cessation rates equal to other forms of NRT.
- *Nicotine inhaler:* trials have shown good long-term abstinence; however, dependence potential is high as it is a quick reinforcer, and there is a risk that smokers will convert to this 'cleaner' form of nicotine inhalation. However, it can be considered a safer form of nicotine use and so, as a form of harm reduction.

Combination nicotine therapies

The nicotine dose delivered by the patch or gum alone may be inadequate for some smokers and they may continue to need to smoke, and/or have withdrawals despite these therapies. Many clinicians supplement nicotine patch therapy with nicotine gum or other forms of short-acting NRT for 'break-out' smoking. Advantages for combined therapy have been demonstrated. There is scope for the combination of patches, wearing several at once, and the combination of patch and other, short-acting forms of nicotine (e.g. inhaled nicotine; see algorithm in Fig. 8.1).

Combination of NRT with other pharmacotherapies

Many dependent smokers do not respond to a single class of pharmacotherapy and a combination may be required. In clinical practice, this is becoming increasingly necessary to bring about cessation of smoking. For example, bupropion may be combined with NRT of any or all types.

Nicotine delivery modes

In order of speed of delivery, risk of vascular effects and risk of dependence:

- Cigarette
- Nasal spray
- Inhaler
- Sublingual tablet
- Lozenge
- Gum
- Patch.

Duration of NRT use

In general, a minimum of 7 weeks use of NRT is recommended to reduce risk of relapse.

- Replacement therapy is a recommended course of treatment rather than an indefinite substitution for smoking behaviour, however very long-term use has shown no evidence of harm.
- There is no evidence that weaning off these therapies is of greater value that simply abruptly stopping. Accordingly a reduction of patch strength (e.g. from 21 mg to 14 mg then 7 mg) is not required.
- Abrupt cessation of 21 mg nicotine patch after approximately 7 weeks of usage will not precipitate withdrawals or relapse.

Contraindications or precautions to the use of NRT

Coronary artery disease and NRT: there is no objective evidence for the risk of nicotine toxicity or adverse effects of NRT in stable ischaemic heart disease. Using any form of NRT is less harmful than smoking. NRT is currently contraindicated in the first 48 hours of acute myocardial infarct or in the setting of recent-onset, unstable angina.

Pregnancy and lactation

It is always preferable that a women stops smoking prior to conception or diagnosis of pregnancy. However, if she continues to smoke it is now considered less harmful to use nicotine-containing products than to continue to smoke.

- Continuous delivery forms of nicotine, i.e. the patch, are generally not recommended as there is a risk of harmful neuronal effects on the fetus.
- Pulsatile nicotine, such as gum or lozenge, is recommended, as the fetus has breaks from nicotine exposure between doses.
- Nicotine is metabolized faster in pregnancy, and so *more* NRT is required in this group of women rather than less, as is commonly believed.

NRT: for common problems see Table 8.2.

Reluctance to use NRT: some smokers are reluctant to use NRT, seeing it as a passive activity or a 'crutch', and may be strongly opposed to the use of any substance, particularly a pharmaceutical product that contains nicotine, in helping them to quit smoking.

Underdosing: there are many misconceptions as to the dosage and absorption of nicotine in NRT. Most smokers achieve plasma nicotine levels when smoking tobacco that are far above those delivered by even the highest doses of NRT. Hence, underdosing is a common problem with NRT.

- 21 mg nicotine patches deliver plasma levels around 10 ng/mL
- 2 mg nicotine gum delivers plasma levels of about 7 ng/mL
- 4 mg nicotine gum delivers plasma levels of about 15 ng/mL

Table 8.2 Other common problems with NRT

Problem	Solution
Hiccups or indigestion with gum	Chew less vigorously
Rash around patch site	Ensure patch site is being rotated
	Can use 1% hydrocortisone cream
Vivid disturbing dreams on patch	Apply new patch prior to sleep or use 16-hour patch
Inhaler seems ineffectual	Breathe in and out from it rather than deep breaths

- This compares with plasma nicotine levels after a cigarette of 40 ng/mL
- The blood levels delivered by nicotine patches and gum are similar with the lozenge and sublingual tablets. Inhaler and nasal spray also deliver lower doses than smoking.

Evidence of underdosing may be:
- concomitant smoking while on patches, gum, or other NRT
- symptoms of nicotine withdrawal while on NRT.

Discontinuation of therapy due to over-assuredness: patients may be tempted to cease NRT once they have achieved a week or two of abstinence from cigarettes.

Remedies
- High levels of nicotine dependence require higher doses of NRT. The 4 mg nicotine gum has been shown to be the most effective of all NRTs in heavily dependent smokers.
- Frequent daily use of short-acting NRTs, e.g. as many gums as cigarettes smoked per day
- The clinician should note the effect NRTs are having on numbers of cigarettes smoked and titrate the NRT accordingly (Fig. 8.1).
  - e.g. if smoker who initially smoked 20 cigarettes per day on a 21 mg nicotine patch has reduced to 10 cigarettes, then the addition of oral nicotine (e.g. gum) or of another whole 21 mg patch may be appropriate. If five cigarettes are now smoked per day then add ½ a patch or less, etc.
  - nicotine inhaler can also be added in this way if few cigarettes are still smoked, or if there are still strong urges to smoke, in a smoker who has maintained abstinence.
- Strongly recommend that patients continue NRT for at least 7 weeks.

Risk of toxicity: toxic levels of nicotine are very rare in smokers, but are more common in those naïve to smoking.
- Nausea is the primary symptom of toxicity.
- Light headedness may also occur.
- There is little to no risk of toxicity in children from oral nicotine products as most would not continue to use these oral forms. Also if oral nicotine products (e.g. gum or lozenge) are swallowed, there is very little absorption. Patches should, however, be kept out of the reach of children

Electronic cigarettes (e-cigarettes)
Some of these products produce a vapour containing nicotine, while others do not. Clinicians and consumers should be well informed when making decisions about these products. To date there has been a vigorous debate amongst those in public health and clinical practice as to whether these products should be readily available or severely restricted.

- There is a potential public health benefit in these products, as they appear to be safer than cigarettes.
- They may be a potential gateway to quitting smoking, though not quitting nicotine. However, at the time of writing, the evidence for their effectiveness as an aid to quitting is, at best, equal to NRT.
- Despite no harm or toxicity to date, their safety is yet to be fully elucidated. Some studies have shown potential cytotoxicity from the many hundreds of flavourings added to the inhaled formula
- These products may prolong dependence.
- There is little to no quality control over the many hundreds of types and their contents.
- Should marketing be restricted or cartridges containing nicotine prescribed?
- There is some evidence that aerosolized nicotine is in the exhaled vapour, thus causing some potential 'passive vaporing'.
- The nicotine in these products is sourced from the tobacco plant.
- There are currently few legal controls over advertising, sales, and distribution of these products. There are fears that using these products will be a significant retrograde step, 'normalizing' smoking and give legitimacy to the tobacco industry.

Other pharmacological interventions: bupropion hydrochloride
Originally developed as an antidepressant, bupropion probably works in reducing desire to smoke by inhibiting reuptake of dopamine and noradrenaline. Bupropion can result in up to 30% quit rates in smokers.

Bupropion is commenced while the smoker is still smoking.

- One 150 mg bupropion tablet is taken for 3 days, then the dose is increased to two 150 mg tablets 8 hours apart each day.
- Smokers may lose a desire to smoke or find smoking unrewarding within a few days after commencement of bupropion.
- A set quit date is recommended by the manufacturers, but some smokers find smoking distasteful prior to their designated day. Cessation should be encouraged if this occurs.

Contraindications for bupropion
These include:
- seizure or history of seizure disorders
- risk of seizures, e.g. CNS tumour, or abrupt alcohol or benzodiazepine withdrawal

- use of a monoamine oxidase inhibitor in last 14 days
- eating disorders.

Effectiveness of bupropion

Clinical experience suggests that:
- about one-third of smokers eligible for bupropion will do well and discontinue smoking
- one-third will seemingly have no effect
- one-third will reduce their tobacco smoking, but not eliminate it.

There is currently no known indicator that best predicts the efficacy of bupropion in smoking cessation for any given smoking patient. Choice of NRT and bupropion hydrochloride is based on medical status; however, patients may find one type of treatment more practical than another.

Duration of treatment
- If no benefit has occurred from bupropion after 2 weeks, discontinue this treatment and attempt use of NRT instead.
- If bupropion has impacted on smoking, it should be continued for at least 7 weeks.
- If there is a reduction in smoking, but cessation has not occurred, NRT can be added (in some form) to eliminate smoking.

Adverse side effects
- Seizures—rare
- Insomnia (can be reduced by taking the second dose of bupropion no longer than 8 hours after the first)
- Sleep disturbance is also a common symptom of withdrawal and may be unrelated to medication.

Other pharmacological interventions: varenicline tartrate

A partial agonist at the $\alpha_4\beta_2$ nicotinic ACh receptor, varenicline reduces the rewarding effects of nicotine.
    Dosage regimen:
- 0.5 mg for the first 3 days.
- 1 mg (taken as 0.5 mg twice daily) for the following 3 days and then 1 mg twice daily until the end of the 12-week treatment.
- Duration of treatment is at least 12 weeks.
- A quit date is set within 2 weeks of commencement of the drug. However, some smokers reduce their smoking prior to this date, but may not completely quit by the set quit date. They should be encouraged to continue varenicline.
- Combining varenicline and NRT can improve outcomes when there is a 'partial' positive effect of varenicline.

Trials have shown good validated long-term abstinence rates, comparable to combination NRTs. Continued use beyond the recommended 12-week time period as a maintenance therapy to prevent relapse has been shown in trials to be effective

Contraindications

Initial post-release reports suggested an increased risk of suicidal ideation with varenicline, and resulted in a black box warning. Some authorities have counselled against its use in individuals at risk of such conditions. However, subsequent more rigorous analyses suggest that these adverse events may be no more common than with any other smoking cessation approach. Accordingly no absolute contraindication to use of varenicline has been agreed on.

Side effects

• Nausea most common (30%) but tends to improve with time.
• Depression, suicidal ideation, and aggression have been reported as side effects. However, evidence suggests that these may be pre-existing symptoms, exacerbated by nicotine withdrawals.

Precautions

• Symptoms of depression or suicidal ideation should be closely monitored (irrespective of the medication) in anyone with a history of depression.
• Dose adjustment is needed in severe renal impairment.

Medications not in widespread use

Glucose or dextrose is a recent and simple innovation to assist smoking cessation based on the increased demand for sweet substances that smokers manifest during the withdrawal phase. It is hypothesized that either the satiation effects of glucose dampen a desire to smoke or that glucose directly affects the neuronal systems involved with nicotine. A few trials to date have shown encouraging outcomes. Weight gain in the placebo controlled trials was increased in those on placebo, rather than those on the active dextrose!

Cytisine, a natural plant-derived chemical, has been used for many decades in Eastern Europe as a cheap and effective smoking cessation product. Its mode of action is as an $\alpha_4\beta_2$ nicotinic ACh receptor partial agonist. It has been known and produced as Tabex® since the 1960s. Since then cytisine analogues have been developed, notably varenicline. Efficacy of cytisine tables (1.5 mg) for smoking cessation resembles that of varenicline (in the order of 30–40% validated abstinence rates) with fewer side effects, and is significantly more efficacious than single forms of NRT. As development of cytosine delivery forms (tablets, patches, or oral strips) continues, this product has the potential to be a widely used pharmacotherapy that may be cheap and easily accessible.

Others: the following medications have been studied in trials, but currently are not recommended as first-line treatment, predominately due to side effects.

• *Clonidine*: clonidine hydrochloride is a presynaptic α_2-adrenergic agonist, which reduces sympathetic activity, mimicking a nicotine effect. Clonidine, an antihypertensive medication, has been used in the treatment of opioid withdrawals and has shown some efficacy in the treatment of nicotine withdrawals. However, there are considerable side effects, particularly the lowering of blood pressure, dry mouth, and constipation. Transdermal clonidine patch has shown some benefit in acute nicotine withdrawals with fewer side effects and considerable relief of cravings, anxiety, and irritability, although it is not favoured as a treatment in smoking cessation.

- *Naltrexone*: opioid antagonistic effects may be helpful in reducing the positive effects of smoking.
- *Mecamylamine*: another blocker of the positive effects of nicotine. However, this antagonist has shown poor efficacy due mainly to side effects. Particularly severe constipation may deter the user.
- *Silver nitrate and silver acetate*: have been used as over-the-counter aversive substances to produce a 'bad taste' while smoking. Not only does lack of compliance interfere with successful abstinence, but continuation to smoke despite the bad taste suggests lack of efficacy.
- *Nortriptyline*: an antidepressant not commonly used for smoking cessation due to the side effects, mainly cardiovascular, which require monitoring. Specialists in smoking cessation have increasingly used this drug successfully, however, in harder-to-treat smokers.

Behavioural interventions

As well as pharmacological interventions, behavioural interventions also play an (almost equally) important role in smoking cessation. Many smokers conceive of their smoking as a pleasurable habit that is too difficult to stop, especially after many years. A focus on the sociobehavioural aspects of smoking cessation is needed in order to better prevent relapse.

- The initial assessment of the smoking (and quitting) history will greatly help provide clues to a patient's needs
- To achieve the behavioural changes that need to take place to bring about permanent abstinence:
  - educate the patient on the nature of nicotine dependence
  - educate about withdrawal symptoms and the time-course of withdrawals
  - encourage and provide evidence-based 'tips' that will help (Fig. 8.2)
  - arrange frequent follow-ups.

Adjust or change pharmacotherapy when needed.

What 'tips' are useful and which may be counterproductive?
Tips that have *not* been demonstrated to be helpful:

- There is no evidence that drinking water alleviates withdrawals, 'flushes' the system of nicotine, or is valuable as a distraction technique.
- Should we recommend total changes in social and environmental contexts? Changes in habits do not necessarily help. Just as treatment for phobias involve the repeated exposure to the cause, cue exposure (the repeated exposure to triggers) has been shown to diminish responses and urges to use. Thus smokers should not avoid situations that may trigger an urge to smoke, such as using the telephone, driving a car, arguments, or even going to a bar or club. Only where there is a significant impact of another drug itself should that behaviour be avoided, e.g. use of alcohol or cannabis, or exposure to someone else's tobacco smoke.

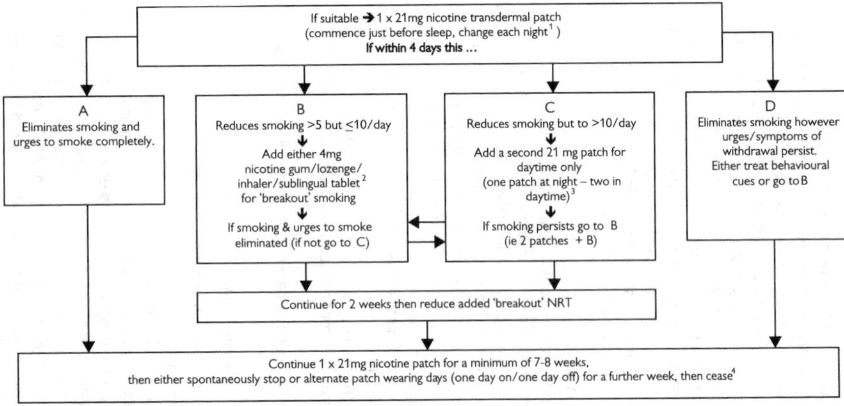
If suitable ➔ 1 x 21mg nicotine transdermal patch
(commence just before sleep, change each night[1])
If within 4 days this ...
A
Eliminates smoking and urges to smoke completely.
B
Reduces smoking >5 but ≤10/day
Add either 4mg nicotine gum/lozenge/ inhaler/sublingual tablet[2] for 'breakout' smoking
If smoking & urges to smoke eliminated (if not go to C)
C
Reduces smoking but to >10/day
Add a second 21 mg patch for daytime only
(one patch at night – two in daytime)[3]
If smoking persists go to B
(ie 2 patches + B)
D
Eliminates smoking however urges/symptoms of withdrawal persist.
Either treat behavioural cues or go to B
Continue for 2 weeks then reduce added 'breakout' NRT
Continue 1 x 21mg nicotine patch for a minimum of 7-8 weeks,
then either spontaneously stop or alternate patch wearing days (one day on/one day off) for a further week, then cease[4]

CONTRAINDICATIONS: 1) PREGNANCY OR LIKELIHOOD (other NRT suitable but not patch)
2) RECENT CARDIOVASCULAR EVENT (within 48 hours)

1. Applying patch just before sleep allows the slow rise of nicotine overnight – the likelihood of first cigarette of the day 'urge' is strongly diminished.
2. Either 4mg nicotine gum or lozenge depending on patient choice. Inhaler or sublingual tablet can be used if the patient needs faster reinforcement.
3. No evidence of toxicity. Consider reducing concentrations if nausea occurs.
4. There is no evidence for wearing (or reduction) of patch strengths

Fig. 8.1 Combination NRT algorithm for hard-to-treat smokers.

Adapted from *Journal of Smoking Cessation*, 1(1), Renee Bittoun, 'A combination NRT algorithm for hard-to-treat smokers', pp. 3–7, Copyright (2006), with permission from Cambridge University Press.

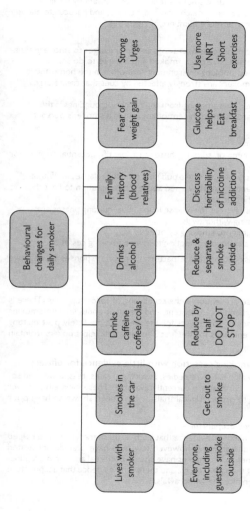

Fig. 8.2 Tactics to assist quitting.

- Do not recommend cutting down or nicotine 'fading' (weaker cigarettes) as dependent smokers tend to compensate by inhaling deeper and extracting as much or more nicotine, and particulate matter through stronger or more numbers of cigarettes.

Social context

Cue conditioning often leads to cravings and strong urges to smoke in situations where smokers have often smoked and are free to do so.

- Well-established smoking environments are often in the home and it is there that smokers are strongly affected by cues that create urges to smoke.
- Eliminating their own smoking from the home surroundings is the first step towards extinguishment of cravings in a smoker's personal surrounds.

Relapse prevention

Refer to assessment of smoking history to identify potential triggers for relapse.

- Note that lapses (even a single puff) become full relapses in 95% of cases, so patients must be warned about the temptation to limit their smoking to 'the odd puff'.
- Three main risk factors for relapse in the initial quitting phases are:
  - overwhelming withdrawals
  - close proximity to smoking by others
  - increasing alcohol consumption following smoking cessation.

Longer-term risk factors are a pattern of poor responses to negative life events.

Follow-up

Implicit in relapse prevention is the scheduling of follow-up visits. There is evidence that scheduled, consistent, and frequent enquiries into smoking status and efficacy of treatments for the weeks immediately post quitting with continuing enquiries for the first 3 months will help smokers maintain abstinence.

Methods for smoking cessation with little evidence for efficacy

There are many alternative remedies, including creams, teas, drops and so-called wonder cures that are currently available. These have either never been subjected to proper clinical trials or have been shown to have poor efficacy.

Hypnotherapy and acupuncture

There is much anecdotal evidence that both of these therapies have helped many smokers quit smoking; however, few trials have ever demonstrated positive outcomes. Some studies have shown both real and sham acupuncture points elicit the same results, and there is no evidence that acupuncture has any effect on nicotine withdrawals.

Weaning off nicotine by reduction of numbers of cigarettes or of nicotine content

Many smokers have felt comforted by the notion that by reducing the number of cigarettes they smoke per day or reducing the intake of nicotine by smoking so-called milder cigarettes would assist them in quitting smoking. A heavily dependent smoker is most likely to titrate the nicotine content required so that either more cigarettes are smoked when the concentration of nicotine is lowered, or deeper inhalations are made as compensation for reducing the number of daily cigarettes smoked. Each of these responses raises blood CO levels. However, if strict smoking criteria are adhered to, that is a regimented daily reduction, this method may still have some positive outcomes.

Harm reduction/palliation

Smoked nicotine intake is suppressed when on NRT and, correspondingly, particulate matter and harmful CO intake are reduced. Accordingly, harm reduction is a reasonable and safe option to consider in smokers unwilling or unable to quit. It is less harmful to smoke while using NRT than smoking without it. Reducing smoking in this manner may also be a gateway to quitting. Temporary abstinence is common where smokers use NRTs in situations where smoking is banned, e.g. airports and workplaces. This is safe and should be encouraged as a harm-reduction strategy. Health groups around the world advocate 'a cutting down to quit' regimen that involves daily alternating smoking a cigarette with any form of NRT such as gum, lozenge, sublingual tablet, or inhaler. The formula called NARS (nicotine-assisted reduction to stop) has shown good unintentional long-term quitting rates.

Benefits of using NRT for temporary abstinence
- Relieves cravings and other withdrawal symptoms
- Reduces cigarette consumption and prevents compensatory smoking
- Smokers may learn that they can manage without tobacco for several hours, which may increase motivation and confidence to quit altogether

Prevention

The international Framework of Tobacco Control (FTC) formulated by the World Health Organization sets out clear targets that individual countries can achieve in order to reduce tobacco promotion and use. To date, more than 150 countries around the world are signatories to this document.
- In many developed countries, the decline in prevalence of smoking has followed antismoking media campaigns, tobacco price increases, bans on promotion of tobacco, restricted smoking in the workplace, and the advent of pharmacotherapies to aid in smoking cessation.
- As well as these tobacco control interventions used to reduce the level of smoking, there needs to be a better understanding of the complex nature of tobacco smoking itself so that doctors and other healthcare professionals can more effectively intervene to reduce the prevalence.

Further reading
Aubin HJ, Luquiens A, Berlin I. (2014). Pharmacotherapy for smoking cessation: pharmacological principles and clinical practice. *Br J Clin Pharmacol* 77:324–36.
Fiore MC, Jaén CR, Baker TB, et al. (2008). *Treating Tobacco Use and Dependence: 2008 Update*. Clinical Practice Guideline. Rockville, MD: U.S. Department of Health and Human Services. Available at: http://www.ncbi.nlm.nih.gov/books/NBK63952/

Alcohol

Introduction *152*
Epidemiology *153*
Pharmacology *154*
Pathophysiology *156*
The spectrum of use and misuse *158*
Core clinical syndromes *162*
Natural history of alcohol use disorders *167*
Screening and brief intervention for unhealthy alcohol
   consumption *169*
Comprehensive assessment of alcohol use disorders *175*
Diagnosis and management of alcohol intoxication *184*
Overview of management of alcohol dependence *186*
Diagnosis and management of alcohol withdrawal *187*
Ongoing treatment of alcohol dependence *200*
Complications of unhealthy alcohol use: their
   assessment and management *214*
Harm reduction/palliation in alcohol use disorders *231*
Alcohol drug interactions *232*

Introduction

Alcohol use is widely accepted in many countries but contributes to a significant burden of harm worldwide. Drinking can range from low-level and low-risk use through to hazardous use, harmful alcohol consumption, and severe alcohol dependence with loss of control over consumption, and a compulsion to drink despite experiencing clear harms from drinking. In alcohol dependence there is a prominent physiological drive to consume alcohol. It develops over many months or years. The classical syndrome of alcohol dependence, if untreated, typically shows a progressive or chronic relapsing course. It can cause great harm both to the drinker and their family and community. Alcohol-dependent people identified in the community by epidemiological surveys may have a different course, particularly when it is less severe (e.g. just meets the criteria for diagnosis). The spectrum of hazardous use, harmful use, alcohol use disorder, and alcohol dependence is termed 'unhealthy alcohol use'.

In most countries, primary care practitioners can offer a range of interventions/treatments for unhealthy alcohol use. In some countries, addiction specialists are also available. In this section we describe the range of treatment options, both in generalist and more specialist settings.

Treatment has developed considerably over the past decade and its effectiveness and cost-effectiveness has been established in many studies.

Treatment may include a menu of options such as:

- withdrawal management (detoxification) procedures
- medications for relapse prevention
- psychological therapies, including brief interventions
- supportive therapies
- engagement with self-help (or mutual help) groups.

Most patients with alcohol dependence can abstain from alcohol for short periods and may do so without treatment or support. However, without treatment 70–90% of patients with well-established alcohol dependence will relapse within the first year. The prognosis with treatment is better, with just under half (30–40%) likely to relapse within 12 months. At 10 years, approximately 30–40% of those with treated alcohol dependence are abstinent.

Epidemiology

Alcohol is among the top five risk factors for years lost from death or disability worldwide. It ranks first in the 15–49-year age group.

In many countries, approximately 15% of hospital in-patients have a disorder that is directly related to excess alcohol consumption; a further 15% may drink above recommended limits or have other alcohol-related problems. In the family practice setting, up to one in six patients may have evidence of a risky alcohol use or an alcohol use disorder.

Overuse of alcohol may cause harm by the acute effects of intoxication, and these harms may be apparent even in the young, infrequent, or episodic drinker:

- Alcohol is associated with up to 80% of suicides and deaths from fire, half of murders, and 30% of fatal road traffic accidents.
- Alcohol is a common factor in injuries of every type—at home, at work, on the roads, and near water.
- In young men there is a linear association between excess alcohol consumption and risk of death, especially from violent causes.
- Because of its disinhibiting effect, it is also often involved in crime.

Long-term alcohol use above recommended limits is a risk factor for a wide range of common conditions, including:

- hypertension, liver disease and cancers.
- depression and anxiety
- cognitive impairment

Alcohol also accentuates the risk of liver damage from other causes such as obesity and hepatitis C. Many of the public are not aware of these risks from long-term consumption.

While there is some evidence of specific health benefits from low level drinking in middle-aged or older adults (with reports of reduction of ischaemic heart disease and improved insulin sensitivity), these are offset by increases in risk of chronic diseases, such cancers from relatively low levels of consumption. Also, episodic heavy drinking is associated with acute risks, including arrhythmias.

Alcohol use disorders occur across a wide range of cultures, and in any social class and age group. However:

- Those with mental illness or who are disadvantaged may be at greater risk.
- Alcohol use disorders peak in adults in their 20s and 30s, so when complications, chronic disability or death occur, they do so in relatively young people.
- There are both genetic and environmental influences on the risk of developing alcohol dependence.

Because of the high prevalence and impact of alcohol use disorders, accurate diagnosis and management of unhealthy alcohol use, particularly in the early stages, are an important part of every clinician's work. Access to timely help minimizes medical and social costs and increases the likelihood of good outcomes.

Pharmacology

Ethyl alcohol or ethanol is water-soluble and readily absorbed from the upper small intestine (80%) and to a lesser extent (20%) from the stomach. Peak blood concentrations are reached after 30–60 minutes. Absorption is delayed by food or drugs which delay gastric emptying. It is accelerated by acidity (including added orange juice) or aeration of alcoholic beverages (the latter distending the stomach).

Alcohol is widely distributed throughout the body. Volume of distribution is roughly equivalent to total body water. As women have a lower proportion of body water and a higher proportion of fat than men, they have higher blood alcohol concentrations (BACs) after ingestion of equivalent amounts of alcohol.

Metabolism occurs mainly in the liver, but a smaller amount of ethanol is also metabolized in the stomach wall (gastric first-pass metabolism). Ethanol is primarily broken down by the enzyme alcohol dehydrogenase to acetaldehyde. This step is rate limiting. Women have 20% lower gastric alcohol dehydrogenase activity than men.

A healthy 70 kg person metabolizes approximately 10 g ethanol (about 1 standard drink) per hour (approximately 0.015 g/100 mL or 15 mg %) BAC per hour.

Acetaldehyde is, in turn, metabolized by aldehyde dehydrogenase to acetate which enters the Krebs cycle, and is ultimately oxidized to carbon dioxide and water (Fig. 9.1).

Some individuals, especially those of Japanese and Chinese origin, have a sub-functioning form of the aldehyde dehydrogenase enzyme so experience higher levels of acetaldehyde for any given alcohol intake. This leads to adverse effects (as seen with the disulfiram reaction), including flushing, headaches, and nausea after small amounts of alcohol. Those who have the variant allele have a much lower risk of alcohol dependence.

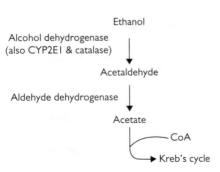

Fig. 9.1 Metabolism of ethanol.

A CYP2E1 cytochrome P450-dependent liver microsomal ethanol oxidizing system (MEOS) also metabolizes a smaller amount of ethanol (3–5%) in healthy subjects. This system may be induced in chronic daily drinkers and alcohol-dependent individuals.

As a result of oxidation of alcohol, hydrogen equivalents are produced, which fuel several subsidiary reactions leading to the production of lactic acid, ketone bodies, and neutral fats. Metabolism of alcohol also leads to depletion of glutathione, induction of oxidative stress, and the generation of free radicals, which can damage cell membranes.

A small percentage (2–3%) of alcohol is excreted unchanged in the urine, expired air, and sweat. This can be detected in breath, urine, or by transdermal alcohol assays.

Pathophysiology

Neurobiology of alcohol effects and dependence

Alcohol has strong reinforcing properties and rewarding effects including euphoria and anxiolysis. The mesolimbic dopamine 'reward' system in the brain (ventral tegmental area, nucleus accumbens, amygdala, and prefrontal cortex) is believed to be involved in these effects.

Pharmacologically, alcohol is a CNS depressant/sedative. These effects are due to:

* potentiation of $GABA_A$ receptor-mediated inhibitory function in the brain
* at higher concentrations, inhibition of glutamatergic N-methyl-D-aspartate (NMDA) excitatory function.

Endogenous opioids, which are released by alcohol, mediate some of the rewarding effects of alcohol, in part by accentuating dopamine release.

Other systems involved in alcohol effects or alcohol dependence include:

* serotonin: a relative deficiency of serotonin (5HT) has been reported in young males with early-onset alcohol dependence
* hypothalamic–pituitary axis and noradrenaline systems: during withdrawal there is considerable over-activity of central and peripheral noradrenaline systems.

Alcohol dependence develops as a result of chronic excessive ingestion of alcohol that leads to several adaptive neurochemical and physiological changes, a process known as 'neuroadaptation':

* With ongoing exposure, the brain attempts to compensate and restore glutamate function by decreasing the number of $GABA_A$ receptors and increasing the number of NMDA receptors, leading to tolerance.
* Once drinking stops, the relative deficit of $GABA_A$ and excess of NMDA function explains the hyperexcitability of the alcohol withdrawal syndrome.

Alcohol-dependent individuals are often magnesium depleted. As magnesium is the brain's natural glutamate antagonist, magnesium depletion, in conjunction with the relative over-activity of the NMDA system during alcohol withdrawal, can increase brain excitability and so predispose to withdrawal seizures. Magnesium deficiency may also impair thiamine utilization.

Pathophysiology of acute complications

Alcohol intoxication causes impaired coordination and judgement, and slowed reaction time, leading to increased risk of injury. The disinhibition associated with intoxication means individuals may also take risks they would otherwise avoid, e.g. unprotected sex or drug-taking. Some are more likely to become violent. Intoxication may also leave a person vulnerable and less able to protect him- or herself, e.g. from sexual or physical assault or fraud.

Severe intoxication can result in acute electrolyte disorders and risk of cardiac arrhythmias.

Because of its central depressant properties, acute alcohol overdose can result in coma (with risk of aspiration) and risk of death from respiratory depression, particularly when taken with other CNS depressants.

Pathophysiology of organ damage

Chronic excessive alcohol consumption causes damage to a wide range of organs. These harms are thought to result from several mechanisms:

- Acetaldehyde (the main product of metabolism of ethanol):
  - is a highly reactive molecule with potential to cause oxidative harm; this can cause direct cell damage and may contribute to increased risk of cancers
  - can form adducts with proteins, which can then be the subject of an immune attack
  - can combine with small molecules, including amine neurotransmitters, to produce compounds with brain activity, e.g. salsalinol—that may contribute to dependence and withdrawal.
- Ethanol:
  - increases membrane permeability. This includes increased absorption of endotoxins from the gastrointestinal tract
  - impairs thiamine absorption and utilization; thiamine deficiency may result in a range of neurological and other organ disorders.

Also see sections on each complication.

Further reading

Koob GF. (2013). Theoretical frameworks and mechanistic aspects of alcohol addiction: alcohol addiction as a reward deficit disorder. *Curr Top Behav Neurosci* 13:3–30.

Koob GF, Buck CL, Cohen A, et al. (2014). Addiction as a stress surfeit disorder. *Neuropharmacol* 76:370–82.

Lim SS, Vos T, Flaxman AD, et al. (2012). A comparative risk assessment of burden of disease and injury attributable to 6 risk factors and risk factor clusters in 21 regions, 1990–2010: a systematic analysis for the Global Burden of Disease Study 2010. *Lancet* 380: 2224–60.

NICE (2010). *Alcohol-Use Disorders: Diagnosis and Clinical Management of Alcohol-Related Physical Complications*. Clinical Guideline 100. London: NICE.

Nutt DJ. (2014). The role of the opioid system in alcohol dependence. *J Psychopharmacol* 28:8–22.

The spectrum of use and misuse

What are safe levels of drinking?

Guidelines for drinking limits are typically based on epidemiological data on the association between alcohol use and long-term or short-term harms. Guidelines may take into account:

- the levels of drinking at which risk of harm begins to increase above the risk for non-drinkers or light drinkers, and/or
- a threshold risk level, for example the level of drinking at which the lifetime risk of a complication exceeds 1/100.

Excessive drinking on a one-off or regular basis has clear risks for health.

Low to moderate consumption (e.g. up to 1 or 2 drinks/day for a man and 1 drink/day for a woman) has been reported to have specific benefits to health in middle-aged and older people (e.g. reduced risk of ischaemic heart disease and diabetes). However, from a relatively low level of consumption there is at the same time an increased risk of other adverse effects (e.g. increased risk of cancer), and at higher levels there is increased risk of cardiac arrhythmias or cardiomyopathy, as well as the unmasking of a propensity to dependence. Accordingly health professionals do not suggest that abstainers commence drinking.

Alcohol can have teratogenic effects and many countries recommend abstinence if pregnant or likely to become pregnant.

Recommended limits for drinking vary around the world, but there is a general consensus on the need for a low level (Table 9.1). Such limits have fallen in recent years as further epidemiological data become available, such as the association between alcohol and some cancers at relatively low levels of consumption.

What is a standard drink?

A standard drink or unit is a concept used to communicate drinking guidelines and to assist in assessing drinking. Units are defined differently in different countries but one unit is typically equivalent to approximately 10 g of ethanol (Table 9.2), though in the US and Canada, a standard drink is around 14 g, while in Japan it is closer to 20 g.

Accordingly it is important to consider amount of ethanol in grams when interpreting international literature. In many developing countries there is no agreed standard drink size.

Beverages such as wine have tended to become higher in alcohol content over recent decades, so standard drink volumes have reduced accordingly.

Alcoholic beverages are often consumed in sizes larger than the 'standard' drink. For example:

- The standard 'small' glass of wine served in the UK is now 175 mL of 12.5% ethanol (by volume) and so equals 2.1 × 8 g units. One unit would be only 80 mL.
- Many commonly sold alcoholic beverage containers in Australia hold about 1.5 Australian standard drinks (e.g. 1 can of beer = 375 mL of 4.8% ethanol = 1.4 × 10 g standard drinks).

Table 9.1 Examples of recommended maximum drinking limits from around the world (in g ethanol)*

Recommended limits for	Adult male			Adult female			Source
	Per day —regular (any occasion)	Per week		Per day —regular (any occasion)	Per week	Pregnancy (breastfeeding)	
UK	[16 g]	112 g		[16 g]	112 g	Avoid alcohol if pregnant or planning pregnancy	Department of Health, UK
Ireland	[25 g]	170 g		15 g	110 g	Best for a pregnant woman not to drink	Department of Health, Ireland
Canada	41 g	204 g		27 g	136 g	No alcohol if pregnant, planning to be or breastfeeding	Canadian Centre on Substance Abuse
USA	28 g (56 g)	196 g		14 g (42 g)	98 g	It is safest to avoid alcohol altogether	Dietary Guidelines for Americans
Australia	20 g (40 g)	140 g		20 g (40 g)	140 g	Not drinking is the safest option if pregnant or breastfeeding	National Health and Medical Research Council
NZ	30 g (60 g)	210 g		20 g (40 g)	140 g	Abstinence is the safest option if pregnant or breastfeeding	Alcohol Liquor Advisory Council

*Square brackets indicate that a guideline was calculated from other information provided, rather than set out directly.

(Continued)

Table 9.1 (Contd.)

Recommended limits for	Adult male		Adult female		Source
France	30 g	[210 g]	30 g	[210 g]	Ministry of Health, Youth & Sports
Germany	24 g	[120 g]	12 g	[60 g]	Federal Centre for Health Education
Japan	40 g	280 g	20 g	140–280 g	Ministry of Health, Labor & Welfare
India	20 g	[140 g]	10 g	50 g	National Drug Dependence Treatment Center (NDDTC), All India Institute of Medical Sciences

Under 'Source' column notes: France — 'Avoid alcohol altogether'; Germany — 'No alcohol from the beginning'; Japan — 'Avoid alcohol consumption of any amount'; India — 'Any level of drinking is absolute no-no'.

China: no minimum drinking age, drinking guidelines, or official standard drink sizes were identified.

Square brackets indicate that a guideline was calculated from other information provided, rather than set out directly.

- Home-poured drinks may be 50% or more larger than the standard drink size. For example, heavy drinkers may consume spirits in 200 mL servings, rather than the standard 30 mL nip.
- It is possible to buy 500 mL cans of strong (8–9%) lager (beer) in the UK, each delivering 4 units of alcohol.

Table 9.2 Examples of standard drink sizes from around the world

Country	Standard drink (SD) size
	(in g ethanol)
UK	8
Ireland	10
Canada	14
USA	14
Australia	10
NZ	10
France	10
Japan	20
Germany	10

China has no standard drink size
India: no information found.

Core clinical syndromes

Intoxication

The effects of alcohol depend on the level of tolerance in the drinker. At low BACs, alcohol causes euphoria and has a disinhibiting effect. At higher levels it impairs coordination and at BACs above 0.2 g/100 mL (43 mmol/L) it can depress consciousness.

In the non-tolerant drinker, BACs above 0.3 g/100 mL (65 mmol/L) are associated with risk of death from respiratory depression (Table 9.3).

Table 9.3 Levels of impairment in non-tolerant drinkers by blood ethanol concentration

| Signs and symptoms | BAC in novice drinkers | | |
	mmol/L*	g/100 mL*	mg/100 mL
Euphoria, disinhibition, garrulousness, impaired attention, impaired judgement	6.5	0.03	30
Increased risk of accidents, injuries, violence	10.9	0.05	50
Dysarthria, ataxia, confusion, disorientation	32.6	0.15	150
Increased risk of falls, fractures			
Altered state of consciousness, stupor, blackouts	43.5	0.20	200
Inhalation of vomitus, asphyxiation, coma, death	65.2–108.7	0.30–0.50	300–500

* 1 g% means 1 g/100 mL. To convert to mmol/L, divide by molecular weight of ethanol (46 g/mol = 0.046 g/mmol).

So 1 g per 100 mL = 10 g per litre = 10g/(0.046 g/mmol) per L = 217 mmol/L.

Non-dependent alcohol use disorders

Hazardous alcohol use

A pattern of alcohol consumption that increases a drinker's risk of experiencing harms to health.

Harmful alcohol use (ICD 10)

A pattern of alcohol consumption that is already causing health problems to the drinker (including psychological problems such as depression, alcohol-related accidents or physical illness).

Alcohol abuse

Alcohol abuse is a term used in previous versions of DSM, but not in DSM-5. It was used to describe drinking that is causing repeated social harms to that individual and/or to others (e.g. drink-driving, relationship problems) or repeated drinking in situations that place the individual at physical risk. In DSM-5, alcohol abuse is subsumed under the term alcohol use disorder.

Alcohol dependence (ICD 10)

Alcohol dependence is the clinical term used (in ICD) to describe a person who has become 'addicted' to alcohol. Alcohol dependence is defined as a cluster of psychological, behavioural, and cognitive symptoms fuelled by an inner drive to a repetitive pattern of drinking of alcohol. It tends to be self-perpetuating, typically develops over many months or years, and if untreated commonly shows a progressive or chronic relapsing course. The diagnostic features are outlined in Table 9.4. It corresponds to moderate to severe alcohol use disorder in DSM-5. The colloquial term 'alcoholism' is typically used by the public to refer to someone with severe alcohol dependence or severe alcohol use disorder.

Establishing whether a person is dependent or not on alcohol is clinically important, as it determines the goal and methods of treatment.

- Dependent drinkers show an impaired capacity to control their drinking, and may experience withdrawal symptoms on cessation of alcohol. They should aim for a goal of abstinence and will usually need support and treatment to achieve this goal.
- Individuals with non-dependent alcohol use disorders, on the other hand, will often be able to cut down on their drinking with less support or treatment, some even requiring only a 'brief intervention'.

See Fig. 9.2.

Alcohol use disorder (DSM-5)

In DSM-5, the previous categories of 'alcohol abuse' and 'alcohol dependence' used by DSM were integrated into a single 'alcohol use disorder' (AUD) with mild, moderate, and severe subclassifications. Anyone meeting two of the 11 criteria in a 12-month period receives a diagnosis of AUD; the severity grading is based on the number of criteria met.

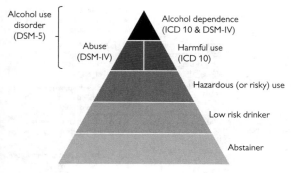

Fig. 9.2 The spectrum of alcohol use and misuse.

Table 9.4 Criteria for a diagnosis of current alcohol dependence (ICD 10) or alcohol use disorder (DSM-5)

	Alcohol dependence (ICD 10)	Alcohol use disorder (DSM-5)
Threshold / timeframe	3+ criteria present together at some time during the past 12 months	2+ criteria occurring within the past 12 months
Impaired control	Difficulty in controlling alcohol use in terms of its onset, termination or level of use	1) Alcohol is often taken in larger amounts or over a longer period than intended 2) Persistent desire or unsuccessful attempts to cut down or control alcohol use
Craving/compulsion	A strong desire or sense of compulsion to drink alcohol (craving or compulsion)	3) Craving, or strong desire or urge to use alcohol
Salience (Drinking 'taking over' life)	Progressive neglect of alternative pleasures or interests because of alcohol use; or increased amount of time necessary to obtain or take alcohol or recover from its effects	4) Recurrent use resulting in failure to fulfil major role obligations at work, school and home 5) Much time spent seeking alcohol, drinking, or getting over alcohol's effects
		6a) Persistent or recurrent social or interpersonal problems caused or exacerbated by the effects of alcohol 6b) Important social or work or recreational activities reduced or given up because of alcohol
Tolerance	Increased amounts of alcohol required to achieve the desired effects (originally produced by lower doses)	7a) A need for markedly increased amounts of alcohol to achieve intoxication or desired effect 7b) A markedly diminished effect with continued use of the same amount of alcohol
Withdrawal or withdrawal relief	Withdrawal symptoms on cessation or reduction of alcohol intake; or using alcohol to relieve or prevent these	8a) Withdrawal is manifested by the characteristic withdrawal syndrome for alcohol 8b) Alcohol is taken to relieve or avoid withdrawal symptoms

(Continued)

Table 9.4 (*Contd.*)

	Alcohol dependence (ICD 10)	Alcohol use disorder (DSM-5)
Continuing use despite harm	Persistence of alcohol use despite clear evidence of overtly harmful consequences	9) Continued alcohol use despite having persistent or recurrent social or interpersonal problems caused or exacerbated by effects of alcohol
		10) Alcohol use is continued despite knowledge of persistent or recurrent physical or psychological problem likely to have been caused or exacerbated by alcohol
		11) Alcohol use in situations in which it is physically hazardous
Number of criteria for a diagnosis	Dependence: 3+	Alcohol use disorder: Mild: 2–3 Moderate: 4–5 Severe: 6+

The alcohol withdrawal syndrome

The alcohol withdrawal syndrome is a cluster of symptoms involving CNS hyperactivity, which occurs when an alcohol-dependent person ceases to drink or markedly reduces their level of consumption (Table 9.5). Not all dependent drinkers experience physical withdrawal symptoms and, when present, withdrawals may range in severity from mild to severe, mirroring the severity of alcohol dependence.

- Simple alcohol withdrawal is typically self-limited, involving overnight insomnia and morning 'edginess', which lasts a few hours or until the first drink of the day.
- In more severe cases, symptoms may increase in severity over the next 48–72 hours, and include anxiety, tremor, sweating, tachycardia, increased temperature, and pulse.
- In the most severe cases, withdrawal symptoms progress to delirium (delirium tremens), a life-threatening illness if not identified and treated early (see Diagnosis and management of alcohol withdrawal, p. 188, p. 189).

Table 9.5 Diagnostic criteria for the alcohol withdrawal syndrome

ICD 10	DSM-5
1. Clear evidence of recent cessation or reduction of alcohol use after repeated and usually prolonged and/or high levels of alcohol use	1. Cessation or reduction in alcohol use that has been heavy and prolonged
2. Symptoms and signs compatible with an alcohol withdrawal syndrome : Psychological disturbance: anxiety irritability agitation sleep disorders Physical symptoms/signs: sweating tremor tachycardia raised BP raised temperature nausea or vomiting	2. Two or more of the following developing within several hours to a few days after ceasing or reducing alcohol use: a) autonomic hyperactivity—sweating, tachycardia b) increased hand tremor c) insomnia d) nausea or vomiting e) transient visual, tactile or auditory hallucinations or illusions f) psychomotor agitation g) anxiety h) generalized tonic–clonic seizures

Further reading

American Psychiatric Association (2013). *Diagnostic and Statistical Manual of Mental Disorders* (5th ed). Washington, DC: American Psychiatric Association.

World Health Organization (1992). *The ICD 10 Classification of Mental and Behavioural Disorders. Clinical Descriptions and Diagnostic Guidelines*. Geneva: World Health Organization. Available at: http://www.who.int/substance_abuse/terminology/ICD10ClinicalDiagnosis.pdf (See Chapter V, subsection on 'Mental and behavioural disorders due to psychoactive substance use'.)

Natural history of alcohol use disorders

In countries where drinking is prevalent, alcohol consumption typically starts in the teenage years.

- Episodic consumption is a common pattern and this has become increasingly heavy in the late teenage years in many countries.
- In the mid 20s the quantity consumed per occasion typically starts to diminish and the frequency of drinking may increase.
- Approximately 15–20% of adults consume alcohol in a risky way. Of these, around one-third progress to alcohol dependence, with most of the others reducing their consumption to low risk levels by their 30s.

Approximately 5% of the population in Western countries have alcohol dependence. There may be some fluctuation between dependence and (non-dependent) risky drinking in non-treatment seeking populations.

Prognosis for alcohol dependence

- Once well established, alcohol dependence tends to progress without treatment and typically follows a chronic relapsing pattern.
- During relapse, following periods of abstinence, there is rapid reinstatement to the previous levels of drinking and dependence (reinstatement; 'back where they started').
- Individuals with established dependence who are seen in treatment settings rarely manage to reduce their drinking to low-risk levels.
- People in the general community with lower levels of dependence may be more likely to do so.

When individuals with alcohol dependence in a public sector facility were followed over 10 years with relatively little formal intervention:

- 30% achieved stable abstinence
- 40% continued to drink heavily
- 30% had a progressive downhill course and died within this period.

In those unable to achieve long-term abstinence, alcohol dependence typically follows a chronic relapsing course. Maintaining long-term abstinence can be very challenging.

A variety of forms of treatment has demonstrated short- to medium-term success, and many drinkers report great assistance from mutual aid programmes, such as AA. Treatment is associated with a reduction in alcohol-related problems in 60% of dependent drinkers.

Among persons with alcohol dependence attending comprehensive public sector treatment programmes (prior to the advent of pharmacotherapies) the prognosis improves, with:

- 45% achieving long-term abstinence ± intermittent relapses
- 35% showing a less favourable course with periods of abstinence interspersed with periods of heavy drinking
- 20% showing a progressive downhill course which appears unresponsive to treatment.

Among private sector facilities, higher rates of recovery over 10 years (50–80%) are claimed, although in some cases, dependence is less severe.

No long-term follow-up figures are yet available for modern treatments for alcohol dependence that include pharmacotherapies, but early outcome figures suggest these are likely to have shown further improvement.

The highest risk of relapse occurs in the first 3 months after cessation of drinking, with the risk reducing thereafter for up to a year. Without pharmacotherapy, the majority (70–80%) of those accessing treatment for alcohol dependence relapse within the first year. The use of pharmacotherapy is associated with a reduced risk of relapse, but this may, nevertheless, still be as high as 40–60% despite strong motivation.

It should be noted that any remission provides the individual with physical and psychological relief from drinking, and provides relief to family, friends, and supporters.

Alcohol dependence and mortality

The presence of complications of alcohol use, e.g. alcohol-related liver disease can greatly shorten the life span (see specific complications, pp. 214–30), e.g.:

- Alcohol-related cirrhosis has a mortality rate of 50% at 5 years (70% among those who continue to drink heavily; 20% among those who abstain).
- Of those with alcohol-related cardiomyopathy, 60% die within 3 years.
- Alcohol dependence complicated by depression, psychosis, or suicidal behaviour also has a worse prognosis. The risk of suicide is 50 times greater in alcohol-dependent individuals compared with the general population.
- Other common causes of death are acute trauma, particularly motor vehicle accidents, accidental injury, drowning, and homicide.

Further reading

Dawson DA, Grant BF, Stinson F, *et al.* (2006). Recovery from DSM-IV alcohol dependence: United States, 2001–2001. *Addiction* 100:281–92.

Weisner C, Matzger H, Kaskutas LA. (2003). How important is treatment?. One-year outcomes of treated and untreated alcohol dependent individuals. *Addiction* 98:901–11.

Screening and brief intervention for unhealthy alcohol consumption

Introduction

Hazardous alcohol use is much more common than alcohol dependence. Screening for unhealthy alcohol consumption, and provision of brief intervention, is among the most effective and cost-effective of preventive approaches for what is one of the leading causes of preventable death. The best evidence for efficacy of brief intervention among those identified by screening is in primary care settings, though screening has also been conducted in a range of other settings such as the ED, trauma units, and universities and colleges. The purpose of screening is to identify those with hazardous or harmful use for the purpose of counselling them to achieve reductions in use that could prevent adverse health consequences.

Screening for what?

The target of screening ('unhealthy alcohol use') is any alcohol use that risks or has already caused health consequences (Table 9.6).

Screening tests

The best screening tests are brief questions (or questionnaires) that can be readily incorporated into routine clinical work. The briefest and easiest to interpret is a single item (Box 9.1). Questionnaires should be asked verbatim.

Use of the first three consumption items of the Alcohol Use Disorders Identification Test (AUDIT-C) has been well validated in primary care settings (Box 9.2).

Table 9.6 Unhealthy alcohol use

Hazardous use: any alcohol use that risks health consequences:
- Any use:
  - in pregnancy
  - when driving or working with machinery
  - when taking medications that interact with alcohol
  - certain medical conditions, e.g. hepatitis C
- Repeated use of amounts of alcohol that pose a risk to health:
  - definitions of risky amounts are decided on a population basis and vary internationally*
- Use with social consequences, but that does not fulfil criteria for a diagnosis (also known as 'problem use')

Harmful use (ICD 10)/ mild AUD (DSM-5)

Dependence (ICD 10) /moderate to severe AUD in DSM-5. The more severe form is also colloquially known as 'addiction'

*see Table 9.1, p. 159 for guidelines on recommended maximum drinking limits

Box 9.1 Single screening question for unhealthy alcohol use

- How many times in the past year have you had five (*four for women*) or more drinks in a day?
- The question may be preceded by 'Do you sometimes drink beer, wine or other alcoholic beverages?'
- A response of one or greater indicates unhealthy use.
- Note: different thresholds are sometimes used for the number of drinks, depending on standard drink size and national guidelines.

Box 9.2 The AUDIT-C

1. How often did you have a drink containing alcohol in the past year?
   Never (0 points)
   Monthly or less (1 point)
   Two to four times a month (2 points)
   Two to three times per week (3 points)
   Four or more times a week (4 points)
2. How many drinks containing alcohol did you have on a typical day when you were drinking in the past year?
   0 drinks (0 points)
   1 or 2 (0 points)
   3 or 4 (1 point)
   5 or 6 (2 points)
   7 to 9 (3 points)
   10 or more (4 points)
3. How often did you have six or more drinks on one occasion in the past year?
   Never (0 points)
   Less than monthly (1 point)
   Monthly (2 points)
   Weekly (3 points)
   Daily or almost daily (4 points)

Scoring varies according to standard drink size and local needs:
- In the US, a total score of 4+ for a man or 3+ for a woman is used to indicate unhealthy use.
- In the UK, if a patient scores 5+ then they are then asked to complete the remaining seven questions of the AUDIT (see p. 600–1).
- Note that a US standard drink is 14 g and a UK standard unit is 8 g

Specialized questionnaires exist for evaluating adolescents, the elderly, and pregnant women. However the AUDIT-C or a single item enquiry (p. 170) are likely to be adequate for most screening purposes.

- For pregnant women, it is important to identify any use, by asking 'Do you sometimes drink beer, wine, or other alcoholic beverages?'
- For adolescents ask:
  - 'In the past year, on how many days have you had more than a few sips of beer, wine, or any drink containing alcohol' and
  - 'If your friends drink, how many drinks do they usually drink on an occasion?'
  - Friends drinking more than three drinks (two for girls) or any drinking by the patient suggest the need to discuss use.

Higher scores on screening tools (e.g. 7–10 on AUDIT-C, or 8+ on the single screening question) suggest dependence, and need for more detailed assessment.

Assessment
Additional interview should determine if dependence (or DSM-5 moderate to severe AUD) is present because for such patients, intervention is more urgent and they may require further options such as pharmacotherapy and referral to specialized counselling services and mutual help groups (pp. 200–13).

Biological markers of alcohol
Blood or urine tests can help identify recent or regular unhealthy alcohol use; however, none is sufficiently sensitive (or specific) to accurately detect the full spectrum of unhealthy use (pp. 179–82 and Table 9.8).

The blood tests include:
- gamma-glutamyl transferase (GGT), aspartate aminotransferase (AST), and erythrocyte mean cell volume (MCV) and carbohydrate-deficient transferrin (CDT). These can reflect consumption of alcohol over recent weeks. CDT is more sensitive and more specific (fewer 'false positives') but is also more expensive
- alcohol metabolites such as serum phosphatidylethanol (PEth) and urine ethyl glucuronide (EtG) can identify use in the last few days. These show promise for screening, but as yet none is in common use.

Brief intervention
What is a brief intervention?
Brief intervention typically includes 5–20 minutes discussion of drinking. It usually includes the following components (Boxes 9.3 and 9.4):

> ### Box 9.3 Summary of components of brief intervention
> The components of brief intervention can be summarized using the acronym: 'FLAGS':
> - Feedback: on problems experienced
> - Listen: including to readiness to change
> - Advice: unequivocal advice to change drinking
> - Goals: negotiate goals
> - Strategies: discuss practical methods for achieving goals.

Box 9.4 Brief intervention: examples of components
- Feedback:
  - 'Your score on the questionnaire (AUDIT-C) suggests that your drinking may be harming your health'
  - 'What you have told me about your use of alcohol suggests your health is at risk'
  - 'I am concerned about you because of the risks you are experiencing as a result of the amount you are drinking'
- Listen :
  - Reflectively listen, including to patient's readiness to change
- Advice (should be clear):
  - Precede advice by asking permission ('is it OK if I give you some advice about your drinking?') and by asking what the patient thinks of the feedback you just gave
  - 'My best medical advice is that you cut down to 1–2 drinks a day at most'
  - Then ask what the patient thinks of the advice. Is it applicable? Could they do it?
- Goal setting:
  - 'There are a number of options. What would you prefer? To abstain? To cut down? To how much?'
- Strategies: discuss practical methods for achieving goals
  - For drinkers who are dependent (only): 'Would you consider seeing a specialist? A medication? These help some of my other patients in your situation'
  - 'Can you think of a way you can say 'no' to the (next) drink? Some people say 'I'm getting fit' or 'doctor's orders'.

The discussion of drinking should be done empathically (listening and demonstrating to the patient that you have listened) and with recognition that sometimes confidence (self-efficacy) needs to be supported (say 'I think you can make this change').

Reflective listening helps patients feel that they have been heard, and it helps them make changes. Repeat or rephrase what they have said: 'It sounds like you are worried you might be drinking too much.' To help patients initiate change, e.g. when the patient says something about their intent to change, say 'So, you are going to cut down'; 'You feel you really need to quit.'

Advice and goal setting should take into account severity of the problem, and readiness to change. Find out if they think their alcohol use risks harm or is a problem. Readiness to change can be assessed by asking 'On a scale of 1–10 how ready are you to make a change in your drinking?' or 'How important it is for you to cut down or quit?' or 'How confident are you that if you wanted to cut down that you would succeed?' For low number responses, follow the question with 'What would it take to increase that score?'

One reason to assess readiness is to determine how best to counsel the patient. A patient who does not think their use is hazardous and is not considering change is in the 'precontemplation' stage. One considering change is in 'contemplation' and one planning to or making a change is in the 'determination' or 'action' stage of readiness to change. The style of counselling can be adapted to the patient's current stage.

General appearance
A person with unhealthy alcohol consumption may not show any physical evidence of this. This is why alertness to the possibility of unhealthy alcohol use, and opportunistic enquiry, is valuable.

Goal of the brief intervention
The goal of the brief intervention depends in part on the severity of the drinking, and on patient preferences and readiness to change.
- For patients who are not dependent (e.g. hazardous or harmful alcohol use/mild AUD): reducing to within recommended limits is appropriate. If an individual has experienced harmful consequences, a brief period of abstinence may be useful; monitoring progress is important to gauge achievement of goals.
- For patients with alcohol dependence (moderate to severe AUD): the best goal is abstinence, but if the patient rejects such a goal, a trial of cutting down is reasonable (it can be very educational for the patient).
- Abstinence is also the best goal for those who have been unable to cut down, women who are pregnant or trying to conceive, children and young people, people with a health condition or medication that precludes drinking, prior harms of drinking and those with a family history of an alcohol disorder.

Strategies
Discuss practical steps that the individual can use to achieve their goal. These might include:
- avoiding certain circumstances where they are likely to drink to excess (or drink at all, for those aiming for abstinence)
- sources of support, including websites (see Further reading and p. 628)
- for those who are dependent on alcohol and ready to change, consider medication, referral for specialized counselling and encouragement to attend a mutual aid groups like Alcoholics Anonymous or SMART Recovery®
- for all, a menu of options is better than only one.

Does it work?
In the primary care setting, where the advice/brief counselling is offered by the primary care clinician, drinking is reduced, on average, by about three to four drinks a week, and about 10% fewer patients are drinking in a hazardous fashion a year later. Some studies and meta-analyses demonstrate decreased days of subsequent hospitalization. On a population basis these effects are large, though one should not be surprised if effects in individuals are small.

There is some evidence for efficacy in ED settings, but less evidence in hospital settings probably in part because the context is less conducive to it, repeat intervention isn't usually done by the same clinician, and severity of drinking problems may be greater. Nonetheless, there are additional reasons to identify any alcohol use in patients, even beyond identification of hazardous use for the purpose of delivering a brief intervention with a goal of less hazardous use. Other reasons include appropriate diagnosis of symptoms of medical and mental illnesses, and safer prescribing of medications that might interact with alcohol.

Is it acceptable to patients?

Doctors worry that patients will resent them asking about alcohol consumption; however, surveys have shown that patients expect to receive advice from their doctor on drinking and other lifestyle issues and respect their doctor as a source of such health information. Many are unaware they are placing their health at risk and are willing to learn how to optimize their health.

It is the responsibility of health practitioners to arm patients with the information they need in order to make informed decisions about health, and to support and encourage them when they wish to make changes to their drinking. On the other hand, it is important to acknowledge the individual has the right to choose their own lifestyle.

Further reading

Kaner E, Bland M, Cassidy P, et al. (2013). Effectiveness of screening and brief intervention in primary care (SIPS trial): pragmatic cluster randomized controlled trial. BMJ 346:1–14.

Miller WR, Rollnick S. (2013). Motivational Interviewing: Helping People Change (3rd ed). New York: Guilford Press.

NICE. Alcohol_Use Disorders: Preventing the Development of Hazardous and Harmful Drinking. Public Health Intervention Guidance No 24. London: NICE.

O'Donnell A, Anderson P, Newbury-Birch D, et al. (2014). The impact of brief alchol interventions in primary healthcare: a systematic review of reviews. Alcohol Alcohol 49:66–7

Saitz R. (2005). Clinical practice. Unhealthy alcohol use. N Engl J Med 352:596–607.

Comprehensive assessment of alcohol use disorders

Assessment is the first step in the management of alcohol use disorder. It helps build a therapeutic relationship with the patient, establish the diagnosis, and plan appropriate management. This is particularly relevant where there are clues to alcohol misuse. It also indicates the type of assessment that would be undertaken by a specialist practitioner or treatment agency. It includes the assessment of intoxication, of dependence on alcohol, risk of withdrawal, or complications of alcohol use.

General principles of taking an effective alcohol and drug use history have previously been described (pp. 69–70), including effective interviewing styles.

The history

The alcohol history

Start with a history of recent drinking, noting the following:

- Home-poured drinks are often larger than a standard drink and it is necessary to ask the glass size and the level of drink in the glass.
- If the patient mentions one type of alcohol (e.g. beer), ask about other forms (e.g. wine and spirits).
- Enabling the patient to feel comfortable about admitting to heavy drinking will help elicit a more accurate response: e.g. 'How often do you get through a carton (case) of beer?' Or, if you suspect heavy drinking, and the patient appears reluctant to put a figure to the amount consumed: 'Would you get through 20 drinks per day?'
- If the patient is having difficulty recalling their alcohol use a 'retrospective diary' style approach can be useful. Work backwards from the current time. 'What have you had to drink before you came here today? What were you doing yesterday, what did you drink then? What were you doing the day before… what did you drink then? …' etc., for up to a week. Pinning drinking to events assists recall.
- It can be helpful to elicit a typical heavy drinking day, timetabling consumption from the time of waking to time of going to bed.

Is the patient dependent on alcohol?

Where the patient has experienced clear alcohol withdrawal, you can be confident that they will fulfil criteria for a diagnosis of alcohol dependence (or moderate to severe AUD in DSM-5).

Where clear evidence for dependence has not emerged, the ICD or DSM criteria can be operationalized into questions to clarify the diagnosis (see Table 9.7 and pp. 590–9).

Does the patient experience alcohol withdrawal?

Check for overnight alcohol withdrawal: e.g. insomnia or morning tension that resolves with the first drink (see p. 187 for assessment of alcohol withdrawal).

Time of last drink: to assist in predicting or assessing the timing and severity of any withdrawal.

Tridimensional approach to assessment

1. Intake:
   • Type of alcoholic beverage
   • Quantity (e.g. number of standard drinks per day/week)
   • Frequency
   • Pattern (episodic or daily drinking)
   • Duration of excessive consumption
   • Time of last drink
   • Periods of abstinence previously
2. Dependence:
   • Impaired control
   • Craving/compulsion
   • Salience
   • Tolerance
   • Withdrawal
   • Continuing use despite harm
3. Consequences:
   • Medical
   • Psychiatric
   • Social.

Table 9.7 Eliciting evidence of dependence on alcohol

ICD criterion	Question
Impaired control	How easy is it for you to avoid or stop drinking, if you have something important on?
Craving/compulsion	If you don't have alcohol around, do you think about it a lot?
Drinking 'taking over' life	What does your typical day involve?
Tolerance	How much do you need to drink before you feel unsteady on your feet?
Withdrawal or withdrawal relief	How do you feel in the morning when you wake up, before your first drink?
Persistent use despite awareness of harm	[If necessary, clarify if the patient was aware that any reported harms were linked to their drinking]

Note: see diagnostic criteria for dependence or moderate to severe AUD in Table 9.5, p. 166).

Overview of lifetime drinking history

Some simple questions can elicit an overview in the dependent drinker:

- 'Over the last 10 years, how many years overall have you been drinking daily?'
- 'What is the longest time that you've had dry?'
- 'How did you achieve this?'

In most cases, in the initial history an overview is required rather than great detail.

Complications of drinking

- Dependent or heavy drinkers should be asked about any liver disease (alcohol-related or other)
- The general medical history acts as a screen for history of complications in any system.

Desire to change drinking

If this does not emerge spontaneously in the interview, it should be explored:

- Elements of motivational interviewing can be used to assess the desire to change and at the same time, may help develop motivation in the ambivalent patient: e.g. 'What do you like about your drinking? What problems does it cause you?'
- 'Have you thought about changing your drinking?'
- 'Have you ever tried to change your drinking?'

Current and past treatment for alcohol use disorders

- For example, 'Have you had help for your drinking before?'
- Past medications, counselling (and type of counselling), engagement with AA or other support.

History of other substance use (prescribed, alternative, licit and illicit)

As described in Chapter 5 (p. 70), assessing benzodiazepine use is particularly important, because of cross-tolerance with alcohol. Benzodiazepine use or withdrawal can complicate alcohol dependence or withdrawal.

Medical history

History should include all body systems, to elicit systems affected by alcohol, thus providing an overview of health including coexisting conditions that can be affected by alcohol (see Complications of alcohol, pp. 214–30).

Psychiatric history

This should include depression, anxiety, any admissions to psychiatric hospitals.

- Screen for depression and anxiety in particular. Where present, assess their nature and severity, including how much they interfere with function.
- Check for suicidal ideation: does it ever get so bad you think of harming yourself? Any previous episodes?
- Relationship to drinking: was depression/anxiety a problem before you started drinking regularly? If there has been a past remission from drinking: What was your depression/anxiety like when you had been dry for 6 months/12 months?

Other current medications
These give an indication of health, and of potential alcohol drug interactions.

Family history: of alcohol or drug problems.

Social history and context
Current living arrangements/social setting:
- Do other people at home drink heavily? Do key friends and family drink?
- Employment status

Forensic history: history of drink driving, assaults.

Physical examination

In many people with alcohol use disorders, signs may be minor or non-existent.

General Appearance
- Facial telangiectasia, facial puffiness and erythema, and coating and furrowing of the tongue, parotid enlargement, rhinophyma, rosacea.
- Conjunctival injection
- Obesity, especially truncal
- Poor self care

Cardiovascular
- Hypertension (associated with harmful drinking, or withdrawal)
- Tachycardia (in withdrawal, blood loss)
- Tachyarrhythmia, atrial fibrillation, heart failure, cardiomyopathy.

Respiratory
- Chronic airways disease—due to concomitant smoking (important when sedation is to be considered)
- Infections, pneumonia (impaired immune system)
- Aspiration pneumonia.

Gastrointestinal
- Tender epigastrium—gastritis
- Cutaneous signs of liver disease—spider naevi on face, upper trunk and arms, liver nails
- Dupuytren's contracture
- Palmar erythema
- Gynaecomastia, loss of body hair
- Hepatomegaly—of variable degree may occur in patients with fatty infiltration, alcoholic hepatitis, fibrosis, and cirrhosis
- Splenomegaly, ascites, distended abdominal wall veins
- Check for asterixis if hepatic encephalopathy is suspected
- Testicular atrophy, hirsutism in females
- Excessive bruising related to thrombocytopenia, coagulopathy
- Protein calorie malnutrition

Musculoskeletal
- Gout
- Muscle wasting with proximal myopathy

Endocrine disorders
- Pseudo-Cushing's syndrome
- Hypogonadism (in males)

Skin
- Psoriasis
- Acne rosacea.

Neurological
- Pupil size (e.g. if possible head injury)
- Ophthalmoplegia (diplopia), nystagmus, ataxia, confusion (e.g. in Wernicke's encephalopathy, other intracerebral pathology; also see pp. 95–7 for assessment of the intoxicated or confused patient).
- Cerebellar signs (predominantly truncal ataxia with gait disturbances)
- Evidence of alcohol-related brain damage; frontal lobe impairment, memory loss, and cognitive impairment
- Peripheral neuropathy
- Mental state examination (pp. 73–6).

Laboratory tests that are commonly used

(See Table 9.8, and Table 9.12.)

When to do blood tests in assessing alcohol use and its complications
Several physiological markers are available to gauge recent alcohol use. For individuals drinking more than 40 g ethanol or more a day, or those where complications of drinking are suspected, blood tests should be ordered to help assess recent drinking and/or the physical harms of alcohol, particularly the presence of alcohol-related liver injury (see Table 9.11).

Because of the relatively low prevalence of significant liver damage even in heavy drinkers (20–25%), liver enzymes may be normal in a majority of cases seen in family practice. Alcohol can cause significant health and social problems without any detectable liver enzyme abnormality, particularly in persons under 30 years of age.

Accordingly, in pre-test counselling the patient should be advised that in many cases the blood tests will be normal, even where there are major social or psychological problems from alcohol, or when long-term health is at risk. The tests are often done to check for evidence of significant liver damage. This warning helps prevent the patient from feeling that normal results negate the clinician's advice about changing their drinking.

In cases presenting to a family practice or outpatient clinic blood tests usually include:
- *Biochemical screen:* EUC, LFTs (enzymes, albumin, bilirubin)
- FBC
- INR/APTT in heavier drinkers (see Table 9.11).

Table 9.8 Laboratory tests used to assess alcohol use

Investigations	Results	Interpretation and comments
Blood alcohol	Raised with recent intoxication	Recent alcohol consumption. Urine alcohol levels stay positive longer than blood levels
		Passive breathalysers provide a breath alcohol reading on those not capable or willing to blow into a breathalyser. High correlation between breath and blood alcohol. Occasional 'false' positives from mouthwash or handwash.
FBC	Macrocytosis	Increased red cell volume (MCV) in 20–30% of heavy drinkers in the community and 50–75% of heavy drinking inpatients
	More sensitive among women, and drinkers aged > 30 years	Due to direct toxic effect of alcohol on the bone marrow and in a minority, folate deficiency
	Long half-life of 60 days after reduction/ cessation of drinking (red cell survives 120 days)	Other causes of macrocytosis include:
		Folate or B_{12} deficiency, including through malabsorption
		New red blood cells (reticulocytosis): e.g. bleeding, haemolysis
		Bone marrow disorders
		Hypothyroidism
		A range of medications, in particular anticonvulsants (phenytoin)
		Smoking
Liver tests:		
GGT	Elevated	Elevated in only 30–50% of heavy drinkers in the community and 50–80% of medical in-patients
	More sensitive among men, and > 30 years of age.	GGT is the most sensitive of the traditional markers
	Half-life of 2 weeks with abstinence if no underlying liver disease	Other causes of elevation:
		liver & biliary diseases
		diabetes
		pancreatitis
		hypertriglyceridaemia
		wide range of medications e.g. anti-convulsants (phenytoin)
		NSAIDs
		Smoking

Table 9.8 (Contd.)

Investigations	Results	Interpretation and comments
AST & ALT	Elevated Half-life of 2 weeks with abstinence if no underlying disease	Transaminases are relatively insensitive: only 20% of those drinking 60g+ of ethanol in the community have elevated results Raised levels tend to reflect histological change/impairment of hepatocyte cell membrane integrity AST and ALT levels are high, and typically less than GGT. AST/ALT ratio > 2 is indicative of alcohol as a cause of the test abnormality
Electrolytes, urea, creatinine	Increased serum uric acid	Gout may be precipitated by alcohol consumption
Cholesterol	Increased HDL cholesterol	An incidental finding rather than one of major diagnostic value
Carbohydrate deficient transferrin (CDT)	Raised ratio of transferrin with reduced carbohydrate content in comparison to total transferrin Half-life of 17 days with abstinence	Isoforms of serum transferrin which are lower in carbohydrate content increase with regular heavy drinking Higher specificity than liver enzymes, and higher sensitivity in dependent drinkers GGT and CDT may be elevated in different drinkers to those who experience CDT elevation, so can be used together False positives in advanced cirrhosis of other causes, and in primary biliary cirrhosis. Available in some centres only and more expensive than liver enzymes
Ethyl glucuronide (EtG) (urinary)	Raised with consumption in last 1–3 days Detection period depends on level of consumption	Only available in some centres Occasional 'false' positives with mouth or hand washes

Other laboratory markers for recent alcohol consumption are used in research settings, but are not broadly available. These include the ratio of 5-hydroxytryptophol: 5-hydroxyindoleacetic acid (5HTOL:5HIAA); phosphatidyl ethanol (PEth) and fatty acid ethyl esters (FAEE).

In those presenting with confusion, with significant alcohol withdrawal, or with complications, a wider range of laboratory tests may be indicated (for investigations for delirium, see p. 96; for alcohol withdrawal, pp. 189–90; for complications, pp. 215–21).

When elevated at baseline, GGT results are useful in monitoring progress and in providing feedback and encouragement to the patient who is doing well. In those without underlying liver disease, GGT and transaminases typically return to normal in the 4–6 weeks following abstinence. MCV takes up to 4 months to return to normal.

Other laboratory markers for recent alcohol consumption e.g. CDT are available in some centres. CDT has better specificity than GGT, though there are still causes of false positives (see p. 180). Like GGT it has a half-life of just over 2 weeks.

Other tests such as urine ethyl glucuronide (EtG); blood levels of phosphatidylethanol (PEth) or fatty acid ethyl esters (FAEE); or the urinary ratio of 5-hydroxytryptophol: 5-hydroxyindoleacetic acid (5HTOL:5HIAA) are available in some centres. These have also been used in workplace settings, and in monitoring impaired health professionals or drink drivers. They measure consumption in recent hours or days.

Further reading
Niemelä O, Alatalo P (2010). Biomarkers of alcohol consumption and related liver disease. *Scand J Clin Lab Invest* 70:305–12.

Establishing a diagnosis
Having taken a history, performed a physical examination, and ordered any necessary investigations, it is important that a formal diagnosis is reached in relation to the alcohol use disorders and any complications.

Diagnosing whether or not the person is dependent on alcohol is particularly important. Presence of dependence determines the treatment plan, e.g. whether the goal needs to be abstinence and the potential need for withdrawal management and for relapse prevention strategies.

The diagnosis should include:
- Diagnosis of the alcohol use disorder—whether:
  - non-dependent hazardous or harmful drinking (ICD 10)/mild AUD (DSM-5) or
  - alcohol dependence (ICD 10)/moderate or severe AUD (DSM-5)
- Diagnoses of any complications of this:
  - Medical
  - Neuropsychiatric
  - Social
- Diagnosis of antecedent or coexisting conditions (physical, neuropsychiatric, and relevant major social stressors):
  - Including diagnoses of other substance use disorders
  - Major antecedent factors or factors perpetuating ongoing drinking may be listed.

Assessment and diagnostic schedules
A range of formal diagnostic and assessment instruments are available to assist in assessing level of dependence (or severity of an AUD). Most are not required for routine clinical practice, but can be useful research tools. Also some specialist clinical services routinely use such tools to provide a quantified measure of patient characteristics and needs.

Diagnostic schedules provide structured assessment of ICD or DSM criteria for alcohol use disorders. Examples include the:
- CIDI (Composite International Diagnostic Interview)
- SCAN (Schedules for Clinical Assessment for Neuropsychiatry)
- DIS (Diagnostic Interview Schedule)
- AUDADIS (Alcohol Use Disorder and Associated Disabilities Interview schedule)

Assessment tools include those which are comprehensive, e.g. the ASI (Addiction Severity Index), and those which are brief, e.g. the 10-item AUDIT (Alcohol Use Disorders Identification Test). Assessment instruments are also used for quantifying aspects of AUD such as alcohol-related problems, withdrawal states or dependence severity. Other examples include:

- SADQ (Severity of Alcohol Dependence Questionnaire); and the
- Alcohol-Related Problems (ARP) Questionnaire
- CIWA-Ar (Clinical Institute Withdrawal Assessment of Alcohol Scale, revised)
- AWS (Alcohol Withdrawal Scale).

Scales for assessment and monitoring of alcohol withdrawal can be clinically valuable in monitoring patient progress (see pp. 606–16), particularly where more than one clinician is involved in patient care.

For further details on assessment and diagnostic instruments, see Chapter 27.

Diagnosis and management of alcohol intoxication

Alcohol intoxication varies from just perceptible to life-threatening. In this section the assessment and management of more severe intoxication is described.

Assessment

Alcohol intoxication is a differential diagnosis in patients presenting with abnormal mental states, confusion, ataxia, or coma. It may be complicated by overdose with other drugs, e.g. benzodiazepines, opioids, tricyclic antidepressants, paracetamol, stimulants, and Ecstasy.

The person presenting in an intoxicated state may also have other medical or surgical illnesses such as head injury, Wernicke's encephalopathy, hypoglycaemia, electrolyte disturbances, hypoxia, hepatic encephalopathy, or intoxication with other alcohols (methanol or ethylene glycol) which are often missed.

Assess and monitor:
- Vital signs—temperature, BP, PR, breathing
- Neurological observations:
  - Glasgow coma scale—hourly
  - mental state should be monitored for features not consistent with intoxication alone, e.g. confusion, disorientation, anxiety, panic, psychosis, suicidality
- Breath or blood alcohol levels
- Urine drug screen.

Management

Severe alcohol intoxication or alcohol poisoning can be a life-threatening condition, particularly in a non-tolerant individual.

If the patient is drowsy, confused, or has reduced level of consciousness:
- General supportive measures, to ensure that vital signs are stable and monitor airways, breathing and circulation
- Protect from falls/aspiration.

If the patient is unconscious, in addition:
- Place in coma position to avoid aspiration
- Assisted respiration may be necessary
- Avoid prolonged immobility to prevent rhabdomyolysis
- Maintain fluid balance and urine output; give intravenous fluids and replace electrolytes/magnesium/glucose as necessary.

> Always give thiamine parenterally before the administration of glucose solutions where there is a suspicion of chronic heavy alcohol use, to avoid precipitating Wernicke's encephalopathy.

When the patient improves:
- If intoxication was acute (e.g. in a young person), provide brief intervention
- If intoxication was part of a chronic alcohol problem:
  - Place on alcohol withdrawal scale
  - Review need for treatment for alcohol dependence
  - Discuss/arrange follow-up at the alcohol and drug services.

Examination of the confused patient

While confusion and disorientation occur in non-tolerant individuals at blood alcohol levels over 33 mmol/L (150 mg/dL or 0.15 g), these symptoms may occur at lower doses for those with other vulnerabilities (e.g. the elderly, those with pre-existing brain disorders, those taking sedative medication). In these vulnerable individuals confusion may take days or weeks to clear. Medical conditions need to be excluded. These may mimic or coincide with severe intoxication. Medical illnesses may also be masked by intoxication.

Exclude other causes of confusion or impaired level of consciousness, including head injury, metabolic abnormalities, hypoglycaemia, hypoxia, infection, poisoning with other agents, and Wernicke's encephalopathy (pp. 95–7).

In a person with probable alcohol dependence (moderate to severe AUD), consider a diagnosis of Wernicke's encephalopathy (p. 224, pp. 225–6) until proven otherwise. A raised GGT or collateral history may be the only indication of a covert alcohol problem, so remain alert to this possibility.

Overview of management of alcohol dependence

Alcohol dependence (moderate or severe alcohol use AUD) is characterized by impaired control over drinking. Fewer than 5% of dependent drinkers who seek residential treatment are able to return to controlled drinking. Accordingly, dependent drinkers are advised to abstain from alcohol. They usually need access to significant treatment and support to achieve sustained abstinence and to prevent relapse(s).

Although the ideal goal of treatment for alcohol dependence (or moderate or severe AUD) is abstinence, this is not always possible or acceptable to the drinker in the short term. Sometimes an interim goal of one month's abstinence may be acceptable, after which the patient may have observed enough benefits of abstinence that they may be prepared to extend this period. Continued follow-up with repeated advice incorporating motivational interviewing techniques is important.

Treatment includes a range of steps, for which the clinician and/or patient are responsible. The patient's family and those around can assist in providing appropriate support.

The 10 key components of management of alcohol dependence

1. Information and education. Motivational interviewing can be used to improve the chance of stopping drinking
2. The patient must then reach a point of acceptance of the need to stop drinking and develop commitment to abstinence
3. Management of alcohol withdrawal (i.e. detoxification), if not already completed (pp. 190–1)
4. Pharmacotherapies—to reduce relapse
5. Psychological/psychosocial therapies: e.g. cognitive, behavioural, 12-step facilitation; family counselling can be considered
6. Management of medical, psychiatric, and social complications or co-morbidity
7. Support from family and friends (and for family)
8. Mutual support groups/12-step fellowship
9. Continual care/follow-up (residential rehabilitation in some cases)
10. Personal, lifestyle, and environmental change.

If the patient continues to relapse after all these steps have been taken, referral to a rehabilitation unit or therapeutic community may be considered.

Diagnosis and management of alcohol withdrawal

The alcohol withdrawal syndrome is a cluster of symptoms involving CNS hyperactivity, which occurs when an alcohol-dependent person ceases to drink or markedly reduces their level of consumption. This can occur when a dependent drinker either chooses to stop or cut down on drinking, or is prevented from drinking by an illness or lack of availability of alcohol.

Not all dependent drinkers experience physical withdrawal symptoms and, when present, withdrawals may range in severity from mild to severe, mirroring the severity of alcohol dependence.

Simple alcohol withdrawal is typically self-limited, involving overnight insomnia and morning 'edginess', which lasts until the first drink of the day. In more severe cases, symptoms may increase in severity over the next 48–72 h, and include anxiety, tremor, sweating, tachycardia, increased temperature, and pulse (Fig. 9.3). In the most severe cases, withdrawal symptoms progress to delirium (delirium tremens; see Fig. 9.3), a life-threatening illness if not identified and treated early (see Diagnosis and management of alcohol withdrawal, p. 188, p. 189).

The severity of alcohol withdrawal increases with:
- older age
- high levels of consumption and increased duration of drinking (duration of current drinking episode, and total)
- coexisting medical disorders
- concurrent sedative (benzodiazepine) dependence
- recent anaesthesia
- malnutrition
- past history of alcohol withdrawal or seizures.

Where withdrawal is anticipated and treated early, complications should be rare. However, some patients present to the health service already in advanced withdrawal or with complications.

Features of the alcohol withdrawal syndrome

Mild to moderate withdrawal typically has:
- onset: 6–24 hours after the last drink
- peak: 24–48 hours after the last drink
- duration: 3–7 days.

Clinical features
- Sweating
- Tremor
- Tachycardia
- Raised blood pressure
- Raised temperature
- Apprehension, anxiety, irritability, agitation, insomnia.

- Nausea
- Vomiting
- Alcohol withdrawal seizures
- may occur in 2–5% cases of withdrawal
- Seizures may herald the onset of delirium tremens.

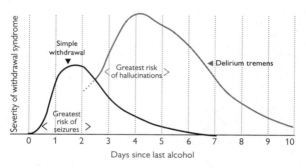

Fig. 9.3 Typical course of alcohol withdrawal.

Rating and monitoring the alcohol withdrawal syndrome

Regular monitoring of alcohol withdrawal is important. Two scales are commonly used to rate the severity of key features; these are the Alcohol Withdrawal Scale (AWS) and the Clinical Institute Withdrawal Assessment for Alcohol, Revised Version (CIWA-Ar; see Chapter 27, pp. 608–11).

Both are rating scales, rather than diagnostic instruments, and a variety of other medical or psychiatric conditions can cause elevated scores.

Delirium tremens

Delirium tremens ('the DTs') represents a very severe alcohol withdrawal syndrome (e.g. typically AWS score ≥15 or CIWA-Ar ≥20). It occurs in about 5% of patients in alcohol withdrawal, often in those who are medically compromised and/or with a long history of dependence. If good screening and treatment policies are implemented, DTs should occur rarely when alcohol withdrawal is adequately treated. DTs is still seen when patients present in a state of advanced withdrawal.

Delirium tremens is a potentially life-threatening condition (Box 9.5). Before the days of effective sedation and ready access to intravenous fluid replacement, the mortality rate was 35%. Effective diagnosis and management should reduce this in the modern world to under 1%.

Box 9.5 Delirium tremens

(I.e. severe alcohol withdrawal.)
- Onset: 48–72 hours after the last drink (may occur up to 5 days after)
- Duration: 3–10 days
- Generally preceded by other signs of alcohol withdrawal
- Seizures may herald the onset of delirium tremens.

Clinical features

As per severe alcohol withdrawal:
- Autonomic hyperactivity: tachycardia, sweating, tremor, hypertension, fever
- Severe anxiety, marked agitation
- Dehydration, electrolyte imbalances may be present.

Plus:
- Clouding of consciousness/delirium (disorientation and confusion, fluctuating mental state); symptoms often emerge at night-time
- Hallucinations: typically visual or tactile
- Paranoid delusions
- Cardiovascular collapse may occur.
  Untreated delirium tremens has a mortality of up to 35%.

Differential diagnosis of the alcohol withdrawal syndrome

A range of medical disorders may mimic or coexist with alcohol withdrawal. Coexisting medical conditions should be identified and treated concurrently. In particular, infection, hypoxia, gastrointestinal bleeding, Wernicke's encephalopathy, hepatic encephalopathy, head injury, subdural haematoma, metabolic disturbances, and concurrent benzodiazepine withdrawal should be considered (also see Chapter 6 (pp. 85–101) and Box 25.4 (p. 556).

Investigations for the alcohol withdrawal syndrome

Investigations are directed to:
- exclude metabolic imbalances
- assess recent alcohol use
- assess evidence of any co-morbid or complicating medical conditions (also see Tables 9.8 and 9.11)
- detect conditions which may mimic or exacerbate withdrawal, or be precipitated by withdrawal.

Tests which are of particular importance in assessment and management of alcohol withdrawal are:
- FBC: e.g.:
  - Low Hb (anaemia, recent bleed)
  - Leucocytosis (occult infection)
- INR: liver function; if INR is increased and albumin reduced, this may influence the choice of sedatives, e.g. oxazepam may be preferred
- biochemistry:
  - EUC to detect dehydration, hypokalaemia, or hyponatraemia

- serum magnesium levels (hypomagnesaemia)
- blood glucose—hypoglycaemia or hyperglycaemia
- LFTs : low albumin (chronic liver disease)
- AST/ALT ratio >1.5 (acute alcoholic hepatitis)
- BAC—if withdrawal signs and symptoms are present with relatively high BAC, withdrawal is likely to worsen as BAC falls
- urine drug screens—if suspicion of other drug use, e.g. stimulant or benzodiazepine use
- *if clinically indicated*, tests to exclude other pathology, e.g.:
  - brain CT or MRI—head injury, subdural haematoma.

At what BAC should treatment for withdrawal be considered?
  Treatment for withdrawal is typically based on symptoms and signs, and history of past withdrawal experience.
- Do not use BAC results as a primary guide to determining withdrawal management.
- If the patient is tolerant to BACs exceeding 65 mmol/L (0.3 mg/dL), withdrawal signs may occur at a relatively high BAC (e.g. 33 mmol/L or 0.15 g/dL and treatment should commence).
- When the BAC is more than 33 mmol/L (0.15 mg/dL) caution should be used in initiating sedation. It is advisable, if withdrawal is apparent at BACs >33 mmol/L (>0.15 mg/dL) to discuss management with an addiction medicine specialist or experienced internal medicine physician.
- A benzodiazepine (e.g. diazepam) is generally administered for withdrawal management when signs of this are evident.
- However, if a person has a history of complicated withdrawal (e.g. seizures, DTs) prophylactic diazepam should be considered, once the person is no longer clinically intoxicated.

(Note: for breath alcohol: 32.6 mmol/L=150 mg/dL=0.15%.)

Management of the alcohol withdrawal syndrome

Management varies according to whether it is a simple and mild withdrawal or a more severe or very severe withdrawal (delirium tremens). An accurate alcohol history at the time of presentation, including presence and severity of dependence, past experience of withdrawal ± seizures, and the time of last drink, can allow earlier treatment and prevention of complications, and selection of the best location for withdrawal management.

Management and monitoring
- Skilled nursing is key to management. Nurse the patient in a quiet, dimly lit room and, if needed, provide reassurance and regular reorientation.
- *Regular monitoring*: all patients in withdrawal, or at risk of withdrawal (e.g. suspected of drinking 60 g or more of ethanol per day) should be monitored regularly with an appropriate withdrawal scale, e.g. the AWS

(Alcohol Withdrawal Scale) or CIWA-Ar (Clinical Institute Withdrawal Assessment of Alcohol Scale, revised) (see pp. 608–11).
- In the general hospital setting, monitoring is typically every 2–4 hours
- In the home or outpatient setting, monitoring might be daily.
- For severe withdrawal/delirium tremens monitor more frequently, e.g. 1–2-hourly.

When to monitor for alcohol withdrawal

Monitoring with the AWS or the CIWA-Ar, 2–4-hourly is recommended for those patients:
- Drinking 60 g or more ethanol per day for several years
- With a previous history of alcohol withdrawal
- Presenting with a high BAC without signs of intoxication
- With a history of seizures and suspected heavy drinking.

Note that the alcohol withdrawal scale is *not* a diagnostic instrument.
Other medical and psychiatric conditions and withdrawal from benzodiazepines may result in similar clinical signs.

Sedation

For simple, uncomplicated alcohol withdrawal (e.g. AWS <5 or CIWA-Ar <10), rest and reassurance may be all that is required. However, if the alcohol withdrawal scale rating reaches or exceeds the threshold (AWS ≥5 or CIWA-Ar ≥10) administer regular benzodiazepines, titrated against the withdrawal scale. Benzodiazepines have been shown to reduce withdrawal symptoms, and prevent complications such as seizures and delirium tremens.

Individuals with a history of seizures may need prophylactic sedation before withdrawal features reach the withdrawal scale threshold.

Table 9.9 gives examples of benzodiazepine regimens that may be administered, depending on the severity of withdrawal syndrome. The dose can be titrated according to the patient's response.

Diazepam is used in many countries. An equivalent regimen using chlordiazepoxide is often preferred in the US and the UK, because it is thought to have less of a predisposition to dependence than diazepam.

Diazepam loading may be required for patients whose withdrawal score is rising despite the diazepam doses shown, or for those who present, or are detected in, severe withdrawal that does not respond to this regimen.

Some clinical units prefer an individualized symptom-triggered approach for use of benzodiazepines based on evaluation of AWS or CIWA-Ar scores at 15-minute to hourly intervals until symptoms are controlled and then at 4–6-hourly intervals.

Typically the maximum dose of diazepam should not exceed 120 mg in 24 hours. If more diazepam is required, seek specialist advice. However, provided that there are no concurrent problems (see Precautions, pp. 193–4) and a specialist has first been consulted, up to 240 mg diazepam may be administered in the first 24 hours.

Table 9.9 Examples of benzodiazepine dose regimens for management of alcohol withdrawal

Severity of alcohol withdrawal	Diazepam regimen	Chlordiazepoxide regimen	Frequency of monitoring
Mild e.g. AWS <5; CIWA <10	• Nil	• Nil	• 1–4 times daily
Moderate e.g. AWS 5–9; CIWA 10–14	• 5–20 mg orally • 3–4 times per day • reduce by 5–10 mg each day to zero over 5–7 days	• 10–20 mg every 6 hours • reduce gradually to zero over 5–7 days	• 4-hourly
Severe e.g. AWS10–14; CIWA 15–19	• Diazepam loading: 20 mg orally every 2 hours until patient calm and mildly sedated; then • Regular dosing of 10–20 mg orally every 6 hours; with supplementary doses of 10–20 mg if required until patient is calm and mildly sedated; • Then reduce by 5–10 mg a day to zero over 5–7 days.	• 30–40 mg orally • every 6 hours • reduce gradually over 7 days	• 2-hourly
Very severe / delirium tremens e.g. AWS≥15 CIWA ≥20	• Diazepam loading: 20 mg orally every 2 hours until patient calm and mildly sedated; or • IV diazepam 10 mg slowly, repeat after 30 min if necessary • If IV diazepam is required, nurse patient in a high dependency or intensive care unit • Once stable, continue regular oral dose regimens as described for severe withdrawal	• Day 1: 40 mg every 6 hours; • additional doses of 10–20 mg (to a total of 40 mg extra) as required • Day 2: 40 mg every 6 hours • Day 3: 30 mg every 6 hours • Day 4: 25 mg every 6 hours • Days 5–7: 20 mg, 15 mg, and 10 mg every 6 hours respectively • Days 8–10: 10 mg every 8 hours, 12 hours, and at night respectively	• Every 15–60 min

> ### Delirium tremens is a medical emergency
> Intravenous benzodiazepines may be required, and if so, the patient should be nursed in a high dependency or intensive care unit.
> Once the patient is stabilized and able to take oral medications, they can resume the oral dose regimens described in Table 9.10.

Other sedation regimens are sometimes used, including a regimen with sublingual lorazepam for patients who are nil by mouth.

Where there is suspicion of drug seeking behaviour, clinical signs are used in preference to self-reported symptoms, in titrating the sedation regimen.

> ### Precautions in use of benzodiazepines
> - In patients with chronic airflow limitation without respiratory failure, the dose of diazepam should be either be reduced or a shorter acting benzodiazepine, e.g. oxazepam, be considered. Monitor oximeter readings before and after each dose of benzodiazepine.
> - If there is respiratory failure, *do not* sedate in a general ward. Urgent referral to a high dependency or intensive care unit is recommended.
> - In patients with cirrhosis and hepatic decompensation (e.g. encephalopathy, ascites, jaundice), diazepam may worsen hepatic encephalopathy. In such cases, give short-acting benzodiazepines, e.g. oxazepam 15 mg every 2 hours to a maximum of 45 mg, then review.
> - Do not administer benzodiazepines for more than 1 or 2 weeks (to avoid the risk of dependence).
> - Do not discharge patient with a full prescription for benzodiazepines
>   - unless there is coexisting benzodiazepine dependence, in which case a tapering dose regimen may be required, often with regulated dispensing of benzodiazepines (see pp. 321–2)
> - In the elderly or those with alcohol-related brain damage, too much diazepam can result in falls or exacerbate confusion.
>   - If there is disorientation without significant tremor or sweating, consider haloperidol rather than diazepam.

Supplements
- Fluids and electrolytes: correct dehydration and fluid and electrolyte imbalance particularly hypokalaemia (e.g. with potassium supplements 80–240 mmol/day). In patients with little food intake prior to withdrawal, consider risk of refeeding syndrome.
- If there have been periods of prolonged immobility, which may cause rhabdomyolysis and acute kidney injury, check CPK; rehydrate and monitor fluid balance, turn regularly.

- Correct hypomagnesaemia with magnesium aspartate 500 mg orally 2–4 times a day with meals.
  - Magnesium is an essential co factor in thiamine-dependent enzyme systems and low magnesium levels may result in failure to respond to thiamine therapy.
  - Magnesium is contraindicated in renal failure.

Additional medication
- Antipsychotic medication: If the patient remains agitated or has hallucinations administer:
  - haloperidol 2.5–5 mg orally and repeat 3–4 times a day if necessary
  or
  - olanzapine 2.5–5 mg orally, then repeated three to four times a day. Olanzapine has a lower risk of extrapyramidal side effects.
- Small doses of clonidine or propranolol may be useful in patients with uncontrolled hypertension.
- Exclude, and treat, concurrent medical and/or psychiatric conditions.

Give prophylactic thiamine
Vitamin deficiency, particularly thiamine deficiency, is common in alcohol-dependent patients. The increased metabolic demands of withdrawal may precipitate Wernicke's syndrome.

Prophylactic thiamine should be given to all individuals requiring withdrawal management. *Do not administer intravenous glucose solutions before this is done.*

Alcohol can impair the absorption of oral thiamine, and if medical management of alcohol withdrawal is required, parenteral thiamine should be given, unless contraindicated.
- IM thiamine has a very low incidence of anaphylactic reactions and can be used in non-hospital settings. Some authorities recommend the availability of an 'anaphylaxis bag' in these settings.
- In the hospital setting, IV may be preferred to reduce discomfort, but be aware of (low) risk of anaphylaxis.
- Administer prophylactic thiamine (at least 100 mg) intramuscularly or intravenously once daily for 3–5 days then orally thereafter.
  - In the UK, this comes in the form of one pair of high-potency Pabrinex® ampoules, each pair containing 250 mg thiamine.

Prevention of Wernicke's encephalopathy
- Administer thiamine in a dose of at least 300 mg thiamine per day orally or at least 100 mg IM for 3–5 days:
  - In the UK: a pair of high-potency Pabrinex® (B-complex vitamin) ampoules is used. Each pair contains 250 mg thiamine
- Follow with oral thiamine 100 mg daily
- Multivitamins daily orally.
- Give thiamine before IV glucose or other carbohydrate load.

If the patient is judged to be at high risk of developing Wernicke's (e.g. with malnutrition, vomiting, or poor oral intake), then treat with higher doses of IM or IV thiamine such as 100–300 mg daily.

Note that these guidelines are for *prevention* of Wernicke's encephalopathy. Higher doses are used for *treatment* of suspected or diagnosed Wernicke's encephalopathy (p. 225).

Alcohol withdrawal seizures

Alcohol withdrawal seizures account for 10–40% of all adult seizure presentations to an ED. In general alcohol withdrawal seizures occur in 2–5% of alcohol-dependent individuals, approximately 6–48 hours after cessation of drinking and the peak risk of a seizure is at 12–24 hours.

In elective or predicted alcohol withdrawal, early benzodiazepine treatment typically prevents the occurrence of a withdrawal seizure. In well managed medical detoxification units, the prevalence of seizures should be less than 1%. The seizures are classically single, generalized, grand mal tonic-clonic convulsions without focal features and associated with loss of consciousness. Sometimes there will be a number of seizures over a period of 3–4 days. Rarely, status epilepticus will supervene.

- Once individuals have experienced a withdrawal seizure they are at increased risk of developing seizures during subsequent episodes of alcohol withdrawal.
- The risk of seizure is proportional to the level of alcohol consumption and increases with subsequent episodes of alcohol withdrawal.
- The risk of seizures increases in those with a history of idiopathic epilepsy, head injury or concurrent benzodiazepine dependence. Alcohol withdrawal lowers the seizure threshold for such disorders.
- The seizure may occur early before the full range of features of alcohol withdrawal becomes apparent.
- Seizures may herald the onset of delirium tremens, with up to 25% of cases without active treatment going on to develop delirium tremens.

Assessment of alcohol withdrawal seizures

For a first seizure the regular seizure 'work-up' is recommended to exclude organic disease or a structural lesion. Investigation is particularly important if seizures are atypical, e.g. multiple or focal seizures.

A first or atypical seizure work-up

This includes:
- EUC and serum calcium and magnesium
- Blood sugar
- FBC
- BAC; plasma and urine drug screen.
- Head CT scan or MRI
- EEG.

Management of alcohol withdrawal seizures
Patients with seizures should be admitted for monitoring and treatment, particularly if there is a history of benzodiazepine use.

Diazepam (or chlordiazepoxide) as described for the treatment of alcohol withdrawal (p. 191, p. 192) will prevent seizure activity. If seizures are thought to be due to or exacerbated by benzodiazepine withdrawal, higher doses of benzodiazepines may be required and should be followed by a tapering dose regimen (see Management of benzodiazepine withdrawal, p. 320).

Long-term prophylactic anticonvulsant therapy (e.g. phenytoin) is ineffective in preventing recurrences of a withdrawal seizure. If a patient is already on phenytoin or another anticonvulsant (e.g. for diagnosed epilepsy), blood levels should be taken to assess patient compliance and the anticonvulsant continued in the usual dose during the withdrawal period, and reviewed subsequently.

In some countries, anti-epileptics such as carbamazepine are used as prophylactic treatments during alcohol withdrawal, particularly if patients are at risk of seizures

There is an increased risk of future withdrawal seizures if drinking continues after a first withdrawal seizure, so the patient should be advised that future attempts to stop drinking should be managed in hospital. The issue of safety with driving also should be considered (pp. 573–4).

Further reading

Bråthen G, Ben-Menachem E, Brodtkorb E, *et al.* (2005). EFNS guideline on the diagnosis and management of alcohol-related seizures: report of EFNS task force. *Eur J Neurol* 12:575–81.

Charness ME, Simon RP, Greenberg DA. (1989). Ethanol and the nervous system. *N Engl J Med* 321(7):442–54.

Hoffman RS, Weinhouse GL. (2015). Management of Moderate and Severe Alcohol Withdrawal Syndromes. UpToDate®. Available at: http://www.uptodate.com/contents/management-of-moderate-and-severe-alcohol-withdrawal-syndromes

Lingford-Hughes AR, Welch S, Peters L, *et al.* (2012). BAP updated guidelines: evidence-based guidelines for the pharmacological management of substance abuse, harmful use, addiction and comorbidity: recommendations from BAP. *J Psychopharmacol* 26:899–952.

Education and follow-up after alcohol withdrawal in hospital

Prior to discharge from hospital, ensure the patient understands that they have experienced an alcohol withdrawal syndrome. If they are not yet familiar with it, explain the nature of dependence, and why a goal of abstinence is necessary (i.e. that if they drink, it will mean loss of control and rapid reinstatement of heavy drinking). If they have had withdrawal seizures they should be warned not to drive for a proscribed period (pp. 573–4).

Discuss ongoing care with the patient and negotiate a plan. Patients can be given the choice of various treatment options for relapse prevention and to enhance motivation (pp. 207–11), and encouraged to access several of these. Most alcohol-dependent patients are offered pharmacotherapies for relapse prevention before they leave hospital (pp. 200–2).

An important part of a successful treatment regimen involves continued follow-up and support. Typically, a dependent patient is offered an appointment with a specialist drug and alcohol unit where available, where the management can draw on a multidisciplinary team including medical officer, nurse/nurse specialist, psychologist, and social worker. Wherever possible a member of the team can meet the patient in hospital, to assist with engagement and subsequent attendance at follow-up.

Some family doctors have considerable experience in managing alcohol dependence, and can link the patient with private or public psychology services. Discuss the management plan with the patient's family doctor.

Elective alcohol detoxification

Alcohol withdrawal may be managed electively. This is generally referred to as 'detoxification'. Detoxification is a planned process which allows alcohol-dependent patients to cease drinking in the most comfortable and least distressing manner. It can remove a barrier to cessation of drinking and, in the management of alcohol dependence, it is the first step towards a goal of abstinence and recovery. The emphasis is on preventing a withdrawal syndrome developing or if one does develop, to minimize its symptoms and ensure that adverse consequences, especially DTs, are avoided.

Detoxification may be medicated or non-medicated depending on the anticipated severity of alcohol withdrawal. It can be conducted on an ambulatory or in-patient basis.

Settings for alcohol detoxification

Where to manage elective detoxification

Where detoxification takes place depends on the severity of alcohol dependence and past history of withdrawal, the presence or absence of concurrent medical conditions, and also on what local facilities are available.

The severity of the alcohol withdrawal syndrome is increased by:
- older age
- greater duration and amount of alcohol consumption
- concurrent sedative (especially benzodiazepine) use/dependence
- recent anaesthesia
- in malnourished patients or those with severe vomiting or diarrhoea.

Patients with the above features are best detoxified in a hospital or in a specialist detoxification unit.

Criteria for undertaking home/ambulatory detoxification
Home (ambulatory) detoxification may be attempted if:
- the patient has mild to moderate alcohol dependence
- the doctor and healthcare worker have easy access to the patient and can review the patient on a daily basis
- the patient lives with a supportive partner or family
- low risk of complications:
  - no past history of severe withdrawals or delirium tremens
  - no past history of withdrawal seizures or epilepsy
  - not on multiple medications
- not misusing multiple psychoactive substances
- no concurrent medical or psychiatric problems (including suicidal ideation; psychosis or cognitive impairment) which may place the patient at risk.
- the patient is not vomiting or malnourished.

Management of detoxification in the home/ambulatory setting
- Daily supervision either by nurse or doctor
- Encourage a quiet and safe environment
- Advise patient of likely signs and symptoms of alcohol withdrawal, and when they should seek assistance
- Monitor daily using a withdrawal scale.
  - With treatment, the score on AWS should remain <5 or on CIWA-AR should remain <10
- Sedation: benzodiazepines can be used to reduce withdrawal symptoms; however the safety of their use needs to be maximized and the following precautions taken:
  - The patient should be assessed as reliable to use according to directions and should fulfil the criteria for home detoxification
  - Daily dispensing wherever possible. The patient is reviewed, then given that day's medications.
- Patients should be warned about potential risks of benzodiazepines, in particular:
  - Unsteadiness and possible falls. They should not drive while taking benzodiazepines.
  - Sedation: withhold a dose if sedated, and cease benzodiazepines if drinking resumes
  - Dependence with continued use: benzodiazepines are for short-term use only (not more than 1 week) because of their potential for tolerance and dependence.

Treatment regimens
Diazepam 10 mg four times a day orally typically for 2 days, reducing daily to zero over the next 3–6 days (see Table 9.10).

In the UK, other benzodiazepines with long half-lives (e.g. chlordiazepoxide) are administered. They may pose a lower risk of diversion to the black market as they have lower street value than diazepam and have a lower potential for dependence.
- Thiamine 100 mg daily orally for a month, or indefinitely if the patient resumes drinking:
  - Initial parenteral (IM) doses should be considered, particularly if the patient's diet has been suboptimal or in where malabsorption of thiamine is suspected (e.g. vomiting or heavier consumption)
- Ensure good nutrition and give oral multivitamins
- Ensure that patient is well hydrated and correct any identified electrolyte imbalance and low magnesium levels
- When doubt exists over abstinence, check breath alcohol levels.

When transfer to hospital is required
If the AWS or CIWA-Ar score rises rapidly or if the patient develops withdrawal seizures, agitation that is difficult to control, or hallucinations, transfer to hospital should be undertaken.

With the dosage regimen in pp. 198–9 (and if necessary two extra 10 mg doses of diazepam on each of the first 2 days) withdrawal symptoms should be controlled, and the withdrawal rating scales should largely stay below the

Table 9.10 Examples of home/ambulatory benzodiazepine regimens for management of alcohol withdrawal

Time period	Oral diazepam regimen (Australia)*	Oral chlordiazepoxide regimen (UK)
Days: 1 & 2	10 mg every 6 h	15–20 mg every 6 h
Days: 3 & 4	5 mg every 6 h	10 mg every 6 h
Days: 5 & 6	5 mg morning and at night	5 mg every 6 h
Day 7	5 mg at night	5–10 mg at night
Day 8	Cease	Cease

* Titrate dose according to the history and to the response of the individual patient. Withhold if sedated or if drinking resumes.

required thresholds. If the rating scales are not able to be maintained below those thresholds, transfer to hospital.

When a 'detox unit' is needed or preferred
Some drinkers find it easier to stop drinking in a 'detox centre' or specialist alcohol treatment unit, where they are provided with a supportive environment, and are away from ready availability of alcohol.

Other drinkers may be unsuitable for home withdrawal management because of severe dependence or unsuitable home environment (see earlier-listed criteria for home detoxification).

Ongoing treatment of alcohol dependence

Pharmacotherapies to reduce the risk of relapse

Pharmacotherapies aim to prevent relapse or lapse and/or to maintain abstinence from alcohol. They may do this through reducing craving and the internal drive to drink or by reducing the reward of drinking. In the case of disulfiram (Antabuse®), aversive pharmacotherapy provides negative reinforcement for any slip-up.

Pharmacotherapies are typically prescribed for relapse prevention after acute alcohol withdrawal is over, usually 5–7 days after the last drink. This helps clarify whether any symptoms, such as nausea, are due to alcohol withdrawal or due to the medication. However, recent evidence suggests a role for starting naltrexone while the individual is still drinking, to reduce the desire for alcohol. They are usually prescribed for 3–18 months.

Pharmacological treatments are best prescribed in conjunction with a comprehensive behavioural modification psychosocial programme. Regular follow-up and psychosocial support is necessary, and monitoring can assist with earlier assistance with relapse. One-to-one counselling can be provided, with referral to a psychologist, self-help group, and/or other support networks as required.

Naltrexone

Naltrexone is a mu opioid receptor antagonist. It is thought to act by blocking endorphin-mediated pleasurable effects of alcohol, which tends to reduce heavy drinking and craving for alcohol.

In randomized controlled trials, oral naltrexone 50 mg/day delays time to relapse to heavy drinking and reduces the number of heavy drinking days, and increases percentage of days abstinent. The effect size is typically small to moderate (number needed to treat: nine), but effects may be greater in those with a strong family history (which may be a marker for those the Asn40Asp polymorphism of the mu opioid receptor gene).

If a drinker is already abstinent, and is taking naltrexone, it is important to advise them to continue the naltrexone if they should slip up to drinking. The naltrexone should be continued for a period to see if it assists in reducing quantity consumed. Some studies also demonstrate benefit of starting naltrexone even in dependent drinkers who are still consuming alcohol.

Once-monthly, injectable extended-release naltrexone shows promise, but is not yet widely available. Naltrexone implants are under study, but have not been approved pending confirmation of consistent blood levels.

Metabolism: oral naltrexone is absorbed from the gastrointestinal tract, metabolized in the liver to 6 beta naltrexol and excreted in the urine. The 24-hour+ duration of action enables once-daily dose administration.

Side effects: gastrointestinal side effects are relatively common (nausea, diarrhoea), particularly in the first week of treatment. Fatigue and headache are sometimes reported. Dose-related hepatotoxicity can occur, but at recommended doses is very uncommon.

Naltrexone may be commenced at half dose (25 mg) for the first few days to reduce side effects, then increased to the full dose of 50 mg daily.

Duration of treatment: the first 12 weeks after cessation, but may extend to 12 months or longer if found helpful.

Contraindications
- Pregnancy
- Need for opioid analgesics to manage pain
- Opioid dependence: naltrexone can precipitate severe withdrawal
- Severe hepatic impairment
- Severe renal impairment.

Precautions
- When opioid pain relief is required:
  - Discontinue for at least 72 hours before elective surgery.
  - Patients on naltrexone should carry a card warning that they are on an opioid antagonist in case of need for emergency analgesia. In such an emergency, regional anaesthesia, general anaesthesia or non-opioid analgesics can be used for pain relief.
  - When opioids are required in an emergency, greater than normal doses of opioids are required to achieve pain relief. This carries the risk of bronchoconstriction (presumably due to release of histamine). The patient should be closely monitored in a setting equipped and staffed for cardiopulmonary resuscitation.
- Periodically monitor liver function because of risk of dose-related hepatic impairment.

Nalmefene

Nalmefene is a newer mu opioid antagonist and partial kappa agonist, which is structurally related to naltrexone. Although the traditional goal of treatment of alcohol dependence/moderate or severe AUD is abstinence, the goal of nalmefene treatment is reduced drinking. It is recommended for use on an 'as needed' basis in high-risk situations as part of a targeted dosing strategy for patients who continue drinking at high to very high risk levels after an initial assessment/brief intervention. A reduction in heavy drinking days by 60–70% has been reported with 62% patients completing 1 year of therapy. Nalmefene is not yet approved in Australia and the US but is available in Europe.

Dose: one tablet (18.6 mg of nalmefene hydrochloride dehydrate) 1–2 hours before the anticipated time of risky drinking. Maximum of one tablet/day.

Side effects, precautions and contraindications are similar to naltrexone. Nalmefene is generally well tolerated.

Further reading

Franck J, Jayaram-Lindström N. (2013). Pharmacotherapy for alcohol dependence: status of current treatments. *Curr Opin Neurobiol* 23:692–9.

Lingford-Hughes AR, Welch S, Peters L, *et al*. (2012). BAP updated guidelines. Evidence-based guidelines for the pharmacological management of substance abuse, harmful use, addiction and comorbidity: recommendations from BAP. *J Psychopharmacol* 26:899–952. Available at: http://jop.sagepub.com/content/26/7/899

Maisel NC, Blodgett JC, Wilbourne PL, *et al*. (2013). Metaanalysis of naltrexone and acamprosate for treating alcohol use disorders: when are these medications most helpful? *Addiction* 108:275–93.

Acamprosate (calcium acetylhomotaurinate)

Meta-analyses demonstrate that acamprosate is significantly superior to placebo in increasing periods of abstinence and preventing relapse.

Mechanism of action: acamprosate is thought to reduce the craving induced by alcohol withdrawal by modulating NMDA receptor transmission and resetting the balance between that stimulatory transmission and inhibitory $GABA_A$ transmission. This decreases the hyperglutamatergic states associated with alcohol withdrawal, increasing beta endorphin in those with high alcohol intake and, possibly modulating the hypothalamo–pituitary–adrenal axis.

By compensating for the neurobiological derangement produced by alcohol withdrawal, acamprosate is useful for 'relief drinkers' i.e. patients who drink to overcome withdrawal symptoms (negative reinforcement). Accordingly it is less useful for episodic heavy drinkers.

Acamprosate is slowly absorbed from the gastrointestinal tract over a period of 4 hours. Peak concentrations are reached after 5–7 hours and steady state levels are achieved after 7 days.

Acamprosate is not metabolized significantly in the liver, and is excreted unchanged in the urine. The elimination half-life of acamprosate is between 13–28 hours.

Dose: acamprosate 333 mg tablets 2 tablets three times per day if body weight ≥60 kg; this dose is reduced to 2 tablets twice daily if body weight < 60 kg. Because of the three times a day dosage, patient adherence to the regimen is often low.

Side effects: diarrhoea, nausea, vomiting, skin rash, reduced libido.

Precautions: use with caution in patients with renal impairment as accumulation of acamprosate may occur.

Contraindications: renal failure

Further reading

Anton R, O'Malley S, Ciraula D, *et al*. (2006). Combined pharmacotherapies and behavioural interventions for alcohol dependence: the COMBINE study, a randomized controlled trial. *JAMA* 295:2003–17.

Kalk NJ, Lingford-Hughes A. (2012). The clinical pharmacology of acamprosate. *Br J Clin Pharmacol* 77(2):315–23.

Kranzler HR, Van Kirk J. (2001). Efficacy of naltrexone and acamprosate for alcoholism treatment: a meta-analysis. *Alcohol Clin Exp Res* 25:1335–41.

Mason B, Ownby R. (2000). Acamprosate for the treatment of alcohol dependence: a review of double-blind, placebo-controlled trials. *CNS Spectrums* 5(2):58–69.

Rösner S, Hackl-Herrwerth A, Leucht S, *et al*. (2011). Acamprosate for alcohol dependence. *Cochrane Database Syst Rev* 9:CD004332.

Disulfiram (tetraethythiuram disulphide)

Mechanism of action:

Disulfiram (Antabuse®) irreversibly inhibits aldehyde dehydrogenase, the enzyme that converts acetaldehyde to acetate, and leads to accumulation of acetaldehyde after drinking of alcohol. Acetaldehyde is a noxious compound and this unpleasant reaction acts as a psychological deterrent to drinking (aversive therapy). Inhibition of enzyme activity occurs within 12 hours and lasts more than 5 days.

The disulfiram-alcohol reaction includes flushing, headache, palpitations, dyspnoea, nausea, hypotension, prostration, and ECG changes. It varies in intensity between individuals and usually occurs within 10 minutes and peaks at 20–30 minutes, and lasts for 1–2 hours. The reaction can be caused even by small amounts of alcohol inadvertently taken in cough mixtures, sauces, or dressings of food, etc. The reaction is severe enough to have the individual bed-bound while it lasts, and sometimes hospitalization is required.

This form of aversive therapy is effective in motivated and reliable patients who are well supported and who participate in a comprehensive treatment programme, and where dosing of disulfiram is under close supervision. The patient must be able to understand and consent to the use of the medication and be able to remember what will happen if he or she drinks alcohol. Supervised daily dosing by a clinic, pharmacy or family member can play an important role in treatment.

Side effects: drowsiness, tiredness, confusion, peripheral neuropathy and rarely psychosis, optic neuritis, and hepatitis. Transient headache, impotence, acneform eruption, allergic dermatitis, gastric upset and metallic or garlic taste have also been reported during the first 2 weeks of therapy.

Contraindications: psychosis, ischaemic heart disease, severe renal or hepatic disease, and hypersensitivity to thiuram derivatives (pesticides; rubber); pregnancy, nursing mothers, cognitive impairment which impedes understanding of or recall of the medication's effect.

Drug interactions: metronidazole, isoniazid, phenytoin, long-acting benzodiazepines, anticoagulants.

Precautions: patients need to abstain from alcohol for at least 1 day before administration of disulfiram (or longer if the individual has consumed more than 24 'standard' drinks in the past day) and for at least 1 week after cessation of treatment.

Disulfiram is currently available as 200 mg tablets. Dose is initially 100 mg/day for 1–2 weeks increasing to 200 mg/day for 6 weeks to 6 months (maximum dose 300 mg, i.e. one and a half tablets). Duration of treatment is determined by its degree of success and patient preference. Some patients decide to stay on lifelong treatment.

While disulfiram implants have been trialled, to date sustained and consistent blood levels have not been achieved.

Occasionally a patient finds they can drink on disulfiram with few effects. If this occurs, the dose can be increased to 300 mg. If still not effective in deterring drinking, disulfiram should be ceased.

Baclofen

A GABA$_B$ receptor agonist used in the treatment of spasticity, baclofen may reduce craving and consumption in alcohol dependence. Baclofen appears to suppress alcohol-mediated dopamine release. Because of its limited hepatic metabolism, it is well tolerated in patients with liver disease.

Dose: given in three divided doses, intially 15–30 mg/day and increased in a stepwise way up to 150 mg daily.

Side effects: sedation, dizziness, headache, rash, urinary difficulties.

Precautions: Wean off baclofen gradually to avoid withdrawal syndrome (confusion, anxiety, seizures, delusions, hallucinations and delirium).

As baclofen is eliminated renally, use with caution in patients with renal disease.

Sodium oxybate

Sodium oxybate is the sodium salt of gamma-hydroxybutyrate (GHB). It stimulates GABA$_B$ receptors, mimicking the effect of alcohol. It is used in some countries for treatment of withdrawal and for relapse prevention in alcohol dependence.

Dose: 50 mg/kg/day; may be increased to 100 mg/kg/day in three divided doses.

Adverse effects: vertigo, drowsiness, toxicity in overdose.

Precautions: Because of risk of misuse, avoid in high risk patients (e.g. with psychiatric or addiction co-morbidity). Avoid in epilepsy.

Topiramate

This anticonvulsant has shown promise in decreasing alcohol intake, but side effects may be a barrier. It may reduce glutamatergic function and enhance GABA$_A$ receptor activity or modulate impulsivity.

Dose: titrate up to 150 mg twice daily, with a starting dose of 25 mg twice daily.

Side effects: sedation, unsteadiness, paraesthesia, headache, dizziness, depression, anxiety, cognitive impairment, glaucoma. Topiramate may lead to weight loss, which may be of advantage to some obese patients. It is contraindicated in pregnancy.

Pregabalin and gabapentin

The GABAergic drugs, pregabalin and gabapentin, have shown promise in alcohol dependence relapse prevention.

Others

Several medicines are under investigation, including those which target the stress response to alcohol dependence, such as CRF (corticotropin releasing factor) antagonists and α1-adrenergic antagonists (e.g. prazosin).

Ondansetron, a 5HT$_3$ antagonist and anti-emetic, may reduce alcohol consumption in early onset alcohol-dependent males with LL genotype serotonin transporter 5HTT.

Selective serotonin reuptake inhibitors (SSRIs) may assist in treatment of alcohol dependence with co-morbid depression. However, SSRI may worsen outcomes in early onset alcohol dependence, and have been reported to create new alcohol dependence so caution is needed.

Further reading

Franck J, Jayaram-Lindström N. (2013). Pharmacotherapy for alcohol dependence: status of current treatments. *Curr Opin Neurobiol* 23:692–9.

Law FD, Nutt DJ. (2012). Drugs used in the treatment of the addictions. In *New Oxford Textbook of Psychiatry* (2nd ed), pp. 7–10. Oxford: Oxford University Press.

Lingford-Hughes AR, Welch S, Peters L, *et al.* (2012). BAP updated guidelines: evidence-based guidelines for the pharmacological management of substance abuse, harmful use, addiction and comorbidity: recommendations from BAP. *J Psychopharmacol* 26:899–952.

Pani P, Trogu E, Pacini M, *et al.* (2015). Anticonvulsants for alcohol dependence. *Cochrane Database Syst Rev* 4:CD006754.

Table 9.11 A comparison of the clinical use of naltrexone, acamprosate, and disulfiram in treatment of alcohol dependence

	Naltrexone	Acamprosate	Disulfiram
Mechanism of action	Inhibits effects of endogenous opioids at mu receptor sites	Inhibits excitatory glutamates at NMDA receptor.	Inhibits aldehyde dehydrogenase
	Anti-craving agent: Useful for the 'reward drinker"	Anticraving agent—useful for the 'relief drinker"	Aversive therapy—as a deterrent to drinking
Mode of administration	50 mg once daily, can start on half dose for up to 1 week	Two tablets (333 mg each) every 8 hours with meals (omit lunchtime tablets if <60 kg body weight)	One tablet (200 mg) daily. May increase to maximum 400 mg daily—requires close supervision
When to commence	Generally recommend to wait until withdrawal complete	One week after the last drink (or when withdrawal complete)	At least one day after the last drink
Adverse effects	Nausea, diarrhoea, fatigue headache Hepatotoxicity (dose-related)	Diarrhoea Skin eruptions Mild sedation is occasionally reported	Alcohol/disulfiram interactions: avoid medicines containing alcohol; wait at least 2 weeks after ceasing disulfiram before drinking alcohol Complications at higher than recommended doses include: drowsiness psychotic reactions peripheral neuropathy, optic neuritis, hepatitis, impotence, dermatitis. Cardiovascular events in susceptible individuals

Table 9.11 (*Contd.*)

	Naltrexone	Acamprosate	Disulfiram
Contraindications	Acute hepatitis; advanced liver disease		Advanced liver disease
	Need for opioid analgesia (e.g. chronic pain)		Hypersensitivity to thiuram derivatives (rubber); severe myocardial disease/ischaemic heart disease, psychotic states
	Opioid dependence (may precipitate severe opioid withdrawals)		Drinking in the last 24 h: may precipitate a disulfiram-alcohol; interaction
	Advanced renal disease	Severe renal impairment	Renal disease
	Pregnancy	Pregnancy	Pregnancy
	Suicidality		
Precautions	Monitor liver function	Monitor renal function	Monitor liver function. If drinking continues check supervision. If drinking then persists, cease
Drug interactions	Opioid analgesics—blocked		Metronidazole
	Illicit opioids—precipitated withdrawal in opioid dependence		Isoniazid
			Phenytoin
			Anticoagulants

* Some drinkers consume alcohol primarily for the pleasurable effects—'reward drinkers'. Others drink primarily to relieve symptoms of protracted withdrawal, such as 'relief drinkers'. There is a spectrum of behaviour in between the two extremes, and considerable overlap.

Choosing and combining medications

There is currently only limited evidence on which medication to choose and when to combine them.

Naltrexone offers the considerable advantage of once-a-day dosing, although it may have gastrointestinal side effects. Naltrexone may also offer particular advantages for dependent drinkers who have less physiological withdrawal, including those who drink episodically or in binges, as it reduces the reward of drinking. It may be particularly beneficial in drinkers with a strong family history of AUD.

Acamprosate tends to have fewer gastrointestinal side effects, and can be used in those who need to take opioid analgesia. However, patient compliance with treatment may be a problem because of the three-times-a-day dosing. It may offer advantages for drinkers with higher levels of physiological dependence, and particularly those who have a persistent low-grade anxiety or insomnia after alcohol withdrawal.

A combination of acamprosate with naltrexone can be used, particularly in patients with severe dependence or where monotherapy has failed. Either or both of these can also be combined with disulfiram.

Pharmacotherapy should always be instituted as part of a comprehensive treatment programme including approaches to assist patient adherence to the medication regimen (see Psychosocial interventions, pp. 207–11).

There are not yet clear data on how long medication should be continued. As risk of relapse is greatest for the first 3 months, then gradually reduces over 12 months, most clinicians would suggest continuing for up to 12 months if there is suggestion of benefit. If the client reports significant benefit, or shows sustained good outcomes with few side effects, many clinicians would advise continuing the medication indefinitely. Further research is needed into any potential risks from long-term use of these medications.

Psychosocial interventions for alcohol use disorders

Psychosocial interventions are a key ingredient in the treatment for alcohol use disorders, with a good evidence base for effectiveness. Interventions range from simple brief advice for hazardous drinkers identified by screening in primary care, through to intensive psychosocial interventions delivered in residential rehabilitation settings for people with more severe alcohol dependence (severe AUD) and complex needs. There is therefore a need to tailor the nature and intensity of psychosocial interventions to the individual's presenting needs.

Context and setting

Psychosocial interventions are delivered in a variety of settings and contexts by a range of professionals. Brief interventions can be delivered in primary care by general practitioners, practice nurses, or counsellors with relatively minimal training (pp. 169–74). A stepped care approach may be helpful in this context, within which patients who do not initially respond to a brief intervention can be referred to a more experienced practitioner for more intensive intervention. For those with moderate or severe alcohol dependence, psychosocial interventions will often be delivered by a trained professional in a specialist alcohol treatment service or counselling agency.

For the drinker with alcohol dependence (severe AUD), psychosocial intervention may be part of a wider treatment programme which includes case management, medical interventions such as alcohol detoxification, and prescribing of relapse prevention medications (e.g. acamprosate, naltrexone, pp. 200–2).

Professionals delivering psychosocial interventions can include nurses, counsellors, psychologists, medical practitioners or occupational therapists. While a range of health and welfare practitioners will use elements of psychosocial interventions, formal counselling or other psychosocial interventions should be delivered by practitioners who have appropriate training and competence where available. Such professionals should also receive supervision from a more experienced therapist and be guided by an intervention manual.

Interventions are typically delivered in a community-based or outpatient setting, but can also be part of a residential programme of care such as residential rehabilitation or in prisons. Interventions can be delivered individually, in a group therapy context, or in the context of couples or family therapy. Increasingly psychosocial interventions are being delivered through books, DVDs, self-help manuals, Internet- or smartphone-based applications, achieving greater accessibility to the target population.

Care coordination and case management
The aim of both care coordination and case management is to ensure that patients receive the appropriate elements of care and interventions through regular clinical review. Case management is the more intensive approach which involves comprehensive assessment and regular monitoring of progress and risks, as well as ensuring that other professionals involved in the patient's care provide interventions in a timely and coordinated manner. Case management is an effective psychosocial intervention in its own right and is necessary to ensure effective delivery of a complex programme of care. This has been taken a step further by employing assertive outreach methods for patients with particularly complex needs and poor social circumstances who are difficult to engage.

Specific psychosocial interventions
A wide range of psychosocial approaches has been developed for treatment of alcohol use disorders. These are based on a range of underpinning psychological theories of the nature of the underlying condition being treated. Behavioural interventions are based on the principle that alcohol dependence is a learned behaviour which is amenable to behavioural modification. Cognitive interventions are more concerned with the role of thinking and cognition in the prevention of relapse. Social approaches focus more on interactions with the social environment such as social networks and social skills. Twelve-step approaches are based on the principles of Alcoholics Anonymous. Comprehensive reviews of the research on psychosocial interventions have concluded that while several psychosocial interventions are more effective than no intervention, there is little difference in effectiveness between active interventions.

Brief interventions
Brief interventions (pp. 169–74) have effectiveness in the context of opportunistic screening for unhealthy drinking, e.g. in primary healthcare settings. Patients with alcohol dependence generally require more intensive psychosocial interventions, although it should be noted that many achieve recovery without recourse to professional support.

Motivational enhancement therapy (MET)
This involves encouraging the patient to explore their drinking and the impact is has on their life to encourage self-change. There is often a discrepancy between a patient's desire to drink alcohol and the negative consequences it has on their health and social functioning. Motivational techniques include expressing empathy, developing discrepancy, avoiding arguments, rolling with resistance, and supporting self-efficacy. Motivational interviewing techniques can be used by the clinician as part of assessing and

engaging patients. A formal MET programme is usually conducted over four to six sessions.

Cognitive behaviour therapy and coping skills training

This approach focuses on the patient's thoughts and feelings in helping them to identify and cope more effectively with triggers (or high-risk situations) that can lead to relapse. This can include developing and rehearsing relapse prevention strategies, such as coping with craving or avoiding high-risk situations. In later stages of therapy, lifestyle changes are encouraged to develop positive alternatives to drinking and maintain abstinence. Formal CBT programmes typically involve delivery as a 12-session intervention over a 3-month period.

Cue exposure treatment

When alcohol-dependent patients who are trying to remain abstinent come into contact with cues, such as places where they used to drink or the sight of their favourite drink, this can precipitate an intense craving for alcohol. This in turn can trigger relapse. The main method of cue exposure is to expose the patient to alcohol cues in a safe environment, such as a hospital, with the aim of extinguishing the conditioned response to alcohol cues, and increase the patient's confidence in resisting the temptation to drink. It is at present more of an experimental than a mainstream therapeutic approach.

Contingency management

This is another behavioural approach which uses a system of incentives (usually small financial rewards) to reinforce abstinence or adherence to other psychosocial or pharmacological intervention. This has been shown to be effective in the substance misuse field but is only beginning to be employed in the alcohol treatment context with some evidence of positive effects.

Social network and community reinforcement interventions

People with alcohol dependence are often engaged in social networks which reinforce continued drinking and/or are isolated from positive social contact supporting abstinence. Social network therapy aims to enhance the patient's social networks to provide positive social support for abstinence. Community reinforcement is a similar approach which engages the patient's family, social, community, vocational, and leisure contacts to provide reinforcement to alter drinking behaviour. This includes elements of contingency management.

Self-help/mutual aid

Alcoholics Anonymous (AA) is a self-help movement in which people with alcohol dependence support each other to achieve recovery through mutual aid. Other organizations such as SMART Recovery® (i.e. self-management and recovery training; founded on the principles of CBT) have also been developed. While these organizations typically operate independently of the health and social care system, professionals have a role in helping people with alcohol dependence to engage with available local resources.

AA has operated internationally since the 1950s and is based on the 12 steps and 12 traditions of AA (see p. 627). There is a large number of active AA groups worldwide where it is possible to attend and obtain support at regular meetings. A 'sponsor' system allows those who have achieved more stable recovery to support others at an earlier stage in the process. In addition there are more specific AA groups catering for particular populations, e.g. women, young people, those with a particular sexual orientation, ethnicity or language. Similar support is available to families of people with alcohol dependence through AlAnon. It is helpful for professionals working in this field to attend and observe AA or SMART meetings to gain a better understanding of what is offered in order to inform patients of the potential benefits.

General principles

Several principles are important in the delivery of all psychosocial interventions.

- Confidentiality: therapists should respect the patient's right to confidentiality and conduct therapy in a private setting.
- Respect: therapists should respect the preferences of the patient and treat them in a non-judgemental manner.
- Communication and listening: therapists should check that they have understood the patient and the patient understands them by regular summary and feedback in the course of therapy.
- Empathy: therapists should have the capacity to recognize and respond to the emotions experienced by the patient.

Some therapists consistently achieve better outcomes than others. Important therapist factors include their level of training and skill in delivering the interventions, and their empathy and ability to form an effective 'therapeutic alliance' with the patient. Therapists working with patients who have more complex needs will require a higher level of training and competence.

Twelve-step facilitation (TSF)

Although AA helps many people, often patients disengage from AA at the end of a designated treatment period such as detoxification. TSF has been designed as a psychosocial intervention delivered by professional therapists to enhance engagement with AA, both within the designated treatment episode and into the longer-term aftercare phase.

Family interventions

Family interventions recognize both the impact of the individual's drinking on the family, and the potential of family members to support the individual's recovery. Family-based interventions take two forms. The first is involvement of the family directly in the patient's therapy, either in couples therapy, where both partners are present, or the whole family. Couples therapy depends on it being both safe and appropriate for the partner to be involved, bearing in mind the role of domestic violence. Family therapy is more commonly used in treating adolescents, and can be extended to the young person's wider social network in, e.g. multidimensional family therapy. The second area is the provision of therapy and support to the family members themselves. Often family members experience a wide range of psychological and social problems as a consequence of the alcohol-dependent patient's behaviour. In addition, families are often unclear about the best ways to help the affected family member. Both of these issues warrant interventions for family members in their own right.

Intensive day programmes

Where patients have more complex needs or lack social support, intensive day programmes, operating 5–7 days per week, can provide intensive psychosocial support in the community at a lower cost than residential rehabilitation. For most patients a community-based programme will be more cost-effective than a residential programme.

Children and young people

Special considerations are required for psychosocial interventions for this population. Greater harm is likely to be caused by heavy drinking in young people and they are more likely to experience psychiatric comorbidity and social problems than adults. A number of specific approaches have been developed for this group including multisystemic therapy, multidimensional family therapy, and brief strategic family therapy. All of these approaches have been developed to manage the wide range and complexity of problems experienced by heavy drinking adolescents, who often also misuse drugs. As a general principle it is important to closely involve families in the treatment of children and adolescents as part of the treatment programme, and there should be a lower threshold for both more intensive interventions and residential programmes in this group (see pp. 494–5 for further detail on management of children and adolescents).

Further reading

Miller WR, Wilbourne PL. (2002). Mesa Grande: a methodological analysis of clinical trials of treatments for alcohol use disorders. *Addiction* 97:265–77.

NICE (2011). *Alcohol Use Disorders: Diagnosis, Assessment and Management of Harmful Drinking and Alcohol Dependence*. Clinical Guideline 115. London: NICE.

Residential or in-patient treatment (excluding detoxification)

This treatment approach provides a safe and supportive environment for patients with complex needs and who lack social support in the community to receive psychosocial interventions. Also, patients with severe alcohol dependence who have repeatedly relapsed despite comprehensive out-patient treatment/rehabilitation, may require a more intensive in-patient residential treatment programme, lasting several weeks or months (see Box 9.6).

Box 9.6 Suggested criteria for residential treatment

- Completion of comprehensive assessment and diagnosis
- Failure to respond to out-patient treatment or unable to comply with this treatment
- Lack of social support including homelessness, unstable living environment, surrounded by other heavy drinkers
- Co-morbid psychiatric or medical complications, or malnutrition
- Rural domicile with no out-patient services
- Severe life crises
- Coexisting severe drug dependence.

Residential treatment programmes address the same issues and many use a similar range of treatment approaches to community-based treatment programmes, including pharmacotherapies, psychological therapies, psychosocial interventions, and self-help, 12-step, or other therapeutic approaches. There remain some centres that have kept their traditional focus almost exclusively on 12-step facilitation and fellowship.

In addition to providing food and shelter and some 'time out' in a safer environment, residential treatment programmes provide a structured daily routine, staff-directed programmes, and daily activities.

For most patients, residential rehabilitation achieves an equivalent outcome to similarly intensive community-based programmes, while at the same time being considerably more costly. Accordingly, it has been recommended that residential programmes be reserved for people who lack social support, including those who are homeless, who live in rural areas, those in crisis, or who have physical or psychiatric disorders, where attendance at an intensive community programme would be impractical or inappropriate.

Some rehabilitation centres will accept self-referred clients or referrals from primary care, and in some regions phone services are available to advise on the location of appropriate treatment services. Other residential rehabilitation services only accept referrals from specialist out-patient or inpatient alcohol treatment services.

Individuals with impaired cognitive function and a record of disruptive behaviour, e.g. through severe personality disorder or poorly controlled schizophrenia, may be particularly in need of residential treatment facilities, however not all centres are able to accept such individuals. Also, persons with significant medical disorders, such as advanced cirrhosis, may pose challenges in finding a suitable location for treatment.

Drinkers with major psychiatric or medical problems or with alcohol-related brain damage who are unable to look after themselves may require longer-term care either in residential facilities or in a nursing home (also see Guardianship, p. 587).

Continuing care

Alcohol dependence, once it requires clinical care, typically behaves as a chronic relapsing condition. It responds to persistent and consistent treatment, which is delivered with understanding and enthusiasm. It is inappropriate to consider treatment as consisting only of intensive 2–3-week periods of hospital (residential) therapy, without attention to the future. The relationship between the treatment service and the patient needs to be maintained over the long term.

Alcohol-dependent patients should be advised that if they drink, this typically leads to loss of control and return to heavy drinking (reinstatement), often with a progressive downhill course. Accordingly, the clear goal of treatment should be abstinence from alcohol. The patient should be encouraged to return early for assistance if relapse occurs.

Aftercare is essential. The nature of the continuing care will vary widely from person to person. It may consist of:
• pharmacotherapy, using, e.g. naltrexone or acamprosate for 3 months to 2 years, and regular follow-up with a medical practitioner, often in conjunction with a psychologist or other clinical colleague

- regular participation in individual or group counselling, e.g. at a specialist alcohol treatment agency, which may initially be on a weekly basis
- participation in mutual support groups such as AA, or in other community-based group-based therapeutic approaches such as the CBT-based Smart Recovery®
- regular follow-up by the patient's general medical practitioner, primary care nurse, psychologist, or counsellor
- regular follow-up by a medical or other specialist on alcohol treatment.

Good communication between the patient's general practitioner and specialist alcohol treatment team assists with providing quality care.

Complications of unhealthy alcohol use: their assessment and management

The complications of drinking may result from acute intoxication or chronic excessive drinking. Alcohol affects almost every system of the body and the risk of chronic alcohol-related organ damage increases with increasing levels of alcohol intake and with duration of drinking, particularly when drinking has continued for 5 years or more. Alcohol also causes and exacerbates a range of mental health conditions.

Acute complications

Acute complications of alcohol consumption may be medical, neuropsychiatric, or social.

Medical

- Coma and respiratory depression: alcohol intoxication is a potentially lethal condition because of the risk of respiratory depression in non-tolerant drinkers. Many young people in particular present to the ED with an acute 'overdose' of alcohol or 'alcohol poisoning' (for management see pp. 184–5).
- Drug overdose (accidental or suicidal): the risk of respiratory depression is increased if alcohol and other CNS depressants such as benzodiazepines or opioids are taken at the same time. Aspiration pneumonia may complicate severe intoxication.
- Trauma: intoxication predisposes to accidents particularly in episodic heavy drinkers, e.g. motor vehicle accidents, acts of violence, falls, and fractures (ribs/long bones); subdural haematoma may occur after head injury. In some countries there may be a medico-legal requirement to measure a blood alcohol level in people involved in a motor vehicle accident who are presenting for treatment. For example, in Australia all drivers in motor vehicle accidents who present to hospital must have a specially collected blood sample sent for forensic testing (see Drink driving, pp. 564–5).
- Burns.
- Drowning.
- Sexual risk-taking, and consequent risk of HIV and other STIs and unwanted pregnancy.
- Upper gastrointestinal bleeding from gastritis, oesophagitis, Mallory–Weiss tear or when alcohol is taken in conjunction with NSAIDs.
- Acute pancreatitis (p. 220).
- Atrial fibrillation may be induced by an acute excessive consumption of alcohol during an acute alcoholic binge in an otherwise healthy heart—the 'holiday heart' syndrome. Alcohol is a common cause of atrial fibrillation in people under the age of 65 who are otherwise healthy.

Neuropsychiatric

- Alcohol intoxication.
- Amnesic episodes (alcohol-induced blackouts; memory blackouts):
  - A period of anterograde amnesia during heavy drinking. These occur when a high blood alcohol interferes with the acquisition and storage

of new memories (i.e. the person cannot remember what they did after the onset of intoxication)

- The person may appear intoxicated, but there are no observable cognitive abnormalities; they may find him/herself in unknown surroundings on recovery
- Realization of amnesic episode occurs on recovery.
- Subdural haematoma: secondary to head injury, particularly if there is coexisting thrombocytopenia. May be overlooked if the patient is intoxicated.
- Confusion and disorientation occur at a BAC of around 0.15 g/100 mL in healthy, non-tolerant drinkers, but can occur at relatively low BACs in vulnerable individuals, such as the elderly. (See p. 96 for differential diagnosis.)
- Strokes: excess alcohol, especially episodic heavy drinking or binge drinking, is a risk factor for haemorrhagic strokes.
- Acute nerve pressure palsies, especially of the brachial plexus ('Saturday night palsy').
- Suicide attempts: because of its disinhibiting effect, and its effect on mood (depression), alcohol is commonly associated with suicide attempts.

Social

Acute intoxication can cause a range of social problems often arising from disinhibited behaviour or from short-term neglect of alternative responsibilities. Alcohol intoxication may trigger other substance use or gambling, or may impair judgement as to when to stop. Gambling losses in turn may trigger drinking.

Chronic complications

Complications of longer term, unhealthy alcohol use may also be classified as medical, psychiatric, and social. Here we provide an overview, together with an account of the laboratory investigations typically undertaken as part of the assessment (Table 9.12). Further details of the clinical features and management are provided in pp. 221–3 and pp. 224–7.

Alcohol-related liver disease

Alcohol-related fatty liver:

- Often asymptomatic; may present with right hypochondrial or mid-abdominal discomfort
- When uncomplicated, liver tests may be normal or there may be isolated GGT elevation (Table 9.8)
- Abstinence over a period of 2–3 months should lead to normalization of liver function tests.

Alcoholic hepatitis:

- May be asymptomatic or present with jaundice and/or abdominal pain.
- Elevations of GGT and AST and ALT, with AST/ALT ratio of >2, and ALT and AST levels usually no more than 250 U/L
- Albumin may be low and bilirubin raised.

Table 9.12 Laboratory tests used in assessing suspected complications of unhealthy drinking

Investigations	Results	Interpretation and comments
FBC	Low Hb	Anaemia, e.g. nutritional, due to gastrointestinal blood loss, haemolysis in cirrhosis, or bone marrow suppression.
	Macrocytosis	Heavy drinkers. MCV. Most commonly moderately elevated MCV. Reflects alcohol toxicity on erythrocyte precursors.
		Less commonly, associated with B_{12} or folate deficiency, reticulocytosis or chronic liver disease
		Anticonvulsants may cause slight increase
	Microcytosis	Iron deficiency secondary to overt or silent GI blood loss
	Red cell abnormalities	Spur cells or other red cell abnormalities in advancing liver disease
	Raised WCC (leucocytosis) Reduced WCC (leucopenia)	Infections secondary to poor self-care or reduced T cell function, lung infections secondary to smoking
		Pancytopenia in advanced liver disease
	Reduced platelets (thrombocytopenia)	Falling platelets may be a warning sign of advancing cirrhosis with or without hypersplenism; liver is a source of thrombopoietin; in advanced liver disease there may be pancytopenia.
		Toxic effect of alcohol on megakaryocytes
Electrolyte, urea creatinine	Hyponatraemia; hypokalaemia	Dilution; suppression of antidiuretic hormone
		Urinary potassium loss and loss of muscle bulk
Minerals	Reduced magnesium	Alcohol impairs absorption and increases urinary excretion
		Low Mg may lower seizure threshold or result in failure to respond to thiamine in WE/WKS
	Zinc deficiency	
Blood sugar	Raised	Reversible insulin resistance with repeated heavy drinking
		Diabetes as a consequence of pancreatic damage
	Low	Consumption of alcohol on an empty stomach

Table 9.12 (Contd.)

Investigations	Results	Interpretation and comments
LFTs	Elevated GGT	Heavy drinking; liver disease; diabetes; pancreatitis; anticonvulsants (phenytoin)
	AST and ALT	AST/ALT ratio of >2 is indicative of alcohol as a cause of the liver disease, rather than immune or viral hepatitis
		Where ALT elevation predominates, consider hepatitis B or C as a possible coexisting diagnosis
		In uncomplicated alcoholic hepatitis, levels are usually 100–300 U/L
		Where ALT or AST exceeds 300 U/L consider other causes of liver disease
	ALP elevated	Suggests chronic fibrotic liver disease or tumour
	Albumin reduced	Reduced synthetic function, or dilution in fluid overload/ascites
INR APTT	Raised Raised	Reduced production of clotting factors in advancing cirrhosis
Serology for viral hepatitis		In assessing differential diagnosis and/or additive factors in cirrhosis, particularly if there is a past history of injecting drug use (hepatitis C), or patient born in a country with high prevalence of hepatitis B
Alpha fetoprotein	Raised	Elevated in some cases of hepatocellular carcinoma, as a complication of cirrhosis
Serum B_{12}/folate	Low serum folate	Reduced absorption of folate, nutritional deficiency. Causes macrocytosis.
	Low serum B_{12}	Nutritional deficiency, reduced absorption. Causes macrocytosis
Serum amylase/lipase	Elevated	Acute pancreatitis.
CPK	Raised	Traumatic muscle necrosis, acute myopathy or acute rhabdomyolysis — especially if recent coma
		Increased risk of acute kidney injury
Beta hydroxybutyric acid; lactic acid	Raised	In alcoholic ketoacidosis there is elevated beta hydroxybutyric acid and lactic acid, and a large anion gap. Blood sugar is often low or low normal, but may be slightly elevated
Urine drug screens		May help detect other drug use, especially in a person with altered consciousness. Results may not be available for hours or days

Alcoholic cirrhosis:
- In the majority of cases presents with features of hepatic decompensation, but may be asymtomatic.
- As hepatic synthetic function falls, albumin may fall and bilirubin rise, while the INR (or prothrombin time) becomes prolonged
- Falling platelets may be a warning sign of worsening liver damage
- In advanced liver disease there may be pancytopenia.

Liver cell cancer:
- Complicates 15% of cases of cirrhosis
- Elevations in ALP and GGT are expected
- α-fetoprotein will become elevated in a proportion of cases
- In patients with cirrhosis, monitor with α-fetoprotein and abdominal ultrasound twice yearly.

Table 9.13 Other investigations for assessing complications of unhealthy alcohol use

Investigation	Finding	Interpretation/comment
Abdominal (liver spleen) ultrasound	Altered texture or organ size	Can give an indication of the presence of cirrhosis (irregular texture, altered size) and secondary splenomegaly. Fatty liver and cirrhosis give rise to increased echotexture but ultrasound cannot definitively diagnose cirrhosis. A screen for hepatocellular carcinoma
Fibroscan	Increased liver rigidity with cirrhosis	Can help gauge the severity of cirrhosis
Abdominal CT	Altered texture or organ size	Evidence of abnormal or changing liver size and texture or secondary splenomegaly. Evidence of hepatocellular carcinoma
Liver biopsy*	Nature of liver disease	Not routinely indicated. If diagnosis is uncertain or to stage the severity of liver disease
Endoscopy	Varices, reflux, gastritis, oesophagitis	All newly diagnosed cirrhotic patients should have an endoscopy to determine if varices are present, to allow prophylactic therapy to reduce risk of bleeding
Abdominal X-ray	Calcification in the pancreas	Chronic pancreatitis

(Continued)

Table 9.13 (Contd.)

Investigation	Finding	Interpretation/comment
Chest X-ray	Pneumonia, TB	Aspiration pneumonia following heavy intoxication; lobar pneumonia secondary to smoking; increased risk of TB in alcohol dependence (decreased T-cell function, poor living conditions) If a chronic heavy smoker (e.g. lung hyperinflation on chest X-ray) be cautious in use of benzodiazepines in alcohol withdrawal
	Cardiomegaly, pulmonary oedema	Cardiomyopathy.
Oximeter readings, blood gases	Chronic airways limitation, hypoxia, respiratory acidosis	If a chronic heavy smoker with coexisting chronic airways obstruction /pneumonia. Look for hypoxia, particularly in the confused or sedated patient, or where benzodiazepines are to be administered
ECG	Atrial fibrillation	Alcohol-induced atrial fibrillation secondary to acute intoxication or to cardiomyopathy
Cardiac echo	Four-chamber dilatation and hypokinesis with low ejection fraction	Cardiomyopathy
Brain CT	Space-occupying lesion; atrophy	Important to detect possible subdural in a person with decreased level of consciousness; differential diagnosis of first withdrawal seizure or atypical seizure; assessment of reducing level of cognitive function
MRI	Ventricular enlargement, widespread cortical atrophy and a thinner corpus callosum	Can be useful in differential diagnosis of reducing level of cognitive function
EEG		To help differentiate epilepsy from alcohol withdrawal seizure; rarely status epilepticus can cause a persistent and fluctuating delirium

* Where there is no suspicion of a cause of liver disease other than alcohol, liver biopsy is rarely required. Biopsy can assist with differential diagnosis or establishing the relative impact of coexisting causes of liver disease, and when there is lack of improvement of LFTs, despite documented abstinence from alcohol.

Acute pancreatitis
- Acute pancreatitis, when severe, is a medical emergency.
- Investigations for suspected acute pancreatitis should include serum amylase and lipase levels, electrolytes, plain X-ray of the abdomen, chest X-ray, and abdominal ultrasound.
- CT abdomen and blood gases are usually undertaken subsequently.

Chronic pancreatitis
- Usually presents with abdominal pain or pancreatic insufficiency
- Stool tests for faecal fats (steatorrhoea)
- Plain X-ray abdomen (pancreatic calcification)
- Abdominal ultrasound
- CT abdomen
- Refer to gastroenterologist; may require endoscopic retrograde cholangiopancreatography (ERCP) or surgery.

Alcohol-related brain damage

Harmful alcohol consumption and dependence are associated with morphological changes in the brain. Structural imaging studies (CT, MRI) have shown reductions in grey and white matter volume, especially in the frontal lobes. These effects may be mediated by repeated intoxication and withdrawal. They are more pronounced in the ageing brain and in women, and are partially reversible with abstinence, particularly in younger individuals. The mechanisms underlying reversibility are not fully understood. Disruption of white matter tracts has also been reported, particularly in the frontal and temporal regions, and may be caused by excessive extracellular and intracellular fluid accumulation. Again, the ageing and female alcoholic brains appear to be more susceptible to these changes

An MRI brain scan of an alcohol-dependent subject, compared with a scan of an age-matched healthy control, will typically show evidence of ventricular enlargement, cortical atrophy, and a thinner corpus callosum (Fig. 9.4).

Functional imaging

Functional neuroimaging studies show that alcohol affects brain function. Alcohol dependent patients show more activity in response to alcohol-associated cues in parts of the mesocorticolimbic dopamine system than do healthy controls. Light drinkers show more activation in the ventral striatum whereas, in heavy drinkers, activation is more prominent in the dorsal striatum reflecting a 'switch' to more compulsive drinking. Cue-exposure interventions have been shown to alter fMRI cue-reactivity in alcohol dependent patients, suggesting that neuro-imaging may have role in monitoring the effects of both psychological and pharmacological treatments.

PET and SPECT studies have reported lower glucose metabolism in cortical and subcortical regions of the alcoholic brain compared with controls.

Control Man (31 years old)   Alcoholic Man (33 years old)

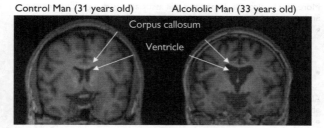

Fig. 9.4 Structural brain damage in an alcohol-dependent patient compared to an age-matched healthy control.

Reproduced from *Alcoholism: Clinical and Experimental Research*, 35(10), Bühler M and Mann K, Alcohol and the Human Brain: A Systematic Review of Different Neuroimaging Method, pp. 1771–1793, Copyright (2011), with permission from John Wiley and Sons.

Further reading

Bühler M, Mann K. (2011). Alcohol and the human brain: a systematic review of different neuro-imaging methods. *Alcohol Clin Exp Res* 10:1771–93.

Management of medical and neuropsychiatric complications of chronic unhealthy alcohol use

Alcohol-related organ damage is often multifactorial in aetiology and clinicians and patients must deal with all issues to ensure recovery occurs. These factors include nutritional, immunological and vascular processes. The basis for the treatment of all alcohol related medical conditions still remains abstinence from alcohol, without which all other therapeutic interventions will fail.

Every relevant support must be provided to patients advised to significantly reduce or abstain from alcohol. These include counselling, medical monitoring, and the use of pharmacotherapies pp. 200–13.

Alcohol-related liver disease

For every type of alcohol-related liver disease, abstinence is the basis for any management strategy. Unless alcohol intake is ceased, liver disease will progress in most patients.

Alcoholic fatty liver is almost always benign in itself and often asymptomatic. It resolves after 2–3 months abstinence from alcohol.

Alcohol-induced hepatitis: elevation of ALT and AST indicates a degree of hepatocyte necrosis and thus alcohol related hepatitis.

- In a majority of patients this is a mild process. It is underdiagnosed and abstinence leads to improved hepatic function.
- Liver enzymes should be monitored regularly to confirm that abstinence over a period of 3–6 months has led to normalization of liver function tests.

More severe alcoholic hepatitis is still associated with significant morbidity and mortality.

- Severity should be assessed using the Maddrey discriminant function (MDF) or MELD score.
  - If MDF is >32, steroids and or pentoxyphylline should be used as they have proven benefit in this condition.
- Consultation with a gastroenterologist or other physician is indicated, and in some cases intensive care is required.

Alcoholic cirrhosis: the management of alcoholic cirrhosis commences with abstinence from alcohol.

- All efforts should be made including the use of pharmacotherapies such as baclofen and in some cases, disulfiram.
- Active management of the complications of cirrhosis reduces risk of death while the liver inflammation and function improve.

Active treatment includes:

- Ensuring an adequate dietary input, including encouraging evening protein intake.
- Prophylactic beta blockade or nitrate administration and/or variceal banding in those with portal hypertension to minimize risk of variceal haemorrhage.
- Ascites is managed by salt restriction, fluid restriction, as appropriate and diuretic therapy used carefully to avoid intravascular volume depletion and the risk of hepatorenal syndrome. Repeated paracenteses may be required.
- Portal systemic encephalopathy responds well to lactulose; rifaximin is now increasingly available with documented benefit where lactulose is not tolerated.
- The use of albumin to correct hypoalbuminaemia is increasingly being addressed as this may reduce risks of infection, hepatorenal syndrome and ascites.
- Patients with cirrhosis should be monitored twice yearly with AFP and abdominal ultrasound screening for hepatocellular carcinoma.

Management of other liver disease, complicated by alcohol use

All liver diseases are aggravated by the use of alcohol. Injecting drug users are at markedly increased risk of contracting hepatitis C, B, and D, and they are also at risk of direct drug-related toxicity. Alcohol consumed at hazardous levels will increase the rate of progression of liver disease in patients with hepatitis C and B by altering viral replication, influencing immune function and causing direct hepatic injury. Patients should be warned of these potential additive harmful effects and advised to reduce or cease alcohol use. Monitoring the effects of alcohol ingestion on LFTs is an excellent way of determining with patients how much they can safely drink.

Other gastrointestinal

Acute and chronic pancreatitis are well recognized in alcohol-dependent patients. Abstinence from alcohol is the key management approach once the acute problem has resolved.

Acute pancreatitis is best managed in a surgical or medical unit used to dealing with this condition as new approaches are regularly being trialled. Pain in acute pancreatitis may require high doses of opioids for a short period but patients should not be discharged with PRN opioids as this raises risk of longer-term opioid dependence. As morphine may cause spasm of the sphincter of Oddi, pethidine or other narcotic agents are preferable.

Chronic pancreatitis also requires input from specialist units. This condition is associated with a high rate of opioid dependence, so avoid these agents for long-term use. Regularly evaluate for evidence of complications and treat pancreatic insufficiency and diabetes as relevant.

Cardiovascular disease

Alcohol-related hypertension: alcohol is a common cause of (or contributor to) hypertension. Hypertension responds less well to antihypertensive agents if the patient continues to drink excessively and generally improves with abstinence or when alcohol is markedly reduced.

Alcoholic cardiomyopathy: requires a broad approach to management, which is best supervised by a cardiologist. Abstinence from alcohol is key, as with continued heavy drinking 80% die within 3 years. Medical management will require the use of agents directed at improving cardiac function, controlling arrhythmias, anticoagulation and relieving fluid overload. Thiamine 200 mg daily is recommended and ensuring normal levels of Mg, Zn, Se is also important.

Diabetes complicated by alcohol misuse

Diabetic patients should exercise caution when drinking, particularly those on insulin (regular heavy drinking reversibly increases insulin resistance) and oral hypoglycaemic agents (risk of hypoglycaemia) and biguanides (risk of lactic acidosis). Patients on sulfonylureas may experience unpleasant disulfiram-like reactions when they drink alcohol.

Haematological disorders

- Anaemia of chronic infection : treat cause, e.g. tuberculosis
- Microcytic anaemia: treat cause of bleeding, e.g. gastritis, oesophageal varices, coagulopathy in severe liver disease
- Macrocytic (megaloblastic) anaemia: cease excess alcohol. Ensure nutritious diet; B_{12} or folate supplementation
- Leucopenia: due to immunosuppression; portal hypertension/ hypersplenism
- Leucocytosis: treat concurrent infections
- Thrombocytopenia: due to cirrhosis/hypersplenism and toxic effect on bone marrow.

Rhabdomyolysis and myoglobinuria

From 'long lie' associated with heavy intoxication. Management includes:
- rehydration
- renal dialysis where appropriate.

Malignancies

Alcohol use increases the risk of developing a number of malignancies.

Neuropsychiatric complications

Wernicke's encephalopathy

Wernicke's encephalopathy is an acute reversible neuropsychiatric condition which occurs as a result of thiamine deficiency. It occurs mainly but not exclusively in individuals with alcohol use disorders who are malnourished and in those with malabsorption or repeated vomiting and diarrhoea.

Thiamine is an essential co-factor for many enzymes in the glycolytic and pentose phosphate pathways, and thiamine deficiency is due to low thiamine intake, impaired thiamine absorption, or impaired thiamine utilization.

Wernicke's encephalopathy can present during the course of alcohol withdrawal or DTs, or while the individual is still drinking. It is characterized by one or more symptoms/signs from the classical triad:
- Oculomotor abnormalities:
  - Nystagmus
  - Ophthalmoplegia: paralysis or weakness, most commonly affecting lateral or upward gaze, often with diplopia (i.e. effects on external recti, e.g. sixth nerve palsy)
- Cerebellar dysfunction (ataxia)
- Confusion of recent onset (disorientation, inattention, poor responsiveness).

However, the full triad of symptoms is seen in only 16–20% of cases and the diagnosis is often missed. Patients with Wernicke's encephalopathy may present with nausea, vomiting and confusion, and rarely, hypothermia, hypotension, and coma.

Autopsy studies show that Wernicke's pathology is 20 times more common than the classical triad, and is seen in 12.5% of people who misuse alcohol and in 0.4–2.8% of the general population.

Wernicke's encephalopathy is difficult to differentiate from, and often coexists with, other causes of confusion/delirium (pp. 95–7). It is therefore commonly underdiagnosed, untreated, or inadequately treated.

Wernicke's encephalopathy constitutes a medical emergency with an estimated mortality of 10–20% if untreated. It is easily reversible with the timely administration of adequate doses of parenteral thiamine.

Most patients who do not recover promptly within the first 48–72 hours develop Korsakoff's syndrome with irreversible memory loss (pp. 226–7).

There should be a high index of suspicion of Wernicke's encephalopathy/Wernicke Korsakoff syndrome (WE/KS) in patients with alcohol use disorders. Consider a diagnosis of Wernicke's encephalopathy in any confused patient with an alcohol use disorder until proven otherwise.

Investigations for Wernicke's encephalopathy

Where Wernicke's encephalopathy is clinically suspected, treatment with high-dose intravenous thiamine should commence before any investigations are carried out.

Treatment is generally safe and inexpensive and the consequences of delaying treatment can be lifelong disability.
- FBC, urea and electrolytes, LFTs, coags, thyroid function tests, blood glucose levels, serum.
- Magnesium, B_{12}, folate and other tests as required to differentiate from other causes of delirium (p. 95, pp. 95–7, p. 96).

- While low blood thiamine or thiamine pyrophosphate levels and low erythrocyte transketolase activity (ETKA) support the diagnosis of WE/WKS, these are typically not done because it is important not to delay treatment while awaiting the results.
- A normal CT brain does not rule out the diagnosis of WE. A brain MRI supports the diagnosis by showing structural changes in the brain in the area of the hippocampus, mammillary bodies, mammillothalamic tract and thalamus.

Management of suspected or established Wernicke's encephalopathy
NB: Wernicke's encephalopathy is a medical emergency.

In a hospital setting, always treat with intravenous thiamine. Parenteral administration is needed as alcohol interferes with thiamine absorption. In addition there are often medical complications of drinking, e.g. gastritis, vomiting, which may impair absorption. As little as 5% of an oral dose of thiamine may be absorbed in alcohol dependence. If intravenous thiamine is not possible, as a temporary measure use intramuscular thiamine.

In addition, oral multivitamin preparations should be given daily.

There is not clear evidence on the optimal dose of thiamine and no universally accepted guidelines.

Guidelines for the treatment of patients with suspected or established Wernicke's encephalopathy
- At least 500 mg thiamine IV (or IM), three times daily, for 5 days:
  - In the UK this is given as at least two pairs of ampoules (i.e. 4 ampoules) of high-potency B-complex vitamins IV (Pabrinex®)
  - Administer IV thiamine (e.g. Pabrinex®) in 100 mL normal saline over 30 minutes.
- If no response to therapy is observed after this time, discontinue.
- If a response is observed, continue with 250–300 mg thiamine (e.g. one pair of Pabrinex® ampoules) daily for another 5 days, or longer if improvement continues.
- Follow with oral thiamine and multivitamin supplementation thereafter and as an out-patient.
NB: for patients with enduring ataxia, polyneuritis or memory disturbance, high-potency vitamins should be given for as long as improvement continues

---

Precautions in treating Wernicke's encephalopathy
There is a small risk of anaphylaxis with intravenous thiamine, therefore, slow intravenous administration in 100 mL normal saline over 30 minutes is recommended. There should be ready access to appropriate resuscitation measures. IM thiamine preparations have a lower incidence of anaphylactic reactions than IV preparations, at 1 per 5 million pairs of ampoules of Pabrinex®, which is far lower than many frequently used drugs that carry no special warning.

It is imperative that parenteral thiamine is given before a dextrose drip, as a carbohydrate load has the potential to precipitate or exacerbate Wernicke's encephalopathy.

- Ensure that the patient is kept well hydrated and that any electrolyte imbalance is corrected.
- Ensure that serum magnesium levels are normal because magnesium is an essential co-factor in many thiamine dependent enzyme systems and low magnesium levels may result in failure to respond to thiamine therapy.
- Exclude, and treat, any other cause of confusion/delirium (Table 6.1 and pp. 95–7) which may coexist with WE/WKS.

Other harmful effects of alcohol on the central nervous system
Chronic alcohol-related brain damage

- *Korsakoff's syndrome* (persistent alcohol-induced amnestic confabulatory neurocognitive disorder): this is a sequel to untreated or inadequately treated Wernicke's encephalopathy. An estimated 20% of individuals with KS will require long-term institutionalized care
  - Clinical features: it is a largely irreversible condition characterized by short-term memory loss, severe difficulty learning new information with rapid forgetting, and compensatory confabulation. Cued recall is better than spontaneous recall. Long-term memory is typically preserved. Korsakoff syndrome is difficult to differentiate from other causes of dementia and; in some individuals features of Korsakoff's overlap with cortical pathology (with cortical atrophy and ventricular dilation, especially involving the frontal lobes.
  - Symptoms of Wernicke's encephalopathy may be mixed with those of Korsakoff's syndrome as a result of repeated episodes of clinical or sub clinical thiamine deficiency (Wernicke Korsakoff syndrome).
- *Frontal lobe syndrome*: cognitive deterioration following years of heavy drinking, which may be heavy episodic drinking. It is characterized by disinhibition, defective conceptualization and abstract thinking, impaired organization and strategic planning, concreteness of thought, poor appreciation of social cues, personality change and, in advanced cases perseveration and long tract signs. Imaging shows cerebrocortical degeneration and cortical atrophy (see p. 221). It is important to define type of brain damage and exclude other treatable causes. There may be slight regeneration with abstinence, but most changes are irreversible.
- *Cerebellar degeneration*: occurs after more than 10 years of excessive drinking and typically affects the vermis leading to truncal ataxia, unsteadiness and gait disturbances, dysarthria, uncoordinated movements, blurred vision and frequent falls. It is usually found in association with other cerebral injury but in some patients ataxia predominates. Treatment involves abstinence, thiamine, nutritional supplementation, and walking aids
- *Marchiafava–Bignami syndrome*: a rare disorder which involves demyelination of the central part of the corpus callosum and adjacent subcortical white matter and has a poor prognosis. As it is generally seen in malnourished alcohol-dependent persons, abstinence and nutritional supplementation is recommended. It should be managed in a specialist neurological setting.

- *Central pontine myelinolysis:* a rare demyelinating disease of the pons seen in alcohol-dependent patients following rapid correction of hyponatraemia. Patients present with quadriplegia and pseudobulbar palsy.

Management of chronic alcohol-related brain damage

Ensure any reversible factors are treated. For treatment of Wernicke's syndrome, see pp. 225–6.

The degree of brain damage can be assessed by referring to a neuropsychologist. Patients with marked alcohol-related brain damage (or those with coexisting severe psychiatric or medical problems) may be unable to care for themselves and require long-term care or supervision or placement in a residential unit, nursing home, or dementia unit. In milder cases, support either at home or in a community location by community health services is possible. Provision of information and support to carers is important.

Abstinence from alcohol is important to preserve residual cognitive function, but can be challenging to achieve. Abstinence will arrest the progression of alcohol-related brain damage and may lead to gradual improvement in some neuropsychiatric functions and brain scan results.

Ensuring adequate nutrition and supplementing this with thiamine 100 mg daily is recommended plus multivitamins orally daily. Where facilities are available, memory retraining in an appropriate environment and familiar surroundings can be attempted, though the degree of recovery is likely to be small. Memory retraining techniques—resource books for carers, memory books, memory joggers—can be used. A structured environment with lifelong support or supervision may be required.

It can be very challenging to find a satisfactory placement for these individuals. Assistance from the social work team, specialist addiction services, or psychiatric, geriatric, and neurology teams may be valuable.

In some cases legal provisions may need to be invoked to assist with controlling finances (see pp. 586–7).

Other neurological complications

Peripheral neuropathy: with glove and stocking tingling and numbness, sensory impairment and absent ankle jerks. Hypersensitivity of soles of feet may be an early sign.

Abstinence and thiamine plus management of the patient with significant sensory loss are critical. Some recovery may occur with abstinence for over a year.

Further reading

Best Practice BMJ Evidence Centre (2001). *Wernicke's Encephalopathy.* BMJ Publishing Group 2001. Available at: http://best practice.bmj.com acs.hen.com/best practice monograph/405

Caine R, Brathen G, Ivashynka A, *et al.* (1997). EFNS guidelines for diagnosis, therapy and prevention of Wernicke's encephalopathy. *Eur J Neurol* 17:1408–18.

Sechi GP, Serra A. (2007). Wernicke's encephalopathy – new clinical settings and recent advances in diagnosis and treatment. *Lancet Neurol* 6:442–55.

Thomson AD, Cook CCH, Touquet R, *et al.* (2002). The Royal College of Physicians report on alcohol: guidelines for managing Wernicke's encephalopathy in the accident and emergency department. *Alcohol Alcohol* 39(6):513–21.

Thomson AD, Marshall EJ, Bell D. (2013). Time to act on the management of Wernicke's encephalopathy in the UK. *Alcohol Alcohol* 48:4–8.

Fetal alcohol spectrum disorders

There remains a tragic reality in many communities of mothers delivering more than one child affected by this disorder, the most common preventable form of brain injury in infants (see pp. 514–17). Every effort needs to be made to educate the profession and the public about this condition. Affected children and families may need considerable support.

Psychiatric complications of alcohol misuse

Alcoholic hallucinosis and alcoholic paranoia

Both disorders can develop during a drinking bout, can begin during alcohol withdrawal or can occur within several weeks of the cessation of drinking. They occur in a state of clear consciousness (i.e. the patient is not delirious). These disorders are likely to completely resolve, within a few days or several weeks if alcohol is discontinued. However, the patient may need admission and short-term antipsychotic medication if there are high levels of distress or concerns about safety.

Depression

With prolonged heavy drinking, around 80% of individuals will develop depressive symptoms, and around 30–40% of individuals will have symptoms resembling a major depressive episode. In most cases, the depressive symptoms improve significantly after about 3 weeks of abstinence, even without antidepressant medication.

In about 20% of patients, the depression is not alcohol-induced and requires treatment with antidepressant medication.

Key indicators that the depression may not be alcohol-induced are:

- the patient has had symptoms of major depression during significant periods of abstinence in the past (at least 4 weeks or more)
- the initial onset of depression clearly occurred before the onset of heavy drinking
- there is a strong family history of mood disorder
- the patient is still clinically depressed after 4 weeks or more of abstinence.

Patients with ongoing untreated depressive symptoms are more likely to relapse after treatment for their alcohol problem, so concomitant treatment of both disorders is required. Treatment for depression can include counselling to address lifestyle problems (including relationship problems, unemployment, bereavement, or other losses), cognitive behaviour therapy and antidepressant medication if the depression is moderate to severe.

Antidepressant medication should be selected on the basis that it is unlikely to potentiate the effects of alcohol, such as the selective serotonin reuptake inhibitors (SSRIs), venlafaxine, moclobemide, or reboxetine. The patient should be reminded that medication is unlikely to be effective if they continue to drink heavily. With continued drinking the patient may need to consider medication to reduce the cravings for alcohol, such as acamprosate. While naltrexone also reduces cravings to drink, it can sometimes exacerbate depression and should be used cautiously, ensuring the patient's mental state is monitored closely.

Anxiety

Symptoms of uncomplicated alcohol withdrawal can mimic anxiety and panic disorder. Withdrawal anxiety and its associated symptoms respond to short-term treatment with diazepam, as well as supportive care.

Once detoxification from alcohol is completed, many individuals will experience a protracted post-withdrawal phase. This may last for some months and symptoms may look like an anxiety disorder. Almost any form of anxiety can occur for 3–12 months after drinking has ceased, including generalized anxiety, panic attacks, and social anxiety. The patient should be reassured that the symptoms are likely to abate or reduce over time without treatment. Cognitive behavioural techniques may be helpful in managing the symptoms.

Approximately 25% of patients will have a history of an anxiety disorder preceding heavy drinking, and may need medication for this during recovery. Ideally treatment of the anxiety disorder should be started after drinking has stopped but in many cases this is not possible. Initiation of an effective antianxiety treatment, especially an SSRI, can help get the anxiety under control, thus allowing drinking cessation. Benzodiazepines may have a place, but only in specialist settings, because the risk of misuse of dependence on them is high (see BAP treatment guidelines, below).

Further reading

Lingford-Hughes AR, Welch S, Peters L, *et al.* (2012). BAP updated guidelines: evidence-based guidelines for the pharmacological management of substance abuse, harmful use, addiction and comorbidity: recommendations from BAP. *J Psychopharmacol* 26:899–952.

Help with social and legal complications of alcohol use disorders

The majority of people with alcohol use disorders experience social problems associated with their drinking. These include relationship breakdown, employment problems, and financial strain. A significant portion will also experience legal problems, e.g. relating to drink driving or violent offences. In addition to those who have social and legal problems secondary to their alcohol use, some individuals with AUDs had major primary social stressors which placed them at increased risk of developing problem drinking. This may include, for example, individuals who are in domestic violence relationships. Whether social problems are primary or secondary to drinking, the resulting stress may increase the risk of relapse to heavy drinking. Accordingly it is important to look at the patient in their family and community context, and provide assistance where possible.

Provision of stable housing can be a key factor in assisting with achieving and maintaining abstinence. If a social worker is not available, the clinician may be able to guide the drinker towards an agency that assists with accomodation. Sometimes such agencies can link clients with complex needs (e.g. mental health problems or brain damage) with supported accommodation.

Financial pressures are common. A range of services may be available via local charitable organizations to help those in financial need: these can include financial counsellors, emergency financial aid, free meals, or other practical assistance.

The extent of government support varies by country and region, but as well as social benefits schemes, such as unemployment or sickness benefits, innovative programmes are sometimes available. For example, in parts of Australia, individuals with debt to the government can 'work off' their debt by attending training or counselling.

Where a doctor is asked to certify whether a dependent drinker is suitable for a government-paid disability pension, this requires careful weighing up of the factors which may impair the individual's ability to work (including presence of any alcohol-related brain damage) against the benefits to the individual that employment can provide, including connection with society, self-esteem, and prevention of boredom, which can itself be a trigger to drinking.

Where the individual is facing legal charges, in some countries free legal aid services are available to those in financial need.

Relationship counsellors can be of assistance for stress between partners or within families, though addressing the drinking itself is typically key to an improvement in the relationship.

Where family violence is involved, linking the victim with a domestic violence support group or service can be important. Some counselling programmes also exist for the perpetrators of violence.

Clinicians must be mindful of their responsibilities to monitor any risk to children who may be either victims of abuse or neglect, or who may be traumatized by witnessing family violence. Clinicians may need to notify child protection agencies (pp. 575–9) and also may be able to informally increase the child's ability to access a safe haven or support.

Harm reduction/palliation in alcohol use disorders

In some cases a dependent drinker cannot or will not cease drinking. In other cases, a drinker may take several attempts before they are able to achieve a sustained period of abstinence. In these cases the clinician should consider what can be done to reduce the harms to the drinker, their family and community.

Thiamine can be taken daily to reduce the risk of neurocognitive impairment, though the patient should not be lulled into a false sense of security by believing it eliminates the risk. In those with established cognitive impairment, long-term supervision may need to be organized (see p. 227).

The clinician has a duty of care to consider the safety of any children who are in the care of the drinker, and to consider their safety on the road or in the workplace (Chapter 26, pp. 575–9).

Some heavy drinkers will agree to limit the risk associated with their drinking, e.g. by leaving their car keys at home, or only drinking when their children are in the care of a responsible adult for the night. Others are unable to commit to this. The safety of the drinker in relation to driving should be assessed and action taken if the risk of repeated drink driving seems high (see section on drink driving, pp. 564–9). It is the responsibility of the treating clinician to consider the safety of any children under the care of the drinker (pp. 575–9).

Living with a dependent drinker can be an extremely difficult experience. Several agencies (volunteer and professional) offer support to the family and children of dependent drinkers. Mutual support is available through Al-Anon (for adult family members) and Alateen (for teenagers).

Alcohol drug interactions

When prescribing any medication to a person with an alcohol use disorder, potential impacts of their drinking must be considered.

Acute alcohol consumption may inhibit a drug's metabolism by competing with the drug for the metabolizing enzymes, thereby prolonging and enhancing the drug's availability, and increasing the risk of side effects. Chronic alcohol consumption may induce drug metabolizing systems, thus decreasing the drug's blood level.

Alcohol's sedative effects can add to the sedative effects of another drug. Great caution and adequate safeguards must be employed when prescribing a potentially addictive drug such as benzodiazepines to an out-patient who has been alcohol dependent (Table 9.14).

Table 9.14 Alcohol–drug interactions

Medication	Type of interaction
CNS depressants: Benzodiazepines Barbiturates Phenothiazines Tricyclic antidepressants Antihistamines Opioids Anaesthetic agents	Acute alcohol consumption potentiates the sedative effects of CNS depressants, particularly in the elderly. It may also reduce opioid tolerance, so enhancing the risk of overdose death.
Oral hypoglycaemic agents: Sulfonylurea compounds	Diabetics on sulfonylureas should be advised not to drink Acute alcohol ingestion prolongs availability of hypoglycaemic agents with risk of hypoglycaemia Hypoglycaemia may also occur with poor dietary intake or depletion of glycogen stores Chronic alcohol consumption decreases the availability of hypoglycaemic agents with risk of hyperglycaemia
Antipsychotic medication: Phenothiazines	Acute alcohol consumption increases sedative effects, impairs coordination and may result in liver impairment
Anticonvulsants: Phenytoin	Acute alcohol ingestion can cause sedation

(Continued)

Table 9.14 (*Contd.*)

Medication	Type of interaction
Inhibitors of gastric alcohol dehydrogenase: Cimetidine	Raise BAC—at low doses of alcohol (uncertain clinical significance at higher doses)
Oral anticoagulants: Warfarin	Acute alcohol ingestion increases risk of haemorrhage
	Chronic alcohol consumption decreases anticoagulant effects.
Non-narcotic analgesics: Aspirin, NSAIDs Paracetamol	Increased risk of GI bleeding
	Chronic alcohol consumption increases risk of liver damage with paracetamol overdose

Further reading

Lingford-Hughes AR, Welch S, Peters L, et al. (2012). BAP updated guidelines: evidence-based guidelines for the pharmacological management of substance abuse, harmful use, addiction and comorbidity: recommendations from BAP. *J Psychopharmacol* 26:899–952.

Marshall EJ, Humphreys K, Ball DM, et al. (2010). *The Treatment of Drinking Problems: A Guide for the Helping Professions* (5th ed). Cambridge: Cambridge University Press.

McCaul ME, Petry NM. (2003). The role of psychosocial treatments in pharmacotherapy for alcoholism. *Am J Addict* 12:S41–S52.

Soyka M, Chick J. (2003). Use of acamprosate and opioid antagonists in the treatment of alcohol dependence: a European perspective. *Am J Addict* 12:S69–80.

Cannabis

Introduction and epidemiology 236
Chemistry, pharmacology, and pathophysiology 237
Core clinical syndromes 240
Physical and neuropsychiatric sequelae 242
Natural history 244
Policy and prevention 244
Clinical assessment and diagnosis 245
Brief interventions 246
Management of intoxication and withdrawal 246
Management of cannabis use and dependence 247
Management of complications 248

Introduction and epidemiology

Of all the psychoactive substances generally classified as illicit, cannabis (marijuana) is the most commonly used. Naturally produced cannabis comes in the form of the dried leaves and the flowering heads of the marijuana plant, *Cannabis sativa*. Typically, cannabis is smoked in a water-cooled pipe (a 'bong') or as a small hand-rolled cigarette ('joint'). It is often combined with tobacco which increases its flammability. It can be eaten in the form of cake or cookies.

- An estimated 160 million adults worldwide (4% of the adult population) smoke it in any one year.
- In many Western countries, half the population aged 20–40 years report having smoked cannabis at least once in their lives, 25–30% in the past year, and 15–20% over the past month.
- Most people who smoke cannabis do so experimentally, intermittently, or casually. Around 11% of young people become harmful or dependent users. In the EU, 1% of all adults are cannabis dependent.
- Cannabis use is particularly common among young people, often being the first drug (apart from alcohol, tobacco, and caffeine) which they use. This raises concerns because of the vulnerability of the developing brain to its deleterious effects.
- Cannabis contains around 100 chemicals unique to the plant which are called 'cannabinoids'. There is a wide variation in the combination of cannabinoids in different types of cannabis.

In addition to *C. sativa*, other species of the hemp plant such as *C. indica* are smoked. Varietals and subspecies and hybrids of these two species have been developed. The *C. indica* derivatives often have small leaves and give off a foul odour (hence the colloquial name 'skunk'). Cannabis grows especially well in warm, wet climates. The natural form is known as plantation or 'bush' cannabis. Increasingly, it is grown hydroponically, in greenhouse conditions, and this has the advantage (for producers) of producing more crops per year, and often cannabis of a higher potency.

Hashish is made from the plant's resin. It is sold in solid pieces, and usually mixed with tobacco and smoked. Hashish oil is the most concentrated form and is typically spread on tobacco and smoked.

In recent years, cannabinoid analogues have been synthesized. More than 400 of these compounds are now recognized, and they have distinct pharmacological effects, with an especially high prevalence of psychotic phenomena described. These synthetic cannabinoids tend to be smoked by existing cannabis users. In many countries they are not classified as illicit drugs and are sold as 'spice'. Individual compounds have particular brand names; examples are Supernova, Northern Lights, Kilimanjaro Sky, K2, Kronik, Ash, and Black Label.

Chemistry, pharmacology, and pathophysiology

- There are more than 100 naturally occurring cannabinoids.
- They interact with cannabis receptors, which are distributed throughout the CNS (principally CB_1 receptors) and the gastrointestinal tract (mostly CB_2 receptors).
- Principal biologically active ingredient of cannabis is delta 9-tetrahydrocannabinol (Δ9-THC).
- Next commonest ingredient is typically cannabidiol, which has several effects opposite to those of Δ9-THC.
- These two (and some other active cannabinoids) produce the desired psychological effects of cannabis smoking.
- Δ9-THC produces the more vivid and hallucinatory experiences; cannabidiol causes a relaxed sensation and may have antipsychotic effects counterbalancing the effects of Δ9-THC.
- An explanation for the more psychotomimetic and deleterious mental effects of new forms of cannabis (e.g. 'skunk') is that they contain little, if any, cannabidiol so the actions of Δ9-THC are not attenuated.
- 'Skunk' and sinsemilla cannabis (the latter derived from the unfertilized and seedless heads of the female plant) may have a THC concentration several times that of naturally grown cannabis (up to 18%).
- The pharmacological effects of synthetic cannabinoids are more closely related to those of Δ9-THC than to cannabidiol.

Many claims are made about the potency of various forms of cannabis (Table 10.1). There appears to have been a gradual increase in potency of forms of cannabis that are most commonly smoked. This may be related to varietals and hybrid forms, promotion of growth by hydroponic, greenhouse technology, and early cropping, which prevents loss

Table 10.1 Δ9-THC content of different preparations of cannabis

	Approximate THC content (depends on the plant, soil, sunlight, humidity)
Marijuana plant:	
leaves and stem	0.5–5%
buds and heads	7–15%
sinsemilla (unfertilized female flowering heads)	10–18%
Hashish (resin from top of plant)	2–20%
Hash oil (concentrated hashish extract)	15–50%

of potency due to oxidation during storage. In addition, there is evidence that the typical dose per occasion has increased in recent years.

Cannabis receptors have naturally occurring (endogenous) ligands, such as anandamide. These substances are synthesized in the CNS from membrane phospholipids and neuronal depolarization appears to influence such synthesis. The endogenous cannabinoids act on cannabis receptors (both in presynaptic and postsynaptic locations), and in doing so influence second messenger processes involved in learning and memory. The CB_1 and CB_2 receptors have quite different functions and locations. The main cannabis receptor is the CB_1 type, which is located in areas in the brain involved with mood and memory. The psychological effects of Δ9-THC are mediated through CB_1 receptors (the effects are lost in mice where these receptors have been deleted (knock-outs) and the effects of THC are blocked by selective CB_1 receptor antagonists such as rimonabant. The gastrointestinal effects of cannabis appear to be mediated by CB_2 receptors.

Absorption, distribution, and breakdown of cannabis

- Cannabinoids are rapidly absorbed from the alveolar membrane in the lungs.
- After smoking, plasma levels of cannabinoids are detectable in 2 minutes, with peak levels typically reached in 10–20 minutes.
- Highly fat-soluble compounds, which distribute into body fat stores and fatty organs such as the brain.
- Have a biphasic elimination profile: the first phase lasts about 30 minutes, and reflects redistribution of cannabinoids into fat stores.
- The second, elimination, phase lasts 20–80 hours (sometimes more) and reflects the metabolic clearance of cannabis in the liver and excretion of water-soluble metabolites through the kidneys.
- THC is metabolized mainly in the liver to 11-nor-THC-9-carboxylic acid.
- Metabolites may be detected in the urine weeks after a single joint or up to 3 months after repeated daily use because of the large amount of cannabinoids that reside in body fat stores, from which they gradually leak out.

The very enduring presence of inactive cannabis metabolites is detectable in urine screens, so individuals may be found 'drug positive' weeks after the effects of cannabis have worn off (these generally disappear within a day). Cannabis use is thus an easy target for drug testing which in some situations (e.g. prisons) has the perverse effect of encouraging use of shorter-acting, but more dangerous drugs, such as synthetic cannabinoids, heroin, ketamine, or GHB.

Pharmacological effects

After cannabis is smoked the effects last approximately 2–4 hours, sometimes more, depending on the dose. When taken orally, the effects are delayed but may last longer, for up to 12–24 hours. The effects vary with the setting, but typically include:

- euphoria, relaxation, sleep (in some cases anxiety or restlessness)
- floating sensations, lightness of limbs, depersonalization

- altered perception of time, temporal disintegration
- rapid flow of ideas, talkativeness
- loosening of associations, fragmented thinking
- disturbed memory
- conjunctival injection (red eyes)
- tachycardia
- elevations in blood pressure
- increased appetite (the 'munchies')
- dry mouth
- fall in intraocular pressure
- antiemetic effect.

Pathophysiology

PET studies show that cannabis increases blood flow to parts of the brain that mediate mood and decreases blood flow to areas associated with attention and cognition. Some of the effects of cannabis may be due to the release of dopamine (DA) in striatal and prefrontal cortical regions.

Cannabis dependence likely reflects adaptive changes in receptor function as withdrawal can be precipitated by antagonists such as rimonabant. Conversely, drugs combining THC and cannabidiol in equal proportions such as nabiximols (Sativex®) may reduce the severity of withdrawal symptoms in the short term.

Therapeutic uses of cannabis

There are several therapeutic uses of cannabinoids, for which there is evidence of efficacy. These include:
- as an antiemetic (during chemotherapy or radiotherapy)
- as an appetite stimulant (in HIV/AIDS patients)
- in the relief of glaucoma
- for spasticity and pain in certain neurological disorders, such as multiple sclerosis, spinal cord injuries, and movement disorders.

Nabilone is a synthetic cannabinoid that is licensed for the first two indications in the US and some other countries.

Currently there is a wide variety of disorders being researched (including cancer and obesity) for their responsiveness to various cannabinoids.

Medical marijuana

The term 'medical marijuana' is generally used to refer to the flowering heads of the marijuana plant or its crude extracts, which have not been processed pharmaceutically. These products are generally not recognized or approved as medications by regulatory authorities (such as the US Food and Drug Administration), but legislation has been passed in several countries and US states allowing individuals to smoke cannabis under medical prescription. Prescriptions are issued predominantly for pain disorders and for psychological difficulties such as anxiety and insomnia. The rationale for prescribing a smoked product is dubious.

Core clinical syndromes

Acute cannabis intoxication

This is seen after smoking a high dose of cannabis, and occasionally after seemingly small doses in susceptible people. Common features are as follows:

- *Anxiety and panic attacks*: the most common adverse emotional reactions with acute intoxication. Most often reported in naïve users and more common in those with a pre-existing anxiety disorder. Such cannabis-induced panic attacks last no more than 5–8 hours, but the user may feel as if they are losing control or going mad during that time.
- *Dysphoria*: there may be a period of lowered mood, which is usually mild, brief, and self-limiting.
- *Suspiciousness and paranoia*: unusual when naturally grown cannabis is smoked but more common with subspecies or synthetic compounds. Can heighten the feeling of fear and loss of control. May occur in healthy individuals with no past or family history of psychotic disorders.
- *Perceptual distortions*: unusual somatic or visual sensations may be experienced. These may be reported up to a week after an episode of cannabis use.
- *Visual and auditory illusions or hallucinations* (may contribute to paranoid experiences).
- *Loss of insight*: there may be associated paranoia; also occurs with persistent cognitive impairment.
- *Cognitive impairment*: cannabis intoxication commonly results in impaired or at least altered attention, concentration, learning, and memory.
- *Psychomotor impairment*: increased risk of accidents because of impaired psychomotor performance, as well as altered concentration and attention.
- *Confusion and delirium*: confusion and delirium are more common with large doses of high-potency cannabis. Clinical features include confusion, persecutory delusions, hallucinations (auditory and visual), emotional lability, panic, and there may be depersonalization and derealization.

The intoxicating effects of cannabis are typically short-lived, relatively benign, and recovery is usually complete within a week of ceasing cannabis. The psychotic features such as paranoia and hallucinations may resemble some aspects of a psychotic illness, but they are transient in nature and fully resolve as intoxication clears. Perceptual distortions may occur for several weeks; they are sometimes described as flashbacks. However, because cannabis has a long half-life, the experience is not strictly speaking occurring in abstinence, so cannot be called a flashback.

Death from overdose of smoked cannabis has not been described but deaths have occurred due to violence or accidents. There is an increased risk of motor vehicle accidents, though cannabis (unlike alcohol) tends to produce inhibited, rather than disinhibited driving behaviour.

Non-dependent (hazardous/harmful) use of cannabis

Cannabis may be used on a single occasion experimentally in teenage and young adult years, or periodically at parties or other social occasions. No adverse effects are apparent with such infrequent use. Use of cannabis in the 16–30-year-old age group approaches normative in some countries where more than 50% of young people have tried it at least once. In the absence of a known threshold for harm, hazardous or 'risky' cannabis use is difficult to define scientifically.

Harmful cannabis use refers to repeated use of cannabis causing physical or mental harm. This can include repeated episodes of clinically significant intoxication. A common example of physical harm is recurrent bronchitis and other chest infections.

Cannabis dependence

Chronic regular daily use may extend up to 14–16 hours of continual smoking per day. The patient may be intoxicated for much of this period. A proportion of regular chronic users will exhibit features of dependence, including:

- tolerance
- poor control over use
- unsuccessful attempts to stop or cut down
- cannabis taking a higher priority over other aspects of life
- continued despite clear evidence of harm (e.g. chest infection)
- withdrawal symptoms on cessation of use (in some cases).

Cannabis withdrawal syndrome

The withdrawal syndrome occurs in some cannabis-dependent individuals when they cease cannabis use. The exact prevalence is not clear, but may be as high as 20% of regular heavy users. Symptoms of acute withdrawal start approximately 4 hours after cessation of cannabis, peak at 4–7 days, and last 2–3 weeks (see Box 10.1). Protracted milder withdrawals symptoms may last several weeks. Cannabis withdrawal can be precipitated by the CB_1 antagonist rimonabant.

Box 10.1 Clinical features of the cannabis withdrawal syndrome

- Lethargy
- Irritability
- Restlessness, anxiety
- Insomnia
- Mood changes
- Reduced appetite
- Muscle spasm
- Headache.

Physical and neuropsychiatric sequelae

Medical complications

These include:

- increased risk of accidents, including motor vehicle accidents, especially if alcohol is also consumed
- impaired pulmonary function, recurrent bronchitis, worsening of asthma, cancer of the lungs (from carcinogens in cannabis and tobacco smoke).

Neuropsychiatric complications

In addition to the acute intoxicating effects of cannabis, long-term use can lead to persistent psychiatric, neuropsychiatric, and cognitive impairment.

- *Anxiety and panic attacks*: these are the most common adverse effects and occur two to four times more commonly in long-term cannabis users than in the general population.
- *Depression*: following the euphoria usually experienced with cannabis intoxication, there may be a period of lowered mood, which is usually brief and self-limiting. Longer-lasting depressive symptoms are now recognized, and recent studies have established that the prevalence of depression is raised in long-term cannabis users, many of whom are cannabis dependent.
- *Paranoia*: cannabis intoxication may be associated with mild levels of suspiciousness, paranoia, and loss of insight, and these can occur in healthy individuals with no past or family history of psychotic disorders. Persistent paranoia occurs in cannabis-related psychosis (see p. 243). Paranoia is a more common acute effect of cannabis which is high in THC and low in CBD (often varieties called skunk or sinsemilla).
- *Delirium*: this may occur in acute cannabis intoxication, especially when high-potency cannabis has been smoked. Clinical features include confusion, paranoid (and often persecutory) delusions, auditory and/or visual hallucinations, emotional lability, panic, and sometimes depersonalization and derealization. Recovery is usually complete within a week of stopping cannabis. Persistent delirium is described but is rare.
- *Amotivational syndrome*: an 'amotivational syndrome' has been long described in long-term cannabis users. It comprises lack of motivation, apathy, social withdrawal, and lethargy, and there is often impaired memory and concentration. It may be due to the effects of chronic intoxication, and some dispute its existence as a discrete entity. It may improve or resolve with abstinence, unless it reflects other factors, such as personality dysfunction and other substance use.
- *Cognitive impairment*: cannabis intoxication commonly results in impaired attention, concentration, learning, and memory. Regular cannabis use can also lead to often subtle cognitive impairments—in memory, attention, organization, and integration of complex

information. There is usually improvement in cognitive function with cessation of cannabis use, but persistent impairment is described even with abstinence of a year or more.

Acute psychosis

There is ongoing controversy about the existence of this syndrome. Several authors have described acute psychotic episodes occurring in clear consciousness following cannabis use, and more commonly after heavy use or those with long-term use and/or cannabis dependence. The psychotic episodes are characterized by rapid onset, with a relatively benign course, and usually recovering completely within a week of abstinence even without antipsychotic agents. There is no evidence of confusion or delirium.

Psychotic features may comprise predominantly affective-like symptoms (of a manic or hypomanic type), or those resembling a schizophreniform psychosis (with auditory or visual hallucinations, delusions, and sometimes incoherent speech).

Chronic psychosis

There is also considerable debate about whether cannabis use can induce a chronic psychosis, including schizophrenia. The following might represent a consensus:

- In patients with schizophrenia, cannabis use may trigger a relapse of the disorder and may exacerbate existing symptoms even when the patient is otherwise stable on medication.
- Regular heavy users of cannabis may suffer repeated, short episodes of psychosis and be in a lingering, subpsychotic state; however, the psychotic symptoms will abate once cannabis use cease.
- Cannabis use may precipitate psychotic symptoms in an individual who is in the prodrome of schizophrenia or has a high genetic or other susceptibly to it; COMT and AKT1 polymorphisms have been implicated.
- Cohort studies indicate that cannabis users have a 2- to 4-fold increase in the relative risk for developing schizophrenia. Eliminating cannabis use in those at risk would reduce the incidence of schizophrenia by 8–15%.
- Cannabis alone probably does not cause schizophrenia but it is an important component of a constellation of risk factors for it.

Social complications

- Among adolescents, impaired performance at school and earlier school leaving
- Reduced academic achievement in young people generally
- Delinquency (in adolescence it may be difficult to distinguish the behavioural changes and moodiness of adolescence from the effects of cannabis use)
- Impaired job performance, unemployment
- Financial problems
- Relationship problems, family problems
- Criminal activity and legal problems.

Natural history

Information is scant on the natural history of various levels of cannabis use.
- Cannabis use typically begins in the mid to late teens, and is most prevalent in early adulthood.
- Most cannabis use is irregular, with very few users engaging in long-term daily use.
- About 10% of those who ever use cannabis become daily users, and another 20–30% use weekly.
- Of those who have cannabis dependence, about 50% are still smoking regularly at 5 years.
- Smoking cannabis for up to 30–40 years is well recognized.
- Transitions in life roles, such as entry into full-time employment, getting married, or having children, are associated with reductions in or cessation of use for many people. The largest decreases are seen in cannabis use among males and females after marriage, and especially during pregnancy and after childbirth in women.

Policy and prevention

Although cannabis is considered a less harmful drug than many, people (particularly young people) with a family history of substance dependence or mental illness such as schizophrenia or psychosis are best advised to avoid it.

Everyone should be informed about the potential neuropsychiatric complications of cannabis use.

Those using cannabis should be advised about the risks of driving while under the influence of cannabis, particularly if it is used in combination with alcohol.

There have been major global changes in regulation of cannabis in recent years. These include medical marijuana being available in 20 US states, some parts of Europe, and being fully legalized in 2014 in Uruguay and two US states.

Clinical assessment and diagnosis

History

As part of the history of substance use (see pp. 69–70), enquire about the three dimensions of cannabis involvement, as follows:

Use
- What is smoked? Cannabis leaf (low potency), the more potent flowering heads ('bud')?
- How is it produced? Naturally grown, hydroponically grown?
- Or are particular forms smoked (e.g. skunk, sinsemilla) or synthetics?
- How is it smoked? As a joint, or using a bong or pipe?
- How much is smoked per occasion/per day? Quantify in 'cones', grams, or ounces: 1 ounce = 28 grams; 1 gram = 15 cones.
- How many hours in a day do you feel the effects (are 'stoned')?
- How frequently is it smoked? Daily, or episodically?
- Is there a pattern to its use, e.g. at weekends only?
- What is the duration of smoking? Months, years, decades?
- When was the last smoke?

Dependence
- Do you experience withdrawal symptoms (indicates dependence)?
- Have you continued to smoke cannabis despite problems?
- Is cannabis use taking over your life?
- Are you affected ('stoned') for more than 4–6 hours per day regularly? (Suggests dependence).

Complications:
- History of respiratory illnesses.
- History of psychiatric illness and possible relationship to cannabis use.
- Social, occupational, and legal problems.

Taking a family history of cannabis (and other substance) use and a family history of psychiatric illness are also important.

Examination

Clinical examination may be normal, but the following may give clues to cannabis involvement:
- Conjunctival injection (red eyes).
- Tachycardia, raised blood pressure.
- Signs of chronic obstructive airways disease.

Mental state examination may reveal anxiety, panic, depression, confusion, paranoid ideation, and (in heavy users/ those with cannabis dependence), features of psychosis (see pp. 73–6).

Laboratory investigations

Cannabis is lipophilic and can be detected in plasma for up to a month. In some countries, blood and/or saliva are tested to determine competence to drive.

Brief interventions

Cannabis users who are non-dependent, but smoking cannabis in a hazardous or harmful way can be offered a brief intervention based on the FLAGS acronym:

- *Feedback:* on any medical, neuropsychiatric, or social harms experienced as the result of cannabis use.
- *Listen:* to the patient's response—does the patient want to quit using?
- *Advice:* convey clear medical advice, e.g. the potential medical, neuropsychiatric, and social complications of cannabis use and the benefits of not smoking cannabis (important particularly for young people).
- *Goals:* set goals tailored according to the individual patient's response.
- *Strategies:* set out strategies to achieve the goals. Offer follow-up to determine progress and offer support.

Management of intoxication and withdrawal

Cannabis intoxication

Intoxication should be managed conservatively in a quiet environment with reassurance and food intake (e.g. chocolate, coffee).

Withdrawal management (detoxification)

Most people who smoke cannabis can stop without the need for medical involvement. However, in those who have developed cannabis dependence, the occurrence of a withdrawal syndrome often stops attempts at ceasing within a few days. The cannabis withdrawal syndrome is an unpleasant experience, particularly as it tends to increase in severity over the first few days (peaking at 6–8 days) and it may be more than a month by the time it resolves. Providing information about the nature of withdrawal symptoms and their time course is a key component of intervention. Standard psychological interventions such as motivational interviewing and behavioural rescheduling are helpful.

Medication is often necessary to manage the withdrawal syndrome. The most effective agents are cannabinoid agonists e.g. nabiximols (Sativex®). Otherwise, the evidence base for withdrawal management is small. Various treatments are used in clinical practice:

- Benzodiazepines (e.g. diazepam 5–10 mg every 6 hours for 7–10 days and ceasing by 14 days) improve insomnia but do not consistently relieve other withdrawal symptoms.
- A low dose of a sedating antipsychotic agent (e.g. quetiapine 50–100 mg as the extended-release form mid evening) may be prescribed to assist sleep and can improve appetite; no improvement in mood is reported. The patient should be warned that the first dose might cause significant sedation and to contact the prescriber if that occurs.
- Mirtazapine 15–30 mg at night also helps with insomnia, but does not appreciably relieve dysphoria.

Management of cannabis use and dependence

There is no known dividing line between safety and harm for cannabis use, and so the level of use at which some intervention is appropriate is not established. For people with likely hazardous cannabis use or harmful use, a brief intervention is appropriate (see p. 57 and p. 246). For patients with cannabis dependence and/or established cannabis-related disorders, more formal management is appropriate. Indeed, cannabis dependence is the primary reason for 28% of new referrals to drug services in the EU, second only to heroin (41%). The key components of management are listed in Box 10.2.

Box 10.2 Ten steps for managing cannabis dependence

1. *Information and understanding*. Provision of information and written materials to help the patient develop an understanding of the nature of cannabis dependence and related harm.
2. *Acceptance and engagement*. The patient will need time to digest the information and consider his/her goals. The use of motivational interviewing may be helpful to induce commitment to change, and develop commitment to cease use
3. *Initiating treatment and detoxification*. See p. 246 for details of withdrawal management.
4. *Pharmacotherapy*. There are no medications of established benefit for the ongoing treatment of cannabis dependence. The CB_1 antagonist rimonabant has not been approved for use. Cannabis agonists (e.g. dronabinol, Sativex®) are currently being evaluated.
5. *Psychological therapies*. These are the primary approaches to management of cannabis dependence, and focus on relapse prevention. The evidence base supports cognitive behavioural therapy and motivational enhancement therapy for up to four sessions; other therapies are currently being evaluated.
6. *Comorbid disorders*. Underlying or complicating mental illness is particularly important to identify. Consider referral to a psychiatrist.
7. *Family and social support*. Treatment of the patient should occur where possible within the family or social context. Parents will usually need education about cannabis use and support to help the family engage with the user and facilitate cessation of use.
8. *Self-help organizations*. Self-help (mutual help) groups such as Marijuana Anonymous (MA) are a valuable resource in some areas.
9. *Aftercare*. Offer follow-up.
10. *Lifestyle and environmental changes*. Help the person identify whether their usual way of doing things might have contributed to their cannabis problem. Identify potential changes to aspects of daily life, home, and environment. Avoiding cannabis or other substance-using people and toxic places will be important, together with a regular routine for life, exercise, work, and interests.

Management of complications

Management of acute mental disorders

Mostly this entails confirming the diagnosis of a cannabis-related disorder, and reassuring the patient (where this is possible) that this is the cause. Acute mental disorders will usually start to abate in 5–8 hours.

- For acute anxiety, a benzodiazepine may be prescribed in the short term.
- Depressive symptoms will need to be assessed as to the likely cause, whether an underlying mood disorder, a cannabis-induced syndrome, or symptomatic of another disorder. Detoxification and review is important prior to considering the place of antidepressants or therapy.
- Psychotic disorders will also need to be assessed as to likely cause and relationship with cannabis use. Detoxification is necessary, combined with appropriate antipsychotic medication.

Management of persisting mental disorders

Psychosis associated with cannabis use can be managed by reducing level of use over time. Harm reduction may be achieved in those not able to reduce by switching from higher THC brands to lower, especially those higher in CBD. In some cases, antipsychotics may be indicated.

Further reading

Advisory Council on the Misuse of Drugs (2008). *Cannabis: Classification and Public Health.* London: UK Home Office.

Allsop DJ, Copeland J, Lintzeris N, et al. (2014). Nabiximols as an agonist replacement therapy during cannabis withdrawal. *JAMA Psychiatry* 71(3):281–91.

Budney A, Hughes A. (2006). The cannabis withdrawal syndrome. *Curr Opin Psychiatry* 19:33–238.

Curran HV, Morgan CJA. (2014). Desired and undesired effects of cannabis on the human mind and psychological well-being. In Pertwee R (ed) *Handbook of Cannabis*, pp. 647–60. Oxford: Oxford University Press.

Moore THM, Zammit S, Lingford-Hughes A, et al. (2007). Cannabis use and risk of psychotic or affective mental health outcomes: a systematic review. *Lancet* 370:319–28.

Morgan CJA , Duffin S, Hunt S, et al. (2012). Neurocognitive function and schizophrenia-proneness in individuals dependent on ketamine, on high potency cannabis ('skunk') or on cocaine. *Pharmacopsychiatry* 45:269–74.

Morgan CJA, Schafer G, Freeman TP, et al. (2010). Impact of cannabidiol on the acute memory and psychotomimetic effects of smoked cannabis: naturalistic study. *Br J Psychiatry* 197:285–90.

Nutt DJ, Nash J. (2002). *Cannabis—An Update.* London: Home Office Publications. Available at: http://www.drugs.gov.uk/ReportsandPublications/Communities/1034165905/Cannabis_update_1999to2002.pdf

Rawlins M. (2008). *Cannabis: Classification and Public Health.* London: Home Office Publication. Available at: https://www.gov.uk/government/uploads/system/uploads/attachment_data/file/119174/acmd-cannabis-report-2008.pdf

Opioids

Introduction and epidemiology 250
Pharmacology of opioids 251
Pathophysiology 256
Natural history of opioid use disorders 256
Core clinical diagnoses 257
Complications of opioid use 259
Identification and brief intervention for opioid misuse 263
Assessment and management of opioid overdose 264
Management of opioid withdrawal 267
Assessment 272
Management of opioid dependence 275
Harm reduction/palliation 293
Prevention 293
Summary 293

Introduction and epidemiology

- Illicitly used opioids represent the third most common form of illicit drug use worldwide. Illicit use includes the use of illegal drugs and the unapproved use of pharmaceutical opioids (see Box 11.1 for examples).
- In most high-income countries, less than 1% of the population has used illicit opioids in the past year. This ranges from 0.1% in Japan and Sweden, 0.5% in countries such as Australia and New Zealand, to 0.9% in the UK and the US.
- Illicit opioid use attracts much public concern because of the tragedy of the many deaths from overdose or other complications.
- Overall, illicit opioids contribute less to the global burden of disease than do licit substances, such as alcohol and tobacco (0.8% as compared with 4% for alcohol and 6% for tobacco).

Dependence on illicit opioids is a serious disorder. It causes considerable suffering to the drug-dependent individual and to those around them.

Dependence (addiction) and its related consequences impose sizeable challenges to the broader community in terms of health and social problems, especially the spread of hepatitis B, C, and HIV infection, criminal activities and resultant incarceration, and economic and social consequences.

Some opioid users take only heroin, others use illegally obtained methadone (orally or injected) and prescribed opioids (orally or parenteral). If opioids are not available, many use alcohol or benzodiazepines to control their withdrawal symptoms. The use of prescription opioids in the US has outranked heroin in recent years.

Box 11.1 Examples of opioids

- Morphine
- Methadone
- Buprenorphine (Subutex®; Suboxone®)
- Oxycodone
- Pethidine

- Codeine
- Diacetylmorphine (heroin)
- Fentanyl
- Pentazocine
- Hydromorphone
- Dextropropoxyphene

Pharmacology of opioids

Opioids all act on opioid receptors in the CNS to produce analgesia and varying amounts of euphoria and sedation. This group includes both naturally occurring compounds such as morphine, an alkaloid of opium obtained from the poppy plant *Papaver somniferum*, and related synthetic chemicals, such as buprenorphine.

Opioids act on different opioid receptors to produce the following effects:

- mu (μ) receptors: euphoria, sedation, analgesia, miosis, reduced gastrointestinal motility, respiratory depression and physical dependence
- kappa (κ) receptors (principally within the spinal cord, basal ganglia, temporal lobes): drowsiness, dysphoria
- delta (δ) receptors: analgesia, cardiovascular effects (hypotension, bradycardia).

Stimulation of mu (and possibly delta) opioid receptors is involved in reward systems (see Neurobiology of dependence, pp. 48–51). In mice that have the mu receptor 'knocked out', the rewarding effects of opioids are abolished, but the analgesic effect of delta receptor agonists may be retained.

Heroin (diamorphine)

Heroin is highly lipid-soluble (Fig. 11.1), and crosses the blood–brain barrier more rapidly than morphine or other opioids. Within 1–2 minutes after IV heroin there is a characteristic 'rush' associated with warm flushing of the skin. Heroin is metabolized in the liver and also in the brain to active metabolites 6-monoacetyl morphine and then morphine. Hence, heroin is a pro-drug of morphine. Heroin may be taken by mouth; other common routes of self-administration inhalation of heroin smoke—'chasing the dragon'.

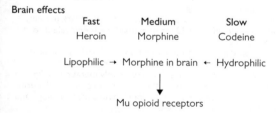

Brain effects

Fast	Medium	Slow
Heroin	Morphine	Codeine

Lipophilic → Morphine in brain ← Hydrophilic

↓

Mu opioid receptors

Fig. 11.1 Heroin and codeine are 'pro-drugs' of morphine.

Morphine

Morphine is the principal opioid used therapeutically. In its oral form there is a high first-pass effect and so for a therapeutic effect, the oral dose should be higher than the parenteral dose. Morphine is metabolized by conjugation in the liver, but one of the major metabolites, morphine-6-glucuronide, is also a mu receptor agonist and is used as an analgesic. The glucuronide metabolites are water-soluble and are excreted in urine.

Codeine

Codeine is also a pro-drug of morphine, being converted to it by CYP2D6. People with low functioning CYP2D6, as a result of block-ade with drugs such as paroxetine, will get less effect from codeine. Conversely, rapid metabolizers will get greater effects perhaps with dangerous consequences. A case is described of a rapid metabolizing woman who was taking codeine for pain and breastfeeding her baby where the baby died of morphine toxicity. Deaths of children post tonsillectomy have been linked to the use of codeine for analgesia.

With repeated administration, tolerance develops to most opioid effects, except miosis and constipation, and withdrawal may occur on cessation of use. Cross-tolerance is the norm among the opioids as they share a common target receptor.

Methadone

Methadone is a long-acting synthetic opioid mu receptor agonist with properties similar to morphine and other opioids. It was first developed in Germany in the 1940s as an analgesic and is available in the form of tablets or as a syrup or solution. Methadone tablets are used for the relief of pain, while methadone syrup and solution are indicated for the treatment of opioid dependence.

Methadone:

- Has a much longer plasma half-life than morphine (mean 22 hours, range 15–32 hours, versus 2 hours for morphine) and this permits once-daily supervised dosing.
- However, it is sometimes misused or diverted to the black market.
- On single dose, the effect of 30 mg of methadone is equivalent to 15 mg of morphine.
- It is well absorbed after oral administration, and reaches a peak at about 4 hours, and readily crosses the blood–brain barrier.
- 90% is bound to plasma proteins. It is extensively metabolized by N-demethylation and cyclization in the liver, and excreted in the urine and bile. Some of the details of methadone's neuropharmacology and metabolism remain poorly defined.
- Rifampicin and phenytoin accelerate the metabolism of methadone by inducing cytochrome P450 enzymes and may precipitate withdrawal symptoms. In contrast, fluvoxamine decreases the metabolism of methadone and may result in symptoms of opioid intoxication.

Buprenorphine

Buprenorphine is a high-affinity, partial agonist at the mu receptor (Fig. 11.2) and an antagonist at the kappa receptor. It competes with and displaces heroin or methadone from the mu receptor sites and is sometimes referred to as a mixed agonist–antagonist. Because of its low intrinsic activity and 'ceiling effects', it has lower risk of respiratory toxicity and, thus, is relatively safer than either heroin or methadone.

Buprenorphine is more potent than either heroin or methadone:

- The smallest sublingual dose of buprenorphine (0.4 mg) is equivalent to 10 mg morphine (intramuscular injection), and 2 mg of sublingual buprenorphine is equivalent to 30 mg oral methadone.
- A ceiling effect limits its respiratory depressant effects at higher doses, as described later in this topic.

Buprenorphine is highly lipophilic and slowly released from fat stores:

- It undergoes extensive first-pass metabolism and, hence, needs to be given sublingually (though depot preparations and patches are under development).
- Onset of action occurs within 30–60 minutes.
- Peak plasma levels are reached in 1–2 hours and the half-life is approximately 20–70 hours (average 35 hours).
- Steady state levels are achieved in 3–7 days.
- Duration of action is dose dependent and ranges from 4 to 12 hours for low doses to 48–72 hours for high doses.

Buprenorphine undergoes enterohepatic circulation. Metabolism is by hepatic microsomal enzyme systems, CYP3A4 and by conjugation with glucuronic acid. Most (70%) is excreted in the faeces and the rest in the urine.

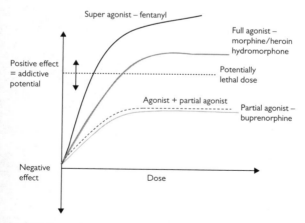

Fig. 11.2 Mu agonist types.

Characteristics of buprenorphine
- More potent than morphine or methadone per mg (up to 30×)
- Good sublingual absorption (60%+) in most patients
- Poor gastric absorption and high first-pass metabolism (only 10% of dose enters systemic circulation)
- Partial agonist at the mu opioid receptor that reduces risk of overdose if abused
- High affinity for the mu opioid receptor blocks access of other opioids to the mu receptor so reduces 'on-top' use
- Half-life (including active metabolite) from one to several days as dose increases
- If there has been recent use of other opioids, buprenorphine can displace them from opioid receptors, precipitating a withdrawal reaction in dependent users due to its high affinity and lower activity at the opioid receptor.

Table 11.1 compares the pharmacology of three important opioids.

Table 11.1 Comparison of the pharmacology of three opioids

	Heroin	Methadone	Buprenorphine
Receptor	Mu agonist	Mu agonist	Partial mu agonist Kappa antagonist
Administration	IV	Oral usually. May be given in reduced dose, IM or subcutaneously when a person is nil by mouth	Sublingual
Peak plasma levels	1–2 min	2–4 h	1–2 h
Plasma half-life	2 h	22 h	Approx. 36 h (20–72 h, increases with dose)
Onset of effect	Minutes	30–60 min	30–60 min
Peak effect	1–2 min	3–6 h	1–4 h
Duration of effect	4–5 h	16–30 h dose dependent	12 h, low dose 72 h, high dose
Liver metabolism	Hydrolysis	MEOS CYP3A4	MEOS CYP3A4 Conjugation
High first-pass metabolism	Yes	No	Yes
Drug interactions	MAOIs Sedatives	MAOIs Sedatives Protease inhibitors CYP3A4 inducers: Phenytoin Rifampicin Carbamazepine CYP3A4 inhibitors: Fluvoxamine	MAOIs Sedatives Protease inhibitors Antimycotics Ca channel blockers Macrolide antibiotics

Pathophysiology

- In contrast to the widespread toxic effects of alcohol, the pathological effects of opioids are limited. These effects reflect the pharmacological effects of the parent drugs and their metabolites. There are no metabolites with inherent tissue-toxic effects as are seen with alcohol.
- The acute complications of opioid toxicity are directly related to pharmacological effects that include sedation, and in severe cases, respiratory depression and overdose death.
- Release of histamine may occur through degranulation of mast cells. Leakage in endothelial cell vessel lining may lead to pulmonary oedema.
- Contraction of smooth muscles occurs with acute opioid use. With chronic use, the opposite of the acute effect tends to occur with smooth muscle becoming hypotonic, leading to risk of gastroparesis.
- Opioids decrease bowel motility and both illicit and prescribed opioid misuse can cause chronic and sometimes severe constipation.
- The dry mouth resulting from opioid use chronically results in dental decay. This is because saliva has antibacterial properties. In addition, heroin-dependent individuals rarely prioritize dental care, because of the preoccupation with drug use.
- Many of the medical complications of illicit heron use are complications of unsafe injecting practices, e.g. viral or bacterial infections (pp. 273–4).

Natural history of opioid use disorders

A high proportion of people who use illicit opioids become dependent on them This may lead to a dependence syndrome (ICD 10 or DSM-IV) or (in DSM-5) an opioid use disorder.

The development of dependence can be relatively rapid, after 6–8 weeks of regular use, or may follow years of intermittent use. Once dependent, users may struggle to control their use for substantial proportions of their lives.

There is a high morbidity and mortality associated with dependence. Some of the complications of illicit opioid use are due to the drug itself (death from overdose, dependence); however, its illegal nature and resulting high cost greatly contribute to the social harms of illicit opioid use. As injection of illicit opioids is in most cases not medically supervised and is often hurried to avoid detection, a large number of medical complications may ensue, and blood-borne virus infection occurs (in particular hepatitis C) in the majority of dependent heroin injectors.

Core clinical diagnoses

A person may use illicit opioids but not meet criteria for an ICD or DSM diagnosis. These individuals are described as either using or misusing the illicit opioid(s). Alternatively, an individual may meet the criteria for a diagnosable drug use disorder, either in the past 12 months (current) or in the past.

Harmful opioid use (ICD 10)

Harmful opioid use is a non-dependent opioid use disorder. A person meets the criteria for it if he/she has experienced complications of use, e.g. overdose or hepatitis C infection or injuries from violence associated with purchasing the drug but is not dependent on opioids.

Opioid use disorder (DSM-5)

An individual has an opioid use disorder if he/she uses opioids repeatedly and meets two or more of the following criteria (according to the DSM-5):

- Impaired control over use (using in larger amounts or over a longer period than intended)
- Great deal of time spent in obtaining, using, or recovering from effects of the opioid
- Craving/compulsion to use
- Unsuccessful attempts to cut down on opioid use
- Preoccupation with opioid use to the neglect of other responsibilities
- Continued opioid use despite having persistent or recurrent personal or social problems caused by the effects of opioids
- Social, occupational, or recreational activities given up because of the opioid use
- Recurrent opioid use in physically hazardous situations
- Tolerance: *need for increased amounts to get desired effect or less effect from using the same amount* (e.g. an opioid user first may have only inhaled the drug; after some time they find they need higher doses and then may revert to injecting to get the desired effect. Injectors may increase their use from a 'half a quarter' a day up to 1 g (street gram) per day or, in financial terms, from US$ 50 per day to hundreds of US$ per day)
- Withdrawal or use of opioids to prevent or relieve withdrawal: the physically dependent user typically describes withdrawal symptoms or feeling 'sick' when they are overdue for their next dose of opioid, with low energy, runny nose, aches, and pains (see later in topic).
- Persistent use despite clear evidence of physical or psychological adverse consequences.

Individuals who meet two or three criteria have a mild disorder, four or five criteria a moderate disorder, and six to eleven a severe disorder.

Opioid dependence (ICD 10)

Opioid dependence is diagnosed when three of the following features have occurred together at the same time during the previous 12 months:

- A strong desire or sense of compulsion to use opioid drugs
- Difficulties in controlling opioid use in terms of its onset, termination, or levels of use
- Progressive neglect of alternative interests because of opioid use or increased amount of time necessary to use opioids or recover from their effects
- Tolerance, such that increased doses of opioid are required in order to achieve effects originally produced by lower doses
- A physiological withdrawal state when opioid use ceases or is reduced, as evidenced by the characteristic withdrawal syndrome or use of opioids with the intention of relieving or avoiding withdrawal symptoms
- Persisting with opioid use despite clear evidence of overtly harmful consequences

Opioid withdrawal syndrome

Simple opioid withdrawal after physiological dependence has occurred, with or without the presence of an opioid use disorder, resembles a flu-like illness, and simple withdrawal is not life-threatening. Symptoms include low energy, aches and pains, rhinorrhoea, sneezing, yawning, lacrimation, sweating, piloerection, tremor, dilated pupils, nausea and vomiting, abdominal cramping, and diarrhoea. Insomnia, psychic distress, and craving for opioids are prominent (see pp. 267–71 for assessment and management of opioid withdrawal).

Complications of opioid use

Acute complications

Complications may be experienced by those who use opioids by oral, injection, or inhaled routes.

Opioid overdose

This is relatively common among heroin and other opioid users especially after intravenous use and a cause of death from respiratory depression; even controlled use of heroin is associated with marked drops in oxygen saturation. (See pp. 264–6 assessment and management of overdose.)

Medical complications of injecting opioid use

Complications of injecting opioid use may arise from:
- the pharmacological effects of the opioid (e.g. overdose)
- adulterants and contaminants in the drug (unknown potency, purity and sterility)
- unsafe injecting practices including needle sharing
- social complications related to the illegal nature and high cost of drugs.

Complications related to contaminants and adulterants

Illicit heroin is typically non-sterile and the potency is unknown. It may be contaminated or 'cut' with a variety of substances, usually added to reduce the cost to the dealer of pure heroin, and so increase their profit. The user may experience unexpected pharmacological or toxic effects. Particulate matter may result in emboli.

Acute heroin reaction (rare): an acute reaction or allergic reaction to pyrogenic material or contaminants in the illicit drug preparation. It is more common with heroin than with other illicit drugs. The acute heroin reaction is typically associated with sudden-onset severe occipital headache, fever, tremor/shaking (occasionally with rigors), tachypnoea, leucocytosis, and may lead to non-cardiogenic pulmonary oedema, cyanosis, coma, and death from respiratory depression.

Complications relating to unsafe injecting practices

Infections: injecting illicit drugs and sharing of injecting equipment places individuals at risk of infections with a variety of agents including blood-borne viruses (hepatitis C, B, and HIV), as well as bacteria and fungi.

Bacterial infections: these are common and may become systemic and life-threatening. In cases of high unexplained fever, or chronic fever, in an IDU, always consider endocarditis or another hidden focus of serious infection.

> *Do blood cultures in all febrile IDUs.*

Bacterial infections are most commonly caused by *Staphylococcus aureus*. They also may be caused by *Streptococcus viridans*, *Clostridium*, or other organisms. Presentations may be local, distant, or systemic and include:
* local infections:
  * abscess, cellulitis
  * septic thrombophlebitis
  * necrotizing fasciitis (mainly with *Clostridium* following subcutaneous injection), necrotizing ulcers.
* embolic or distant infection:
  * metastatic abscesses
  * bacterial endocarditis—mainly *Staphylococcus aureus*. Also *Streptococcus viridans*, *Pseudomonas aeruginosa*. May affect the tricuspid valve or mitral or aortic valves
  * osteomyelitis, septic arthritis
* septicaemia and disseminated infections (mainly streptococci).

Viral infections: IDUs are at risk of one or more blood-borne virus infections, and in particular hepatitis C, B, and HIV.

Hepatitis C: injecting drug use is responsible for 90% of cases of hepatitis C in the developed world. Hepatitis C is associated with acute hepatitis and with a significant burden of chronic liver disease, including cirrhosis and hepatocellular carcinoma. In most countries, the majority of chronic regular IV drug users will be infected with hepatitis C (e.g. 65–70% and higher in countries without ready access to sterile injecting equipment). Hepatitis C has high infectivity. It is spread not only by sharing of needles and syringes, but also by sharing of other injecting equipment (e.g. spoons used for dissolving the drug, swabs, and tourniquets). In addition, putting injecting equipment down on a bench or other surface which may have been contaminated by another users' blood, can potentially lead to infection.

Hepatitis B: hepatitis B is less common than hepatitis C, but evidence of present or past infection is found in 30–50% of regular users. It is most commonly acquired through unsafe injecting practices or unprotected sex. Most people clear the infection.

HIV: in some regions (e.g. many parts of Asia and former Soviet Union states) HIV infection in IDUs is a common complication, with consequent risk of spread to other segments of the community. In other countries, such as Australia and some states in the US, with active harm reduction measures such as needle syringe services and availability of opioid maintenance treatment, the prevalence of HIV in IDUs has remained low (<5%).

Fungal and other infections: particularly common is *Candida albicans*.
* Distant or systemic infection including endocarditis, fungal ophthalmitis.
* Illicit injection of diverted sublingual buprenorphine tablets increases the risk of blood-borne or mouth organisms, including *Candida*.

Vascular complications
- Vasculitis, vascular damage
- Vascular spasm due to local trauma of injecting
- Inadvertent or deliberate injecting into arteries, can be associated with distal ischaemia
- Embolism, strokes
- Aneurysms:
  - Arteriovenous aneurysm
  - Mycotic aneurysms
  - Pulsatile pseudoaneurysms (caused by vascular injuries, *S. aureus* is the main pathogen).

Other medical complications of opioid use

Pulmonary complications
- Infections: including tuberculosis, pneumonias—due to poor living conditions, nutrition, and self-care, associated smoking of tobacco, cannabis and of crack cocaine
- Lung complications may follow inhalation of opioids
- Atelectasis
- Pulmonary emboli, pulmonary infarction (from septic thrombophlebitis or coincident cocaine use)
- Non-cardiogenic pulmonary oedema (heroin)
- Pulmonary granulomas (from insoluble additives).

Sexually transmitted infections: chlamydia, syphilis, gonorrhoea, etc., may be acquired through unprotected sex, either as part of sex work to raise money for drugs, or when under the influence of drugs (e.g. sedated with heroin, alcohol and/or benzodiazepines; or increased libido with concomitant stimulant use).

Rhabdomyolysis: may result from pressure following prolonged unconsciousness with heroin (and/or benzodiazepines, alcohol). May lead to acute renal failure if not diagnosed and appropriately treated.

Dental complications: as opioids (illicit or prescribed) dry the mouth, and bacteria which cause decay can reproduce more readily. Combined with poor dental hygiene, this often leads to severe decay, acute or chronic pain, and dental infections.

Constipation: for individuals with opioid use disorder and for patients on opioid maintenance regimens, constipation may be a troublesome complication. Occasionally reduced bowel motility becomes a medically serious complication with gastroparesis or intestinal pseudo-obstruction.

Renal disease: glomerulonephritis or interstitial nephritis may occur with injecting drug use (an uncommon though severe complication).

Psychiatric complications

Depression and anxiety: individuals with opioid use disorder are five times more likely than the general population to have a depressive disorder. As with the general population, these rates are higher in women than men. The rates of anxiety disorders are about three times higher than the general population. Because opioid users are more likely than the general population to be exposed to traumatic events (particularly physical assault), they also have an increased risk of post-traumatic stress disorder. Self-medication of PTSD symptoms with opioids is well recognized.

Protracted abstinence syndrome: after acutely withdrawing from heroin or other opioids, individuals with physical dependence on opioids often continue to feel uncomfortable for up to 6 months. This protracted withdrawal syndrome varies from a vague sense of feeling abnormal to symptoms of low-level lethargy, insomnia, irritability, depression, anxiety, reduced self-esteem, and exaggerated stress reactions. This may be accompanied by mild physiological changes in blood pressure, respiration, and temperature. These symptoms leave the ex-user vulnerable to drug cravings and relapse.

Social complications

The social complications of opioid use disorder are typically considerable:
- While acutely intoxicated the user is vulnerable and may become the victim of violence, sexual abuse, or theft.
- Chronically, because heroin and other opioids for non-medical purposes are illegal and high cost, many users are drawn into crime (drug dealing, theft, etc.) or sex work to make money.
- Many users become victims of violence through association with the illicit drug and criminal scene.
- A history of imprisonment is common (e.g. either for possession or sale of drugs, or for crimes committed to obtain money for drugs). Long periods of imprisonment may disrupt personal relationships and a criminal record may make finding a job very difficult, even when abstinent from illicit drugs.
- Family problems and/or child neglect may occur.
- Considerable marginalization often accompanies illicit drug use and heroin dependence in particular.

Further reading

Cherubin CE, Sapira JD. (1993). The medical complications of drug addiction and the medical assessment of the intravenous drug user 25 years later. *Ann Intern Med* 119:1017–28.

Gordon RJ, Lowy FD. (2005). Bacterial infections in drug users. *N Engl J Med* 353:1945–54.

Identification and brief intervention for opioid misuse

A significant proportion of the opioid users within the community are not yet seeking treatment. They may have only mild opioid use disorder (e.g. episodically smoking or injecting opioids), or may have moderate to severe disorder, but do not wish to stop use.

While the effectiveness of opportunistic brief intervention is not well established the general principles of brief intervention can be considered when offering assistance.

Feedback Most opioid users are well aware of the harms they have experienced through their use, so any feedback is most often given in the form of empathy rather than new information: e.g. 'I can see that your heroin use has been making your life very difficult'. If no harms have been experienced, the clinician can check if the client is aware of the risks associated with use (e.g. physical dependence, blood-borne viruses in injectors).

Listen To the patient's response—is there any ambivalence about opioid use, which can be capitalized on in a motivational interviewing style approach? Is the individual adamant that he or she wishes to continue using? Has the individual tried to stop many times and is ready for assistance?

Advice Convey your medical advice empathically and non-judgementally. This may include, for example, the reflection that if the individual is prepared to go onto opioid maintenance treatment, his/her life would be simpler—he/she would not have to constantly seek the funds for illicit opioids and his/her prospects of remaining/becoming healthy would be greatly improved. Is he/she aware that methadone or buprenorphine are currently the best proven way to cease illicit opioids?

Goals While the clinician's goal will generally be abstinence from illicit opioids (typically achieved through opioid maintenance treatment), the patient may be unwilling or unable to accept this goal at this point. In that case, the patient and clinician may be able to discuss an interim goal, e.g. for an intermittent user, trying to ensure that opioid use not exceed once weekly; or for the physically dependent user who is not willing to cease, safer injecting practices or attending to hepatitis monitoring or treatment of a co-morbid psychiatric condition.

Strategies If the patient is prepared to accept referral to a specialist addiction treatment centre or other opioid maintenance treatment prescriber, suggest that he/she attend to discuss treatment options. If the patient does not want treatment for his/her opioid use disorder, he or she may still be prepared to discuss harm reduction strategies, or approaches for managing co-morbid or complicating physical or psychiatric conditions. It is always important to offer further assistance if or when the patient wishes to change his/her opioid use. Also, if the patient does not want opioid maintenance treatment or naltrexone treatment, it is important to educate the patient about the poor outcomes likely to ensue without medication assisted treatment: physical and mental health deterioration and social and economic instability.

Assessment and management of opioid overdose

Opioid overdose is a life-threatening condition. Take a good medical and drug history if the patient is able to communicate:
- Obtain collateral information if available
- Look for needle track marks
- Look for signs of opioid overdose—typical signs include pin-point pupils and slowed respiration.

Clinical features of opioid overdose

Symptoms
- Nausea, vomiting in opioid naïve individuals
- Drowsiness.

Physical signs
- Stuporose
- Cool moist skin
- Slow deep respiration (2–7/min)
- Hypothermia
- Bradycardia
- Hypotension
- Pin-point pupils (may be dilated if there is brain damage)
- Coma
- Risk of death from respiratory depression.

NB The classic triad in opioid overdose are: unconsciousness, apnoea, and pin point pupils. Generalized seizures may occur in pethidine overdose. Morphine overdose may occasionally be associated with a confusional state, with agitation and, in some cases, psychosis.

Resuscitation

General supportive and symptomatic measures :
- Maintain 'ABC':
  - Airway: Ensure it is patent
  - Breathing, O_2/monitor and maintain oxygen saturation, using artificial respiration if necessary
  - Circulation.
- Administer antidote: administer naloxone 0.4–2 mg IV or, if IV access not available, IM, subcutaneously, or intranasally with atomizer.

For heroin or other short-acting opioid overdose:
- Initial dose 0.4 mg; naloxone has a short half-life the patient may lapse back into a coma.
- Constant observation is essential and it may be necessary to repeat the dose after 15–20 minutes, and then every 30–60 minutes until the level of consciousness is stable.

- Alternatively, nalmefene, which has a much longer half-life than naloxone, can be administered at doses of 0.5 to 1.0mg/kg without as much need for repeated dosing.
- Naloxone is sometimes given outside the hospital. Patients should then go to hospital for observation as opioid withdrawal symptoms may occur.
- If high doses of naloxone are administered quickly to reverse overdose in an opioid-dependent person, a withdrawal reaction may be precipitated, and result in angry and difficult behaviour.

In some centres 'take-home' naloxone ampoules are made available to patients with opioid use disorder so that in the event of an accidental overdose, family or friends can administer the antidote before the emergency services are called. Naloxone can also be administered intranasally by bystanders with use of a nasal atomizer which can be dispensed with the naloxone.

For methadone overdose: methadone has a long half-life (approximately 20 hours). Thus, in cases of methadone overdose, repeated doses of IV naloxone 0.4–2 mg or a 24-hour infusion may be required and the patient should be monitored for up to 72 hours. Alternatively, nalmefene can be used as described earlier.

For buprenorphine overdose: while overdose of buprenorphine by itself is uncommon, there is a possibility of overdose if patients use heroin concurrently in larger than usual doses after ceasing buprenorphine and/or use benzodiazepine or other sedative drugs in association with buprenorphine.
- Buprenorphine has a long half-life and, in rare instances of overdose, the patients should be monitored for more than 72 hours.
- Vasopressor agents may be required.
- Naloxone is of limited usefulness in the treatment of buprenorphine overdose as buprenorphine is not easily displaced by naloxone because of buprenorphine's high affinity for the mu receptor. The dose of naloxone may have to be increased to 15–20 times and assisted ventilation may be required.

Other measures in the management of opioid overdose
- Give IV fluids.
- In rare cases of non-cardiogenic pulmonary oedema, treat as for pulmonary oedema.
- If the patient does not respond to naloxone, and a combination of opioids and benzodiazepine overdose is suspected, consider careful addition of the benzodiazepine antagonist flumazenil (0.5–2 mg by slow IV infusion).

   Warning: flumazenil may precipitate a withdrawal syndrome in benzodiazepine-dependent patients.
- Exclude medical complications of injection drug use (see pp. 259–61), and treat complicating or concurrent medical conditions. Exclude polysubstance overdose: many opioid overdoses also involve alcohol and/or benzodiazepines.

- Exclude other causes of coma: e.g. head injury, metabolic diseases, electrolyte abnormalities.
- Urine drug screen should be obtained with dispatch: although results will typically only be available once the overdose is resolved, they indicate the extent and range of substance use at the time of overdose, which may inform future management.

Further assessment

If the patient is able to provide any history, or if collateral information is available (e.g. from ambulance officers, general practitioner, family or friends), try to assess recency and type/range of drug use (including alcohol), and typical pattern of drug use. Once overdose has resolved and consciousness is fully restored, a full history can be taken, including substance use (recent and usual), medical and psychiatric history (pp. 69–70). A psychiatric assessment is important where there is suspicion of a suicidal intent.

Education and advice

Once overdose has resolved and consciousness is fully restored, provide education and advice about the complications of opioid use, particularly in combination with alcohol, benzodiazepines, and other CNS depressants. Offer referral to an addiction treatment programme for ongoing treatment, support, and encouragement, and/or discuss other agencies and self-help groups.

Management of opioid withdrawal

The intensity of withdrawal symptoms varies with the severity, duration of use, and level of health of the individual. Typical and uncomplicated opioid withdrawal is not life-threatening.

Withdrawal symptoms occur within hours of cessation of heroin (see Table 11.2). The symptoms of opioid withdrawal resemble a flu-like illness with aches and pains, rhinorrhoea, nausea, and vomiting. Insomnia and strong cravings for opioids may be distressing.

Table 11.2 Onset and duration of opioid withdrawal symptoms

Drug	Onset	Peak effect	Duration
Heroin	4–6 h	18–72 h	5–10 days
Methadone	24–48 h	3–4 days	2 to several weeks
Buprenorphine	2–3 days	5 days	Several weeks

Features of opioid withdrawal

Physical symptoms
- Rhinorrhoea
- Sneezing
- Lacrimation
- Sweating
- Hot and cold flushes
- Piloerection ('cold turkey')
- Abdominal cramps
- Nausea, vomiting, diarrhoea
- Bone and muscle aches and cramps.

Neuropsychiatric symptoms
- Insomnia
- Restlessness, anxiety, irritability, agitation
- Depression
- Intense 'craving' ± drug-seeking behaviour.

Physical signs
- Yawning, rhinorrhoea, lacrimation, sneezing
- Tremor
- Fever (low grade)
- Skin:
  - Sweating
  - Piloerection ('cold turkey')
- Cardiovascular system:
  - Tachycardia, hypertension (mild)
- CNS:
  - Restlessness, agitation
  - Dilated pupils.

Management of opioid withdrawal

- An opioid withdrawal syndrome does not necessarily require hospitalization.
- This is appropriate where there is intercurrent illness, severe vomiting, pregnancy, or concurrent benzodiazepine or alcohol dependence or withdrawal.
- Opioid withdrawal can mostly be managed on an ambulatory basis.
- An important question is whether cessation of opioids is a desirable goal, or whether opioid agonist maintenance is to be preferred. *Because of the lowered tolerance that results from detoxification, there is a high risk of subsequent overdose if and when opioid use resumes.*
- Consider whether cessation of opioid use is appropriate or whether agonist maintenance is to be preferred.
- It is not necessary for an opioid user to complete withdrawal from opioids before commencing opioid maintenance treatment.
- If an individual does not wish to have maintenance treatment, or if this is not appropriate or locally available, three options are set out in sections p. 269 to p. 270 for withdrawal management ('detoxification').
- In most cases, tapering doses of buprenorphine treatment provides the simplest and most effective management of withdrawal symptoms. It provides greater rates of completion of detoxification than does symptomatic treatment alone or having a medication-free regimen (going 'cold turkey').
- Buprenorphine provides swifter and safer relief of withdrawal symptoms than methadone because the dose can be increased relatively swiftly, and weaning off buprenorphine also tends to be quicker and easier.
- If buprenorphine is not a feasible option, methadone may be more appropriate (e.g. coincident acute severe pain where methadone may facilitate control of pain; or recent history of long-acting opioid use, where buprenorphine may precipitate a withdrawal reaction).
- In the US, methadone can only be used for treatment of opioid withdrawal in federally licensed opioid treatment programmes. The exception is that any opioid can be administered (not prescribed) over a period of 72 hours while arranging to transition a patient who is in opioid withdrawal into more comprehensive treatment.
- In some countries, rapid or ultra-rapid detoxification using naltrexone is sought by members of the public, often through private treatment providers. The ultra-rapid technique has been demonstrated to have an unacceptable high rate of complications without any better outcomes than seen with simple outpatient withdrawal. Thus, the ultra-rapid technique should not be recommended.
- Whichever of the below-listed options for management of opioid withdrawal symptoms is chosen, general supportive measures such as reassurance, rest, hydration, and good nutrition are useful adjuncts.

Monitor regularly with an opioid withdrawal scale (see Chapter 27).

Short-term detoxification or withdrawal therapy by substitution with small to moderate doses of either methadone or buprenorphine may be used. Buprenorphine typically provides more rapid relief of withdrawal symptoms as doses can be increased more rapidly. However, there is a risk of precipitated opioid withdrawal if buprenorphine is administered too early after use of opioids.

Option 1: Tapering with buprenorphine:

- Before initiation of buprenorphine treatment, wait until at least 12–24 hours after the last dose of heroin or other short-acting opioids or 48–72 hours after low-dose methadone (up to 30 mg methadone per day) until opioid withdrawal signs can be clearly and objectively observed in order to avoid precipitating withdrawal.
- After waiting for the above-mentioned period (day 1), prescribe 4–8 mg sublingually, unless the patient is on high doses of other psychotropic drugs when the dose may need to be limited to two 2 mg doses.
- Sublingual administration is vital, whether in the form of tablets or film; the preparation should dissolve in 5–10 minutes.
- Depending on whether the patient is taking other psychotropic drugs, increase dose by 4–8 mg per day (i.e. 6–16 mg on day 2, and 8–24 mg on day 3).
- From day 4 or 5, depending on response, reduce by 2–4 mg/day to zero.
- If a slow reduction is desired, the dose may be reduced by 2 mg/day down to 8 mg, then by 0.8 mg/day. Once the dose has reached 2 mg reductions may be by 0.4 mg steps.
- In the US, 2 mg is the lowest dosage form available. An alternative strategy is to dose 2 mg every other day or every third day for a few days to a few weeks prior to stopping entirely.
- While recently buprenorphine has been commenced 24 hours after higher doses of methadone (30–60 mg), precipitated withdrawal symptoms are more likely following higher doses.

Option 2: Tapering with methadone:

- There is no need to wait for a prescribed period after the last dose of another opioid before commencing methadone. However, it is important to ensure that there are no signs of opioid toxicity and it is preferable to wait for a withdrawal syndrome to appear.
- Give 20 mg methadone syrup/solution orally on day 1, and further doses of 10 mg 4 and 8 hours later if there are current signs of opioid withdrawal.
- Give 20–40 mg methadone on days 2 and 3.
- From day 4 reduce by 5 mg every day to zero.
- Reduction may be slower if desired.

Note: short-term detoxification does not confer the benefits obtained from longer-term opioid maintenance treatment for relapse prevention, and there is a *high risk of relapse after detoxification with increased risks of death from overdose*. Exposure to medications and to treatment staff in an outpatient or inpatient detoxification setting may encourage later engagement with maintenance therapy. Supervised withdrawal (short-term detox) may also be reasonable if the ultimate plan is to treat a patient with naltrexone.

Option 3: Clonidine (or lofexidine) plus symptomatic treatment

Simple opioid withdrawal symptoms may require no treatment. However, if symptoms are distressing, the following regimen may be instituted:

- *Diazepam:* 5–10 mg orally nocte (or in some cases every 6 hours) for 3–4 days and then taper off over 2–3 days (for insomnia, anxiety, restlessness). Daily dispensing is recommended to reduce the risk of misuse.
- *Hyoscine butylbromide:* 20 mg orally 6-hourly (for abdominal cramps).
- *Loperamide:* if diarrhoea is a problem, give two tablets initially, then one tablet after each unformed stool (maximum four tablets/day) or atropine sulphate: diphenoxylate (Lomotil®) two tablets, three to four times a day.
- *Clonidine:* 150–300 mcg orally (or in some countries lofexidine is used instead) three to four times a day reduces opioid withdrawal symptoms. Clonidine and lofexidine decrease central sympathetic outflow by stimulating central presynaptic inhibitory alpha-2-receptors on the noradrenaline neurons. As they can lower blood pressure, regular monitoring is necessary. If diastolic pressure is lower than 60 mmHg before any dose, omit that dose. Reduce clonidine/lofexidine in a stepwise fashion over a period of 1 week. A small test dose of 50 mcg with monitoring of blood pressure is advisable prior to administering the full dose of clonidine.
- Hydroxyzine or other sedating antihistamines may be used to help with insomnia.
- Ondansetron 4–8 mg every 6 hours PRN for nausea/vomiting.

Note: quinine bisulfate is no longer routinely recommended for the treatment of muscle cramps because of the risk of thrombocytopenia.

Accelerated 'rapid detoxification' or 'ultra-rapid opioid detoxification (UROD)' induced by naltrexone

Naltrexone, a specific mu opioid antagonist that acts by competitively blocking opioid receptors, can precipitate opioid withdrawal if administered soon after use of heroin or other opioids.

- To shorten the period of detoxification, strategies have been used where naltrexone is administered to induce opioid withdrawal either under general anaesthesia ('ultra-rapid opioid detoxification') or light sedation (rapid detoxification).
- The resulting severe opioid withdrawal symptoms are treated symptomatically with clonidine, antiemetics, and sedatives.

- Detoxification is then typically followed by 6–12 months of maintenance treatment with naltrexone to prevent relapse.
- While abstinence rates of more than 60% have been claimed, there is currently insufficient evidence of efficacy or safety to endorse this form of treatment as routine for opioid dependence.
- Naltrexone-induced withdrawal may be severe with vomiting, confusion, agitation, delirium, and depression. The risks of prolonged anaesthesia or sedation are significant themselves.
- As it is associated with greater risks than conventionally treated (or, indeed, untreated heroin withdrawal), in rapid detoxification is employed only as part of formal ethics-approved studies or in selected private clinics. It is not standard practice in most mainstream drug and alcohol treatment units and as noted earlier, it is not recommended.

Sometimes patients and families have unrealistic expectations that rapid (or, indeed, any form of acute) detoxification may 'cure' their opioid dependence in one step. As with all substance dependence, management of the withdrawal syndrome is just an early step in achieving the desired outcome of long-term abstinence. Relapse prevention remains the main challenge.

Assessment

As described in the Chapter 2, comprehensive assessment should include taking a thorough history.

History

Opioid use history: amount, frequency, route, recency, and duration of opioid use

- Quantity of heroin is often described in street grams, quarters (approximately 0.25 g) or points (approximately 0.1 g). In some parts of the US, quantity of heroin is defined by number of 'bags' used. Each bag is generally considered to be 0.05–0.1 g. As the purity of heroin varies, these weights are only very approximate guides to the amounts used.
Patients using primarily prescription opioids can usually describe the type, dosage strength, and number of pills they are using.
- Money spent on heroin or other opioids provides not only an indication of amount being used, but also the likely social impact of use.
- Frequency of use—number of 'hits' per day, number of days per week.
- Route: oral, injected, or inhaled?
- Recency: when was the last hit? Are you 'hanging out' or 'sick' (withdrawing) now?
- Duration of use: age of first use, age when use became daily. Since that time, how many years have you used and how many have you been 'clean' (abstinent from heroin)?

Presence of dependence: in particular, does the individual experience withdrawals between doses of heroin or other opioids or if heroin or other opioids run out?

Types of treatment tried

- What was the longest period of abstinence? How did the patient achieve this?
- What treatment has the patient tried? Why did relapse occur?

Complications of heroin or other opioid use

- In particular, viral hepatitis status (hepatitis B, C) and HIV status: When was the patient last tested? Has the patient been vaccinated against hepatitis B? What are the LFTs findings?

Other drug use history

Including illicit and prescribed; in particular ask about benzodiazepines. Also, alcohol and tobacco use/dependence.

Other medical and psychiatric history

- Past hospitalizations
- Screening questions for mental health disorders, such as 'are you bothered much by anxiety or depression? Have you ever had treatment for a mental health disorder?'

Family history/brief social history: ask if a partner or close friends use heroin.

Medications.

Physical examination
Look for signs of intoxication or withdrawal, and consistency of physical signs with the history of recent drug use. Check for signs of complications of opioid injecting, such as vein damage, stigmata of liver disease, cardiac murmurs.

Laboratory tests
- FBC
- EUC
- LFTs (isolated elevation of ALT suggests chronic hepatitis C infection; levels may fluctuate)
- Serological investigation for blood-borne viruses (see later in topic)
- Tests for STIs
- Urine drug screen—is useful both at initial assessment and as part of monitoring, as an objective measure of heroin or other drug use
- Other tests as indicated:
  - TFTs
  - CPK
  - BSL.

Other investigations as indicated
- Chest X-ray (e.g. if fever)
- CT head/MRI (e.g. potential intra cerebral infection).

Assessment of viral infections
Assessment of viral infections should be undertaken at the treatment clinic or general practice setting as these patients will often not attend another specialty service while still having problems with injection drug use.

> Offer serological testing for hepatitis C and B, and HIV on all patients with a history of injecting drug use, and where appropriate, tests for STIs. In the US, all patients should be tested for HIV regardless of injecting history and all patients born between 1945 and 1960 should be tested for hepatitis C regardless of injecting history.

- Serology for blood-borne viruses:
  - Hepatitis C: anti-HCV
  - If hepatitis C Ab positive, can periodically test HCV RNA (PCR) to assess if viral replication is occurring
  - If HCV RNA positive, further tests to define genotype and viral load if treatment is considered
  - Hepatitis B: HBsAg, anti-HBs, anti-HBc (see later in topic)
  - HIV: anti-HIV

Pre- and post-test counselling is important, not only to avoid stress, but as an opportunity for raising awareness of the risks of blood-borne virus infection associated with injecting drug use, the need for testing for the presence of infection for up to 6 months after the last episode of injecting and for ongoing monitoring should viral hepatitis be present. However, in the US, pre- and post-test counselling are not required as data show that people sometimes do not get tested or do not come back for their results when counselling is required.

Interpretation of hepatitis C serology

- Hep C Ab positive—current or past infection (60–70% of IDUs are anti-HCV positive)
- HCV RNA (PCR) positive—active replication of virus, infectivity
- Hepatitis C genotype (if treatment is being considered)—treatment efficacy varies by genotype.
- All HCV RNA-positive patients should be informed of the availability and efficacy of treatment and offered referral.

Interpretation of hepatitis B serology

- HBsAg positive—acute or chronic infection with hepatitis B:
  - If HBeAg is also positive there is a high level of viral replication, higher level of infectivity, higher risk of progression of HBV liver disease
- Anti-HBc—exposure to the virus:
  - Where HBsAg is negative, core antibody (IgG) represents past exposure to hepatitis B, with possible ongoing infection
- Anti-HBs positive—reflects immune state secondary to either vaccination or past infection.

IDUs who are not immune to hepatitis B should be offered vaccination.

HBsAg-positive patients should have HBV DNA measured, LFTs undertaken, and those with raised ALT or high viral load referred for possible treatment. Family and sexual contacts should be followed up and tested.

In some cases, liver ultrasound and CT scan may be indicated to assess the severity of viral hepatitis, or the presence of a complication, such as cirrhosis and hepatocellular carcinoma.

Serology for HIV

- Anti-HIV positive—probable HIV infection, confirm with HIV RNA PCR
- If positive, refer to an appropriate specialist for monitoring and consideration for treatment.

Management of opioid dependence

After detoxification alone there is a high rate of relapse to opioid dependence. Tolerance to opioids diminishes after periods of abstinence and so relapse is associated with an increased risk of death from overdose. Therefore, it is most important to consider the long-term management of opioid dependence. Treatment can be described according to the ten key components outlined on pp. 107–12, but with particular emphasis on pharmacotherapy.

Information and education

Advice and education are provided. This may employ the principles of motivational interviewing.

Acceptance and engagement

Let the patient digest the information and advice provided, and consider their current status and available options. For treatment to be successful the patient must then reach a point of acceptance of the need to change their opioid use and to develop commitment.

Initiating treatment: detoxification

Opioid detoxification is rarely indicated in IDUs. It has a place prior to entering a residential programme or therapeutic community. Otherwise it should be employed cautiously, given the evidence for increased morbidity and mortality following detoxification. It may be *dangerous* to try to complete withdrawal before commencing methadone or buprenorphine.

Pharmacotherapy: principles of agonist maintenance

Explain treatment options, including that opioid substitution treatment (with methadone, buprenorphine, or buprenorphine/naloxone) is currently the most effective way to help achieve a goal of abstinence from heroin, resume daily work or other important activities, and avoid or minimize harm associated with injecting drug use.

- Long-acting opioids provide relief from craving and withdrawal symptoms, and allow the patient to escape the domination of illicit opioids.
- The large amount of time previously spent getting money to buy heroin or other opioids, being intoxicated, or withdrawing is now freed up by the use of a single daily dose of a supervised, pure, and long-acting opioid.
- Maintenance opioid treatment of heroin or other opioid dependence results in 70% reduction in opioid use and improved treatment retention compared with non-pharmacological treatments, with 40–50% of patients remaining in treatment at 6 months.
- It avoids the multiple complications of injecting drug use, substantially reduces criminal activity and enables re-engagement in routine life.

Legal and administrative requirements in prescribing methadone and buprenorphine

The legal restrictions on prescribing opioid maintenance treatment vary considerably between countries. In Australia, for example, in order to prescribe methadone or buprenorphine to heroin-dependent patients, medical practitioners must be accredited by the state or territory health department after completing a training course. In addition, each patient who is to commence methadone or buprenorphine for treatment of opioid dependence must be approved by the state authority. This is to prevent the same patient presenting for opioids at more than one service.

In addition:

- In the early stages of maintenance, all doses are supervised at a clinic.
- Once a person is stable, they generally have the option of transferring to pharmacy dosing, and gradually increasing the number of unsupervised ('takeaway') doses per week, to a maximum of four takeaways of methadone per week.
- For buprenorphine/naloxone the number of takeaways can be progressively increased so that a very stable patient collects his or her medication from a pharmacy only once a month.
- If a patient is under the age of 18 years a second opinion from an approved prescriber is necessary in some regions. In some regions, patients under the age of 16 years cannot be prescribed methadone unless court approval is obtained.

In the UK, there are fewer restrictions on prescribing, which can be by trained psychiatrists or GPs. Consumption of the opioid dose is usually monitored at community pharmacies or in specialized clinical drug treatment settings, though stable patients may graduate to take supplies home on a weekly basis.

In the US, physicians must obtain a waiver from the federal Center for Substance Abuse Treatment and the Drug Enforcement Agency to prescribe buprenorphine or buprenorphine/naloxone. Typically the waiver is obtained by completing an 8-hour training course. The physician prescribing the buprenorphine or buprenorphine/naloxone writes a prescription for the medication that the patient obtains at a pharmacy. The physician determines the amount of medication to prescribe. Methadone can only be dispensed from federally regulated opioid treatment programmes. Patients can get take-home doses of methadone based upon their time and stability in treatment with a maximum of 30 take-home doses at one time.

Methadone maintenance

Induction on to methadone maintenance

Informed consent should always be obtained from the patient before entry into an opioid maintenance programme.

- Commence treatment with 20–30 mg methadone orally daily. Maximum starting dose is 40 mg to avoid risk of overdose. In the US, the maximum initial dose is 30 mg.
- An additional 10 mg can be given if the patient shows evidence of withdrawal signs 2 hours after the initial dose.
- If the patient has been abstinent from heroin for a period of time, starting dose should be low (e.g. 10–20 mg).
- Do not administer methadone if patient is drowsy or intoxicated.
- Steady state levels are reached by 5–7 days.

- During the induction phase, patients should be reviewed daily (e.g. by a nurse or doctor).
- Increase the dose of methadone by increments of 5 mg every 3 or 4 days until the patient is stable. Do not give more than 40 mg daily in the first week. Such a dose should relieve cravings and withdrawal.
- Increase gradually to a maintenance dose of 60–80 mg/day to relieve withdrawal symptoms and facilitate their ceasing heroin or other opioid use. However, a higher dose, in the range of 80–120 mg/day, is considered optimum for most.
- Some patients may require considerably higher doses, and if there is ongoing regular heroin or other opioid use, the patient should be given an increased dose of methadone so that any resumption of opioid use is less likely to produce significant euphoria. In addition to increasing the methadone dose it may also be useful to try to address this via behavioural means (e.g. ensuring they have an activity with a non-using friend organized for pay day).
- In some countries, a second specialist opinion is required for doses exceeding 150 mg or 200 mg daily (e.g. this is required in Australia for a dose over 200 mg, but there is no such requirement in the US).
- Approximately 10% of individuals are rapid metabolizers of methadone; standard doses do not achieve therapeutic plasma concentrations.
  - If clinically a patient seems to require a dose greater than 200 mg, firstly measure trough (i.e. before the day's methadone dose is due) and peak (i.e. 3–4 hours after dose) methadone levels, to document that plasma levels are low despite adequate attendance at dosing.
  - An ideal peak to trough ratio is 2:1. Individuals who have a peak to trough ratio of greater than 2:1 are likely to be rapid metabolizers.
  - For rapid metabolizers twice-daily methadone dosing should be considered.
  - If contemplating a single daily large dose, perform an ECG to check for QTc prolongation which is a side effect of methadone. Some rapid metabolizers of methadone may need to switch drugs.
- The patient should be maintained at an adequate dose for an indefinite period. Most patients prefer and do well with ongoing maintenance.

Cessation of methadone

If the patient wishes to cease methadone maintenance treatment:
- First ascertain that the patient has been free of illicit drug and problematic alcohol use for a prolonged period of time (at least 1 year), that any medical or psychiatric disorders are well stabilized, that the patient is engaged in productive activities, and that the patient has adequate social support.
- Then reduce the dose by 2.5–5 mg every 1–2 weeks or slower if necessary, to zero. If there is no need for haste, reducing by 2.5 mg fortnightly often ensures a smooth and relatively symptom-free reduction in dose.

- At this rate it is often only when methadone doses fall below 40 mg that withdrawal symptoms are felt.
- If withdrawal symptoms have become problematic by the time the methadone dose has fallen to less than 30 mg daily, the patient may transfer to buprenorphine maintenance at least 24 hours after the last dose of low-dose methadone (see following section on maintenance).
- Reassure the patient that if at any time the patient becomes uncomfortable, the dosage can be increased and/or the taper can be held at the current dose for as long as necessary. Oftentimes stable patients are satisfied with a dose reduction and do not continue to request coming completely off methadone.

Buprenorphine maintenance

Buprenorphine is a partial opioid agonist with high receptor affinity but low activity, so to avoid precipitating withdrawals, wait at least 8 hours after the last dose of heroin or other short-acting opioids. Longer periods of time are needed following longer-acting opioids.

Induction on to buprenorphine maintenance

- The prescriber must ascertain that the patient is in moderate opioid withdrawal as evidenced by objectively observable signs (not self-reported symptoms) of withdrawal.
- When the patient exhibits observable signs of withdrawal, buprenorphine can be initiated at a dosage of 2–4 mg sublingually. Usually this dosage will begin to alleviate withdrawal signs and symptoms within 30–60 minutes. Additional 2 mg to 4 mg doses can be taken by the patient sequentially throughout the first day to alleviate any residual withdrawal symptoms to a total dose on day 1 of 8–16 mg.
- Note that if the combination preparation Suboxone® is used, the buprenorphine dose is as above; the amount of naloxone in this preparation is 25% of the buprenorphine (i.e. 0.5 mg with 2 mg buprenorphine).
- Thereafter, increase buprenorphine by 2–4 mg daily until the patient is comfortable up to a maximum daily dose of 32 mg/day. Most patients need a minimum of 16 mg. Every effort should be made to achieve a stable dose (no withdrawal symptoms, no cravings, no illicit opioid use, and minimal side effects) within the first several days of treatment.
- *Be very cautious about patients who are taking other psychotropic drugs (prescribed or unapproved).* The above-described induction schedule reduces the risk of CNS interactions which can produce undue sedation, which can (rarely) have fatal results.
- If the prescriber is convinced that no other sedating drugs are being taken, the dose of buprenorphine can be increased if necessary to 32 mg by the end of day 2.
- Patients who have already been withdrawn from opioids and for whom withdrawal signs and symptoms have been documented to have resolved should get an initial dose of 2 mg buprenorphine, with

very gradual dose titration upward to a therapeutic dose to avoid initial intoxication since they may have lower tolerance.

- Clinician experience plays an important role in the success of buprenorphine induction. Clinician discomfort with a new medication and anxiety about precipitating opioid withdrawal in the patient lead to anxiety about buprenorphine induction among clinicians new to buprenorphine prescribing. Patients tend to sense and share this clinician anxiety and they do not do as well.
- Withdrawal in each individual can be estimated by having the patient recall his/her experience of previous withdrawal on a scale of 1 to 10, 1 being no withdrawal and 10 being the worst ever. Moderate withdrawal would be a score of 5–7 and it is generally safe to administer the first dose of buprenorphine at that point.
- The patient should be advised against using heroin, street methadone, or other opioids during the period of dose stabilization. If he/she does, difficulties in dose stabilization and opioid withdrawal symptoms (in the case of buprenorphine) may develop and require symptomatic treatment. Overdose is a risk particularly with the combination of heroin and methadone.
- Side effects of buprenorphine are typically few. Many people report feeling very normal on buprenorphine. Headache and nausea may occur, and may suggest the need for a lower dose. A 'racing' or 'speed-like' effect has been reported with buprenorphine. This tends to resolve with a lower dose.

Cessation of buprenorphine

- If the patient wishes to cease buprenorphine treatment, firstly ascertain that the patient has been free of illicit opioid use and problematic alcohol use for a prolonged period, that any medical or psychiatric disorders are well stabilized, that the patient is engaged in productive activities, and that the patient has adequate social support.
- Then reduce the dose by 2 mg weekly (or more slowly or rapidly as tolerated) to zero.
- To avoid insomnia after cessation of buprenorphine, the final stages of reduction (e.g. once the patient has reached 2 mg daily) can be slowed down to 0.4 mg weekly. In the US, the 2 mg dose is the lowest available. The patient could take 2 mg on alternate days as an alternative to a dose lower than 2 mg.
- For most patients, weaning off buprenorphine is relatively symptom-free when conducted at this pace, although many patients have considerable difficulty moving from 4 mg or 2 mg to zero. These patients can be encouraged to remain on this low dosage as long as needed and consider trying to taper down again sometime in the future.

Advantages of buprenorphine

- Long duration of action:
  - Alternate-day dosing is typically possible, using double the dose, up to a maximum of 32 mg
  - In some patients higher doses (triple dose to a maximum of 32 mg) can used to provide 3-day weekend cover
- Less euphoria
- Less sedation than methadone—'feel more normal' (though not all want to)
- Less severe withdrawals on dose reduction and cessation
- Relatively safe in overdose because of 'ceiling effect', e.g. if accidentally taken by children.

Disadvantages of buprenorphine

- Easy diversion if not properly supervised
- May precipitate withdrawals in opioid-dependent patients (if care is not taken to document observable signs of withdrawal prior to administration of first dose)
- Naloxone is only partially effective in overdose; dose of naloxone may have to be increased to 15–20 times, and assisted ventilation may be required.

Precautions with buprenorphine

Drug interactions

- MAOIs
- CNS depressants: alcohol, benzodiazepines, antihistamines, tricyclic antidepressants, major tranquillizers (additive depressant effect). *Deaths have been reported following the combined use of buprenorphine with benzodiazepines and/or alcohol*
- Hepatic CYP3A4 enzyme inhibitors: slow the metabolism of buprenorphine: protease inhibitors, antimycotics, calcium channel blockers; macrolide antibiotics, fluoxetine and fluvoxamine (particularly the latter)
- Hepatic CYP3A4 enzyme inducers: metabolism is enhanced by phenobarbital, rifampicin, phenytoin, carbamazepine, and cortisol.

Concomitant medical conditions

- As for all opioids: use with caution where there is recent head injury, acute abdomen, or chronic airways limitation
- Significant liver disease.

Concomitant conditions

- Pregnancy: is listed as a contraindication to buprenorphine by the manufacturers some countries but not in the UK, US, and many European countries. There is a growing body of evidence to the safety of buprenorphine if the patient wants to use it.

Contraindications

- Acute intoxication with alcohol or other CNS depressants
- Severe hepatic or renal insufficiency
- The buprenorphine/naloxone product is contraindicated in pregnancy.

Principles of methadone maintenance and buprenorphine maintenance treatment

- Initial doses must be modest (no more than 40 mg with methadone and 8 mg with buprenorphine).
- Approximately four half-lives are needed to achieve steady state trough levels, i.e. about 4–6 days for methadone and may be 5–10 or more days for buprenorphine.
- Drug interactions: methadone and buprenorphine both are metabolized by some common pathways such as cytochrome P450. Fluoxetine and fluvoxamine both inhibit the breakdown of agonist treatments, most substantially with the latter. Metabolism is enhanced by rifampicin, phenytoin, carbamazepine, efavirenz, nevirapine and cortisol. Antiretroviral zidovudine metabolism is slowed by methadone but not by buprenorphine.
- Optimal doses of methadone are typically 80–120 mg. Usually dose is titrated according to clinical response.
- Optimal doses of buprenorphine are typically in the 12–24 mg range. Maximum dose is 32mg for daily or second daily dosing.

Buprenorphine/naloxone maintenance

Buprenorphine/naloxone is a combination tablet or film containing buprenorphine and naloxone in the ratio 4:1. It is taken sublingually in a dose of buprenorphine the same as that of buprenorphine alone. Naloxone, a mu opioid receptor blocker, has extremely poor bioavailability and minimal effect when taken sublingually/orally. It is added to buprenorphine in order to prevent diversion and illicit intravenous use, as naloxone is active when administered intravenously. This means that if the buprenorphine/naloxone combination is injected intravenously, naloxone will to some extent block the effect of buprenorphine, but more importantly it will precipitate withdrawal in opioid-dependent people. In this way diversion to replace street heroin use is reduced. The combination has the advantage of increasing the possibility of unsupervised takeaways. The buprenorphine–naloxone combination is contraindicated in pregnancy, and the need for contraception is required if considering it.

Choosing between methadone and buprenorphine/naloxone

Patients will often have a strong preference as to which form of opioid maintenance treatment they prefer. There is not yet a firm evidence base to guide choice, but clinical practice suggests that:
- methadone may offer advantages to patients:
  - where craving is not adequately relieved with maximal doses of buprenorphine
  - where engagement has been (or is predicted to be) difficult with buprenorphine, e.g. challenging behaviour, severe opioid dependence. The fact that withdrawal is experienced earlier after a missed dose of methadone encourages more regular attendance
- buprenorphine may offer particular advantages to patients:
  - who have a shorter duration of opioid dependence, or less severe dependence
  - who prefer to avoid any sedating side effects
  - who need the flexibility of future takeaway (unsupervised) doses, e.g. for work. Because of the relative safety of the buprenorphine/naloxone formulation, in some regions, in a very stable patient, tablets can be dispensed monthly
  - who are known to be fast metabolizers of methadone or are on medications that will interact with methadone, more than with buprenorphine or who have QTc prolongation with methadone.

Prescribing methadone or buprenorphine for inpatients

If a patient is documented to be already on methadone maintenance, methadone is continued in hospital unless specific contraindications like head injury or unconsciousness are present. It is important to check the date and amount of the last dose given with the dispensing point.
- If oral dosing is impractical, a reduced dose (e.g. two-thirds the oral dose is often given intramuscularly as divided twice-daily doses).
- Patients on methadone who experience acute pain (e.g. with fractures) and who require opiate analgesia will typically need the analgesia in addition to their usual dose of methadone. Forms of analgesia which are not compromised by opioid tolerance, such as tramadol (which has serotonergic, as well as opioid actions), or strong non-steroidal anti-inflammatory drugs (e.g. ketorolac) may provide relief for some patients.
- If a patient has heroin dependence and is not yet on methadone or buprenorphine, they can be offered the option of commencing maintenance treatment while in hospital, provided that a prescriber and dosing point will be available when they leave hospital. Informed consent should be obtained, as per standard induction onto treatment. In the US, such patients could only be offered buprenorphine by a physician approved by the Federal government to prescribe it. They could not be offered methadone unless it is for pain or a federally licensed programme has admitted the patient and is dispensing it. The exception is that any physician can administer an opioid medication for up to 72 hours while arranging to get the patient into more comprehensive treatment.

Follow-up and monitoring for out-patients on opioid maintenance treatment
A nurse, pharmacist, or doctor assesses whether the patient is over-dosed or withdrawing at the time of each supervised dose.

The prescribing doctor reviews the patient on the methadone or buprenorphine programme regularly with urine drug screens as required, initially at weekly intervals. Once stable, the patient is reviewed at monthly to three-monthly intervals. At review, recent drug use is assessed and the patient is examined for fresh needle track marks and signs of opioid intoxication or withdrawal.

In drug and alcohol treatment services a case worker is typically allocated who:
- monitors progress
- provides support, advice, and counselling
- assesses and monitors any concerns in relation to any children under the care of the patient
- assists with (or refers for assistance with) accommodation, employment, and other needs
- provides harm minimization interventions where indicated.

Missed doses of opioid maintenance treatment
As tolerance to opioids can diminish with a period of opioid abstinence, if a patient misses three or more doses of maintenance treatment the dose should be reduced.

Methadone
- Patients who miss three to five consecutive doses need assessment for the extent of intervening opioid use and presence of intoxication or withdrawal. Then the previous dose is usually reduced, as tolerance may have decreased then increased back to the original dose over the ensuing days with careful monitoring.
- If the patient has missed more than five doses, the reinduction strategy needs to be patient specific and should err on the side of caution to avoid inadvertent methadone intoxication or overdose.

Buprenorphine
- Patients who miss one or two doses of buprenorphine may receive the usual dose subsequently (this dose should always be at least 8–12 hours after any heroin use)
- Patients who miss 3–5 days consecutive daily dosing (or of alternative day dosing):
  - If there is no likelihood of precipitated opioid withdrawals (no heroin in the past 8–12 hours, no long-acting opioids in the past 24 hours), the next dose of buprenorphine is administered in a dose of half to two-thirds of the usual dose, up to a maximum of 24 mg. The dose is increased gradually back to the usual dose
  - The patient who has used heroin in the past 8–12 hours should be asked to re-present after more than 4 hours to assess for intoxication or withdrawal.
- Patients who miss more than five consecutive doses require re-induction onto buprenorphine as per the initial induction regimen.

Switching opioid maintenance medications

From methadone to buprenorphine:

• Slowly taper the dose of methadone to preferably less than 30 mg/day (wherever possible not more than 40 mg/day). Maintain on this dose for at least 1 week.

• To avoid precipitating opioid withdrawals, wait 48–72 hours after the last dose of methadone and observe for signs of opioid withdrawal before commencing buprenorphine. Signs of withdrawal may be very subtle in early stages of methadone withdrawal.

Starting dose:

• 2–4 mg buprenorphine as initial dose; withdrawal signs and symptoms should be decreased after 30–60 minutes.

• If so, give additional doses in office or at home until withdrawal symptoms and craving fully abate, usually between 8 mg and 16 mg on day 1.

• Then increase by 2–4 mg/day according to response to maximum of 32 mg/day.

In some centres there have been recent trials of transferring patients from higher doses of methadone to buprenorphine, but in these situations, precipitated withdrawal is likely. Transfers from higher dose of methadone should generally be undertaken by a specialist unit and, in some cases, as an in-patient.

From buprenorphine to methadone:

• Taper dose of buprenorphine to approximately 16 mg/day for several days before transfer.

• Wait at least 24 hours before commencing methadone 20–30 mg/day (maximum daily dose 40 mg).

• Increase by 5 mg methadone every 3–4 days until stabilization is achieved.

Pregnancy

In the latter half of pregnancy, methadone requirements may increase gradually. Then, typically after the baby is born, the dose may need to be reduced somewhat. In each case, dosage is titrated against clinical symptoms.

In the US, buprenorphine is recognized as a reasonable alternative to methadone for use in pregnancy and certainly may be the only option in areas where federally licensed opioid treatment programmes do not exist. Evidence suggests that neonatal abstinence syndrome in infants born to mothers on buprenorphine is not as severe as the abstinence syndrome in infants born to mothers on methadone.

Concurrent benzodiazepine use

Up to 35% of patients in an opioid treatment programme are known to use benzodiazepines. This may emerge via the history or via routine urine drug screen (which should always test for benzodiazepines). The concurrent use of benzodiazepines carries the additional risk of overdose, especially if either drug is used IV.

When a patient is dependent on benzodiazepines, a supervised benzodiazepine reduction regimen may be required once opioid treatment is stabilized (p. 319).

How long should maintenance treatment be continued?

Patients should be on opioid maintenance treatment for as long as is necessary to achieve stability. Not infrequently, achieving recovery from drug addiction and functional stability requires many years. Patients should stay on maintenance as long as they and their physician find it beneficial. Not all patients feel safe to stop opioid maintenance treatment and their self-assessment of risk of relapse is important. Lifelong maintenance is not an unreasonable course.

If the patient has been free from illicit heroin and other opioid and illicit drug use and free from hazardous alcohol use (preferably for at least 1 year), his/her life is relatively stable, and he/she would like to commence reduction of maintenance treatment, a gradual reduction of dose can be planned with the patient. In many centres, a flexible prescription can be written so that the patient has the option to reduce their dose (by a defined amount) when he/she feels comfortable to do so.

Weaning off maintenance treatment

Weaning off methadone

- Slowly reducing the dose to zero may take weeks to several years
- For methadone maintenance—reduce by 2.5–5 mg every 1–2 weeks or slower if necessary to zero
- Ideally, 2.5 mg reduction no more than fortnightly, to minimize withdrawal
- If withdrawal is troublesome despite a slow rate of dose reduction, the patient can switch to buprenorphine
- The switch to buprenorphine is easier if methadone dose has been 30 mg or lower for at least a week.

Weaning off buprenorphine

- For buprenorphine maintenance—reduce the dose by 2 mg weekly down to a dose of 2 mg. The rate of reduction may then be slowed to 0.4 mg weekly, or 2 mg can be taken every other day.

There are typically fewer withdrawal symptoms when weaning off buprenorphine than off methadone.

Heroin maintenance

Trials of heroin maintenance treatment have been undertaken in some centres in the UK. In some countries like the UK and Switzerland, heroin prescription has been a niche treatment for a small number of heroin-dependent individuals. There has been some resurgence of interest in heroin prescription in recent years with findings from controlled trials in Canada, Switzerland, the Netherlands, and now the UK.

NB Opioid maintenance therapy is often called 'opioid substitution therapy' which gives rise to the mistaken idea that the essence of the treatment is to substitute one legal drug for the other illegal drug. In reality the aim of maintenance treatment is to prevent relapse, and relapse is a matter of memory—drug memory. So for maintenance treatment to be successful, patients must be helped and guided to substitute the drug-use memories with non-drug memories by doing non-drug-related activities repeatedly until they becomes habits embedded in their memories that form the basis of their new life. Only then is it possible for them to successfully get off maintenance opioids. The question is often asked when a patient should get off opioid substitution therapy. The answer, simply put, is this: get a life, and then get off.

Dealing with other challenging situations

Detailed guidelines are available to assist with situations such as missed doses, accidental overdosing, and vomited doses

Further reading

Department of Health (England) and the devolved administrations (2007). *Drug Misuse and Dependence—Guidelines on Clinical Management.* London: Department of Health (England), the Scottish Government, Welsh Assembly Government and Northern Ireland Executive. Available at: http://www.nta.nhs.uk/publications/documents/clinical_guidelines_2007.pdf

Lintzeris N, Clark N, Winstock A, et al. *National Clinical Guidelines and Procedures for the use of Buprenorphine in the Treatment of Opioid Dependence.* Canberra: Australian Government Department of Health and Ageing 2006. Available at: http://www.nationaldrugstrategy.gov.au/internet/drugstrategy/publishing.nsf/Content/buprenorphine-guide

NSW Health. New South Wales Opioid Treatment Programme (2014). *Clinical Guidelines for Methadone and Buprenorphine Treatment of Opioid Dependence.* Sydney: Mental Health and Drug and Alcohol Office, New South Wales Health.

Saxon AJ. (2013). Treatment of opioid dependence. In Ko M-C, Husbands SM (eds) *Research and Development of Opioid-Related Ligands*, pp. 61–102. New York: Oxford University Press.

Treatment with an opioid antagonist: naltrexone

Pharmacology

Naltrexone, a mu (and delta and kappa) antagonist, acts by competitively blocking opioid receptors. It possesses no intrinsic opioid-like effects, and there is no risk of dependence.

- Peak plasma levels after oral administration are reached in 1 hour. It is metabolized in the liver to 6-beta naltrexol and excreted primarily in the urine. The half-life of naltrexone is about 4 hours and that of 6-beta naltrexol is 12 hours.

- Unlike naloxone, naltrexone is effective orally and the longer duration of action enables once-daily dosage. Naltrexone is also available in an extended-release intramuscular injection formulation that typically provides mu-opioid antagonism for 30 days and therefore can be given monthly. Administration of this formulation obviates concerns about adherence to oral medications.

Naltrexone is an alternative to methadone and buprenorphine for relapse prevention in opioid-dependent patients who do not want opioid agonist therapy. It is indicated as part of a comprehensive treatment and rehabilitation programme with psychosocial support, individual and family counselling, and follow-up to enhance dosing adherence. It works best in individuals for whom adherence can be made mandatory via negative contingency, such as doctors and pharmacists.

As naltrexone may precipitate severe opioid withdrawal symptoms if taken soon after dependent patients have recently used opioids, treatment should not be initiated until the patient has remained heroin- and opioid-free for at least 7–10 days. This is best achieved by a period of detoxification either in a detoxification unit or at home under professional supervision.

An opioid-free state is verified by urine drug screens and a naloxone challenge test. If signs and symptoms of opioid withdrawal are observed after the challenge, a waiting period of 24 hours is recommended before repeating the challenge. Because of the long half-life of methadone (approximately 20 hours) or buprenorphine (up to 72 hours depending on the dose), a drug-free period for 10–14 days is recommended prior to initiating treatment with naltrexone, although some patients can make the transition more rapidly.

Patient acceptability of naltrexone has been poor, and lack of adherence and high drop-out rates, particularly in the first month of treatment, are commonly encountered. Early experience with the extended-release injection indicates it may have greater acceptability than the oral form. More work is needed to determine how efficacious the injection will be in clinical practice. While on naltrexone, self-administration of heroin or other opioids has little or no effect unless high doses are used.

Precautions with naltrexone
- Patients with chronic pain on opioid analgesics.
- Discontinue for at least 72 hours prior to elective surgery. In emergencies, blockade may be overcome by greater-than-normal doses of opioids, but this carries the risk of respiratory depression and histamine release.

Naltrexone treatment in opioid dependence
- A relapse prevention medication.
- Will precipitate withdrawal if given to people who are physiologically dependent, thus requires detoxification with naloxone challenge to verify absence of physiological dependence before starting treatment.
- Available since the 1970s as a 50 mg tablet that blocks opioid effects for 24–36 hours and must be taken daily.
- Compliance with the tablet has been a major limitation—needs high patient commitment.
- Development of extended-release formulations (Vivitrol®, Prodetoxon®) has attenuated compliance problems in the short term; longer-term adherence remains unknown and is being studied. Naltrexone implants are available in some countries.
- Concerns about increasing risk for overdose—but seem no greater than those associated with detoxification.

- No apparent interactions with antiretroviral therapies.
- Potential for use in correctional facilities likely to reduce risk for relapse and overdose if given before reentry, and may increase enrolment in longer-term treatment.
- Comprehensive treatment and rehabilitation programme with counselling, psychosocial support, and follow-up to enhance compliance likely to improve treatment outcome.

Side effects
- More than 10% patients may complain of non-specific side effects, mainly gastrointestinal symptoms
- Depression
- Anxiety, nervousness
- Low energy
- Headache, joint, and muscular pain
- Hepatocellular injury if used in doses substantially higher than those shown effective and approved for preventing opioid relapse.

Further reading

Bell J, Kimber J, Lintzeris N, *et al.* (2003). *Clinical Guidelines and Procedures for the Use of Naltrexone in the Treatment of Opioid Dependence.* Canberra: Australian Government Department of Health and Ageing. Available at: http://www.health.gov.au/internet/wcms/publishing.nsf/Content/health-pubhlth-publicat-drugpubs.htm/$FILE/naltrexone_cguide.pdf

Krupitsky E, Nunes EV, Ling W, *et al.* (2011). Injectable extended-release naltrexone for opioid dependence: a double-blind, placebo-controlled, multicenter randomized trial. *Lancet* 377:1506–13.

Krupitsky EM, Zvartau EE, Blokhina E, *et al.* (2012) Randomized trial of long acting sustain-release naltrexone implant vs. oral naltrexone or placebo for preventing relapse to opioid dependence. *Arch Gen Psych* 69(9):973–81.

Saxon AJ. (2013). Treatment of opioid dependence. In Ko M-C, Husbands SM (eds) *Research and Development of Opioid-Related Ligands,* pp. 61–102. New York: Oxford University Press.

Woody GE, Metzger DS. (2011) Injectable extended release naltrexone for opioid dependence. *Lancet* 378:664–5.

Psychological therapies

Psychosocial and psychological therapies can be provided to some extent by the treating doctor, but in many cases, referring the patient to a psychologist or counsellor has significant advantages. As well as supportive counselling, a number of specific approaches are commonly employed:

- *Motivational enhancement therapy:* can be used to help enhance engagement with treatment (initially and on an ongoing basis), and to address illicit opioid use.
- *Cognitive behavioural therapy:* e.g. may include increasing understanding and methods for dealing with the triggers to drug use; training to enhance skills in problem-solving, assertiveness, communication, behavioural self-management, relaxation, stress or anger management, or alcohol and drug refusal.
- *Dialectical behavioural therapy* is suitable for patients after an initial course of the above-listed therapies, particularly when unresolved personal issues or personality difficulties are evident.

- A range of other approaches are employed in some centres, such as behaviour modification programmes (e.g. community reinforcement approach; contingency management).

Identification and treatment of co-morbid physical disorders

Comprehensive treatment of patients with opioid dependence requires parallel treatment of medical complications (e.g. of hepatitis C).

Monitoring and management of blood-borne virus infection

Patients often believe that if they feel well there is no need for monitoring or treatment for blood-borne viruses. The patient should be well educated about the value of monitoring as an early warning system should harms or disease progression occur.

Hepatitis C

Patients with chronic hepatitis C infection are generally asymptomatic. If symptoms occur, the main symptom is tiredness or lethargy.

- Any patient who is positive for hepatitis C antibody needs regular monitoring of LFTs (usually twice yearly) and periodic monitoring of HCV RNA, unless he or she has cleared the virus (HCV RNA negative). Viral clearance without treatment occurs in 20–30% of cases.
- Treatments for HCV have improved at a spectacular rate, with sustained viral response rates (SVRs), which equate to viral clearance, rising from 20% in the 1990s to 95% currently with new oral agents. The need for pegylated interferon and up to 12 months of therapy will no longer be an issue for the vast majority of patients. Treatments will be based on oral agents, some of which are already approved in the US, Europe (simeprevir and sofosbuvir), and Australia (simeprevir). Treatment duration may fall to only 8 weeks for some new combinations of oral direct acting antivirals (DAAs). New agents include sofosbuvir, ledipasvir, faldaprevir, asunaprevir, daclatasvir, ombitasvir, paritaprevir, dasabuvir, and ritonavir. One or other of these is prescribed usually in combination with at least one other drug.
- All HCV RNA-positive patients should be informed of treatment availability and efficacy. If HCV RNA remains positive it indicates active replication of the virus as well as infectivity. Such patients should be fully assessed, informed of the state of their liver disease, and encouraged to consider treatment to prevent progression of the disease and further spread of hepatitis C viral infection. Often, the challenge of undertaking treatment is the turning point in their drug using lifestyle. While new drugs appear to work well for all genotypes it is still appropriate to check genotype and viral load in all patients considering treatment.
- Where there is persistent LFT elevation or evidence of declining liver function (e.g. falling platelets or rising INR, even in the presence of normal LFTs), referral to a liver specialist should be particularly prompt.

- Assessment for treatment will usually include liver ultrasound and or CT scan. Liver biopsy still provides much information about liver disease stage and severity but in most countries it is not a prerequisite for treatment. Many units use transient elastography to assess fibrosis stage of HCV.
- All patients with hepatitis C should be advised not to drink alcohol to excess as this aggravates viral hepatitis. There is not clear evidence as to what level of drinking is safe in this condition. Some clinicians advise limiting consumption to half the recommended limit for a healthy person, and ensuring the consumption is not daily.
- Patients should be educated on avoiding spread of hepatitis C (e.g. taking care with blood spills, avoid sharing toothbrush, comb, or razor where there may be microscopic blood transfer).

Hepatitis B

IDUs who are not immune to hepatitis B should be offered vaccination. Patients who are positive for hepatitis B antigen should have an HBV DNA ordered and liver function assessed prior to referral for possible treatment, and their contacts followed-up and tested. Advice on preventing spread should be provided (e.g. vaccination of key contacts, protected sex with non-immune partners).

In people with established cirrhosis, regular monitoring will include 6-monthly abdominal ultrasound and (possibly) AFP, to screen for hepatocellular carcinoma. Treatment and monitoring will be conducted in association with a liver specialist.

HIV

Patients who are positive for HIV Ab should be referred to the appropriate HIV specialist (e.g. immunology or infectious diseases specialist) to assess the need for treatment and for monitoring.

Identification and treatment of co-morbid psychiatric disorders

Depression and anxiety: for some individuals, opioids may be used to self-medicate a pre-existing depression. However, for a significant number, depressive symptoms remit once the individual's opioid problem is treated. This suggests the symptoms may be caused by the stresses and chaotic lifestyle associated with the disorder, as well as the pharmacological instability related to altering states of intoxication and withdrawal.

- As a general guideline, consider starting an antidepressant medication if the depression persists for more than 4 weeks after initiating treatment, or there is a clear history of depression during previous periods of abstinence for 4 weeks or more.
- Depressed patients with hepatitis C require treatment of depression prior to commencing treatment with interferon as untreated or severe depression is a contraindication to treatment.
- Patients with opioid use disorder also have high rates of anxiety disorders and post-traumatic stress disorder which, if present, should be treated. Use of benzodiazepines should be avoided if at all possible for treating these disorders in this population.

Protracted abstinence syndrome: there is no proven effective treatment for symptoms such as insomnia, lethargy, irritability, depression, anxiety, reduced self-esteem, and an abnormal response to stressful experience. The patient should be reassured that the symptoms are normal, and will improve and abate over time. Some patients do have some response to clonidine or hydroxyzine. Cognitive behavioural strategies may be useful to help the individual gain some control over the symptoms. Some patients with pre-existing anxiety or depressive disorders will find these re-emerge once they withdraw from opioids and medication should be instituted in such cases.

Family and social support
Families of users require support, assistance, and advice on how to cope with living/interacting with the user. Families also need information and advice on how to best support and help the user.

Self-help (mutual-help) organizations
Narcotics Anonymous (NA): as with AA for alcohol dependence, NA can be offered to opioid-dependent patients who are seeking to maintain abstinence, particularly those who are not taking opioid maintenance treatment. NA groups have traditionally discouraged opioid maintenance treatment, so patients on opioid maintenance treatment are not generally referred to NA.

Nar-Anon and Nalteen are associated organizations developed to provide education and support for partners and teenage children of drug-dependent patients.

Aftercare
Regular monitoring and support, and the maintenance of a therapeutic relationship are highly important. At follow-up the clinician can regularly reassess the situation (gathering new information, revising diagnoses and treatment plans accordingly).

While the cost-effectiveness of residential inpatient treatment and rehabilitation programmes is subject to debate, residential in-patient treatment programmes are appropriate for some patients who have failed to respond to out-patient treatment, who are polysubstance users (e.g. alcohol and/or benzodiazepines, or chaotic stimulant use), have no social support, and who have co-morbid psychiatric or medical illnesses. Such programmes have demonstrated efficacy.

In addition to providing food and shelter and some 'time out' in a safer environment, residential treatment programmes provide a structured daily routine and staff-directed programmes, and daily activities. Ideally, the programmes should be tailored according to the needs of individual patients.

Patients with severe coexisting psychiatric or medical problems who are unable to look after themselves may require longer-term care either in residential facilities or in a nursing home.

Changes to lifestyle, home, and environment

Many heroin-dependent individuals find they are only able to cease illicit opioid use by reducing or cutting off contact with heroin-using friends.

Re-engaging with activities of normal living (e.g. training, employment, or recreation), helps reduce boredom, improves self-esteem, and reduces the risk of drug use. Simple measures like increasing level of exercise can improve mood and self-esteem, and reduce the risk of relapse. Where the individual has unstable or unsuitable housing, assisting them to address this can have an important impact on drug use.

Further reading

Teesson M, Mills K, Ross J, et al. (2008). The impact of treatment on 3 years' outcome for heroin dependence: findings from the Australian Treatment Outcome Study (ATOS). *Addiction* 103:80–8.

Harm reduction/palliation

It is common for some individuals to continue to inject drugs in the induction phase of opioid maintenance treatment, until adequate doses are reached. Other individuals have great difficulty totally eliminating injection drug use, and sporadic use continues while on treatment. Even while efforts proceed to help the individual cease heroin use, it is important to provide realistic harm-reduction advice.

Patients on methadone maintenance treatment in particular should be warned of the risk of overdose if they use heroin on top of methadone. This risk is further increased by use together with other sedatives such as benzodiazepines and alcohol.

For those individuals who continue to inject (whether or not they have accepted treatment for their dependence), check if they are using clean needles and are aware of the risk of transmission of hepatitis C from other injecting equipment.

Any patient who is not immune to hepatitis B (or currently infected) should be offered hepatitis B vaccination. In pregnant women, defer vaccination till after birth of the baby. Patients with chronic hepatitis C infection, particularly those who are HCV-RNA positive, should be considered for treatment.

Prevention

Control of supply has been the measure most widely used to prevent illicit opioid use. There is evidence that when supply of heroin is reduced (whether by international factors or local controls), rates of heroin overdose decrease. However, some users will switch to use of other opioids and other illicit or licit substances when heroin is less available.

Community education methods are used to attempt to reduce demand for heroin, but evidence for the effectiveness of these is limited.

There has not been a great deal of research specifically into prevention of illicit opioid use, but general measures to reduce the risk factors for illicit drug use are likely to be beneficial: early intervention for children in troubled families, addressing disadvantages in communities, increasing opportunities for individuals at risk to feel connected to and valued by society, and quality treatment of mental health disorders.

Summary

Illicit opioid use often causes deaths and sickness among young people, and opioid dependence typically runs a course of relapse and remission. Any contact of opioid users with the healthcare system can provide the opportunity for engagement with treatment and/or harm reduction services. Treatment has well-documented efficacy. Currently, opioid maintenance treatment is the most effective treatment available. While the person is engaged in treatment, their concurrent or complicating medical conditions (in particular, hepatitis C) and psychiatric conditions can be treated.

Pain and opioids

Introduction 296
Opioids in pain management 297
Epidemiology 299
Assessing opioid addiction in patients with pain 300
Managing pain, managing risk 301
Management of chronic pain and opioid dependence 302
Acute pain management in current or former addicts 304
Issues in service delivery 305

Introduction

Key concepts

Opioid dependence can be a difficult concept to grasp and to identify clinically in the setting of pain, particularly chronic pain. It is defined in ICD 10 as 'a strong desire to take the drug, impaired control over its use, persistent use despite harmful consequences, a higher priority given to drug use than to other activities and obligations, increased tolerance, and sometimes physical withdrawal reactions when drug use is discontinued'.

When there is chronic pain treated with long-term opioids, the clinician may be uncertain as to whether to attribute a patient's preoccupation with opioid use to the increasing doses being taken, and deteriorating function, to their underlying pain, or to the development of opioid dependence (Box 12.1).

Alan Leshner, former Director of the US National Institute on Drug Abuse commented: 'Addiction is not taking lots of drugs; it's taking drugs and acting like an addict.' This applies equally to the diagnosis of opioid dependence (addiction) in chronic pain. In DSM-5 the term 'substance dependence' has been replaced by 'substance use disorder' in part to avoid possible under-treatment of pain due to fear of addiction.

A cardinal feature of the dependence syndrome is the propensity to relapse—to return rapidly to compulsive drug use. Even after many years of drug abstinence, neuroplastic brain changes following drug dependence are not fully reversible, which explains the ongoing risk of relapse in patients with a history of opioid dependence. The risk of precipitating relapse is a concern in managing pain in such patients. It is critically important to re-double efforts of 'recovery' during periods when the use of an opioid is unavoidable for medical reasons.

Box 12.1 Key points to understanding

Be clear about the distinction between physiological dependence on opioids and the *clinical syndrome* of opioid dependence (or addiction). Confusion arises when this distinction is not understood sufficiently. In the setting of pain, it is more useful to monitor patients for behaviours suggestive of opioid dependence, rather than respond uncritically to subjective symptoms.

Opioids in pain management

Opioids are uniquely effective in alleviating the affective component of pain—relieving anxiety and fear—as well as easing pain. However, when used in chronic pain, opioids have limitations, and several observational studies suggest poor functional outcomes in people treated with opioids. Side effects are not rare, and include nausea and vomiting, constipation, increased sweating, and decreased sexual function. In addition, opioid use can cause a syndrome of decreased pain tolerance, increased anxiety, depression, and sleep disturbances. Three factors contribute to this: opioid-induced hyperalgesia, withdrawal, and dependence/addiction.

Hyperalgesia

Opioid-induced hyperalgesia results from activation of specific brain and spinal cord pathways, with increased release of excitatory neurotransmitters and more intensive spinal synaptic transmission. All opioids, including methadone and buprenorphine, lead to a dose-dependent reduction of the pain threshold. Hyperalgesia is reversible with dose reduction or cessation of opioids.

Withdrawal

Withdrawal from opioids includes, among other features, generalized aches and pains, dysphoric mood, disturbed sleep, and craving for opioids. The emergence of withdrawal symptoms between doses causes increased pain ('operant pain') and contributes to a cycle of pain and drug use. This is particularly the case in patients using short-acting opioids. Regular use of long-acting opioids involves less reinforcement and less risk of operant pain than 'as required' usage of short-acting opioids.

Dependence/addiction

It is not known how often a patient with chronic pain, and no prior history of addiction, becomes addicted (e.g. displaying drug-seeking behaviours) as a result of being prescribed opioids. US reports of the risk of addiction in people receiving opioids vary widely, from 2% to 50%, and a recent review estimated 35% of people treated with opioids for chronic pain met criteria for a substance use disorder. However, this reflects in part the fact that many people using prescribed opioids have deliberately sought them, and often their addiction did not arise as a result of being prescribed opioids. If opioids are prescribed to patients with no addiction history, drug-seeking and related behaviours are relatively uncommon, but if prescribed to unselected patients, such behaviours are frequently seen.

Balancing benefit and risk

There is good evidence that opioids are effective for pain relief when used appropriately and in the short term, perhaps up to 3 or 4 months. Beyond that, the benefit/risk ratio begins to shift toward loss of efficacy and increased adverse effects, especially as measured functionally. The longer the opioid use and the higher the dose, the worse the picture becomes, although there will always be some patients who benefit from long-term stable use of opioids for pain and suffering.

The threshold seems to be around 100–120 mg equivalent dose of morphine per day and treatment duration of about 120 days. Certain patients are especially prone to developing problems with prescription opioids. Unfortunately, there is considerable evidence that the majority of prescribed opioids are prescribed precisely to the group of patients who are most likely to have problems with them, the so-called 'adverse selection phenomenon'.

Influences on medical practice

The recent history of the use of opioids for treatment of non-malignant pain can be likened to the 40-year journey in the wilderness! Cicely Saunders' founding of St Christopher's Hospice in the UK in 1967 highlighted the under-treatment of pain and the under-utilization of opioids for relief of pain and suffering. Emphasis on pain relief then began to overshadow the undoubted problems of loss of efficacy over time and the development of opioid dependence/addiction. The WHO issued guidelines for cancer pain relief in 1986 and the 2010 Declaration of Montreal by the International Association for the Study of Pain highlighted the under-treatment of pain.

The medical community began to advocate for pain relief to be regarded as a basic right of patients, and medicolegal cases found in favour of patients whose pain was inadequately treated. Yet concern about inappropriate use persisted. A pharmaceutical company was fined $635 million for claiming OxyContin® was less addictive than other opioid analgesics. The controversy continues, and some medical practitioners continue to prescribe large amounts of opioids for pain treatment while at the same time others face prosecution for over-prescribing opioids.

Epidemiology

Since the early 2000s there has been a steady increase in prescribing of pharmaceutical opioids globally, and also increases in morbidity and mortality related to these drugs. This has affected some countries to the extent there is talk of an epidemic of prescription opioid dependence and misuse. For example, in the US, 2 million Americans are estimated to be dependent on pharmaceutical opioids. Increasing fatal overdoses and dependence arising from use of prescribed opioid analgesics has also been reported in Canada, Europe, Asia, and Australia. The epidemic has been the result of increasing global prescription of opioids, driven by pharmaceutical industry marketing rather than clear evidence of long-term efficacy of opioids in chronic pain. Increased global prescribing has increased the availability of drugs, and the prevalence of prescription drug misuse.

Diversion

There is a latent demand for reinforcing drugs, and there is potential profit to be made throughout the supply chain—from manufacturing and marketing, prescribing, and diverting opioid drugs to the black market. Because potent opioids are tightly regulated, diversion often involves other medications, particularly oxycodone, as these drugs are often subject to lower levels of control. Diversion from opioid substitution treatment (OST) outlets contributes to the total amount of opioids available for purchase in the community.

Factors influencing the likelihood of prescribed opioids being diverted include:

- formulation: e.g. high volume, dilute liquid is less easily diverted than tablets
- availability: diversion of methadone from OST rises in proportion to the amount of unsupervised administration
- availability of heroin: in settings where heroin is plentiful, there tends to be less diversion of prescription opioids
- availability of treatment places: shortage of treatment places increases risk of diversion.

Assessing opioid addiction in patients with pain

The central features of the opioid dependence syndrome are often difficult to identify in patients with pain, especially chronic pain. Features such as (1) a strong desire to take the drug, (2) impaired control over use, (3) persistent use despite harmful consequences, (4) higher priority given to drug use than to other activities and obligations, (5) increased tolerance, and (6) sometimes physical withdrawal reactions may be denied, understated or explained away when the patient's source of opioids is the medical practitioner. (See Box 12.2.)

Some of these behaviours, such as injecting oral medication, indicate a more serious problem than other behaviours such as using up a prescription early. It appears that the number of these behaviours in a patient is an indicator of the severity of dependence. Box 12.3 shows some predictors of misuse.

Box 12.2 Behaviours that suggest dependence/addiction

- Opioid diversion
- Insistence that only opioid treatment will alleviate pain
- Taking doses larger than those prescribed or increasing dosage without consulting the clinician
- Continued requests for dose escalations
- Seeking opioids from different physicians ('doctor shopping')
- Resisting urine drug screening, referrals to specialists, and other aspects of treatment
- Repeatedly losing medications or prescriptions or seeking early refills
- Attempting unscheduled visits, typically after office hours or when the clinician is unavailable
- Appearing sedated
- Misusing alcohol or using illicit or over-the-counter, internet, or other prescribed drugs
- Deteriorating functioning (e.g. problems at home or on the job)
- Injecting (having track marks) or snorting oral formulations
- Obtaining medications illegally (e.g. from multiple clinicians, street dealers), family members, the Internet, forged prescriptions).

Box 12.3 Predictors of misuse of prescribed opioids

- Age (18–25 years)
- Drug or drink driving convictions
- Low socioeconomic status (misuse and diversion)
- Prior opioid abuse
- Prior alcohol and/or substance abuse
- Family history of opioid, other drug and alcohol abuse
- Depression and other psychiatric disorders.

Managing pain, managing risk

Example

A patient with chronic low back pain (three surgical interventions) has been requesting progressively more analgesia, and has reached 760 mg oxycodone daily. The patient says the pain is bad and only oxycodone works. The GP is concerned, the pain specialist is concerned, and the GP notes that the patient has become increasingly estranged from his family.

Comment

In this situation, we have limited information. This is the reality of managing chronic pain—we are usually only aware of what the patient presents to us, and know little of what is going on. From this vignette, we know that:

- the patient is taking high doses of an opioid (equivalent to approximately 2 g oral morphine daily), meaning the patient is highly tolerant and unlikely to be receiving optimal analgesia
- there is poor functioning, reflected in family estrangement and doctors' concern.

There is little doubt that the patient experiences back pain, but also little doubt that the *primary problem is now opioid dependence*. Non-pharmacological management is to discuss the diagnosis of dependence, set realistic objectives of treatment, and explain the rationale for switching to a long-acting opioid. Pharmacological management is to switch from oxycodone to methadone, initially with supervised dosing and slow dose increments to ensure safety during induction (the patient may not have been taking all his prescribed medication) and monitor compliance.

Principles of opioid prescribing

- Single prescriber
- Single pharmacy
- Patient and prescriber sign opioid agreement
- Lowest possible effective dose should be used
- Do not combine opioids with sedative-hypnotics or benzodiazepines unless specifically indicated, and then with increased monitoring
- Routinely assess functional and pain status
- Monitor for medication misuse and compliance (urine drug screening).

The American Pain Society suggests doses of up to 200 mg morphine equivalent per day may be prescribed by generalist physicians. Above this level, referral for specialist assessment should be sought. The British Pain Society Guidelines recommend specialist referral for doses of 120–180 mg or greater (see Table 12.1 for dosage equivalence).

Urine drug screening identifies inappropriate opioid and other drug use in patients with pain more frequently than does clinical assessment.

Management of chronic pain and opioid dependence

Chronic pain is common in people currently or previously addicted, and management of pain in these individuals is of critical importance. Under-treatment of pain and careless prescribing can both precipitate relapse to addiction in abstinent addicts, and can destabilize patients on OST.

Chronic pain management in current or former addicts

The limited efficacy of opioids for chronic pain, and risk of relapse on exposure to opioids, mean that in people who identify as abstinent former opioid addicts, and who are concerned at the risk of re-addiction, it is preferable to avoid opioid analgesics for management of chronic pain.

Former addicts who request opioid analgesics for chronic pain need a careful assessment of their pain, their addiction history and status, and their psychological functioning. If the pain appears something that is likely to respond to opioids, it is prudent that an addiction specialist assesses the patient prior to initiation of long-term opioid therapy. In some cases, the person seeking prescribed opioids may be intending to use the medication for their own purposes, but not necessarily as prescribed. Prescribed drugs are sometimes obtained for intoxication, to avoid withdrawal, or, in places where maintenance treatment with methadone is inaccessible, as an alternative maintenance medication. Even where treatment is accessible, some patients are deterred by the stigma, the loss of privacy, or the rigid rules which may be experienced in treatment programmes, and seek long-term prescriptions on the grounds of pain rather than enrolling in a treatment programme.

Managing pain, managing addiction

Data from clinical trials suggests only modest benefits of opioids over placebo in the management of chronic pain, but there is a substantial evidence base for the effectiveness of highly structured opioid prescribing in managing opioid dependence. Attempting to wean people with established opioid dependence and chronic pain from opioids can be difficult, and continuing long-acting opioids with appropriate safeguards and monitoring is often a pragmatic strategy. It is often unclear whether the primary diagnosis is pain or opioid dependence. Given the lack of certainty in identifying individuals at risk, some authors have recommended 'universal precautions'—using the risk-management strategies applied in addiction treatment (including random urine drug testing) as the default assumption in prescribing opioids long term.

Effective prescribing for pain or addiction requires a clear diagnosis, rationale for treatment, objectives against which to assess effectiveness, monitoring with urine drug screens, and regular review. For people with a sense of loss of control over their pain, or over their drug use, externally imposed structure can be therapeutically useful, and direct observation of administration can be helpful at times.

However, there are also differences in treating pain and addiction. Methadone and buprenorphine, administered once daily in a stable dose, can suppress withdrawal for 24 hours, but do not provide 24-hour analgesia. They are more effective as analgesics if the dose is divided and given at intervals through the day.

High doses of methadone (>60 mg/day) are optimal in treating addiction, where the aim is to induce a high level of opioid tolerance, attenuating the effect of injecting heroin. However, in managing pain, lower doses, and less tolerance, are the preferred strategy.

Table 12.1 Approximate equianalgesic doses of various opioids

Opioid	Oral	Parenteral	Duration of action (hours)
Morphine	30 mg	10 mg	Injection: 2–3 h
Codeine	180–200 mg		Linctus: 3–4 h
Methadone	Acute dosing 30 mg Chronic dosing 7 mg (methadone accumulates—it takes 75 half-lives, or 5–7 days, to reach steady state levels)	In patients on methadone maintenance treatment, give two-thirds of the usual dose in two split doses IM	Syrup/tablet or injection: 6–8 h initially; increases to >24 hours with long-term use
Buprenorphine	0.4 mg	0.1 mg IV or SC	6–8 h
Oxycodone	10 mg	5 mg	3–4 h tabs/injection 12 h SR tab
Pethidine		100 mg IM or IV	2–3 h
Tramadol	100–150 mg	50–100 mg IM or IV	3–6 h
Fentanyl		100 micrograms IM, IV, SC	0.5–2 h lozenge/injection 72 h patch

Acute pain management in current or former addicts

Management of addicted individuals can be difficult as addicted patients are not always open about their addiction. They may be using multiple drugs. Even if they report using heroin, their actual level of tolerance cannot be accurately determined by history, as street drugs are of variable purity. While hospitalized, some addicted individuals may self-medicate, placing themselves at risk of toxicity, drug interactions, and complications of injecting.

- Opioids are not contraindicated in abstinent, former addicts with acute pain. There is a poorly defined, probably small risk that exposure to opioids will trigger relapse to addiction. If possible, this risk should be discussed with the patient who may prefer non-opioid analgesia.
- If opioids are used for pain management in recovering addicts, medication should be transferred to long-acting opioids at the earliest opportunity. Support should be offered during hospitalization, and follow-up arrangements put in place. Such structure helps protect patients against the risk of relapse.
- In patients on OST with acute pain, withdrawal needs to be controlled and analgesia given in addition; this means continuing OST in hospitalized patients and giving additional opioid analgesia as needed. People on buprenorphine undergoing elective surgery should continue their usual dose, and have additional opioid analgesia titrated against response; some may require additional modalities of pain relief.
- In hospitalized heroin users, prescribing methadone can prevent opioid withdrawal complicating management. When initiating methadone in hospitalized patients, or continuing methadone in people whose medication has not been supervised, titrating regular small doses (10–20mg) against response is required. Induction onto methadone is complex due to variable pharmacokinetics. In people who metabolize the drug slowly, methadone accumulates over several days, and a dose which might have been safe on day 1 can be toxic on day 2 or 3. Patients need to be monitored for signs of toxicity during the first week of methadone.
- A non-judgemental stance is necessary for effective assessment and management, which is optimized by access to skilled and experienced addictions staff.
- If prescribing opioid analgesics to abstinent ex-addicts switch from short- to long-acting medications as quickly as appropriate (to minimize reinforcing effects). They may also benefit from additional support during postoperative periods.

Issues in service delivery

Competencies

- Prescribing for chronic pain requires competence, comprising knowledge, skills, and attitudes. Maintenance of competence requires the opportunity to reflect on practice.
- Knowledge includes opioid pharmacology, and principles of managing pain and of managing addiction. Good communication skills are critical in managing pain and associated anxiety, and an empathic, non-judgemental stance is needed in relating to all patients. Clinicians need to be able to recognize and diagnose opioid dependence, to be able to set realistic objectives of treatment, and to monitor and adjust treatment according to response.
- Standardized tools (such as screening questionnaires) have serious limitations, and are not a substitute for competent assessment. The decision of how to manage, and whether to prescribe opioids, needs to be reached in agreement between an appropriately skilled doctor and patient.

Treatment systems

- Effective pain management in complex patients is the result of the interaction between the clinician's competence, and the setting in which he or she works. A competent practitioner working in a chaotic system in which information is not shared can have difficulties achieving safe and effective pain management. A hospital with comprehensive policies and procedures cannot guarantee good care of patients if individual practitioners are not supported in dealing with complex, stigmatized patients.
- Opioid dependence is sufficiently common that all hospitals should have protocols for the management of pain in people identified as opioid dependent. These protocols should deal with history taking, identification and management of withdrawal, continuation of OST in hospitalized addicts, and provision of pain relief in people with current or past addiction. Such protocols are more likely to be useful if supported by training. Ideally, large hospitals should have an addictions consultation-liaison service, to provide training, assess and advise on management of complex patients, and support staff in management. Pain management is likely to be more effective if an acute pain team is available to provide support in complex cases.
- Addiction services need skilled staff familiar with the principles of chronic pain management, able to assess and refer patients appropriately.
- Given the overlap between chronic pain and opioid dependence, pain clinics should not only liaise with addiction services regarding individual patients, but should have access to specialist addiction assessment.

Further reading

Australian and New Zealand College Anaesthetists and Faculty of Pain Medicine (2010). *Acute Pain Management: Scientific Evidence* (3rd ed). Melbourne: ANZCA and FPM.

Chou R, Fanciullo G, Fine PG, *et al.* (2009). Opioids for chronic noncancer pain: Prediction and identification of aberrant drug-related behaviors: A review of the evidence for an American Pain Society and American Academy of Pain Medicine clinical practice guideline. *J Pain* 10:131–46.

Substance Abuse and Mental Health Services Administration (2012). *A Treatment Improvement Protocol. TIP 54 Managing Chronic Pain in Adults With or in Recovery From Substance Use Disorders.* Rockville, MD: SAMHSA.

Benzodiazepines and the other sedative-hypnotics

Introduction and epidemiology 308
Pharmacology 309
Core clinical syndromes 311
Complications of benzodiazepine use 314
Natural history of benzodiazepine dependence 316
Screening and opportunistic intervention 316
Assessment and management of benzodiazepine overdose/intoxication 317
Assessment and management of benzodiazepine dependence and withdrawal 319
Barbiturates 323
'Z' drugs 324
Prevention of benzodiazepine abuse and dependence 325

Introduction and epidemiology

Sedative-hypnotics are CNS depressants which act predominantly on gamma-aminobutyric acid (GABA) A receptors, the main inhibitory system in the brain. The benzodiazepines are numerically and in terms of prescriptions and sales the most important of this group. Several other sedative-hypnotic drugs are available, including the barbiturates, which were in some ways the forerunners of the benzodiazepines, but which have been supplanted for most indications by them. A recently introduced group is the 'z' drugs, which are predominantly prescribed as hypnotics. In some countries, sedative-hypnotics can be purchased in pharmacies. They are also widely available through illicit sources, including through the Internet.

Sedative-hypnotics include:

- benzodiazepines
- barbiturates
- the 'z' drugs (zolpidem, zopiclone, and zaleplon)
- chloral hydrate.

The most commonly used sedative-hypnotics are the benzodiazepines, which were first introduced into clinical practice in the 1960s. Prior to the introduction of benzodiazepines, the most commonly available sedative-hypnotics were the barbiturates and non-barbiturate drugs, such as methaqualone and chloral hydrate. Benzodiazepines, because they are a much safer alternative to barbiturates, are now one of the most prescribed drugs on the market.

In Western societies, it is estimated that around 10% of adults regularly take benzodiazepines. Although in the past decade there has been a reduction of prescription benzodiazepines for day-time use in anxiety treatment, hypnotic use remains quite stable. Self-medication with benzodiazepines is common, particularly by those who are alcohol or opioid dependent, or who misuse psychostimulants. To illustrate this, 35% of medicines obtained by 'doctor shoppers' in Australia are benzodiazepines.

Clinical indications for benzodiazepines are fewer nowadays, given the concern about abuse and dependence. They include:

- insomnia—short-term use only (<2 weeks)
- anxiety/panic attacks—short-term use only, while other appropriate medications (e.g. antidepressants) are initiated; sometimes prescribed for 'breakthrough' acute anxiety symptoms, which are not well controlled by other means
- pre-anaesthetic medication
- seizures/epilepsy—acute use especially to cease seizure activity;
- skeletal muscle relaxation (muscle spasms, e.g. acute back pain)
- management of various withdrawal syndromes
- in certain psychiatric illnesses such as mania and psychosis.

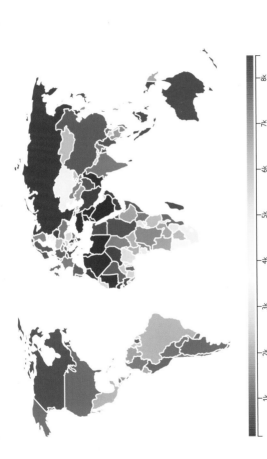

Colour plate 1 Healthy life years lost because of alcohol use globally in 2010 (as age-adjusted DALYs per 100,000 people attributed to alcohol). (See also Fig. 2.1.)

Reproduced with permission from Institute for Health Metrics and Evaluation (IHME). GBD Compare. Copyright (2013), with permission from the University of Washington. Available from http://vizhub.healthdata.org/gbd-compare (Accessed 1 February 2014.)

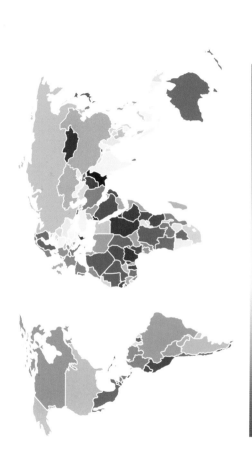

Colour plate 2 Healthy life years lost because of tobacco use globally in 2010 (as age-adjusted DALYs lost attributable to tobacco per 100,000 people). (See also Fig. 2.3.)

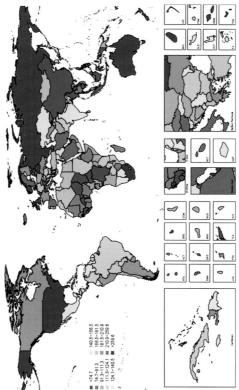

Colour plate 3 (a) Opioid-dependence DALYs per 100,000 persons. (b) Amphetamine-dependence DALYs per 100,000 persons. (c) Cocaine-dependence DALYs per 100,000 persons. (d) Cannabis-dependence DALYs per 100,000 persons. (See also Fig. 2.6.)

Reproduced from *The Lancet*, 382(9904), Degenhardt L, Whiteford H, Ferrari AJ, Baxter A, Charlson F, Hall W, et al. The global burden of disease attributable to illicit drug use and dependence: Results from the GBD 2010 study, pp. 1564–74, Copyright (2013), with permission from Elsevier.

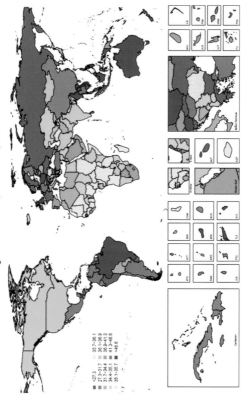

Amphetamine use disorders DALYs per 100,000 people, Age-standardized, Both sexes, 2010

Colour plate 3 (*Contd.*)

Cocaine use disorders DALYs per 100,000 people, Age-standardized, Both sexes, 2010

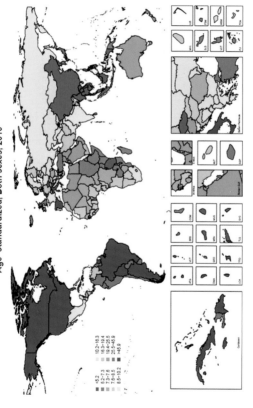

- <5.2
- 5.2–7.3
- 7.3–7.6
- 7.6–8.5
- 8.5–10.2
- 10.2–16.3
- 16.3–19.4
- 19.4–25.5
- 25.5–45.9
- >45.9

Colour plate 3 (Contd.)

Cannabis use disorders DALYs per 100,000 people,
Age-standardized, Both sexes, 2010

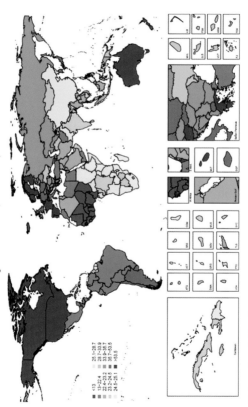

Colour plate 3 (Contd.)

Pharmacology

Benzodiazepines have sedative-hypnotic, anxiolytic, anticonvulsant, amnesia-inducing, and muscle relaxant properties.

They increase GABA inhibition by acting as indirect modulators on the $GABA_A$ receptor, which has specific binding sites for these drugs—the so-called benzodiazepine receptor. There are a number of different sub-types of the $GABA_A$ receptor which are thought to mediate the various actions of benzodiazepines. For instance:

- alpha-1 $GABA_A$ receptors mediate sedation, ataxia, some anterograde amnesia and some seizure protection
- alpha-2 and -3 $GABA_A$ subunits mediate anxiolysis, some anticonvulsant properties, and skeletal muscle relaxation.
- alpha-5 subunits are highly localized in hippocampus and contribute to the amnestic actions.

Benzodiazepines are well absorbed after oral use. A number of benzo-diazepines (e.g. diazepam) are metabolized in the liver to longer-acting active metabolites, e.g. nordiazepam. Eventually, water-soluble compounds are formed, which are excreted in the urine. In the setting of illicit drug use, oral benzodiazepines may be crushed or otherwise prepared for injecting. Very lipophilic benzodiazepines, such as flunitrazepam, are sometimes crushed and insufflated ('snorted').

The duration of action of benzodiazepines depends on the half-life of the parent drug and its active metabolite (see Table 13.1). Because of long half-lives, urine drug screens of long-acting benzodiazepines may test positive for up to several weeks after use.

Side effects of benzodiazepines

- Drowsiness, dizziness
- Tiredness
- Dysarthria
- Ataxia, risk of falls (especially in elderly people)
- Impaired psychomotor performance and reaction time (increased risk of car accidents)
- Poor memory and concentration (can be complete anterograde amnesia for some hours after taking the drug)
- Emotional blunting
- Rarely, paradoxical excitement and disinhibition (particularly in children and elderly).

There is no current evidence to indicate that benzodiazepine use or withdrawal results in permanent structural or functional brain damage except where a period of hypoxia has eventuated.

Short half-life drugs have a higher risk of withdrawal problems with inter-dose and early morning anxiety. Long half-life preparations have more residual daytime drowsiness and cognitive impairment.

Table 13.1 Benzodiazepine half-life and conversion table

Form of benzodiazepine	The dose of that benzodiazepine which is approximately equivalent to diazepam (5 mg)	Approximate $t\frac{1}{2}$ (hours)
Ultra-short acting benzodiazepines ($t_{\frac{1}{2}} < 4$ h)		
Triazolam	0.25 mg	1–3
Midazolam	15 mg	1–3
Short- to intermediate-acting benzodiazepines		
Oxazepam	15 mg	4–15
Lorazepam	1 mg	12–16
Temazepam	10 mg	5–15 (10)
Bromazepam	3 mg	20
Alprazolam	0.5 mg	6–25
Flunitrazepam	1 mg	20–30
Clobazam	10 mg	17–49
Nitrazepam	5 mg	16–48
Long-acting benzodiazepines (includes effects of active metabolites):		
Clonazepam	0.5 mg	22–54
Diazepam	5 mg	20–80
Chlordiazepoxide	10 mg	>50
Flurazepam	15 mg	>50
Clorazepate	10 mg	>50
'Z' drugs		
Zolpidem	10 mg	2.4
Zopiclone	7.5 mg	5.2
Zaleplon	10 mg	1.5

Benzodiazepines with long half-lives should be avoided in patients with hepatic or renal decompensation.

Core clinical syndromes

Benzodiazepine overdose/intoxication

Benzodiazepine intoxication is characterized by:
- drowsiness, confusion
- dysarthria
- ataxia and impaired coordination
- impaired concentration
- respiratory depression
- coma
- death (this is uncommon if benzodiazepines only are taken, but can occur when used in combination with other CNS depressants such as alcohol, opioids).

Non-dependent benzodiazepine misuse

Benzodiazepine misuse/hazardous use

A person may misuse benzodiazepines, e.g. purchase them from illicit sources, use intermittently in supratherapeutic doses, or dissolve oral preparations for use via the intravenous route, but may not yet have developed clear adverse effects or dependence.

Harmful benzodiazepine use (ICD 10)

An individual may experience physical harms from their use of benzodiazepines (e.g. falls in the elderly, accidents, or other complications of injecting benzodiazepines) or mental harm.

Benzodiazepine abuse (DSM-IV)

Benzodiazepine abuse occurs when recurring benzodiazepine misuse results in repeated adverse social impacts, but the individual is not dependent on benzodiazepines. For example, their benzodiazepine use may result from a conscious desire to intermittently use benzodiazepines as 'downers' to overcome excitatory effects of psychostimulants, for the relief of alcohol or opioid withdrawal symptoms, or to relieve insomnia, stress or anxiety (Box 13.1).

> **Box 13.1 Conditions which increase the risk of abuse/ dependence**
> - Insomnia (particularly in the elderly)
> - Chronic pain (with benzodiazepines used for muscle relaxation, insomnia, anxiety)
> - Alcohol dependence (for alleviation of withdrawal symptoms)
> - Opioid dependence (for alleviation of withdrawal symptoms)
> - Psychostimulant abuse/dependence (to reduce or terminate the stimulant effect)
> - Psychiatric illnesses:
>   - Generalized anxiety disorders
>   - Panic attacks
>   - Agoraphobia
>   - Psychotic states
>   - Depression
>   - Antisocial personality disorder.

A high level of awareness of potential benzodiazepine use or misuse is necessary.

Benzodiazepine dependence

Dependence on benzodiazepines may occur after regular, daily use for more than 4–6 weeks, even at therapeutic doses. Two-thirds of benzodiazepine-dependent persons are women. When a person is dependent on benzodiazepines, they will typically:

- experience withdrawal symptoms on cessation or marked reduction in dose (see following section)
- become tolerant to the hypnotic and sedative effects
- have impaired control over use (be unable to stop use when they want to)
- in some cases (usually where use has been at supratherapeutic doses), they may be aware of a strong desire to use benzodiazepines, and may continue to use despite evidence of harms (e.g. falls, accidents, injuries).

Once benzodiazepine dependence has developed, it is difficult to successfully discontinue use.

The benzodiazepine withdrawal syndrome

The benzodiazepine withdrawal syndrome is a cluster of somatic, psychological, and behavioural symptoms (Box 13.2), which arise on abrupt discontinuation or dose reduction of benzodiazepines in a benzodiazepine-dependent individual.

Abrupt discontinuation of benzodiazepines, or tapering off benzodiazepines too quickly, when they are prescribed for insomnia, generalized anxiety disorders, panic attacks, or agoraphobia, may result in either recurrence of the underlying disorder, a rebound of symptoms, or a benzodiazepine withdrawal syndrome. These are difficult to distinguish in clinical practice as they may occur simultaneously or sequentially.

The time course of benzodiazepine withdrawal depends on the half-life of the benzodiazepine used:

- For short-acting benzodiazepines (oxazepam, temazepam, lorazepam), onset of withdrawal symptoms occurs 1–2 days after the last dose, peaks at 2–5 days, and lasts 2–4 weeks or more.
- For longer-acting preparations (diazepam, chlordiazepoxide), onset of withdrawal symptoms occurs later, peaks at 7–10 days, and lasts for 8 weeks or longer. In some cases, a protracted withdrawal phase may last up to 12 months.

The risk of benzodiazepine withdrawal and the severity of the withdrawal syndrome are increased with:

- shorter half-life of the drug, higher doses
- the rapidity of withdrawal
- underlying personality of the patient
- coexisting medical, alcohol, and other drug problems.

Benzodiazepine withdrawal seizures may be serious and life-threatening.

Box 13.2 Benzodiazepine withdrawal syndrome: clinical features

Somatic symptoms and signs

- Sweating
- Tremor, fasciculation
- Muscle pain, stiffness, and aches (limbs, back, neck, jaw)
- Dizziness, light-headedness
- Paraesthesiae, shooting pains in neck and spine
- Palpitations
- Visual disturbances (blurred vision, diplopia, photophobia, vision lags behind eye movements)
- Tinnitus, headache
- Gastrointestinal symptoms: nausea, anorexia, weight loss, diarrhoea (may resemble irritable bowel syndrome). Weight loss is prominent in the long term
- Faintness and dizziness; sense of unsteadiness
- Menorrhagia and breast pain
- Spontaneous orgasms.

Psychological symptoms

- Rebound insomnia, nightmares
- Anxiety, panic attacks
- Irritability, restlessness, agitation
- Poor memory and concentration
- Perceptual distortions—sensory hypersensitivity (light, sound, touch, taste); abnormal sensations, e.g. 'cotton wool' sensations
- Metallic taste
- Distortions of body image
- Feelings of unreality, depersonalization. derealization
- Depression, dysphoria.

Acute brain syndrome

- Confusion, disorientation, and delirium (may be intermittent); a common cause of confusion in the elderly
- Delusions, paranoia
- Hallucinations (visual, auditory)
- Grand mal seizures—occur 1–12 days after discontinuing benzodiazepines. Patients taking high doses (>50 mg diazepam equivalence) are at increased risk of withdrawal seizures

Consider benzodiazepine withdrawals in unexplained seizures in an adult. Grand mal seizures and delirium constitute serious and potentially life-threatening withdrawal symptoms

Complications of benzodiazepine use

Physical complications of benzodiazepine use

- Overdose/intoxication (accidental or suicidal)
- Accidents, injuries
- Complications of injecting oral preparations: As well as the usual risks of injecting drug use, there are added risks when powders or gels intended for oral use are prepared for and used intravenously, e.g. local vascular irritation, and as veins become less accessible, users may deliberately, or accidentally inject into arteries. This may result in particulate matter lodging in peripheral vasculature, resulting in ischaemia and gangrene, and diffuse lung disease.

Note that benzodiazepine dependence and withdrawal represents the most important form of harm.

Neuropsychiatric complications of benzodiazepine use

Memory impairment/anterograde amnesia

There is impaired ability to learn new information. Recall of information learned prior to taking the drug is not affected (indeed, can even be enhanced). Memory impairment is more likely with:

- intravenous administration or high oral doses
- when other sedative agents are used (e.g. alcohol)
- with high potency benzodiazepines (e.g. triazolam).

The sedative and amnestic effects are sometimes used preoperatively or to subdue a victim, and erase the victim's memory of a crime. For example, flunitrazepam has been termed a 'date rape' drug when slipped into the victim's drink (though in the majority of such cases alcohol is the sole or primary intoxicant). The amnesic effect of high-dose benzodiazepines is more commonly an undesired side effect of misuse. Individuals using high doses (e.g. up to 25 tablets as a handful) may commit crimes, while disinhibited, e.g. assault or shoplifting, then not remember this the next day.

With long-term use of benzodiazepines, even with therapeutic doses, the problem is with consolidation of memory, i.e. information of interest is noted and can be recalled immediately, but is not transferred into long-term memory. However, recall of information learned prior to benzodiazepine intake is not affected. This is more likely in the elderly where it may resemble dementia.

Anxiety

During benzodiazepine withdrawal, symptoms resembling an anxiety disorder can occur. The following syndromes are recognized in withdrawal:

- Social phobia
- Generalized anxiety disorder
- Obsessive–compulsive symptoms
- Panic attacks.

It is difficult to distinguish whether these symptoms represent a recurrence of the underlying anxiety disorder currently being treated, or a rebound of symptoms during the benzodiazepine withdrawal. However, withdrawal-related anxiety symptoms are time-limited, improving significantly within a month and disappearing altogether within several months. If the symptoms represent re-emergence of a pre-existing anxiety disorder, they are likely to persist and worsen during the first month post-withdrawal.

Depression

Benzodiazepines have been reported to cause depression or exacerbate existing symptoms of depression. Depression may emerge during benzodiazepine withdrawal and can lead to relapse.

Paradoxical disinhibition

Instead of having the expected calming and sedating effect, benzodiazepines occasionally cause irritability, restlessness, hostility, aggressiveness and violence; rarely, the clinical picture resembles hypomania/psychosis.

Psychosis

Psychotic symptoms in a state of clear consciousness may develop during benzodiazepine withdrawal. These include agitation, aggression, persecutory delusions, and hallucinations (mainly visual) in association with other symptoms of benzodiazepine withdrawal.

Delirium:

This may occur during:
- *benzodiazepine withdrawal:* with confusion, delusions, hallucinations in association with other symptoms
- *benzodiazepine overdose:* with disorientation, confusion, memory impairment in association with reduced level of consciousness, and other signs of benzodiazepine overdose.

Comorbid disorders and complications

Many mental health disorders are seen in patients with benzodiazepine use disorders. Sometimes these are pre-existing or primary disorders, but often they are complications of the benzodiazepine use. Referral to a psychiatrist for diagnosis and management of comorbid disorders is helpful. Psychiatric assessment is much easier once any severe benzodiazepine abuse or dependence is under control, but in some cases concurrent treatment may be necessary.

Pre-existing anxiety disorders will likely need treatment with SSRIs, and often this has to be started to facilitate benzodiazepine detoxification. In some patients, maintenance therapy with benzodiazepines may be necessary. If there is significant depression, this may lead to relapse to benzodiazepine use. It is advisable to stabilize on an antidepressant before attempting to stop the benzodiazepine, although full benefit from such treatment may occur only after the benzodiazepine has finally been ceased.

Natural history of benzodiazepine dependence

Most benzodiazepine use is short term or confined to managing sleep disturbance or otherwise to induce sleep. Approximately 30% of people who start taking benzodiazepines develop dependence on these drugs.

- Benzodiazepine dependence is well described with therapeutic doses of these drugs.
- Of people taking 15–20 mg diazepam (or equivalent) daily for 3 months, 40% experience a withdrawal syndrome when the drug is discontinued (under double-blind conditions), and 70% do so after 6 months' administration. The risk of dependence increases as the dose extends into supratherapeutic ranges.

There is relatively little information on the natural history of benzodiazepine dependence, except that, without intervention, it tends to be long term and there is a tendency to relapse after a period of non-use.

Continuing use is characterized by increased dependence, in common with the ever-present risk of a withdrawal syndrome when supply is interrupted.

The natural history in treated populations varies widely, with abstinence rates of 70% at 1 year being reported in the people prescribed benzodiazepines legitimately and in elderly populations, ranging down to 20% in other studies, and below in street users of these drugs.

Screening and opportunistic intervention

- Routinely inquire whether benzodiazepines are taken for insomnia, stress, anxiety, etc.
- How much is taken, whether daily or intermittently, and for how long.
- Determine whether the patient is using benzodiazepines hazardously or harmfully, or whether the patient is dependent on benzodiazepines.

If the patient is not dependent, but using benzodiazepines in a hazardous or harmful way (amount), the principles of brief intervention can be applied, as described by the FLAGS acronym, i.e.

F   Feedback on problems experienced or likely to be experienced.
L   Listen to readiness to change.
A   Advise patient about the potential risks associated with continued benzodiazepine use, in particular benzodiazepine dependence and withdrawals and recommend change in pattern of use.
G   Negotiate goals.
S   Strategies.

If the patient is benzodiazepine dependent, the principal approach is to encourage stepwise reduction in dose (on an ambulatory basis).

Assessment and management of benzodiazepine overdose/intoxication

History

Where history is possible (from patient, or collateral sources), try to identify:

- how much benzodiazepine was taken and the time it was taken
- usual benzodiazepine dose, its frequency (whether daily or intermittently) and duration—to assess likelihood of dependence and subsequent risk of benzodiazepine withdrawal
- what other substances were taken concurrently (including alcohol, prescribed and illicit drugs, especially other respiratory suppressants such as opioids)
- any major coexisting medical conditions
- any major psychiatric co-morbidity, e.g. depression. Was the overdose suicidal or accidental?
- when the patient is stabilized, a fuller assessment can be completed.

Clinical examination

The patient may be:

- drowsy
- confused
- have slow, slurred speech
- ataxic, poor coordination of movements
- comatose.

Look for signs of head injury and other injuries

Death may result from respiratory depression, more particularly when taken in combination with alcohol and other CNS depressants.

Investigations

Routine baseline investigations include:

- FBC
- EUC
- LFTs
- blood sugar levels
- arterial blood gases (if indicated)
- BAC
- plasma or urine drug screens: will determine if there is polysubstance use
- CT head or MRI (if head injury is suspected).

Management

Simple benzodiazepine overdose is rarely life-threatening, general supportive measures are all that is required. Overdose may be more dangerous when benzodiazepines are used in combination with other CNS depressants (e.g. alcohol, opioids).

- General supportive measures: maintain airways, breathing, and circulation.
- May require assisted ventilation, in mixed overdose with alcohol, opioids, and other CNS depressants.
- If gastric lavage and activated charcoal is considered necessary, take necessary precautions to avoid aspiration.
- The specific benzodiazepine antagonist flumazenil may be given 1–2 mg slow IV infusion over several minutes as this often leads to rapid return to consciousness. As the duration of action is brief and shorter than the benzodiazepine agonists used in the overdose, repeat doses may be required after 1–2 h, so continuous monitoring is also required.

- *Warning*—flumazenil may precipitate a withdrawal syndrome including seizures in patients with benzodiazepine dependence. This risk is increased if other pro-convulsant drugs (e.g. tricyclic antidepressants) have also been taken. It can also precipitate panic attacks.

- Administer parenteral thiamine, particularly if the patient has a concurrent alcohol problem.
- If concurrent opioid overdose is suspected, administer naloxone (see p. 264–5).
- Exclude other causes of coma.

Assessment and management of benzodiazepine dependence and withdrawal

History

Identify the problem by taking a comprehensive drug and alcohol history and psychiatric history (see Chapter 5 for details). Important points include:

- a history of benzodiazepine use, including name of drug, daily amount taken, frequency, and duration of use (see Table 13.1 for details)
- history of features of dependence on benzodiazepines
- time of last use of benzodiazepines—the time of onset of benzodiazepine withdrawal can be predicted by the time of last use and the preparation taken (whether long or short acting)
- coexisting substance use or dependence, particularly alcohol, opioids, and psychostimulants
- psychiatric history and medication taken for the treatment of anxiety, generalized anxiety disorder, panic attacks, agoraphobia, psychosis.

Clinical examination

The physical examination may be largely non-contributory. A thorough mental state examination should be undertaken.

- any history of withdrawal seizures or epilepsy

Investigations

A urine drug screen may be helpful to identify polysubstance use.

Management

Hospital treatment of benzodiazepine withdrawal

- Provide reassurance and support.
- General supportive care, monitor vital signs and mental state every 4–8 hours.
- If the patient has been taking a short-acting benzodiazepine preparation, switch to a long-acting preparation, such as diazepam orally.
- Refer to an equivalence table (see Table 13.1) to convert the dose to diazepam. A general rule of thumb is that the smallest dose form of another form of benzodiazepine is equivalent to 5 mg diazepam.
- On day 1 administer 50% of the stated usual daily dose as the *diazepam equivalent*. If you are certain of the patient's dose, it is permissible to prescribe 80% of it.
- Administer in divided doses for the next 3 days until the patient is stabilized and not showing signs of overt withdrawal.
- On day 5 embark on a gradual step-wise reduction in the daily dose. In hospital this may be 10–15% of the dose every 2–3 days. Titrate the dose and speed of reduction according to response.
- *If significant withdrawal symptoms recur*, slow the reduction or return to the previous dose until patient is stable, then reduce more slowly (e.g. by 2.5–5 mg every 4–5 days) until the drug is ceased.

- When the need for in-patient admission is over, dose reduction may continue as an out-patient. This allows for more gradual weaning off benzodiazepines.
- Limited amounts of benzodiazepines should be dispensed, preferably on a day-by-day basis.

Clinical example

A patient presents for in-patient withdrawal management, having been taking 20 × 30 mg oxazepam tablets every day for 3 months:
- Calculate each oxazepam 30 mg tablet is equivalent to two diazepam 5 mg tablets, so the patient is taking the equivalent of 40 × diazepam 5 mg tablets daily, or 200 mg diazepam
- Reduce this to a starting dose of 50% on day 1, i.e. 20 diazepam tablets daily (100 mg) unless there is strong corroborative information on the dose. This is given as 25 mg four times daily
- Once stable (no tremor, sleeping at night), commence reduction of 10%. This can be titrated slowly according to the patient's response.

Management of severe benzodiazepine withdrawal (with delirium or seizures)

Severe benzodiazepine withdrawal requires urgent action and specialist advice should be sought. May require transfer to a high dependency unit or intensive care unit. Key management steps are as follows:
- Administer diazepam 10 mg by slow IV injection; repeat after 30 minutes if necessary. Alternatively, IV midazolam may be administered
- Consider other potential causes of delirium or seizures, especially alcohol withdrawal, infections (see p. 79, pp. 85–101, p. 556).
- If hallucinations are present, administer olanzapine 5–10 mg orally, or if not available haloperidol 2.5–5 mg IM or orally. Repeat every 4–6 hours if necessary.
- Once the withdrawal syndrome has been controlled, monitor withdrawal symptoms and signs three to four times per day.
- Continue with oral diazepam, generally 40–80 mg daily in three or four divided doses for 2–3 days.
- Once the patient is stable, institute a tapering regimen, reducing the dose of diazepam by 10–15% as described earlier until the dose reaches 20–40 mg/day.

Post-discharge management
- If the patient is still on diazepam at the time of discharge, arrangements need to be made for continuing its gradual dose reduction as an out-patient.
- Involve the patient's GP (family physician) in the ongoing management (provided the patient consents).
- The GP or specialist continues the dose reduction of diazepam and monitors the patient at daily to weekly or fortnightly intervals as required. The patient is gently weaned off diazepam (see later in topic for an out-patient tapering benzodiazepine regimen).
- Organize daily or weekly dispensing of diazepam via a pharmacy or clinic before the patient leaves hospital.

Ambulatory benzodiazepine detoxification

Elective out-patient benzodiazepine detoxification is appropriate for patients with benzodiazepine dependence who do not have a history of severe withdrawal or seizures, who are not concurrently dependent on alcohol or other substances, and who do not have significant concurrent physical or mental illnesses.

Wherever possible, *the starting dose of diazepam should not exceed 40 mg diazepam/day.* Any patient who requires a higher starting dose should have their benzodiazepine reduction commenced by a specialist or as an in-patient. They can then be discharged to an out-patient regimen when the diazepam dose has fallen to 40 mg.

Ambulatory detoxification requires the patient's commitment and close liaison between the medical officer, GP, and psychologist/counsellor. It entails the following:

- Reassure and support the patient, and devise an agreed treatment plan.
- Clarify the patient's understanding of the treatment plan. Some doctors seek verbal agreement while others prefer a signed written agreement of the plan.
- Arrange for frequent dispensing of the medication, sufficient only for 1 day to a week (depending on the patient). Patients generally agree to regulated dispensing, and not to doctor shop or seek benzodiazepines from other sources.
- Arrange for urine drug screens if there is a concern about surreptitious use of other drugs.
- Some countries can provide information to the prescribing doctor about all prescriptions (of publicly subsidized medications) for psychotropic medications. This helps to ensure that the treating doctor is the only source of benzodiazepines.

Tapering diazepam regimen

- Convert the patient's reported usual dose of benzodiazepine to the diazepam equivalent using an equivalence table (see Table 13.1).
- Judge the veracity of the patient's self-report. If the patient is suspected of exaggerating their dose, commence on 50% of the stated dose in diazepam equivalents. If the GP is the only source of benzodiazepines, the starting dose can be 80% of the known dose.
- Once the patient is stable and free from withdrawal, gradually reduce the diazepam dose in a stepwise fashion by 5–10% every 1–2 weeks.
- Titrate dose reduction according to the patient's response, taking into consideration anxiety, the quality of sleep, and presence of tremor.
- If, on dose reduction, withdrawal symptoms recur, maintain at the previous dose until the patient is stable and then continue tapering with smaller dose decrements at longer time intervals, e.g. by 2.5 mg every fortnight. The patient has to be comfortable with, and agree to, the rate of reduction.
- Typically, the final dose reduction steps (e.g. from 10 mg/day onwards) are the most challenging for the patient.

- Reassure the patient that the diazepam dose regimen and dose reductions are prescribed at a rate that minimizes discomfort.
- The medication should be taken 'by the clock' at agreed regular intervals, *not* on an as-required basis in response to insomnia or anxiety. This breaks the pattern of using a chemical solution to stressors.
- Fully weaning off benzodiazepines varies greatly and may take weeks to months. In some severe cases, this may extend to more than a year.
- Psychological treatments are valuable for successful outcome (see later in topic).

Education and information
- Fully inform the patient about the potential side effects of benzodiazepines:
  - Falls (particularly in the elderly)
  - Danger of driving or operating machinery because of risk of accidents, injuries
  - Warn of the risks associated with concurrent use of alcohol, opioids and other CNS depressants
  - Pregnant women should avoid chronic use of benzodiazepines because of the risk of the neonatal withdrawal syndrome.
- Benzodiazepine-dependent patients should not suddenly stop their medication, or reduce their doses too quickly. In general, the withdrawal may be more distressing and life-threatening than continued use.
- Inform the patient fully about the signs and symptoms of benzodiazepine withdrawal. See p. 313.

Psychological therapies
- Practical advice can be provided on good sleep hygiene, such as avoiding caffeine-containing drinks within 6 hours of bedtime, plenty of daytime exercise, avoiding daytime naps, and a relaxing evening routine.
- Explore alternative methods of coping with stress, anxiety, panic attacks or insomnia, e.g.:
  - Relaxation therapy
  - Stress management
  - Meditation
  - Group therapy.
- Explore alternative or adjunctive treatment options:
  - CBT has a useful role during benzodiazepine dose reduction, and the psychologist or other counselling staff can increase the patient's awareness of triggers to benzodiazepine use and alternative ways of coping with these, as well as provide training in relaxation techniques.

Barbiturates

Barbiturates include amobarbital, barbital, butobarbital, phenobarbital, pentobarbital, and secobarbital. Barbiturates bind to the GABA$_A$ receptor and enhance GABAergic transmission. They have a propensity to be fatal in overdose because of their low therapeutic ratio. Since the advent of the safer benzodiazepines in the 1960s, they are less commonly used.

Barbiturate overdose

The great disadvantage of barbiturates is their low therapeutic ratio: the lethal dose may be only four to five times the therapeutic dose and the risk of mortality is accentuated if the person has taken alcohol or another CNS depressant. There is no antidote.

Signs and symptoms of barbiturate overdose
- Lethargy
- Drowsiness
- Coma and death.

Barbiturate-induced coma can resemble a vegetative brain dead state. It is crucial to exclude barbiturate overdose prior to cessation of life support.

Treatment of barbiturate overdose
- General supportive measures: airways, breathing, circulation
- IV fluids
- Alkalization of urine—when phenobarbital or barbital is present.

Barbiturate dependence

Typically seen in people who take barbiturates in doses of more than 500 mg a day on a daily basis for at least 1 month. Abrupt discontinuation in a dependent individual may lead to the barbiturate withdrawal syndrome.

Barbiturate withdrawal syndrome

Barbiturate withdrawal symptoms include tremulousness, sweating, anxiety, agitation, tachycardia, and hypertension in the early stages. If symptoms progress, seizures and delirium become life-threatening.

Treatment of barbiturate withdrawal syndrome
- General supportive measures, regularly monitor pulse rate, blood pressure, and temperature.
- Observe for signs of agitation and barbiturate withdrawal.
- Preferably manage the withdrawal syndrome by repeat doses of phenobarbital 60 mg until the patient is sedated and mildly dysarthric.
- Experience of using phenobarbital in this situation is rare nowadays.
- Many authorities recommend the use of a benzodiazepine:
  - oral diazepam 10–20 mg four times a day
  - reduce gradually by 10 mg every 2–3 days.
- In severe cases, IV diazepam 10 mg may be required and repeat doses every 30 minutes if necessary. Alternatively, midazolam or a barbiturate anaesthetic may be given. Nurse in high dependency unit.
- For hallucinations, give olanzapine 5–10 mg every 6 hours.

'Z' drugs

- Zolpidem is an imidazopyridine hypnotic agent and zopiclone is a cyclopyrrolone hypnotic agent. Both have hypnotic properties similar to those of the benzodiazepines, and their actions are blocked by the antagonist flumazenil. However, they are generally preferred as hypnotics because of better (shorter) kinetics, so are less likely to cause hangover. Although they do have lower dependence potential than classic benzodiazepines but a significant number of cases of abuse or dependence have emerged.
- Zaleplon is an even shorter acting hypnotic that can be used for middle-of-the-night insomnia to get people back to sleep with little risk of hangover if taken more than 4 hours before rising.
- Eszopiclone is the active enantiomer of zopiclone that is licensed in the US and has controlled trial evidence of efficacy with limited withdrawal for 6 months.
- Side effects of zolpidem are increasingly reported even at standard doses and especially at supratherapeutic doses. They include confusion, bizarre behaviour, somnambulance, sleep driving, bingeing on food, and disinhibited sexual behaviour.
- Zopiclone often leads to a metallic taste in the mouth, and may cause blurred vision and palpitations with some hangover sedation.
- If withdrawal symptoms occur on cessation of chronic use, patients may be treated as for diazepam dependence (see pp. 319–22). In commencing a tapering diazepam regimen, one tablet of zolpidem (10 mg) or zopiclone (7.5 mg) is approximately equivalent to 5 mg diazepam.

Prevention of benzodiazepine abuse and dependence

Unless there is good reason, benzodiazepines should be prescribed only for short-term treatment (not more than 2–4 weeks), e.g. for patients with insomnia, anxiety, or for its anticonvulsant or muscle relaxant effects. In patients with incapacitating anxiety, weigh risks against benefits of benzodiazepines and tailor treatment according to the individual patient's needs.

The risks associated with prescribing benzodiazepines in-patients with a history of alcohol and other substance misuse include:

- dose escalation/benzodiazepine dependence/benzodiazepine withdrawals
- diversion to the black market
- doctor-shopping
- drug-related presentations at the clinic
- significant risk of interactions with other CNS depressants such as alcohol, opioids, and cannabis
- negative impact on mental acuity; impaired psychomotor performance
- neuropsychiatric and subtle changes in mood including depressive symptoms.

Minimize prescribing of benzodiazepines.

Benzodiazepines should be avoided in patients with a history of alcohol and substance misuse unless:

- a compelling indication exists to use them (e.g. short-term management of acute alcohol withdrawal)
- there is no good alternative (e.g. treatment has failed with CBT and other medication options).

Further reading

Baldwin DS, Anderson IM, Nutt DJ, et al. (2014). Evidence-based pharmacological treatment of anxiety disorders, post-traumatic stress disorder and obsessive-compulsive disorder: a revision of the 2005 guidelines from the British Association for Psychopharmacology. *J Psychopharmacol* 28:403–39.

Lingford-Hughes AR, Welch S, Peters L, et al. (2012). BAP updated guidelines: evidence-based guidelines for the pharmacological management of substance abuse, harmful use, addiction and comorbidity: recommendations from BAP. *J Psychopharmacol* 26:1–54. Available at: http://www.bap.org.uk/pdfs/BAPaddictionEBG_2012.pdf

Mental Health and Drug and Alcohol Office (2007). *NSW Drug and Alcohol Withdrawal Clinical Practice Guidelines.* Sydney: NSW Department of Health. Available at: http://www.health.nsw.gov.au

Nutt DJ, Malizia AL. (2001). New insights into the role of the GABA(A)-benzodiazepine receptor in psychiatric disorder. *Br J Psychiatry* 179:390–6.

Wilson SJ, Nutt DJ, Alford C, et al. (2010). British Association for Psychopharmacology consensus statement on evidence-based treatment of insomnia, parasomnias and circadian rhythm disorders. *J Psychopharmacol* 24(11):1577–601. Available at: http://www.bap.org.uk/pdfs/BAP_Sleep_Guidelines.pdf

Psychostimulants

Epidemiology and types of psychostimulants 328
Pharmacology 332
Pathophysiology 336
Clinical syndromes 337
Natural history of psychostimulant use 342
Screening and brief intervention 343
Clinical assessment of psychostimulant use disorder 344
Management 348

Epidemiology and types of psychostimulants

Psychostimulants are substances that increase CNS arousal and are typically sympathomimetics, acting like noradrenaline to increase cardiovascular tone and activity. The term psychostimulants refers to both naturally occurring substances and the many synthesized drugs whose primary actions are CNS stimulation.

Naturally occurring psychostimulants have been used by human beings for thousands of years. They include:

• caffeine (a constituent of coffee and tea)
• cocaine (coca leaves)
• betel (areca nut)
• ephedra
• khat.

In addition to plant-based psychostimulants, there are numerous synthetic products, such as amphetamine-type stimulants (ATS) and their derivatives. For more than two decades, many regions around the world have seen ever-increasing production of illicit ATS. They are now the second most commonly used illicit drug after cannabis in both high-income and low-income countries. Much ATS use is attributable to 'instrumental use' to improve productivity.

• An estimated 52 million people worldwide use psychostimulants, primarily ATS substances.
• 75% of those with ATS use disorders live in Asia.
• ATS use disorders are often complicated by consequences such as ATS-related psychosis, predominantly seen among ATS-injecting users and younger populations.
• ATS use disorders occur in all levels of society, although ATS use is most common among younger age groups.
• Cocaine is used less widely, although the prevalence varies greatly with availability from country to country.
• North America and the European countries remain the areas of highest cocaine prevalence, although increasing prevalence is emerging in Oceania and Asia, as economies flourish in the region.
• The emerging synthetic stimulants such as the piperazines and cathinones like mephedrone are very common in Oceania and use continues to increase in Europe and North America.

Prescribed ATS such as dexamphetamine and methylphenidate are prescribed for the treatment of narcolepsy and attention-deficit hyperactivity disorder (ADHD). These and other ATS drugs may be diverted into recreational use. For the clinician, the distinguishing features of consequences and health problems associated with the various psychostimulants are subtle in the initial presentation, whereas variations in longer-term effects may be attributable to the different classes or types of psychostimulants.

Amphetamine and methamphetamine

Amphetamine and methamphetamine are the major psychostimulants used worldwide, with methamphetamine currently predominating. The next most prevalent is 3,4 methylenedioxymethamphetamine (MDMA, or 'Ecstasy,' as it is commonly known). Amphetamines and ATS can be smoked, insufflated ('snorted'), injected, or taken orally, including rubbing on gums. Occasionally, they are taken anally. In some countries (e.g. Australia), a popular route of administration is by injection, but in most of the world, injection is much less common than smoking or oral ingestion (US, Asia, and most European countries).

The reasons for national and regional variations in ATS use are related to historical allegiances to drugs, importation phenomena, legal status and enforcement of laws relating to ATS drugs, as well as to availability of precursors such as pseudoephedrine that enable local-scale manufacture.

The use of ATS drugs produces acute health consequences and long-term problems, often resulting in severe use disorders. Indications of consequences are apparent in increased numbers of patients seeking treatment for ATS-related problems.

The proportion of people in treatment services who have ATS use disorder is:

- 10% in Europe
- 12% in North America
- 20% in Australia and New Zealand
- 21% in Asia
- 36% in much of East and South-East Asia
- 50% in Japan, South Korea, Thailand, Cambodia, and the Philippines.

Saudi Arabia and other parts of the Near and Middle East are emerging as world regions with rapidly increasing ATS problems, particularly involving the use of fenethylline, originally marketed as Captagon® for ADHD and narcolepsy, but long banned in Western countries. Though retaining the name, the illicitly produced Captagon® typically contains other ATS stimulants, including methamphetamine.

MDMA

MDMA or 'Ecstasy' is a chemical analogue of methamphetamine, but with distinct pharmacological effects. It has mixed effects, with hallucinogenic and entactogenic (empathogenic) characteristics that are sought beyond the stimulant and sympathomimetic effects that characterize other ATS drugs.

MDMA use varies widely among countries, with 26 million estimated global users. It occurs in 2.9% of adults in Australia and New Zealand, 1% in North America, and less than 1% in Europe. The primary user population comprises younger people, including adolescents, with 1.5 million European users being 15–34 years of age. In North America, an estimated 1.5% of seniors in high school use MDMA. MDMA is commonly used at 'raves,' concerts, parties, and in the club scene.

Individuals who use MDMA often experience a 'hangover' the day after use. This is characterized by insomnia, fatigue, drowsiness, sore jaw muscles from teeth clenching, loss of balance, and headaches. Given that MDMA is rarely a pure product, many adverse effects may be attributable to substances such as strychnine, PCP, or amphetamine, and much MDMA contains considerable proportions of methamphetamine. In North America, for example, 55% of MDMA seized in the US contained methamphetamine, and 70% of the samples tested in Canada contained methamphetamine.

Cocaine

- Cocaine is a naturally occurring psychostimulant derived from the coca plant, *Erythroxylum coca*, a plant native to South America.
- It is refined into paste, powder, and freebase or 'crack'; these have different modes of usage and different rates of onset.
- Chewing coca leaves occurs only in Central and South America, where the plant is native.
- The crude paste extract is also used almost exclusively in coca-growing countries such as Bolivia, Colombia, and Peru.
- Cocaine hydrochloride powder is the form most commonly used in developed countries; it is insufflated ('snorted') or injected in a solution of water.
- 'Crack' or free-base cocaine is created by mixing powdered cocaine hydrochloride with sodium bicarbonate and allowing it to dry into small 'rocks'. It differs from cocaine powder in rapidity and intensity of effect. Crack is smoked, resulting in very rapid onset of effects. The brief duration of action promotes frequent administration for as long as the drug supply is available, resulting in increased consequences related to the route of administration.

Cocaine's vasoconstrictor and local anaesthetic actions led to its use as a topical anaesthetic, and it is still used in many types of surgery.

Mephedrone and other synthetic stimulants

Synthetic ATS drugs of the cotinine group are referred to as 'designer stimulants,' with the most prevalent of these ever-changing compounds being mephedrone (4-methylmethcathinone) and MDVP (methylene-dioxypyrovalerone), although other forms include methedrone (4-methoxymethcathinone), PMA and PMMA (p-methoxymethamphetamine), butylone (bk-MBDB, beta-keto-N-methylbenzodioxolylpropylamine), flephedrone (4-fluoromethcathinone), and others.

Another set of compounds in this class are the piperazines, originally created as vermicides to treat parasitic infestations, and found useful as antidepressants, with the most common one being BZP (benzylpiperzine). Sale of products containing various combinations of these compounds occurs over the counter in many forms to evade regulation, marketed as plant food/fertilizer, bath salts, and other categories not overtly intended for human use.

Mephedrone and similar substances are not easily manufactured, unlike methamphetamine, which can be produced by simple techniques. Large-scale manufacture occurs primarily in Pakistan, India, and China. The purity of these products is always questionable, occasionally producing medical consequences due to diluents and poor refining resulting in, for example, manganese poisoning. Like other ATS drugs, synthetics occur as powder, liquid forms, tablets, and capsules. To advance their sale, purveyors have often marketed such preparations as 'Ecstasy'.

The routes of administration of the cathinone-based synthetics include all those for the other ATS substance—users orally ingest, snort, inject, or smoke the compounds, producing effects that are similar to the ATS drugs. One difference is the inhalation route, with the substance dissolved in water or other liquid to be sprayed into mouth or nose and inhaled or applied as drops or spray into the eyes.

Little information is available about the cathinones due to their relatively recent emergence and their constantly changing chemical composition. The prevalence of mephedrone use and that of other synthetics is poorly documented in most world regions, including North America. In Europe, the use of mephedrone compounds is very common (preceded only by cannabis, cocaine, and MDMA). The prevalence can change rapidly: in the US, there were no samples of synthetic cathinones presented to poison control centres by the end of 2009, but there were 2639 samples submitted within the next 18 months.

Other stimulants

Khat is a mild intoxicant, which is chewed as the leaf form or drunk as tea. It is used primarily among African and Middle Eastern populations. While not widely appearing in Western countries, the worldwide number of khat users likely exceeds 10 million regular users. Much more common in the regions where the plant is indigenous, khat is appearing among immigrant populations in developed countries.

Ephedra has been used in Asia as a stimulant for centuries. It is also a component of energy pills and diet supplements, relying on the presence of pseudoephedrine. Although prohibited in most Western countries, large production facilities in India, Korea, and China supply quantities for illicit marketing around the world.

Pharmacology

All stimulants cause CNS arousal, excitation, and have sympathomimetic effects similar to noradrenaline. After the acute phase there is typically a phase of dysphoria known as the 'crash' which is of variable severity.

Amphetamines, methamphetamine, and other ATS drugs

The primary action of ATS substances is to activate the release of the monoamines dopamine, noradrenaline, and serotonin from central storage sites in presynaptic nerve terminals, and to a lesser extent to inhibit their reuptake. ATS drugs act as substrates for transporters of these biogenic amines and increase central synaptic concentrations of dopamine, noradrenaline, and serotonin. Noradrenaline release contributes to the sympathomimetic effects, while dopamine elicits central stimulant and rewarding effects, and serotonin is responsible for psychotomimetic effects (see Box 14.1).

Methamphetamine has similar effects to other ATS drugs, but higher brain levels are reached for the same dose, and smoking methamphetamine produces very rapid brain entry, resulting in greater euphoria.

The onset of effect is rapid, occurring within minutes after intranasal administration and even faster after inhalation or intravenous administration. Most amphetamine users take the drug for the 'rush' or 'high' associated with use, but some use amphetamines to stay awake longer (students and truck drivers), to give more energy (e.g. at dance parties), to lose weight (young women), or for increased sexual desire or performance (sex workers). Subsequent to this phase, the person may experience dysphoria and lethargy, a state analogous to a 'hangover' after alcohol consumption.

Box 14.1 Effects of amphetamine type stimulants

Central stimulant effects
- Euphoria
- Increased energy and mental alertness
- Insomnia
- Nervousness or anxiety
- Reduced appetite and weight loss
- Enhanced self-confidence
- Increased libido
- Increased body temperature
- May precipitate psychosis.

Sympathomimetic effects
- Tachycardia
- Raised blood pressure
- Sweating
- Dilated pupils, blurred vision
- Tremor.

ATS substances are metabolized in the liver by cytochrome P450 enzymes to active metabolites. Methamphetamine is partly converted to amphetamine and amphetamine to 4-hydroxyamphetamine. Depending on the pH of the urine, a significant proportion is excreted unchanged by the kidneys. As renal excretion is increased in acidic urine, overdose can be treated by acidifying the urine. Urine drug screen results can remain positive for 2–4 days after use.

3,4-Methylenedioxymethamphetamine (MDMA, Ecstasy)

MDMA is typically taken for its euphoric and stimulant effects, and for generating feelings of closeness with others (a 'hug drug'). It used to be prescribed as an appetite suppressant or to induce a state of improved empathy and consciousness during psychotherapeutic sessions.

Like the other ATS drugs, MDMA releases central monoamines such as dopamine, noradrenaline, and serotonin by reversing the action of their transporters, particularly the serotonin transporter. MDMA also inhibits tryptophan hydroxylase, the rate-limiting enzyme in serotonin synthesis, which is followed by acute depletion of central serotonin levels. The acute release of central serotonin is profound and may lead to permanent serotonin depletion with chronic use.

MDMA is usually taken orally but can be injected. Typically, MDMA is taken as one or two tablets at weekly to monthly intervals, but occasionally several tablets are taken consecutively. Onset of effect occurs within 30 to 60 minutes and peaks at 90 minutes. Duration of effect of a typical dosage is approximately 8 hours. MDMA is metabolized in the liver to an active metabolite, methylenedioxyamphetamine (MDA) (see Box 14.2).

Cocaine

Cocaine is similar in structure to amphetamine sulphate, but is more potent. Cocaine inhibits the reuptake of dopamine, noradrenaline, and serotonin from the synaptic cleft by blocking the transporters of these biogenic amines. Cocaine is thought to produce its rewarding effect primarily by increasing dopamine concentrations in the nucleus accumbens. The block of the noradrenaline transporter produces the sympathomimetic effects.

Box 14.2 Pharmacological effects of MDMA

CNS stimulation
- Euphoria
- Increased alertness and energy
- Diminished appetite
- Heightened empathy and feelings of closeness (entactogenic)
- Psychedelic/hallucinogenic effects (high doses).

Sympathomimetic effects
- Tachycardia
- Hypertension.

The onset of euphoric effect of cocaine is rapid, occurring within minutes, and within seconds when inhaled via smoked administration as in crack. Duration of effect is short, approximately 30–90 minutes depending on the mode of administration. Because of its short duration of intense euphoria, cocaine is at times used repeatedly, in a binge pattern over several hours, which places the user at increased risk of toxicity and side effects (see Box 14.3).

Cocaine is metabolized by cholinesterase mainly in the liver to an inactive demethylated metabolite benzoylecgonine and ecgonine methyl ester. A small proportion (1–2%) is excreted unchanged in the urine. Metabolites can be detected in blood or urine for 36 hours and in the hair for weeks to months after use.

Concurrent use of cocaine and alcohol produce cocaethylene, a longer-acting metabolite that can have more pronounced and prolonged stimulant and cardiotoxic actions. Many of the acute complications of cocaine tend to result from over stimulation of the CNS sympathomimetic effects and/or vasospasm.

Table 14.1 summarizes some of the pharmacological properties of some psychostimulants.

Box 14.3 Pharmacological effects of cocaine

CNS stimulation

- Intense euphoria
- Increased energy, hyperactivity, excitability
- Enhanced confidence and libido
- Increased performance of repetitive tasks
- Insomnia
- Increased risk of aggressive, violent, erratic, and high-risk behaviours
- Potential for drug-induced psychosis.

Sympathomimetic and vasoconstrictor effects

- Tachycardia
- Hypertension
- Vasoconstriction
- Local anaesthetic effects (via stereo-isomer procaine present in cocaine).

Table 14.1 Time course of pharmacological action of psychostimulants

Psychostimulant	Onset of action	Duration of effect
Amphetamines (ATS)	Within minutes for IV use, ~20 min for oral use	8–36 h
Methamphetamine	Within minutes for IV or smoking, ~20 min for oral	8–36 h
MDMA	30–60 min for oral	8–9 h
Mephedrone, BZP, and other synthetics	30–45 min for oral 15–30 min for insufflated	2–3 h
Cocaine	½–2 min for IV use 5–10 sec for smoking 1–3 min for intranasal	Up to 90 min Up to 20 min Up to 90 min

Mephedrone and other synthetic stimulants

Mephedrone and the other cathinones increase serotonin and dopamine in the nucleus accumbens, more so than ATS drugs. The half-life associated with typical dosages appears brief compared to ATS drugs, requiring frequent repeat administrations—similar to cocaine use.

Whereas users may ingest 1 gram of mephedrone in a session, more potent forms such as the p-methoxyamphetamines (PMA and PMMA) require only 10 mg dosage, thus resembling methamphetamine in their potency.

The non-regulation of benzylpiperazine (BZP) in New Zealand until 2008 (long after most countries banned its production and sale) led to widespread use in that country. BZP toxicity was documented in a majority of ATS-related presentations, with complications from polydrug use, often involving MDMA and alcohol, being associated with the majority of serious side effects such as toxic seizures, prolonged seizures, and respiratory and metabolic acidosis.

Other stimulants

Ephedra and khat produce CNS effects and increase heart rate and blood pressure. Acute effects resolve within hours. Ephedra and ephedrine are noradrenergic. Consumption of large quantities of khat, mechanistically similar to the other cathinone drugs, produces thirst, hyperactivity, reduced appetite, and sleep disturbance, with depression occurring after extended use sessions. Khat may cause delusions and hallucinations, and long-term use may result in negative effects on nervous, respiratory, circulatory, and digestive systems.

Pathophysiology

Many acute side effects and complications of psychostimulant use are attributable to their sympathomimetic effects. The additional vaso-constriction with cocaine use is responsible for complications such as peripheral ischaemia, myocardial infarction, cerebral haemorrhage, ischaemic stroke, and bowel ischaemia. Vasoconstriction may threaten placental blood supply.

Following acute ATS intoxication, there is a 'crash'; this is attributed to acute depletion of neurotransmitter stores (as well as exhaustion from excessive activity). Chronic use of psychostimulants seems to have a long-term effect on neurotransmission. Positron emission tomography (PET) studies in chronic methamphetamine users demonstrated a reduction in dopamine transporter concentration suggesting a loss of dopamine projections. This reduction was significantly associated with the duration of use and the severity of persistent psychiatric symptoms.

MDMA causes inhibition of antidiuretic hormone (ADH). In response to hyperthermia, sweating, and dehydration (from the drug and from increased physical activity during parties and raves), large amounts of water may be consumed. The resulting hyponatraemia may be exacer-bated by ADH inhibition. Water intoxication and hyponatraemia may lead to cerebral oedema and, in rare cases, death.

MDMA may have permanent neurotoxic effects on serotonergic nerve terminals that are involved in memory and regulation of mood. Chronic serotonin depletion may result in cognitive impairment, sleep disorders, anxiety states, depressed mood, impulsiveness, and hostility. There is conflicting evidence on whether this damage to serotonergic neurons is permanent, but MDMA users need to be warned of these potential risks.

Clinical syndromes

Acute stimulant intoxication

Stimulant use initially results in euphoria, alertness, and increased libido. Modest doses elevate the pulse and blood pressure and produce vasoconstriction. The effects are greater with increased doses and greater frequency of use and include dilated pupils, sweating, dizziness, tremor, fever, rapid breathing, racing pulse, and elevated blood pressure. Continued use of psychostimulants may cause tremor and muscle contractions, and sustained use of moderate doses will result in fatigue, poor concentration, and depression. Rambling speech, headache, transient ideas of reference, and tinnitus are common during intoxication, and extreme cases can present with paranoid ideation, auditory hallucinations, and tactile hallucinations. Exaggerated anger and aggressive behaviour may occur. Irritability, emotional lability, and suicidality may be present (see Boxes 14.4–14.7).

Box 14.4 Features of ATS (amphetamine and methamphetamine) intoxication

General
- Nausea, vomiting
- Jaw clenching/grinding (bruxism)
- Stereotypic movements/formication (scratching, excoriations)
- Hyperthermia.

Sympathomimetic effects
- Tachypnoea
- Sweating
- Dilated pupils, blurred vision
- Tachycardia
- Hypertension
- Cardiac arrhythmias
- Cardiovascular collapse.

CNS stimulation
- Restlessness, hyperactivity
- Agitation
- Anxiety, panic attacks
- Insomnia, sleep disorders
- Twitching
- Seizures
- Cerebral haemorrhage, stroke.

Psychiatric complications
- ATS-induced psychosis (resembles paranoid schizophrenia)
- Depression during the 'crash phase': suicidality.

Box 14.5 Features of MDMA intoxication

General
- Fatigue
- Nausea
- Dry mouth
- Restlessness
- Insomnia
- Jaw clenching (bruxism)
- Hyperthermia.

Cardiovascular system (sympathomimetic effects)
- Hypertension
- Tachyarrhythmias
- Asystole
- Arteritis, vasculitis
- Cardiovascular collapse.

Gastrointestinal system
- Hepatotoxicity.

Musculoskeletal
- Muscle cramps
- Rhabdomyolysis.
- Dehydration (sweating)
- Water intoxication and hyponatraemia (excess water to overcome dehydration; exacerbated by inappropriate ADH secretion).

Renal
- Acute kidney injury (secondary to rhabdomyolysis).

CNS
- Restlessness in the legs
- Transient gait disturbance
- Increased tactile sensitivity
- Impaired memory and learning
- Cerebral haemorrhage (or cerebral oedema due to water intoxication and hyponatraemia).

Neuropsychiatric
- Agitation
- Hallucinations/psychosis
- Hyponatraemia in combination with hypoglycaemia and/or hypokalaemia suggests PMA toxicity.

Box 14.6 Features of cocaine intoxication

General
- Fatigue
- Nausea
- Dry mouth
- Restlessness
- Insomnia
- Bruxism
- Hyperthermia.

Cardiovascular system
- Tachycardia
- Hypertension
- Tachyarrhythmias
- Myocardial infarction
- Peripheral ischaemia, gangrene.

Respiratory system
- Dyspnoea, tachypnoea (non-cardiogenic pulmonary oedema, pulmonary infarction)
- Haemoptysis: pulmonary infarction and or haemorrhage (due to vasoconstriction).

Gastrointestinal tract
- Abdominal pain, bloody stools, bowel ischaemia, bowel infarction (due to vasoconstrictor effect)
- Hepatic ischaemia, hepatic necrosis (due to vasoconstrictor effect).

Musculoskeletal
- Muscle cramps
- Rhabdomyolysis.

Renal
- Acute kidney injury (secondary to rhabdomyolysis).

CNS
- Tics and other stereotyped muscle activity
- Seizures
- Intracranial haemorrhage
- Ischaemic stroke
- Cerebral vasculitis.

Neuropsychiatric symptoms
- Paranoia, paranoid psychosis
- Violent and erratic behaviour
- Hypomania, mania
- Perceptual disturbances, depersonalization
- Confusion
- Delirium.

Box 14.7 Features of intoxication with mephedrone and other synthetic stimulants

General
- Nausea, vomiting
- Jaw clenching/grinding
- Stereotypic movements/formication (scratching)
- Hyperthermia.

Sympathomimetic effects
- Tachypnoea
- Sweating
- Dilated pupils, blurred vision
- Tachycardia
- Hypertension
- Cardiac arrhythmias
- Cardiovascular collapse.

CNS stimulation
- Restlessness, hyperactivity
- Agitation
- Anxiety, panic attacks
- Insomnia, sleep disorders
- Twitching
- Seizures
- Cerebral haemorrhage, stroke.

Psychiatric
- ATS-induced psychosis (resembles schizophrenia)
- Hallucinations.

Acute stimulant overdose

Severe stimulant intoxication is characterized by:
- anxiety and agitation
- paranoia and other features of psychosis
- suicidality
- cardiovascular distress
- may be non-responsive with tonic–clonic seizures.

Hyperthermia associated with psychostimulant effects on the hypothalamus can result in death. Mortality is a risk in stimulant overdose due to cardiovascular complications, seizures, and hypoxia. In addition, pulmonary complications of overdose and high-dose toxicity include chest pain and dyspnoea. Chronic use of psychostimulants often results in cardiopulmonary consequences such as chest pain, hypertension, tachycardia, and dyspnoea. In ATS overdose, pulmonary hypertension and oedema are found in 70% of fatal cases.

Stimulant use disorder

Stimulant use disorder in DSM-5 encompasses what was termed in DSM-IV as stimulant abuse and stimulant dependence. Many users use these drugs intermittently rather than on a daily basis, and may have a binge pattern of use.

- Stimulant dependence (moderate–severe stimulant use disorder) occurs in 40–60% of regular ATS users after an average period of 3–4 years, and in about 55% of regular cocaine users.
- Dependence is more common among male users, in those who smoke or inject the drugs and in those with a history of mental health problems.
- Stimulant dependent users typically consume a large amount of the drug over several days (a binge), going without sleep before ceasing use through physical exhaustion or running out of money. Daily use to avoid withdrawal symptoms may then develop.
- Dependence is less likely to occur with use of MDMA than the other drugs.

Complications of stimulant use disorder are common. They include local and systemic effects of snorting or injecting use, aggression and violence, psychotic symptoms, and the ever-present risk of progression to severe level use disorder and addictive behaviour.

Withdrawal

The withdrawal syndrome from psychostimulants typically has two phases and sometimes a further preliminary phase of residual toxicity. Withdrawal from ATS use typically starts 2–4 days after last use and symptoms peak at 7–10 days, gradually subsiding over several weeks, with dysphoric mood and anxiety persisting for up to 10 weeks. Cocaine withdrawal symptoms typically commence and resolve earlier, starting within a day of cessation, peaking at 4–7 days, and subsiding over 1–2 weeks.

Residual toxicity phase

This consists of continuing stimulant effects, which may include hyper-activity, agitation and paranoid ideation. With long-acting drugs such as the amphetamines, this phase may persist for 1–3 days. Some patients will exhibit continuing psychotic symptoms and a diagnosis of psychostimulant-induced psychosis may be appropriate.

Initial withdrawal phase

This phase is similar to a post-intoxication 'crash' but at a more extreme level. It often follows intense, high-dose use. Common features are:
- dysphoric mood, which may lead to depression and anhedonia
- anergia (the person may lie in bed for several days)
- fatigue and lassitude
- insomnia or hypersomnia
- increased appetite
- craving for drugs.

Delayed withdrawal phase

A characteristic feature of psychostimulant withdrawal (which often leads to relapse), is the delayed (or 'prolonged extinction') phase after the acute withdrawal symptoms have subsided. This extinction phase is analogous to protracted withdrawal symptoms in alcohol dependence and may last 6–10 weeks. Fluctuations in mood and energy levels are common during this phase, with evidence of fatigue, low mood, anxiety, irritability and disturbed sleep. Cravings for stimulants may occur during all phases of withdrawal and contribute to relapse. Mood will gradually normalize if relapse can be avoided.

Natural history of psychostimulant use

The natural history of stimulant use is varied and insufficiently characterized in the literature. Methamphetamine and cocaine are highly dependence-inducing. In some cases dependence occurs after a few weeks of psychostimulant use, although with ATS it more typically develops over 2–3 years. At 3 years 60% of ATS users have developed dependence. The long-term natural history (>10 years) has yet to be fully described.

The course of ATS use disorder is typically a variable one with periods of non-use and periods of relapse to high level use, and the associated sequelae. At 3 years, mortality is 5% with most of the deaths occurring from accidents, suicide, and homicide, and a smaller proportion as a result of blood-borne infections.

As a result of developing physical and psychological consequences of ATS use disorder, many long-term users seek treatment within 8–10 years.

Screening and brief intervention

Routine questioning of patients in primary care settings about illicit drug use can assist early detection of psychostimulant use. Such screening can support intervention, including assistance to stop drug use in those wishing to change, or provision of harm reduction advice for those not yet willing or able to change their stimulant use. While 'SBIRT' (Screening, Brief Intervention, and Referral to Treatment) has become a widely accepted model, very brief interventions for stimulant use disorder seem to be of limited effectiveness. Two to four sessions of 30 minutes each are more effective, but may not be practical in a busy primary care setting.

As for other forms of unhealthy substance use, clinicians can adopt the model used for alcohol use disorders—denoted by the FLAGS acronym—to frame an early intervention for patients with identified stimulant use disorder. This comprises:

- *Feedback:* provide feedback on medical, neuropsychiatric, or social harms, or major risks that are being faced, such as sexual risk-taking, risk of contaminated equipment and stimulants, and the risk of stroke. Be aware that the individual is likely to know many stimulant users who have had no adverse effects.
- *Listen:* consider the patient's responses, readiness to change, and past attempts to change.
- *Advice:* provide clear advice on substance use and its complications. Raise the patient's awareness of medical, neuropsychiatric, and social complications associated with psychostimulant use. Advise patients with a history of mental health problems (anxiety, depression, psychosis) that they should avoid use of stimulants because of the increased risk of precipitating, prolonging, or exacerbating their psychiatric problems. Advice may also include elements of harm reduction.
- *Goals:* the clinician's goal is likely to be abstinence from psychostimulants but the patient may not yet be ready to accept this goal. Motivational interviewing techniques may develop an interim goal such as decreasing frequency of use or reducing the harm from each episode of use.
- *Strategies:* to achieve the goal, suggest practical steps to try to reduce or cease stimulant use. For example, reduce alcohol use if stimulant use tends to occur as a result of alcohol intoxication; limit time or contact with stimulant-using friends; take less money when going out to a party; look for less hazardous ways to get a 'high'. In the case of a person unwilling to change their stimulant use, motivational interviewing techniques can be employed and harm reduction strategies can be discussed.

Clinical assessment of psychostimulant use disorder

History

Drug use history
- Determine all substances being used and check for concurrent use of alcohol, benzodiazepines, cannabis, and opioids
- Record quantities, frequencies, and patterns of drug use (daily, intermittent, binge)
- Duration of use
- Time of last use
- Route(s) of administration.

Psychiatric history
Identify past suicide attempts or ideation, consider stimulant-related complications and co-morbidities (e.g. anxiety, depression, psychosis). History of ADD/ADHD may be associated with subsequent use of ATS as self-medication for symptoms).

Family history
Determine presence in family members of alcohol and other substance use and psychiatric illness.

Physical examination
- General appearance:
  - Weight loss, poor self-care
  - Clenched jaw, bruxism
  - Fractures or other trauma
  - Sweating (or dehydration)
  - Fever, hyperthermia (from dehydration or water intoxication)
  - Repetitive movements
  - Dilated pupils
- Dental:
  - 'Meth mouth': loss of teeth, caries, broken teeth, periodontal disease, (jaw clenching, tooth grinding, ischaemia)
- Nose (with cocaine):
  - White powder in nostrils
  - Rhinorrhoea, sinusitis, epistaxis
  - Nasal septal necrosis
- Skin changes:
  - Needle track marks
  - Thrombophlebitis, cellulitis, skin abscess
  - 'Meth sores': sores and excoriations on face, arms, or legs (in part due to formication)
- Cardiopulmonary:
  - Tachycardia, tachyarrhythmias, hypertension, myocardial infarction (cocaine), heart murmurs/infective endocarditis (from injecting use)
  - Dyspnoea, tachypnoea, infections
  - Pulmonary oedema

- Genitourinary and renal:
  - Jaundice, hepatomegaly, and/or stigmata of chronic liver disease (hepatitis C)
  - Acute kidney injury (secondary to rhabdomyolysis)
- CNS and neuropsychiatric:
  - Seizures, cerebral haemorrhage, stroke
  - Restlessness, disinhibition, erratic behaviour, rapid speech, anxiety, agitation, hypervigilance, aggression, violence, paranoia, psychosis.
  - Depressed or suicidal in the crash/withdrawal phase (p. 341).
  - Infections
  - Sexually transmitted infections (STIs), HIV/AIDs.

Diagnosis and formulation

As for other substance use disorders, the diagnostic concepts of stimulant use disorders have been changed in DSM-5. The ICD system continues to have Substance Dependence as the central diagnosis. In ICD 10 it requires the presence of three of the following six criteria occurring repeatedly over the previous 12 months:

- Loss of control: awareness of an impaired ability to control use
- Craving or compulsion to use
- A significant amount of time usually spent in drug use and associated activities, to the detriment of other aspects of their lives
- Tolerance: requiring higher doses of the drug (often several grams per day) to achieve the desired affect
- Withdrawal: a withdrawal syndrome on cessation or reduction of use or relief or prevention of withdrawal by daily use to avoid withdrawal symptoms
- Continued and persistent use despite clear evidence of harm.

The DSM-5 criteria are listed below. The presence of 2–3 of the 11 items points to mild use disorder, 4–5 to moderate, and 6+ to severe. The definition is: 'A pattern of amphetamine-type stimulant use or cocaine use leading to clinically significant impairment or distress, as manifest by at least 2 of the following occurring within a 12-month period':

1. The stimulant is often taken in larger amounts or over a longer period than was intended
2. A persistent desire or unsuccessful efforts to cut down or control stimulant use
3. A great deal of time is spent in activities to obtain, use, or recover from the effects of the stimulant
4. Craving, or a strong desire or urge to use the stimulant
5. Recurrent stimulant use resulting in a failure to fulfil major role obligations at work, school, or home
6. Continued stimulant use despite persistent or recurrent social or interpersonal problems caused or exacerbated by the effects of the stimulant
7. Important social, occupational, or recreational activities given up or reduced because of stimulant use
8. Recurrent stimulant use in situations which are physically hazardous

9. Stimulant use is continued despite knowledge of a persistent or recurrent physical or psychological problem likely to have been caused or exacerbated by the stimulant
10. Tolerance, as defined by either of the following:
    a. A need for markedly increased amounts of the stimulant to achieve intoxication or desired effect
    b. A markedly diminished effect with continued use of the same amount of the stimulant
       Not applicable to individuals taking stimulants as medically prescribed
11. Withdrawal, as manifested by either of the following:
    a. The characteristic withdrawal syndrome for the stimulant
    b. The stimulant (or a closely related substance) is taken to relieve or avoid withdrawal symptoms.

Making the diagnosis

Determining the diagnosis of stimulant use

- Does the individual use stimulants without evidence of current harms?
- What are the physical, psychiatric, and social complications of psychostimulant use?
- Is the patient's pattern of stimulant use resulting in consequences and behaviours above the threshold to support a diagnosis of use disorder?
- Is the patient's pattern of stimulant use resulting in consequences that are social harms but the patient otherwise does not meet use disorder criteria?
- Is the patient physiologically compelled to use, indicated for example, by the amount of stimulant required to get an effect increasing?
- Is the patient able to stop stimulant use when desired or necessary?
- Is the patient aware of stimulant-related harms but continues to use?
- Is there history of overdose or complications from injection use?

Routine laboratory investigations

- FBC, EUC, LFTs, TFTs, BSL
- Serological tests for HIV and hepatitis
- Screen for STIs
- Urine drug screen (for cocaine, request plasma benzoylecgonine, the demethylated metabolite of cocaine, as cocaine itself has a variable and short half-life)
- Urine tests at 500 ng/mL cut-off for ATS drugs (e.g. MDMA and methamphetamine) are confirmed by gas chromatography at 250 ng/mL cut-off; note that the confirmation of methamphetamine requires an additional measure of 100 ng/mL of amphetamine. Hair samples can detect ATS substances for up to 90 days.

Other investigations

- ECGs to exclude arrhythmias in toxicity
- Cardiac enzymes, troponin levels if ischaemic heart disease is suspected (cocaine) PK to exclude rhabdomyolysis
- Chest X-ray where indicated
- CT or MRI head: if indicated, e.g. to exclude cerebrovascular accidents.

Management

Management of stimulant intoxication and overdose

Psychostimulant toxicity is treated symptomatically. This includes any necessary sedation and supportive measures in a calm, quiet, and soothing environment. There is no medication that counters overdose, as in the case of naloxone for opioid overdose.

Management of ATS intoxication
- Monitor temperature, blood pressure, pulse rate, and respiratory rate at intervals of 2–4 hours.
- Place on ECG monitor if tachyarrhythmias are present or if the patient complains of chest pain.
- Ensure clear airways, breathing, and circulation.
- If hyperthermic, promote cooling.
- Rehydrate and correct fluid and electrolyte disturbances.
- Acidification of urine with ammonium chloride may help speed the excretion of stimulants other than cocaine.
- If the patient is extremely agitated, sedate with benzodiazepines (e.g. diazepam 10–20 mg orally and repeat after 2 hours until the patient is calm and mildly sedated; typical dose of 60–80 mg in the first 24 hours).
- If the patient is violent or otherwise uncontrollable, give IV diazepam (10 mg slowly), titrating dose according to response. This may be repeated after 30 minutes if necessary, and then switch to oral diazepam as above. An alternative is IV midazolam 2.5–10 mg (IV or IM), repeated as necessary after 10 min, and with further doses given according to response up to a maximum of 20 mg.
- A sedating antipsychotic agent (e.g. olanzapine or quetiapine) may be needed in addition to a benzodiazepine (do not give phenothiazines which lower seizure threshold).

In the presence of sustained, extreme agitation, tachycardia, or hypertension due to synthetic stimulants (cathinones or 'bath salts'), the potential contribution of a fluorinated cathinone such as flephedrone in the suspect compound should be considered. These compounds may retard metabolism of other stimulants.

Persistent symptoms may indicate a need for charcoal or gastric lavage.

Management of MDMA intoxication
In addition to measures previously described:
- Emesis or gastric lavage is indicated if the patient has MDMA toxicity from oral intake, is alert, and has taken MDMA less than 4 hours previously
- Rehydrate and correct fluid and electrolyte imbalance, particularly hyponatraemia.

Management of cocaine intoxication
- Any person with chest pain after cocaine use should be admitted for observation and consideration of suspected myocardial infarction.

- Hypertension may be treated with an alpha blocker (phentolamine) or a combined alpha- and beta-adrenergic blocker (e.g. labetalol). Labetalol reverses cocaine-induced increase in blood pressure but has no effect on cocaine-induced coronary vasoconstriction. Alternatively nitroprusside may be used.
- *Do not use beta blockers* (e.g. propranolol) as they exacerbate cocaine-induced vasoconstriction of coronary arteries.
- *Do not use calcium channel blockers* due to seizures related to their use.

Management of intoxication with mephedrone and other synthetic stimulants

In addition to measures previously described:
- Emesis or gastric lavage is indicated if the patient has stimulant toxicity from oral intake, is alert, and has taken the drug less than 4 hours previously
- Rehydrate and correct fluid and electrolyte imbalance, particularly hyponatraemia.

Management of complications of stimulant intoxication

In severe psychostimulant intoxication, acute rhabdomyolysis may occur. This needs to be diagnosed urgently as there is a risk of renal failure (for which dialysis may be required).

Cocaine-induced myocardial infarction is due to increased myocardial oxygen demand, tachycardia, increased blood pressure, and vasoconstriction of the coronary arteries.
- Admit patients who present with chest pain after cocaine use. Risk is highest in the first hour after use.
- Monitor with serial ECGs plus cardiac enzyme and troponin levels for at least 12 hours.
- Administer sublingual glyceryl trinitrate for chest pain and treat as for myocardial infarction but note that cocaine has local anaesthetic effects.
- Avoid aspirin if cerebral haemorrhage is suspected.

Management after stimulant intoxication resolves
- Monitor closely for depression and suicidality
- Protect from risk of self-injury
- Provide brief intervention if use disorder is mild or infrequent at low level
- Offer ongoing treatment or referral for moderate and severe use disorder.

Management of stimulant withdrawal

Persons with stimulant dependence may experience withdrawal upon sudden drug cessation, such as when admitted to hospital for a psychotic episode.

Cessation of psychostimulant use may also be a planned process including inpatient-based detoxification so that withdrawal symptoms can be managed under medical supervision.

To promote successful cessation and abstinence after detoxification, patients must be educated about withdrawal symptoms and their time course. Medications can be provided for withdrawal symptoms, and the patient should be reassured that symptoms will gradually resolve if they remain abstinent from stimulant use.

Managed detoxification is more suited to a clinical setting, but other options may be used for some motivated patients with mild or moderate use disorder and adequate preparation. Uncomplicated stimulant withdrawal may be managed in a supportive home environment, where there is a live-in caregiver and a nurse and/or general practitioner able to visit daily. An alternative is ambulatory detoxification where the patient visits the hospital/treatment centre or physician's office on a daily basis. A supportive, safe, and quiet environment is essential for rest and sleep to begin recovery after cessation.

For patients with established dependence and those with medical or psychiatric complications, withdrawal is best managed in a detoxification unit or hospital setting. The clinical features of stimulant withdrawal may be complicated by withdrawal from coexisting alcohol or other substance use disorder—many psychostimulant users are polysubstance users (particularly alcohol, benzodiazepines, or opioids). Psychiatric comorbidity adds to the complexity of the withdrawal process.

Key aspects of withdrawal management

- *Insomnia and agitation:* short-term benzodiazepines may be prescribed (e.g. diazepam 5–10 mg, three to four times daily); otherwise sedative drugs are unnecessary.
- *Psychosis:* olanzapine 10–20 mg daily.
- *Adequate diet:* because a significant component of the withdrawal syndrome is probably related to neurotransmitter depletion, recovery may be delayed because of anorexia associated with amphetamine use. It may be useful to provide some nutritional supplements or a well-balanced diet rich in monoamine precursors phenylalanine, tyrosine or L-tryptophan, e.g. pumpkin seeds, chocolate, marmite or vegemite, bananas.
- *Cravings:* the '3 Ds' technique may be helpful in managing cravings. This involves:
  - Delay the decision to use or not for 1 hour
  - Distract yourself with some activity during this hour
  - Decide whether it is worth using after the hour is up.
- *Identify comorbid psychiatric disorders:* recognize that the combination of stimulant use and depression places the person at increased risk of suicide.
- *Suicide risk assessment:* should be undertaken regularly if indicated.
- *Antidepressants:* the benefits of antidepressants in managing stimulant withdrawal symptoms are clearer where there is pre-existing depression and when administered 4–6 weeks after cessation. Antidepressants are unlikely to be effective even for pre-existing depression if the person continues stimulant use. Tricyclic antidepressants may place the patient at risk of toxicity overdose if the patient is suicidal. They may cause CNS depression if combined

with other antidepressants. SSRIs may cause the serotonin syndrome if combined with stimulants.
• *After detoxification:* management of withdrawals is the first step to subsequent treatment for stimulant use disorder with pharmacological, psychological, and social interventions, including residential care.

Management of neuropsychiatric complications

Stimulant-induced psychosis
• General supportive measures:
  • Personalize the interaction, using the patient's name
  • Involve compatible staff in interactions
  • Speak quietly and calmly, using non-threatening questions
  • Maintain calming countenance, with limited eye-to-eye contact
  • Listen passively to the patient to allow venting, offering objective support
  • Provide reassurance of safety and well-being while in clinical care
  • Be thoughtful of simple needs that can be satisfied (cup of coffee, snack)
• Addressing severe symptoms to avoid harm to patient or others:
  • Medicate and hospitalize
  • Restraint used in only the most severe cases
• Pharmacological management:
  • Oral medications when feasible include benzodiazepines as the first-line choice, followed by antipsychotics if insufficient response
  • IM or IV medications (benzodiazepines followed by antipsychotics) are used when the oral route is inappropriate or infeasible
  • Local preferences and guidelines should be consulted when available.

Anxiety
• Inform the patient that anxiety is a result of the stimulant and symptoms will subside as the stimulant wears off
• Provide short-term benzodiazepines for acute anxiety.

Depression
• Depression and suicidality may emerge during withdrawal phase; if severe, hospitalize.
• Post-withdrawal depression may persist but usually subsides with abstinence; use benzodiazepines for short-term treatment of agitation and insomnia.
• When depression persists well after withdrawal (~several weeks of abstinence) or when a pre-existing mood disorder is documented, begin antidepressant medications, especially if suicidality is evident.
• Caution should be exercised in prescribing SSRI medication due to potential for serotonin syndrome in the presence of stimulant use.

Serotonin syndrome associated with stimulant use
Serotonin syndrome is a potentially fatal condition resulting from excess central serotonergic activity that may be precipitated when stimulant use

occurs in the presence of SSRI medications or other drugs that increase serotonin levels.

- Clinical features of serotonin syndrome:
  - Autonomic dysfunction; sweating, shivering, diarrhoea, hypertension, dilated pupils, hyperthermia
  - CNS effects: agitation, mental state changes (confusion, hypomania), coma
  - Neuromuscular dysfunction: hyperreflexia, hypertonia, myoclonus, tremor, seizures
- Management of serotonin syndrome:
  - Curtail serotonin agent
  - Provide emergency care and admit to hospital
  - Give benzodiazepines for agitation and seizures
  - Consider cyproheptadine to block serotonin production.

Management of stimulant use disorder

Determination of a stimulant use disorder demands formal treatment, but in many if not most cases, the patient will be resistant to engaging in any or all of the possible treatment modalities. Provide information and education regarding stimulant use and its complications, and inform the patient of treatment options. This may include brief intervention and motivational interviewing. Let the patient digest the information provided and consider their options. The patient must then reach a point of acceptance of the need to develop a commitment to stop stimulant use. Inpatient detoxification may be a necessary first step for cessation of stimulant use and other drug use in polydrug users (see earlier in topic for management of stimulant withdrawal).

- *Pharmacotherapy*: to date, there are no unequivocally evidence-based pharmacotherapy regimens for the treatment of stimulant use disorder. There are several promising pharmacotherapies, described later in this topic. Consider use of antidepressants for chronic co-morbid depression if the patient has ceased stimulants.
- *Psychological therapy*: motivational interviewing, CBT, and other psychological therapies are an important component of any treatment plan for patients with stimulant use disorder. Such services help to attract and retain patients. CBT involves skills training and practice to deal with craving and high-risk situations associated with relapse. Another approach to help prevent relapse is contingency management. It may involve individual counselling by skilled counsellors using manualized therapy protocols or group drug counselling
- *Treatment of co-morbidity*: parallel treatment of underlying physical, and/or neuropsychiatric co-morbidity or complications.
- *Family and social support*: families of patients require support, assistance, and advice on how to deal with the patient and how to access community services, mental health services, and correctional services. Families also need information and advice on how to support and help the patient.

- *Self-help fellowships:* based on fellowship groups (e.g. AA) with abstinence as a goal, weekly 12-step meetings can be effective as ancillary support services in an overall treatment plan. Patients who participate in both formal drug treatment and weekly 12-step meetings have higher rates of abstinence.
- *Aftercare:* treatment is not just a brief one-off; follow-up counselling is crucial, and in the case of relapse to stimulant use, residential care is an important option.
- *Lifestyle and environmental change:* changes at work, home, and the environment are necessary to begin eliminating the drug-using lifestyle and beginning to achieve a meaningful life without drugs.

Pharmacological treatments under study

A variety of medications are under consideration and in clinical trials, although no medication has been approved in any country for treatment of stimulant use disorder.

Similar to methadone or buprenorphine for opioid addicts, psycho-stimulant substitution therapy has been considered for stimulant use disorder. Dexamphetamine, methylphenidate, and phentermine have been examined. Small-scale studies have shown that agonist substitution engages people in treatment and there are some indications of benefit in terms of reduction of psychosocial harm and drug offences. Prescribing psychostimulants as substitution agents is not possible in most countries, however, and regulatory authorization is necessary.

- Disulfiram (approved for alcohol use disorder) acts as a central inhibitor of dopamine β-hydroxylase, causing an increase of dopamine and decreased synthesis of noradrenaline. As a result it may attenuate the cocaine 'high,' thus reducing the desire to use more cocaine; results have indicated some efficacy among patients with the CC variant of the dopamine β-hydroxylase gene.
- Modafinil is a non-stimulating alerting agent used in narcolepsy and other disorders of daytime. Trials have been mixed in showing an effect on stimulant use, as is the case with most other medications. Results show more consistent effects on cocaine use than on methamphetamine use.
- Bupropion, an approved medication for tobacco use cessation, has shown the greatest effect in trials to date, in terms of reducing methamphetamine use in some patients.
- Mirtazapine also recently was shown to have limited effectiveness.
- Naltrexone has consistently yielded positive results in some populations of IV ATS users, but trials of a depot naltrexone in Iceland did not replicate other European work with oral naltrexone.

Among the many drugs that have been tried with little or no success in reducing stimulant use are buspirone, flupentixol, aripiprazole, and vigabatrin. Trials have shown modest effects for topiramate and lobeline, a nicotinic receptor antagonist. Varenicline, another tobacco cessation drug, is under study.

Perhaps the most promising pharmacotherapy to date is a combi-nation of long-acting depot naltrexone plus daily bupropion, including a medication adherence component to assure daily dosing of the oral bupropion. In early research, the combination appears to have a positive effect in a small sample of severe-level methamphetamine users who were required to endorse >20 days of methamphetamine use in the month before enrolment into the trial.

Other directions in treatment include immunotherapies. Binding ATS in the bloodstream to limit its pharmacologic action by means of a 'vaccine' could reduce relapse. Also of interest are anti-ATS antibodies that could bind the drugs to reduce distribution in the bloodstream. To date, no immunotherapy approaches have been shown adequately effective to have received approval from regulatory agencies.

Further reading

Jenner L, Lee N. (2008). *Treatment Approaches for Users of Methamphetamine: A Practical Guide for Frontline Workers*. Canberra: Australian Government Department of Health and Ageing.
Roll JM, Rawson RA, Ling W, et al. (eds) (2009). *Methamphetamine Addiction: From Basic Science to Treatment*. New York: Guilford Press.

Hallucinogens and dissociative drugs

Introduction and epidemiology 356
Chemistry, pharmacology, and pathophysiology 358
Clinical syndromes 359
Management 361

Introduction and epidemiology

Hallucinogens and dissociative drugs are naturally occurring or manufactured substances, which induce illusions, hallucinations, and other psychotic-type symptoms, and may have other psychoactive effects. Historically they were grouped together under the term hallucinogens, but they are now usually regarded as separate classes of psychoactive substances.

Hallucinogens

The hallucinogens are a large and diverse group of substances which occur in many fungi and plants (where they may have evolved as a defence mechanism against herbivores), or which are chemically synthesized. They are sometimes called psychedelic drugs. They include:

- hallucinogens in fungi and truffles; these include psilocybin ('magic mushrooms') and mescaline, which occurs in the peyote cactus
- ayahuasca, which is a plant brew that provides dimethyltryptamine (DMT) in orally active form
- DMT is now being used by itself in smoked form
- hallucinogen-containing seeds, such as those of *Argyreia nervosa* (Hawaiian baby woodrose) and *Turbina corymbosa* (morning glory)
- synthetic hallucinogens such as lysergic acid diethylamide (LSD)
- newer synthetic drugs such as the *N*-methoxybenzyl derivatives of substituted phenethylamine (NBOMes) and tryptamines; many of these are very potent
- miscellaneous hallucinogens, e.g. nutmeg.

Dissociative drugs

These include:

- ketamine (a dissociative anaesthetic)
- phencyclidine (PCP)
- nitrous oxide.

Route of use

- Magic mushrooms are usually taken orally, with the dose varying with the particular mushroom or other fungus.
- LSD is typically taken in the form of a piece of blotting paper impregnated with the drug, which is absorbed transbuccally or sublingually.
- DMT is smoked (on its own for a short but very intense effect). It is inactive orally unless taken with a MAOI, as in ayahuasca.
- The NBOMes are also usually absorbed transbuccally or sublingually, usually via blotting paper. They are largely inactive orally.
- Ketamine is most commonly insufflated ('snorted') or, less commonly but more dangerously, injected.

Prevalence

LSD

- The prevalence in Western countries has varied considerably over recent decades; widespread use started in the mid–late 1960s and, although prevalence and access appear to have declined in the 1980s–2000s, its use in some countries has recently increased.
- Among young adults (15–34 years) in European countries, lifetime prevalence estimates of LSD range from 0% to 5.5%.
- In the US, lifetime prevalence is 6.5% for young adults (to age 25) and 11% in people aged 26 years and over.

Hallucinogenic mushrooms

- Among young adults in European countries, lifetime prevalence ranges from 0.3% to 14.1%, and in the last year from 0.2% to 5.9%.
- In the US, lifetime prevalence is 10–15%, but use in the last year is much lower (at 0.3% to 2.0%).

Ketamine

- Among young adults, the use of ketamine varies widely across the world.
- The prevalence of use is high in China and in some European countries, especially North-West Europe, where it is 2.0–4.5% for lifetime use.
- In the US, the lifetime prevalence of use is approximately 1%.
- In subgroups of young people (e.g. those in the music scene) lifetime prevalence ranges from 2.9% to 62% and for last month use 0.3% to 28%.

Phencyclidine

- Lifetime prevalence among adults aged 26 or more in the US is 3.0%; use in the past year is minimal.

Chemistry, pharmacology, and pathophysiology

These drugs exert most of their hallucinogenic properties by altering brain 5HT (serotonin) function, especially in the cortical and hippocampal regions. They have high affinity for $5HT_2$ receptors and act as agonists or partial agonists at these receptors. Recent studies suggest that the psychedelic 5HT agonists produce different actions on intracellular second messengers or subpopulations of cortical pyramidal cells than do other non-psychedelic $5HT_2$ acting drugs, which probably explains their effects. Many also exert more general monoamine release responsible for sympathomimetic actions.

The typical effects of hallucinogens include the following:

- Psychedelic effects: distortion of thoughts, mood, and sensory experiences, altered perception, and visual, auditory, tactile, and other hallucinations including synesthesia (where senses merge and are experienced together e.g. sounds seen as colours) and out of body and near death experiences
- Confusion and disorientation
- Acute (and usually self-limiting) psychological symptoms such as anxiety, panic, and agitation
- Paranoid ideation, which may be of psychotic intensity
- Ataxia
- Sympathetic stimulation with dilated pupils and elevated pulse rate and blood pressure and occasionally hyperpyrexia and chest pain
- Nystagmus—in some cases
- Dry flushed skin—with some hallucinogens, especially those with additional anticholinergic properties.

Dissociative drugs such as ketamine and phencyclidine can leave people immobile and vulnerable to assault, hypothermia, and accidental injury including drowning.

Clinical syndromes

Acute intoxication

- Effects of acute hallucinogen intoxication reflect the pharmacological effects described in section p. 358.
- Effects are dose dependent, but there is also individual variation in effects, which may also be influenced by the setting and company in which hallucinogen use takes place and whether other drugs have been used.
- Acute use may lead to precipitation of a mental health disorder in those with a predisposition or prodome, or to exacerbation of existing mental health disorders.

Chronic use and dependence

- Dependence does not occur with most hallucinogens, though regular use may be seen despite pronounced tolerance.
- Chronic use can lead to exacerbation of underlying mental health disorders.
- Flashbacks are a characteristic feature of recurrent hallucinogen use.
- Dependence on ketamine is increasingly recognized either as an isolated form of substance disorder or as part of a polydrug-using repertoire. Tolerance with marked dose escalation is not uncommon.

Hallucinogens and flashbacks

- Flashbacks are hallucinations, perceptions, and emotions similar to those experienced during drug intoxication, but which occur in the absence of drug use and often months or years after the last use of the particular drug.
- The most common flashbacks are visual hallucinations, including flashes and trailing of colour, geometric pseudo-hallucinations, perceptions of movement in the peripheral field of vision, after-images, halos around objects, macropsia, and micropsia.
- Flashbacks seldom interfere with the individual's functioning, but can be distressing.
- Flashbacks are more common after a crisis or after using another drug, such as cannabis, stimulants, and antihistamines.
- Flashbacks usually reduce in intensity over time and cease altogether, though up to 50% may experience the symptoms for up to 5 years.

Treatment involves reassurance that the symptoms are not a feature of mental illness and will pass. Occasionally, benzodiazepines are helpful.

Hallucinogen-induced psychosis

- Psychotic episodes are usually transient, self-limiting, and fully resolving, and are related to dose, duration of dosing, and individual vulnerability.
- Visual hallucinations, from simple shapes and bright colours to complex out-of-body and out-of-this-world experiences are characteristic and may be accompanied by persecutory delusions.
- Emotional states may vary from panic to depression to a manic state.

- May retain insight that the symptoms are drug induced.
- Symptoms usually clear within hours to days to weeks depending on the drug taken.
- If psychotic symptoms persist despite abstinence for more than 4 weeks, it probably reflects a pre-existing psychiatric disorder or the development of a *de novo* condition.

Advise individuals of behavioural sensitization (being at risk of experiencing further episodes of substance-induced psychosis after using the drug again, and often at much lower doses).

Hallucinogens and anxiety

- The stimulation and perceptual alterations with hallucinogenic drugs may create anxiety and panic, with the user believing he/she is 'losing his/her mind.' This is one example of a 'bad trip'.
- Reactions such as this are more common in inexperienced users of these drugs, and when the drug is used alone, or in an unfamiliar or unpleasant setting.
- The length of such a reaction is determined by the duration of action of the drug; for LSD it is approximately 8–12 hours.

Users should be advised to prepare for their experience and preferably have a trusted 'non-tripping' person in the vicinity to help if they become distressed. Treatment generally involves guiding a person through their experience and reassuring the individual that their mental state will return to normal once the effects of the drug wear off. If the reaction is severe, a short course of diazepam will reduce anxiety symptoms.

Acute organic brain syndrome

- Can develop due to toxicity or overdose, or as part of a drug-induced psychosis (another example of a 'bad trip').
- Symptoms include disorientation, agitation, delusions, and hallucinations.
- Individuals can sometimes assault others or harm themselves because of bizarre beliefs (e.g. that they can fly).

Chronic organic brain syndrome

Concerns have been raised that hallucinogens might cause permanent brain impairment with reduced abstract reasoning and intellectual functioning, but this has not been confirmed. Evidence of cognitive impairment in ketamine users (possibly reversible after several months of abstinence) has also been recently identified.

Physical sequelae

Physical sequelae are less common and fatal overdose highly unusual. Ketamine can lead to a toxic ulcerative cystitis, which in turn can cause bladder scarring and atrophy. Early symptoms include frequency, dysuria, and lower abdominal pain ('K-cramps') and haematuria. Users should stay well hydrated, avoid alcohol when using, and seek medical advice should urinary symptoms persist. Sometimes cystectomy (surgical removal of the bladder) is required.

Management

Management of acute toxicity

- Supportive reassurance and reorientation. Most effects are self-limiting, lasting 4–12 hours.
- If required, sedation with diazepam: 10–20 mg orally; titrate dose according to response (shorter-acting IM preparations can be used if required).
- Antipsychotics are not typically required and should be avoided when possible, though in some cases may assist in settling acute agitation (e.g. risperidone, olanzapine, haloperidol).
- Treat hyperthermia, hypertension, tachycardia, seizures, and rhabdomyolysis as appropriate.

Further reading

National Institute on Drug Abuse (2015). *Hallucinogens and Dissociative Drugs.* [Online] Available at: http://www.nida.nih.gov/ResearchReports/Hallucinogens/Hallucinogens.html

Lawn W, Barratt M, Williams M, *et al.* (2014). The NBOMe hallucinogenic drug series: patterns of use, characteristics of users and self-reported effects in a large international sample. *J Psychopharmacol* 28(8):780–8.

Morgan, CJA, Curran HV. (2012). Ketamine use: a review. Addiction 107(1):27–38.

Winstock AR, Kaar S, Borschmann R. (2014). Dimethyltryptamine (DMT): prevalence, user characteristics and abuse liability in a large global sample. *J Psychopharmacol* 28(1):49–54.

Other drugs

Caffeine, guarana, and energy drinks 364
Areca nut (Betel/Pan) 367
Khat (Qat) 369
Solvents and inhalants 370
Kava 374
Gamma hydroxybutyrate (GHB) and gamma
  butyrolactone (GBL) 376
Nitrites 379
Anabolic steroid misuse 380
Proprietary and 'over-the-counter' drugs of abuse 383
New psychoactive substances (NPS) 388

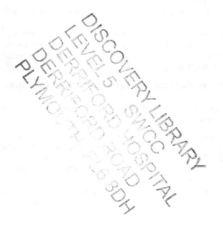

Caffeine, guarana, and energy drinks

Introduction

Caffeine
- Stimulant effects from caffeine have led to its global popularity.
- Beverages remain the major source of caffeine, including coffee, tea, soda, and energy drinks.
- Most caffeine use does not exceed the recommended safe threshold of 400 mg/day for an adult: e.g. 10 × 375 mL cans of cola (~40–50 mg caffeine each), two caffeine tablets (e.g. Vivarin®) of 200 mg each, 5 × 250 mL cups of brewed coffee (approximately 80 mg each, but wide range of caffeine) or 5 cans of a 250 mL typical energy drink (e.g. Red Bull®) each of which has approximately 80 mg of caffeine (see Table 16.1 for recommended limits).

Guarana
Guarana is a popular stimulant which exists as the seeds of the guarana plant, *Paullinia cupana, a* native of the Amazon basin of South America. It contains caffeine, theophylline, and theobromine. Most guarana is sold to industries manufacturing soft and energy drinks, although some is for direct consumption as capsules or for dilution in water.

Energy drinks
- Energy drinks can include a variety of ingredients such as caffeine, guarana, ginseng (*Panax* spp.), taurine, L-carnitine, carbohydrates, glucuronolactone, and vitamins.
- Most also contain sugar, although some come in diet and decaffeinated versions.
- These drinks are mostly used to boost energy, promote wakefulness, maintain alertness, and provide cognitive and mood enhancement.
- Global energy drink consumption has increased, especially in teen and young adult age groups.

Pharmacology and adverse effects of caffeine

Caffeine is:
- an adenosine receptor antagonist that stimulates dopaminergic activity
- a diuretic.

It produces:
- CNS features which may include anxiety, agitation, tremor, confusion, and at high doses seizures
- cardiovascular features which may include tachycardia, palpitations and increased blood pressure
- gastrointestinal features which may include nausea, vomiting, cramping, pain, and diarrhoea.

Table 16.1 Recommended limits for caffeine consumption

The person	Recommended limit
Healthy children (< 12 years old)	2.5 mg/kg body weight
Pregnant women	300 mg/day
Healthy adults	400 mg/day

Source data from Health Canada (2010).

Vulnerable populations

- Among children and youth, energy drink-related visits to US emergency departments doubled from 2007 to 2011.
- Cases of accidental ingestion of caffeine at potentially toxic levels in children under 6 years of age have been reported by poisons control centres.
- Some governments limit caffeine in foods. Australia limits energy drinks to 32 mg/100 mL serving.

Use with alcohol and other drugs

- Drinking energy drinks with alcohol can increase risky behaviour, especially driving behaviour.
- Caffeine has been linked to increased toxicity of other stimulant drugs, including dexamphetamine, cocaine, methylenedioxy-methamphetamine (MDMA), and methylenedioxyamphetamine (MDA). Hyperthermia, cardiovascular events, rhabdomyolysis, and acute kidney injury have been reported.

Clinical syndromes and problems

DSM-5 and ICD 10 contain diagnostic information on problems due to caffeine consumption in energy drinks or other forms (Table 16.2).

Management

- Acute symptoms of caffeine toxicity should be managed by following standard guidelines for care, including ABCs and symptom management. Reports suggest that activated charcoal may limit absorption if treated soon after ingestion.
- Chronic excessive use of caffeine may lead to tolerance, physical dependence, and addiction. Those withdrawing from caffeine should be provided with supportive reassurance and symptom-based treatment.
- Consumers need to know caffeine content to monitor their own consumption.
- Medical advice on safe consumption levels should be sought by persons with chronic diseases.

Further reading

Institute of Medicine (2014). *Caffeine in Food and Dietary Supplements: Examining Safety. Workshop Summary*. Washington, DC: The National Academies Press.

Meredith SE, Juliano LM, Hughes JR, et al. (2013). Caffeine use disorder: a comprehensive review and research agenda. *J Caffeine Res* 3:114-30.

Table 16.2 Diagnosis of energy drink/caffeine-related problems

Diagnostic system	Title and code	Description
DSM-5	Caffeine Intoxication 305.90	Recent high dose of caffeine consumption (>250mg). At least 5 signs/symptoms: excitement, nervousness, insomnia, tachycardia, psychomotor agitation, diuresis, fatigue, restlessness, fasciculation, confused thoughts and speech or gastrointestinal problems. Symptoms are clinically significant or functioning is impaired.
ICD 10	Acute Intoxication due to use of other stimulants, including caffeine F15.0	Dysfunctional behaviour/perceptual abnormalities such as hypervigilance, euphoria, aggression, hallucinations, moodiness or visual/auditory illusions and at least 2 signs (such as psychomotor agitation, tachycardia, vomiting, chest pain, or cardiac arrhythmias).
DSM-5	Caffeine Withdrawal 292.0	After daily caffeine consumption for a long time, and after 24 hours without caffeine, at least 3 signs or symptoms, such as fatigue, headache, irritability, moodiness, low concentration and clinically significant distress or impairment in functioning.
ICD 10	Withdrawal state from other stimulants, including caffeine F15.3	Dysphoric temperament such as sadness and melancholy after cessation or reduction of chronic use and has at least 2 of signs (such as increase in appetite, insomnia/hypersomnia, bad dreams, agitation or desire for stimulants).
DSM-5	Caffeine use disorder	Problematic pattern manifest in 3 of 9 symptoms and clinically significant impairment or distress
ICD 10	Harmful use F15.1	Evidence of identifiable harm from caffeine use for at least 1 month in past 12 months
ICD 10	Dependence syndrome F15.2	3 of 6 symptoms, such as tolerance to, strong desire for, and preoccupation with, occurring repeatedly in past 12 months or for at least 1 month

Areca nut (Betel/Pan)

Epidemiology

- The areca nut is the seed of the areca palm *Areca catechu*. It is often incorrectly referred to as betel nut, but betel refers to the leaf of the plant *Piper betle*, which the nut is often wrapped in. It is the fourth most commonly used psychoactive substance in the world after tobacco, alcohol, and caffeine.
- It is used most commonly within the Indian sub-continent, but is also prevalent in Taiwan and South East Asia, and southern China.
- Historically, areca use has its origins in religious, ceremonial, and social activities, and is purported as having many desirable effects.
- The nut reportedly assists digestion and may be used regularly (daily) by habitués or a social lubricant at social gatherings by occasional users.
- The nut is typically sliced into thin shards and rolled in a betel leaf with slaked lime and a variety of other additives, such as catechu extract and cardamoms to enhance flavour. Commonly tobacco is added to this mix.
- The folded leaf package ('quid') is then chewed. The nut is also marketed in a packaged form as a refined areca product containing a variety of mixtures with and without tobacco, commonly known as pan masala.
- This appears to be the form of areca use most commonly used by Asian immigrants living in Western countries and is popular among children. As a gateway to tobacco use, this practice is potentially significant.

Pharmacology and pathophysiology

- The areca nut contains a number of psychoactive alkaloids, with arecoline being the one present in the greatest quantity.
- It has complex effects upon both parasympathetic and sympathetic nervous systems, reflected in the subjective experience of a mixed of stimulant and anxiolytic effect not unlike tobacco.
- Anecdotally, the nut and arecoline have significant medicinal properties ranging from an antihelminthic and astringent to an aphrodisiac, digestive enhancement, and psychomotor stimulant.

Complications and treatment

- Often chewed with tobacco, areca poses significant health risks to long-term chewers, most notably leucoplakia, and sub-mucosal fibrosis, a progressive scarring condition of the oral mucosa with a high risk (50%) of oral squamous cell carcinoma development.
- Dental practitioners should be alert to this practice and advise on the risk of continued chewing on health and adequate nutrition.
- Concurrent tobacco use should be addressed with nicotine replacement and motivational interviewing.
- A behavioural approach and replacement of the masticatory process with gum may be helpful.
- Dependence may be associated with a mild withdrawal syndrome requiring only symptomatic relief.

Further reading

Burton-Bradley B. (1978). Betel nut chewing in retrospect. *Papua New Guinea Med J* 21(3):236–40.

Trivedy C, Johnson NW. (1997). Oral cancer in South Asia [letter]. *Br Dent J* 182(6):206.

Warnakulasuriya S, Trivedy C, Peters T. (2002). Areca nut use: an independent risk factor for oral cancer. *BMJ* 324(7341):799–800.

Khat (Qat)

Khat (*Catha edulis*) is a perennial shrub indigenous to the Horn of Africa (Ethiopia and Somalia) and the Arabian Peninsula. Like other indigenous substances it frequently accompanies its users when they migrate from their place of origin. Outside its area of propagation, khat is most commonly used among immigrant Somali communities in the UK, Europe, and the US. In recent years, concern has grown regarding the possible adverse effects of khat upon both individuals and their societies.

Preparation and mode of administration

Only the fresh leaves retain their psychoactive potency. Fresh bitter leaves are usually chewed for their stimulant effect (though the leaves may be smoked or infusions prepared), with the extracted juices swallowed and the residue kept within the cheek for some time. This is a relatively slow mode of administration requiring prolonged chewing to provide a relatively mild stimulant effect.

Psychological effects and contextual use

Like other culture-bound substance use such as areca nut, the use of khat has its origins in social, ceremonial, and religious activities. Its mild stimulant effects may promote social interaction, with users reporting increased talkativeness, disinhibition, improved concentration, loss of appetite, and improved stamina. Predominantly used by men, its increasing use by women is sometimes frowned upon.

Pharmacological effects

The main constituents of khat are cathine and cathinone—phenylpropylamines which are CNS stimulants having a similar mechanism of action to amphetamines (through the release of presynaptically stored monoamines) though being considerably less potent. Khat also contains a number of other alkaloids and tannins. Cathinone, the more potent compound, is a very unstable substance that necessitates importation of fresh leaves within 1–2 days of harvesting, before the active components degrade. Cathinone is a classified as a Class 1 drug.

Adverse effects of use

Particularly in its countries of origin, the assessment of the adverse health effects of khat is complicated by poor socioeconomic status of many users. Adverse physical effects reported include oral, gastrointestinal (constipation), hepatic, and cardiac disturbances, as well as those related to accidents whilst intoxicated. Cardiac effects appear related to increases in pulse and blood pressure that may compromise cardiac function in those with underlying disease. Compulsive patterns of use consistent with a dependence syndrome have been described, but there does not appear to be a distinct withdrawal syndrome.

Further reading

Cox G and Rampes H. (2003). Adverse effects of khat: a review. *Adv Psychiatr Treat* 9:456–63.

Solvents and inhalants

Volatile solvent misuse (VSM) is deliberate inhalation of liquid that vaporizes at room temperature and normal atmospheric pressure to induce mental state change.

Volatile substances which are most misused include:
- simple hydrocarbons (acetone, toluene, etc.)
- gases (e.g. butane)
- aerosols (e.g. air freshener, 'poppers')
- glues
- 'others' (e.g. fire extinguishers, correction fluid, petrol, etc.)
- nitrous oxide.

Over 30 different substances are implicated in VSM fatalities. Volatiles are 'legal highs': widely available, relatively cheap, largely legal, easily concealed, with low perceived dependence risk.

Delivery methods
- Use is variably termed to 'huff', 'sniff', 'bag', 'toot', 'buzz'
- Place in mouth
- Sniff container/sleeve/cloth/plastic bag
- Bag/padding over head/face.

Epidemiology
Prevalence
- Varies geographically: in the UK and many parts of Europe lifetime prevalence is 10–12%; 1–2% among 13–15-year-olds. Prevalence similar in males and females; males predominate in treatment populations/ fatalities.
- Nitrous oxide ('hippy crack') second most popular substance after cannabis in 16–24-year age group in UK and several European countries (3–6%)
- Sniffing generally in <30 years, but older age use increasing.
- In several countries (e.g. US, Australia), higher prevalence in rural and remote/disadvantaged communities, including petrol sniffing.

Mortality
- Has declined in many developed countries in recent years, e.g. 46 deaths in UK in 2009 compared with 152 in 1990; 78.5% male.
- One-third VSM deaths in under-20s; in UK 1.1% all-cause mortality among male 15–19 year-olds (and 0.7% in females).
- Scottish deaths disproportionately high (2009).
- Approximately half of deaths involve polysubstance misuse.
- Globally, more 10–14-year-old VSM-related deaths than 'drug abuse' deaths.
- More UK VSM-related under-15s deaths than all other illegal substance misuse combined (2000–2009).

Mechanisms of death (UK: 1971–2009)
- Direct toxic effects on heart (72%).
- Asphyxia (12%).
- Vomit inhalation (8%).
- Accidental trauma (4%).

Suicide
- Most inhalant-related suicides in the UK in 2009 involved helium use (not a volatile solvent but an inert gas):
  - 93% of helium-related mortality appeared to be due to suicide (43 of 46 deaths), compared to 10.9% of VSM-related deaths (5 of 46 deaths).
- Generally, males predominate (70%+), ages 15–75+ years.
- UK VSM-related suicide is falling, but helium-related suicide increased fivefold 2006–2009.
- Male:female suicide ratio higher for VSM-related suicide
- Median age decreasing with time for VSM-related suicide—older age deaths were more likely to be suicide overall (combining both groups), however.

Associations
Crime, antisocial behaviour, criminal justice contact, polysubstance misuse, homelessness, poverty, poor education, gangs, family disruption (low cohesiveness/support, poor relationships, especially father), children in out-of-home care, social exclusion.
- Volatile substances are the most common substance use in 'street children' globally (47% pooled prevalence), before tobacco, alcohol, marijuana.

Natural history
Young people across the social strata may experiment with VSM, but most never progress to regular harmful use/dependence.
- One-fifth develop dependence; many progress to other substances (16% will use Class A drugs).
- VSM more acceptable to younger teens; later tends to be a solitary activity as lowered 'street credibility'.
- No major lifetime usage gender differences; increased male mortality may represent greater risk-taking/'recklessness'.
- As usage continues, increasing polysubstance use, criminality/antisocial behaviour, violence, self-mutilation.
- Older age use increasing.

Pharmacology

VSM causes increased nerve cell membrane permeability, resulting in positive $GABA_A$ modulation, NMDA receptor effects, and increased serotonin release.
- Toluene increases mesolimbic dopamine.
- Volatiles are highly lipophilic (crossing blood–brain barrier easily): rapid onset of effects.

- Volatiles have anticonvulsant, anxiolytic and CNS depressant effect (like alcohol, barbiturates, and similar CNS depressants).
- Withdrawal syndrome is similar to alcohol withdrawal and may occur on cessation of regular, heavy use.

Clinical syndromes

- 'Sudden death sniffing syndrome' (related to catecholamine release causing sudden death, e.g. from arrhythmias).
- Acute effects (<45 minutes): euphoria, disinhibition, disorientation, 'drunkenness', blurred vision, dizziness, slurring, drowsiness, hallucinations, black-outs.
- Later acute effects: hangover, drowsiness, headaches, spots/rashes in oronasal area, black-outs.
- Chronic medical syndromes:
  - Neurological (permanent neurological damage, progressive cognitive decline: ataxia, cerebral atrophy, encephalopathy, Parkinsonism, peripheral/sensorimotor neuropathy, speech problems, trigeminal neuropathy, tremor)
  - Damaged endocrine, GI and reproductive systems, and eyes/ears
  - Skin (burns, dermatitis, hypothermic injury, eczema)
  - Cardiovascular (arrhythmia, fibrosis, ischaemia, ventricular fibrillation)
  - Pulmonary (coughing, wheezing, emphysema, pneumonia)
  - Liver and kidney (toxic damage, failure, hepatorenal syndrome, Fanconi's syndrome)
  - Bone marrow (suppression, anaemia, leukaemia).
- Chronic psychiatric syndromes:
  - Mood disorder/anxiety (up to 45% have lifetime history of mood disorder, 36% anxiety)
  - Personality disorder (up to 45%; antisocial type 36%)
  - Apathy, inattention, insomnia, memory loss, psychosis, suicide.

Management

Immediate

- Treat medical and psychiatric syndromes. Residual volatile stores (fatty tissue) result in prolonged withdrawal state.
- No specific drug treatments, so consider symptomatic withdrawal relief.
- If leaded petrol sniffed, can use chelators in lead toxicity.
- Legal obligations to report to relevant child protection authority.

Longer-term

Given age range and physical health/psychiatric co-morbidity, the general principles for treating children/adolescents apply, including:

- family assessment/intervention
- full physical, mental health, cognitive and polysubstance misuse assessment/treatment
- consider acquired brain injury, and harm reduction approaches to reduce risk
- some agencies offer specific support, e.g. Re-Solv/SOLVE IT in the UK

- increasing recognition by governments and industry of the scale and importance of the problem (e.g. VSM all-party parliamentary group formed in UK in 2013)
- refer on to statutory addiction and/or child services, as indicated.

Prevention

Community measures (prohibition, prevention, and education) vary by country, e.g.:
- Legal measures:
  - Prohibition of sale to under-18s if perceived as for misuse or prohibition of selling under-18s gas lighter fuel; inspectors may 'test' vendors using minors attempting a purchase
  - Laws to address volatile solvent intoxication, e.g. under general law, such as breach of peace
  - UK studies suggest that the 1985 (but not 1999) legislation decreased mortality
  - Notification of children presenting with VSM to child protection agencies
  - Increased controls have been suggested for helium.
- Others:
  - Several Australian communities switched to a non-sniffable petrol ('OPAL'). Evaluations show promising results in reducing VSM, particularly in more remote centres. In some centres, supply control is combined with demand control—diversionary activities which engage young people, with community rehabilitative and educational projects.
  - Product modification involves removing psychoactive substances, adding deterrent agents, or package modification; only the first has produced potentially positive results.

Further reading

Baydala L. (2010). Inhalant abuse. *Paediatr Child Health* 15(7):443–54.

Ghodse H, Corkery J, Ahmed K, *et al.* (2012). *Trends in UK Deaths Associated with Abuse of Volatile Substances, 1971–2009, Report 24.* London: International Centre for Drug Policy, St George's, University of London.

Harris D. (2006). Volatile substance abuse. *Arch Dis Child Educ Pract* 91:ep93–ep100.

Orr KS, Shewan D. (2006). *Review of Evidence Relating to Volatile Substance Abuse in Scotland.* Edinburgh: Scottish Executive.

Wu LT, Howard MO. (2007). Psychiatric disorders in inhalant users: results from the National Epidemiologic Survey on Alcohol and Related conditions. *Drug Alcohol Depend* 88:146–55.

Kava

Kava is an intoxicating drink prepared from the crushed roots of *Piper methysticum* and either water or coconut milk. It is traditionally widely used in South Pacific countries, particularly in ceremonies.

More recently it has been promoted by kava bars, and imported for consumption in other countries, including Australia. In those settings it has been used more heavily and in the absence of traditional controls. In recent years, kava extract has also been sold as an OTC health supplement to remedy anxiety.

Kava's actions include relaxation, 'dreaminess' and sense of well-being. It has anxiolytic, sedative, muscle relaxant, and analgesic properties. Antithrombotic and anticonvulsant effects have been described.

Unlike alcohol, kava is not associated with violence or cognitive impairment during intoxication. However, kava may exacerbate the sedative or intoxicating effects of alcohol.

Pharmacology

Kavalactones, the psychoactive constituents, are found in the resinous plant components and are a group of mostly lipid-soluble lactones characterized by a 5,6-dihydro-A-pyrone ring. Kava's potency has been attributed to the six main lactones: kawain, dihydrokawain, methysticin, dihydromethysticin, yangonin, and desmethoxy-yangonin.

Kava's effects are believed to be mediated via modulation of GABA activity, monoamine oxidase B inhibition, and noradrenaline and dopamine re-uptake inhibition.

Reported adverse health effects of kava

Moderate use of kava appears to be associated with few risks. In heavy use the following complications have been reported:
- Ichthyosis: a characteristic scaly skin rash; one of the commonest complications of heavy kava use (~45% of heavy users and 78% of very heavy users).
- Loss of weight: up to 20% loss of BMI; with loss of appetite in 44% of heavy users.
- Nausea (29% of heavy users), indigestion.
- Elevations of liver enzyme levels in those who drink kava mixed with water. Usually reversible. However fulminant hepatitis has been reported in users of some manufactured remedies containing kava compounds. In these remedies the kava is often prepared using alcohol or acetone rather than water.
- Reaction time and motor skills can be acutely reduced with intoxication.
- Unlike heavy alcohol use, there is no evidence that chronic heavy kava use causes long-term neurological damage.

- Interference with involvement in community and family life, and impact on family and community finances have been reported
- There have been reports of raised cholesterol, lymphocytopenia, increased risk of melioidosis, or sudden cardiac deaths in remote Aboriginal Australians with heavy kava use, but causation has not been established with certainty.

Prevention and treatment

Currently, no specific treatment has been recommended for heavy kava users. Supply control has been the main preventive measure adopted.

Further reading

Clough AR, Jacups SP, Wang Z, et al. (2003). Health effects of kava use in an eastern Arnhem Land community. Intern Med J 33:336–40.

Rychetnik L, Madronio CM. (2011). The health and social effects of drinking water-based infusions of kava: A review of the evidence. Drug Alcohol Rev 30: 74–83.

Sarris JE, LaPorte E, Schweitzer I. (2011). Kava: a comprehensive review of efficacy, safety, and psychopharmacology. Aust NZ J Psychiatry (2011) 45:27–35.

Gamma hydroxybutyrate (GHB) and gamma butyrolactone (GBL)

Also known as G, Liquid Ecstasy, Vitamin G, Grievous Bodily Harm, and Fantasy

Introduction and epidemiology

- Taken by young people, especially in the party, rave, and gay club scene to 'get high' and enhance libido
- In body builders used to increase muscle mass and enhance performance (though evidence minimal)
- Often used with alcohol and other recreational drugs which exacerbate toxicity
- Most commonly used by men in their 20s and 30s.

Clinical use

- GHB is licensed in the US and some European countries (as sodium oxybate) for the treatment of narcolepsy with cataplexy or excessive daytime sleepiness
- As sodium oxybate, it is approved in a small number of European countries for the treatment of alcohol withdrawal and dependence
- May attenuate opiate withdrawal symptoms.

Chemistry and pharmacology

- GHB is a four-carbon fatty acid, naturally occurring neurotransmitter
- GBL is a precursor compound and is rapidly hydrolysed to GHB on exposure to water
- GHB is both a precursor and metabolite of GABA
- GHB binds to endogenous GHB receptors which are widely distributed in the brain especially the pons, hippocampus, cortex, and caudate
- GHB binds to $GABA_B$ receptors and neuromodulates dopamine, opioid, serotonin, and noradrenaline release, and growth hormone secretion
- GHB effects seen after 15–20 minutes, peaking at 30–60 minutes and lasting 3–4 hours
- Rapidly metabolized to H_2O and CO_2 in the lungs
- 2–5% is excreted unchanged in the urine
- Effects prolonged if taken with food and alcohol
- Steep dose–response curve and over half of users report overdose experience.

Preparations

- GBL is a widely used industrial solvent and ingredient of some cleaning and cosmetic products; can be obtained on the Internet, bypassing restriction laws
- GHB typically supplied as a colourless, odourless liquid taken orally
- Usually dissolved in sweet drinks or alcohol to disguise the salty taste.

Measurement
- GHB is detected in the urine up to 12 hours after use
- Since GHB is naturally occurring the limit of detection is set at 10 mg/L
- Concentrations increase with time and temperature and so should be analysed as quickly as possible after collection.

Clinical effects
- Average recreational dose 0.5–5 g
- Effects are comparable to alcohol and ecstasy:
  - euphoria
  - relaxation
  - disinhibition
  - increased empathy
  - enhanced sensuality
  - increased libido
  - increased energy and stamina for dancing.

Risk behaviours
- Increased risk of unsafe sex and BBV infection
- Date rape
- Impaired driving
- Co-ingestion with alcohol and ketamine causes enhanced toxicity.

Intoxication and overdose
The cardinal features of toxicity are rapid onset of drowsiness/coma, associated with respiratory and cardiovascular depression. Preceding nausea and vomiting are common (Table 16.3).

The toxidrome resolves over 3–5 hours but there may be fluctuating recovery with sudden alertness, confusion, and combativeness. Co-intoxicants increase the risk of coma and death.

Management of intoxication
The mainstay of treatment is supportive since no specific antidotes are available. Vital signs and pulse oximetry should be continuously monitored and airway patency maintained. Short-term ventilation may be required.

Table 16.3 Common symptoms and signs of intoxication

Neurological	Headache, dysarthria, ataxia and nystagmus, myoclonus, and seizures
Psychiatric	Anxiety, agitation, disorientation, disinhibition, combativeness, delirium and hallucinations, short-term anterograde amnesia
Gastrointestinal	Nausea, vomiting, and abdominal pain
Respiratory	Dyspnoea, cough, reduced respiratory rate, and hypoxia
Cardiovascular	Chest pain, palpitations, bradycardia, and hypotension

Dependence and withdrawal

- Dependence may develop after 2–3 months of regular use.
- The withdrawal syndrome resembles that of alcohol but onset is more rapid (symptoms can develop within an hour of discontinuation and usually peak within 24 hours).
- Features of delirium tremens are more common.
- Autonomic instability (tremor, sweating, hypertension and pyrexia) is less severe.
- GHB withdrawal symptoms may take up to 2 weeks to resolve.

Management of GHB/GBL dependence/withdrawal

Clinical assessment

- Quantity/frequency/duration of use
- Context of use
- Other drug use
- Abstinent periods
- Previous withdrawal symptom severity
- Medical and mental health history
- Harms/risk behaviours
- Motivation/precipitants for change
- Social functioning/support.

Treatment

- Choice of inpatient or outpatient treatment is guided by severity of dependence (>30 g of GHB or 15 g of GBL or more than thrice-daily ingestion indicates need for inpatient treatment).
- Close monitoring of blood pressure, pulse, respiratory rate, PO_2, and fluid and electrolyte balance.
- First-line treatment is high-dose benzodiazepines (up to 120 mg of diazepam daily) tapered over 7–10 days.
- Baclofen 10 mg three times per day reduces the risk of severe muscle spasms and rhabdomyolysis.
- If symptoms are resistant to benzodiazepines after 24 hours, pentobarbital can be used in an ICU setting.
- Haloperidol is indicated for agitation and psychosis.

Further reading

Goldin M, Bearn J. (2013). *GHB: What Psychiatrists Need to Know*. RC Psych CDP Online Learning Module. Available at: http://www.psychiatrycpd.co.uk/learningmodules/ghbwhatpsychia-tristsneedt.aspx

Gonzalez A, Nutt, DJ. (2005). Gammahydroxybutyrate abuse and dependency. *J Psychopharm* 19(2):195–204.

Nitrites

- Nitrites, principally amyl nitrite ('poppers'), are substances of abuse belonging to the volatile alkyl nitrite family of compounds.
- Inhalation of their fumes (either directly from a bottle or from cotton wool) provides a brief sense of euphoria and sexual arousal.
- Among the clubbing and gay communities, their smooth muscle relaxation and vasodilating properties make them a common component of 'chem sex'.

Epidemiology

- In common use for several decades, with reports from many Western countries regarding their high incidence of abuse, including those in Europe, North America, and Australasia.
- In the UK it is reported that up to 10% of the general population have tried them, and 1% within the last year.
- Rate is higher still within both the 'clubbing' and gay communities.
- In many Western countries they are illegal to sell for human consumption, but nevertheless not illegal to possess. They are therefore often sold for alternative uses such as video head cleaner or room deodorants, and typically easy to purchase either on the high street or online.

Clinical features

- Previously described as low-risk both physically and psychologically.
- Common untoward effects including hypotension, headaches, and potentially significant interactions with sildenafil (Viagra®).
- Visual symptoms secondary to macular pathology ('poppers maculopathy')—reports from the UK, France, Australia, Germany, and Spain.
- These symptoms include symptoms of blurred vision, metamorphopsia (distortion), phosphenes (flashing lights), and fluctuating vision.
- Ophthalmoscopy can show a yellow lesion at the fovea, although this may be very subtle.
- It is not known whether the retinal damage is permanent, although several cases have had long-term reduction in vision.

Further reading

Davies A, Kelly S, Naylor S, et al. (2012). Adverse ophthalmic reaction in poppers users: case series of 'poppers maculopathy'. Eye (Lond) 26(11):1479–86.

Nutt D, King LA, Saulsbury W, et al. (2007). Development of a rational scale to assess the harm of drugs of potential misuse. Lancet 369:1047–53.

Pahlitzsch M, Mai C, Joussen AM, et al. (eds). (2015). Poppers maculopathy: complete restitution of macular changes in OCT after drug abstinence. Semin Ophthalmol 21:1–6.

Anabolic steroid misuse

Introduction and epidemiology

- Anabolic steroid misuse is common in body-builders and professional athletes. They are misused for their muscle-building properties.
- In gay male communities they also have a reputation for instilling a subjective sense of power and dominance.
- Anabolic steroids are also seen increasing use in anti-ageing regimens.
- They have numerous adverse effects both physical and psychological.

True prevalence figures are difficult to obtain because of the illicit nature of this misuse. Lifetime prevalence for males may approach 1%. Highest prevalence rates are seen in male adolescents (up to around 5%) and amongst gymnasium attendees (up to around 25%) and the gay male population.

Methods of use

When used for their anabolic (muscle-building) properties there are three methods widely used:

- Stacking: using oral and injectable steroids in high doses
- Pyramiding: increasing dose and number of preparations taken over a set period and then decreasing slowly to mitigate withdrawal effects
- Cycling: alternating periods of high use (stacking or pyramiding) with periods of abstinence.

Many steroid users consume other drugs to treat steroid-related adverse effects. These include oestrogen antagonists (usually tamoxifen), analgesics, statins, and oral hypoglycaemics.

Human growth hormone is increasingly used alongside steroids. Diuretics may be used to mask steroid misuse. Many misusers look to the illegal but widely available 'Steroid Bible' to guide use.

Pharmacology

Anabolic steroids are compounds chemically related to testosterone and sharing its actions on the body. Testosterone itself is not active orally (high first-pass effect) and it is usually given as 17 A-alkyl substituted molecules (orally active) or parenterally as testosterone esters.

A wide range of steroid compounds has been synthesized. Only a proportion of these is found in bona fide pharmaceutical products and can be detected by standard assays. Different natural and synthetic steroids differ in their relative anabolic and androgenic (virilizing) effects but none is free of the latter.

Pathophysiology

Physical effects

Anabolic steroid misuse is associated with a wide range of important adverse effects. These include:

- elevated lipid profiles
- increased blood pressure
- increased heart size

- sudden cardiac death
- decreased thyroid-stimulating hormone (TSH)
- decreased sperm count
- carcinoma of the liver
- hirsutism
- insulin resistance
- testicular atrophy (clitoral growth in woman)
- gynaecomastia
- prostate hypertrophy
- prostatic carcinoma
- tendon rupture.

Psychological effects

While low doses of anabolic steroids are not normally associated with psychiatric adverse effects, the huge doses used by body-builders and athletes may cause several serious psychological sequelae. These include the following:

- *Aggression:* ('Roid Rage') often severe, provoking violent acts against people or property, often accompanied by irritability and mood instability.
- *Depression:* usually characterized by low mood, insomnia, anxiety and, more rarely, suicidality. Suicide has been widely reported amongst current steroid misusers, and may represent the ultimate outcome of steroid-induced concurrent aggression, depression, and lack of impulse control.
- *Hypomania and mania:* common symptoms include euphoria, grandiosity, over-confidence, irritability, increased libido, and poor judgement.
- *Psychosis* is less common. Symptoms may include paranoid delusions, auditory hallucinations, and delusions of reference.
- *Dependence:* anabolic steroids may provoke endogenous opiate release and dependence is not uncommon. Naloxone can usually be shown to illicit an acute opiate-type withdrawal reaction in heavy misusers. On cessation of misuse, an acute hyperadrenergic state is experienced followed later by depression, fatigue, insomnia, joint pain, anorexia and craving.

Systematic appraisal of the adverse effects of steroid misuse is impossible given its illicit nature. The severity and frequency of all adverse effects are thus impossible to estimate with any accuracy.

Treatment of psychological effects

There are no formal guidelines for the treatment of steroid-induced psychological effects. Some suggestions are given here:

- Aggression: haloperidol, olanzapine, lorazepam
- Depression: standard antidepressants
- Mania: standard treatments
- Psychosis: standard treatments
- Withdrawal: clonidine, lofexidine acutely; antidepressants in the medium term. NSAIDs may be required for muscle and joint pain.

Further reading

Graham S, Kennedy M. (1990). Recent developments in the toxicology of anabolic steroids. *Drug Safety* 5:458–76.

Pope HG Jr, Katz DL. (1988). Affective and psychotic symptoms associated with anabolic steroid use. *Am J Psychiatry* 145:487–90.

Trenton AJ, Currier GW. (2005). Behavioural manifestations of anabolic steroid use. *CNS Drugs* 19:571–95.

See also: http://neptune-clinicalguidance.co.uk

Proprietary and 'over-the-counter' drugs of abuse

Proprietary or 'over the counter' medicines (OTCs) are medicinal products that can be sold to the public without the need for a prescription (Table 16.4). Some are restricted to pharmacies.

Table 16.4 Types of OTC substance misuse

OTC	Effects	Possible adverse effects	Comments
Opioids	See Chapter 11	See Chapter 11	Are available in combination with analgesics, cough and cold remedies. Adverse effects can be related to excessive consumption of these other ingredients
Dextromethorphan	Dissociation, hallucination	Tolerance, tachycardia, nystagmus, ataxia, restlessness, increased blood pressure, nausea, vomiting, dizziness, insomnia, confusion, withdrawal symptoms on cessation. Deaths reported	Misuse reported to be popular in the younger age group
Sedating antihistamines:			
Chlorpheniramine	Euphoria	See comments	In combination with dextromethorphan: tachycardia, increased BP, lethargy, and dizziness
			In combination with dihydrocodeine: convulsions, general acidosis
Diphenhydramine	In some— sleepiness, in others euphoria, hallucinations	Somnolence, sedation, delirium, tremor, coma	

(Continued)

Table 16.4 (*Contd.*)

OTC	Effects	Possible adverse effects	Comments
Dimenhydrinate[a]	Euphoria, hallucinations	Confusion, violence, tolerance, withdrawal symptoms on cessation	
Cyclizine[a,b]	Exhilaration, hallucination	Tachycardia, increased blood pressure, slurred speech, violence, depressed afterwards	Evidence mainly from use in combination with opioids, and from oral rather than IV use
Sympathomimetics (e.g. pseudo-ephedrine, ephedrine)	Stimulation, wakefulness	Tachycardia, hypertension, insomnia, agitation, anxiety, and GI disturbances, psychosis, dependence	Also purchased as precursor substances and not for misuse per se
Laxatives		Electrolyte imbalance reduced bowel muscle tone	

[a]Marketed as antiemetics. [b]When used in combination with opioids such as methadone

Some are only sold from community pharmacies (retail pharmacies), where supervision of a qualified pharmacist is often mandatory. However, many products are available for general sale from non-pharmacy outlets.

In many countries, access to OTCs is subject to regulation based on the level of risk of harm associated with their use. The availability of individual OTCs varies from country to country.

Adverse effects may be due to direct effects of the drug, effects of other ingredients in the OTC product, drug–drug interactions, or route of administration (e.g. insufflation ('snorting') or injecting).

Because many OTCs have the potential to interact with other medicines, or can themselves be misused and cause related harms, health professionals need to be aware of the issue and to include OTC medicine use in medical history taking.

What is OTC misuse?

Misuse can be defined or construed as 'intentional' or 'unintentional'. A more sophisticated classification has been proposed and is illustrated in Table 16.5.

Table 16.5 Types of OTC substance misuse

Type of OTC misuse[a]	Example
1. Inappropriate medical use	Taking the OTC for the wrong indication or at the wrong dose, usually due to lack of knowledge
2. Medication dependence	Where a person starts to take a medication for medical reasons, but use becomes problematic or even dependent
3. Altered body image	E.g. laxative abuse for weight loss
4. Intentional psychotropic abuse	Drug used for a non-medical reason for its 'high'
5. Abuse support	OTCs are used as part of other drug abuse, e.g. in the manufacture of drugs of misuse

[a] 3–5 are generally considered 'intentional' misuse.

Source data from Wills S., *Drugs of Abuse*, Second edition, Copyright (2005), Pharmaceutical Press.

The range of preparations

Opioids/opiates

Many pain remedies contain codeine or dihydrocodeine in combination with non-opioid analgesics (paracetamol and ibuprofen are the most common). Furthermore in the UK, kaolin and morphine mixture is available OTC for the treatment of diarrhoea, and in the UK and New Zealand, Gee's Linctus, a cough medicine which contains squill opiate, is also available; both of these can be abused. These products are often obtained as substitutes when an opioid drug of choice is unavailable. In other cases, individuals may also become dependent on the opioid in the OTC, through overuse. In geographically isolated countries such as New Zealand, where the supply of heroin is irregular, drug users have been known to extract codeine from codeine-containing analgesic OTCs to produce a product known locally as 'homebake'. Opioids are covered in detail in Chapters 11 and 12. However, in addition to problems associated with excessive opioid consumption, there are other risks associated with the use of large amounts of combination OTCs. Excessive paracetamol consumption can lead to fatal hepatotoxicity and excessive ibuprofen consumption can lead to peptic ulcers and bleeding, or renal tubular acidosis.

Dextromethorphan

Dextromethorphan was developed as a cough suppressant, and although structurally similar to opiates, the effects at different doses vary. Abuse appears to be more common amongst adolescents and young adults. When misused at high doses it tends to produce effects such as hallucinations, dissociation, and euphoria. Cessation following chronic use can result in withdrawal symptoms and craving.

Sedating antihistamines

These are generally misused for their ability to cause euphoria and hallucinations, especially at high doses and it is hypothesized that it is their antimuscarinic properties that may be responsible for these effects. The main drugs of concern in this group are believed to be chlorphenamine (chlorpheniramine), cyclizine, diphenhydramine, and dimenhydrinate. There have also been reports of cyclizine being injected, and of its use to enhance the effects of opioids.

Sympathomimetics

Drugs in this class are decongestants and include OTCs which are used as cold and flu remedies. Their active ingredients work as peripheral vasoconstrictors. Some are also centrally active and have mild stimulant properties, thus making them liable to misuse. The use of ephedrine as a performance enhancer in gyms has been reported and it is also used to combat fatigue. Use as a weight loss aid occurs, and products containing this are marketed for this purpose in some countries. Furthermore, ephedrine and pseudoephedrine are sought as precursors for the clandestine manufacture of methamphetamine. Thus, doctors and pharmacists need to be alert to requests for large or repeated quantities of the drugs on their own or in combination products.

Sildenafil

Sildenafil is available OTC in some countries. It is misused to counter the negative impact of amphetamine use on sexual performance, and to increase the length of sexual experience. Potential harms include increased risk of HIV seroconversion as the combination of sildenafil and amphetamine is linked with high-risk sexual behaviour in men who have sex with men, and increased risk of cerebrovascular accident and priapism.

Laxatives

These drugs are misused by people who are trying to lose weight or control their weight, or by those who are concerned with having a regular bowel movement. In the first case, abusers of laxatives tend to be younger females who take these products in the mistaken belief that fewer calories will be absorbed from food and, in the latter case, the group who tend to abuse laxatives are the elderly as many in the Western world believe that a daily bowel evacuation is required to keep healthy. In some, tolerance to the effects of laxatives such as senna results in increasing doses.

Other products

Other products which have been reported to be misused include those containing caffeine, antimuscarinics (e.g. hyoscine), herbal muscle building products, and herbal products containing ephedra (Ma Huang). Indeed, many 'herbal' products contain non herbal ingredients which may be liable to abuse. In addition, other chemicals available OTC from pharmacies have been used in the illicit manufacture or preparation of illegal drugs.

Interventions

Community pharmacists use a number of strategies to avoid or deal with the issue—mainly from a supply reduction perspective, including not stocking the drug, training staff to recognize potential misuse issues, keeping potentially misused substances out of sight, and sharing information with colleagues.

Once a practitioner is aware of OTC misuse or abuse, it may also be possible to intervene from a harm reduction perspective. However, much of misuse/abuse behaviour is likely to be covert and difficult to address or change. In the case of misuse for altered body image, unintentional misuse, and medication dependence, interventions may be more successful. Referral to a GP or drug and alcohol agencies may be appropriate and at a minimum, practitioners should advise individuals about the risks of misuse and overuse where misuse is suspected.

Preventive strategies

Health professionals and professional bodies need to be alert and vigilant. Emphasis is currently on regulation of supply and efforts by pharmacists to avoid selling to known or suspected abusers, but there is still scope to explore the potential for interventions designed to help and support those with OTC abuse problems and to provide treatment for those who want to quit, or who have co-morbidities associated with their misuse. The pharmaceutical industry needs to be aware of the potential for the misuse of OTC products, not just with regard to the ingredients, but also with respect to formulations such as liquid-filled capsules, the contents of which are easy to inject.

Finally, whilst not a major issue from a public health perspective, OTC misuse for some people is highly problematic, sometimes with serious health sequelae, and is something which should not be ignored by health care professionals.

Further reading

Cooper R. (2013). Over-the-counter medicine abuse – a review of the literature. *J Subst Use* 18(2):82–107.

Hughes G, McElnay J, Hughes C, *et al.* (1999). Abuse/misuse of non-prescription drugs. *Pharm World Sci* 21:251–5.

Lessenger JE, Feinberg SD. (2008). Abuse of prescription and over-the-counter medications. *J Am Board Fam Med* 21(1):45–54.

MacFayden L, Eadie D, McGowan T. (2000). Over-the-counter medicine misuse in Scotland. *J R Soc Promot Health* 121:185–92.

Matheson C, Bond C, Pitcairn M. (2002). Misuse of over-the-counter medicines from community pharmacies: a population survey of Scottish pharmacies. *Pharmaceut J* 269:66–8.

Wills S. (2005). *Drugs of Abuse* (2nd ed). London: Pharmaceutical Press.

New psychoactive substances (NPS)

There is a dizzying number of new 'designer drugs' being synthesized, each with a multitude of different street names. Due to analytical difficulties and limited survey data it is difficult to know the extent of use of these drugs but they are available to purchase online and in high street 'head shops'. To evade the law they have been marketed as 'not for human consumption' and as products such as 'bath salts', 'research chemicals', 'herbal incense', and 'pond cleaners'. NPS often try to mimic the effects of traditional illicit drugs and often have analogous chemical structures leading to similar clinical effects. With such a short history of human consumption, the toxic effects of many NPS remain largely unknown or unpredictable.

Basic classification of NPS

There are many ways of classifying NPS, most commonly through their chemical class or their principal pharmacological (psychoactive) effects. Broadly, they can be considered to be stimulant-like, hallucinogen/dissociative-like, cannibis-like, or sedative-like in their actions. Here we adopt a chemical classification as the primary one.

Phenylethylamine derivatives
- Synthetic cathinones (also termed beta-ketonated amphetamines), such as mephedrone, methedrone, and methylenedioxypyrovalerone (MDPV) have similar effects to amphetamine type stimulants (ATS) and act to release presynaptic monoamines.
- Ring-substituted phenylethylamines: 2C- B (2,5- dimethoxy- 4-bromophenethylamine and 2C- I (2,5- dimethoxy- 4- iodophenethylamine) are primarily hallucinogens.
- NBOMes: these are a distinctive group of phenylethylamines, being N-benzyl-oxy-methyl (thus 'NBOMe') or otherwise N-methoxy-benzyl derivatives of previously known phenethylamines such as 2C-I and 2C-B; they also have hallucinogenic effects, and are usually instilled on to blotting paper, like LSD; there are several different NBOMes, of which 25I-NBOMe is the most potent.

Phenylpiperazine derivatives: These include benzylpiperazine (BZP) and are similar to, but milder than, ATS.

Tryptamine derivatives: These include N,N-diallyl-5-methoxytryptamine (5-MeO-DALT), α-methyltryptamine (α-MT); they are structurally similar to serotonin and have hallucinogenic effects similar to LSD.

Synthetic cocaine: This is often much more potent than natural cocaine and can lead to higher rates of vascular complications.

Ketamine derivatives: These include methoxetamine and phencyclidine (PCP) derivatives (e.g. 3-methoxy phencyclidine); these are NMDA receptor antagonists which typically cause dissociative effects that may be longer lasting and more profound than ketamine.

Synthetic cannabinoids: There are pure CB_1 receptor agonists which are generally more potent than Δ^9-THC. They pose a far greater risk of acute harm than natural cannabis, with higher rates of behavioural disturbance and psychotic phenomena. They also appear to have significant sympathomimetic effects. Acute physical harm such as seizures and acute renal and myocardial injury have been reported. More recently, dependence and withdrawal syndromes have been reported among regular users. Some preparations contain compounds with hallucinogenic and/or stimulant properties. See Chapter 10 for more information.

Emerging natural products: Some authorities include naturally occurring compounds found in plants such as *Salvia divinorum* and kratom (*Mitragyna speciose*).

Forces driving production and consumption
- Huge profit margins
- Ease of manufacture by chemically modifying existing psychoactive substances
- Ease of marketing and distribution (predominantly online)
- Evasion of detection in bodily fluids
- May be perceived to be legal and safe by users.

Challenges
- Product variability
- Legal: the law has historically struggled to keep pace with the expansion of chemical analogues
- Analytical: most clinical laboratories are unable to detect EPS in bodily fluids because they cannot maintain a library of 'chemical standards' of the large number of new compounds in circulation
- Unknown and unpredictable toxicology of new derivatives.
- Harm reduction for users.

Further reading
User websites such as http://www.EROWID.com list street names for EPS that can help translate what chemical an individual has taken and expected clinical effects.
www. globaldrugsurvey.com

Polysubstance use

Introduction and epidemiology *392*
Consequences of polysubstance use *395*
Management of polysubstance use *403*

Introduction and epidemiology

Introduction

Substances from a range of chemical and pharmacological classes are used for their mind-altering properties. Both the acute effects and longer-term consequences may differ when substances are combined. Some combinations of substances will potentiate each other, whereas some combinations may result in opposing effects. This chapter considers the patterns, adverse consequences, and management of polysubstance use. It identifies drug use combinations associated with increased risk of morbidity and mortality likely to require medical intervention. These diverse presentations may be complicated by prior psychiatric or medical conditions already requiring treatment. In summary:

- Polysubstance use, rather than use restricted to one particular substance, is increasingly prevalent, especially in young people.
- Combinations of CNS depressants and psychostimulants are popular among many groups of young people.
- Intensive alcohol and benzodiazepine use is a major but often overlooked component of polysubstance use.
- Large increases in prescription and over-the-counter opioid analgesic use are occurring across the developed world.
- Illicit opioid use constitutes the most frequent background against which drug-induced deaths occur.
- Cumulative multiple drug use is associated with poorer physical health, greater likelihood of addiction, and other social and psychiatric problems.
- Polysubstance abuse is a significant predictor of drug overdose.

Definitions and diagnosis

Polysubstance use, sometimes referred to as polydrug use, is the consumption of more than one drug, simultaneously or at different times for either recreational and/or therapeutic purposes.

- Polysubstance use most commonly refers to multiple illicit drug use.
- However, it can include legal substances (most commonly alcohol and tobacco) and both prescription and proprietary (over-the-counter) medication used for non-medical purposes.
- Diagnostic terms that included 'polysubstance' were removed from DSM–5. The individual substance (or group of substances) now needs to be specified. Consistent with the move away from 'abuse' and 'dependence' diagnoses, Substance use disorder (SUD) is now represented on a continuum of severity ranging from 2 'mild' to 11 'severe'.
- Diagnoses of polysubstance use in the ICD system are reserved for when substance use is so indiscriminate that no predominant substance is used. In most cases it is recommended that those who use multiple substances are diagnosed by substance type, with each graded on the basis of severity.

Patterns and prevalence

Types of substances used and drug combinations vary across geographic regions. Risk profiles vary between groups. This reflects differences in socioeconomic circumstances, accessibility, purity, dosing, and patterns of misuse. Local factors, including age group, affects drug use patterns.

- Substance use initiated in *adolescence* is associated with higher probability of drug use in later life, greater difficulties in reducing/stopping, and reflects higher levels of risk behaviours, social exclusion, or deviance. It is important to distinguish experimental from problematic use.
- Expansion of polysubstance use to include stimulants/hallucinogens is often associated with reaching the legal age for club, dance party, and 'rave' attendance. Recent studies report up to 75% of 'rave' attendees use multiple substances (combinations of alcohol, cannabis, amphetamine, notably cocaine, MDMA, GHB, benzodiazepines, ketamine, amyl nitrite ('poppers'), LSD, psilocybin).
- Polysubstance use peaks in the 18–29 age group. In some countries, prescription opioids have become the most commonly abused drug among younger abusers. Unintentional dosing errors and unanticipated drug interactions can lead to acute medical presentation.
- Polysubstance use is pervasive amongst opioid maintenance enrolees (methadone and buprenorphine), and this may persist during pregnancy. Over half report concurrent benzodiazepine use, often sourced from multiple prescribers (doctor shopping) or illicitly. In some countries, almost half report cocaine as the secondary drug of abuse and up to 50% exhibit alcohol-related problems.
- Polysubstance use significantly contributes to the burden of disease amongst people with HIV/AIDS and hepatitis C.
- The elderly are the fastest growing demographic in the developed world. Amongst older patients there is increasing abuse of multiple substances, particularly combinations of alcohol, prescription medication including benzodiazepines and opioids.
- Although the efficacy of long-term opioid treatment for chronic non-malignant pain remains unestablished, large increases in opioid analgesic prescribing continues with prescription medication diversion. More deaths in the US are now attributed to the use of prescribed opioids than to heroin and cocaine use combined.

Major drug combinations to consider are displayed in Fig. 17.1.

Drug use profiles generally fall into a small number of clusters of increasing drug involvement. Latent class analysis (LCA) applied to a wide range of licit and illicit drugs typically reveals three primary 'additive' polysubstance use profiles:

1. a limited range cluster (including alcohol/tobacco/cannabis)
2. a moderate range cluster (adding stimulants, commonly amphetamines and/or cocaine)
3. an extended range cluster (adding non-medical use of prescription drugs, and other illicit drugs).

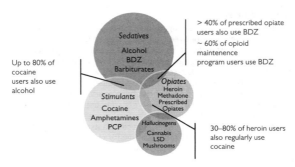

Fig. 17.1 Common drug groups in polysubstance abuse.

Fig. 17.2 shows the three main clusters of drug use identified. Those reporting use of wide-ranging multiple substances have poorer mental health, elevated sexual risk behaviours, and infectious disease prevalence.

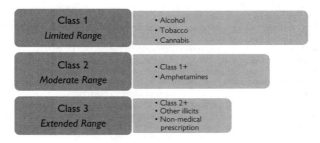

Fig. 17.2 Clusters of multiple substance use in latent class analysis (LCA) analyses.

Consequences of polysubstance use

Reasons for combining drugs
People combine drugs for perceived positive benefits and additive pharmacological effects (Table 17.1). Polysubstance use can occur simultaneously (e.g. alcohol and cannabis), directly mixing (e.g. heroin and cocaine 'speedball'), or sequentially.

Non-acute polysubstance presentations
Non-acute clinical presentations to medical facilities occur in many ways. Polysubstance abuse is usually not apparent to the prescriber. When substance use is identified, attention may be diverted to a single substance. A combination of anxiety, insomnia, and pain are common presenting symptoms. Less frequently 'loss of prescription' prompts attendance. Sedatives including benzodiazepines and opioids are most commonly sought.

Table 17.1 Reasons for combining drugs

Enhanced drug effect	• CNS depressant combinations (alcohol + benzodiazepines + opioids) • Alcohol + cocaine (psychoactive metabolite cocaethylene enhances effects) • Heroin + cocaine ('speedball') • Heroin + amphetamine ('bombitas') • PCP + cocaine ('space basing') • Cannabis + hallucinogens • Cannabis + PCP ('primos') • MDMA + hallucinogens • Alcohol + GHB (gamma-hydroxybutyrate)
Reverse/reduce drug effects	• Sedative use (alcohol/benzodiazepines/opioids) to counteract psychostimulant-induced hyperactive state (agitation, restlessness, insomnia, paranoia) • Benzodiazepine use to relieve anabolic androgenic steroid-induced anxiety/insomnia
Ameliorate withdrawal symptoms	• Sedative use for alcohol/opioid, e.g. benzodiazepines to manage withdrawal symptoms of anxiety and agitation. • Buprenorphine, (partial μ-receptor agonist) to reduce opioid withdrawal (can provoke withdrawal if taken early)
Relieve pain	• Supplementation of prescribed medication: increased dosing/additional alcohol/cannabis/benzodiazepines/proprietary (over-the-counter) medication
Alleviate psychiatric symptoms	• Alcohol/tobacco/cannabis to ameliorate symptoms or prescribed psychiatric medication effects

Acute polysubstance presentations

Management may need to be urgent and decisive. Presentation can be difficult to distinguish from other medical conditions. Some patients may not be capable of giving a coherent history. Multiple substances may have been used; a cluster of certain presenting signs and symptoms ('toxidromes') can point to a specific drug class and can assist diagnostically and with acute management (Table 17.2). Urinalysis may not assist acute clinical management as these tests identify recent drug consumption but give no indication of blood levels or the relationship of drugs to the clinical effects observed. Interactions with alcohol must be considered, including the recognition that stimulants enable users to consume larger quantities of alcohol over longer periods.

Risks associated with particular drug combinations are influenced by:
• characteristics of the user
• presence of tolerance
• health status e.g. hepatic function
• genetic and phenotypic factors
• route of administration (oral, intranasal, intravenous, and rectal)
• drug quantity.

In polysubstance use, adverse interactions occur through several mechanisms, either between drugs with similar effects (pharmacodynamic) or between drugs that alter metabolic enzyme/pathways (pharmacokinetic).

Some key drug combinations and their effects are presented in Box 17.1. Specific toxidromes are shown in Table 17.2.

Box 17.1 Specific combination effects

• Opioids taken with alcohol significantly decrease the ventilatory response to hypercapnia.
• Benzodiazepines + methadone four times more likely to require naloxone/intubation than benzodiazepines + buprenorphine, but the latter can still produce severe overdose effects and deaths.
• β-blockers best avoided in acute cocaine intoxication—may cause an unopposed α-adrenergic effect.
• Opioids + cocaine may amplify negative psychostimulant cardiovascular effects.
• Older drug users often have impaired capacity to metabolize benzodiazepines, and concomitant opioid use (heroin, methadone, buprenorphine) increases risk of respiratory depression.
• Illicit drug intoxication-related cardiac arrest most frequently involves opiates. Associated with poor survival, high incidence of neurological deficit.
• OD risk of buprenorphine low, risk increases if buprenorphine is injected and/or used with other sedatives.
• Polydrug use may mask chronic nitrous oxide (N_2O)-induced vitamin B_{12} deficiency myelopathy.
• Methadone can block HERG K^+ channels and significantly prolong QTc interval. Use of CYP3A4 inhibitors may accentuate this and alter cardiac risk profile.

Table 17.2 Toxidromes

Drug class toxidrome	Presentation	Clinical features		Complications can include:
		Intoxication	Withdrawal	
(1) Sedative-hypnotic				
Alcohol	Stupor/coma	Slurred speech	Abrupt cessation following chronic use: seizures.	Aspiration (pneumonitis)
Benzodiazepines (BDZ)	Confusion	Ataxia		Respiratory failure
Barbiturates	Slurred speech	Impaired memory/attention	Autonomic hyperactivity	
	Apnoea	Confusion/stupor/coma		
(2) Opioid				
Opioids	Altered mental status	CNS depression	Clear sensorium	Respiratory failure
Heroin	Slow shallow breaths	Respiratory depression (hypoventilation with hypercapnia)	Restlessness/yawning	Aspiration (pneumonitis)
Methadone		Miosis	Rhinorrhoea/piloerection	Non-cardiogenic pulmonary oedema
Buprenorphine		Bradycardia	Vomiting/diarrhoea	Rhabdomyolysis
Prescription opioids		Hypotension	Mydriasis	Hypothermia
OTC compound analgesics (NSAID + codeine)		Hypothermia		
		Decreased bowel sounds		

(Continued)

Table 17.2 (Contd.)

Drug class toxidrome	Presentation	Clinical features		Complications can include:
		Intoxication	*Withdrawal*	
(3) Adrenergic Amphetamines/ cocaine/MDMA Ephedrine/phencyclidine PCP	Sympathomimetic effects	CNS: Agitation, euphoria, hallucinations, psychosis Panic/delirium *Neuromuscular:* tremor, hyperreflexia, seizures *Autonomic:* hyperthermia, diaphoresis, mydriasis, flushing *Cardiovascular:* tachycardia Arrhythmias, hypertension Myocardial ischaemia. *Renal:* acute kidney injury *Gastrointestinal:* nausea, vomiting, diarrhoea MDMA may trigger *serotonergic syndrome*	Exhaustion/fatigue Sleep/mood disturbance Anhedonia Myalgia/arthralgia	
Cathinones (β-ketoamphetamines) (ephedrine-like) Mephedrone	Sympathomimetic effects	*Adrenergic/serotonergic effects* including: Hallucinations/agitation/paranoia Psychosis/myoclonus/headache		

(4) Hallucinogenic			
Serotonin-related			
LSD, psilocybin	Depersonalization Disinhibition Hallucinations Psychosis Panic Fever Hyperthermia	Pupillary dilatation Tachycardia/palpations Diaphoresis Uncoordination	
Amphetamine-related			
Cocaine/mescaline	Adrenergic effects	Adrenergic effects	
MDMA (Ecstasy)	Bruxism, Headache, trismus Diaphoresis	Adrenergic effects	
(5) Dissociative			
Dissociative anaesthetics			
Ketamine (N-methyl-D-aspartate glutamate receptor antagonist)	Hyperthermia (>39°C) Hyporeflexia Tremors Tonic/clonic seizures	Nystagmus Tachycardia/ataxia/ Dysarthria, increased salivation	
Phencyclidine (PCP)			Agitated, bizarre behaviour Delirium, psychosis without delirium Catatonia/hypomania with euphoria Analgesic effects of DA, may delay delayed injury detection.

(Continued)

Table 17.2 (Contd.)

Drug class toxidrome	Presentation	Clinical features		Complications can include:
		Intoxication	Withdrawal	
(6) Others				
Cannabinoids (harvested/ synthetic)	Psychological disturbance Disorientation Disinhibition	Miosis Conjunctival injection Tremor Reduced coordination Increased appetite Urinary retention		Agitation Psychosis Hyperemesis
Anticholinergic agents muscarinic receptor blockade Angel's trumpet, Datura spp. mushrooms OTC cold/flu preparations		*Anticholinergic effects* Delirium / psychosis, dry skin/ mucous membranes. Hyperthermia, mydriasis, Loss of accommodation Urinary retention		

(7) Epileptogenic Withdrawal states Alcohol BDZ		
Gamma-hydroxybutyrate (GHB) ('Fantasy')	Somnolence, confusion, hallucinations Not detected on routine urine toxicology	Resembles other CNS depressants; Dizziness/ataxia Hypotonia, myoclonic movements Tonic/clonic seizures 'Sudden awakening'

Above toxidromes can include inhalants (adhesives, aerosols, solvents, nitrous oxide, petrol, cleaning agents, nitrites ('poppers'))

When used without other agents, inhalants rarely present for medical care

Table 17.3 Potential drug interactions with polysubstance use

Opioid ± alcohol ± BZD	• Synergism, facilitates inhibitory neurotransmitter γ-amino-butyric acid (GABA) inhibition: increased sedation, decreased respiration
Methadone + anticonvulsants —phenytoin —carbamazepine + antituberculosis medication —rifampicin + antiretrovirals —ritonavir/nevirapine + antipsychotic —quetiapine	• *Decreased* plasma methadone levels due to accelerated metabolism of methadone(CYP3A4/CYP2D6 *inducer*) may precipitate withdrawal symptoms
Methadone + sedative —diazepam + antidepressant —fluoxetine + antifungal —fluconazole	• *Increased* plasma methadone levels: • decreases metabolism of methadone (CYP3A4/CYP2D6 *inhibitor*) and may result in symptoms of intoxication • Synthetic piperidine morphine analogues e.g. fentanyl, methadone-proserotonergic and combined with SSRI (e.g. fluoxetine) or SNRI (e.g. venlafaxine) can cause serotonin syndrome
Buprenorphine + cocaine	• Cocaine can significantly diminish buprenorphine concentrations
Antiretroviral (ARV) ritonavir + MDMA + GHB	• Inhibitor of CYP2D6 substrates MDMA/GHB
Sedative + telaprevir/ boceprevir (ARV)	• Some sedatives (alprazolam, midazolam) show marked change in AUC when coadministered with some HCV medication (CYP3A inhibitors)

Management of polysubstance use

Once immediate health risks have been treated it is necessary to establish whether detoxification (inpatient/outpatient) is required (refer to other chapters which deal with specific substance detoxification). This will be influenced by the severity/chronicity of dependence, social supports, and the local availability of detoxification facilities.

In-patient detoxification is indicated when severe withdrawal is likely and where chaotic lifestyles make out-patient treatment unlikely to succeed.

Where meta-analyses have been conducted, psychosocial treatments for polysubstance misuse demonstrate only modest efficacy. Single-substance psychosocial treatments for alcohol, tobacco, cannabis, and stimulants are effective; as are pharmacological treatments for alcohol, opiates, and tobacco. It is unclear if treating multiple substances sequentially is more effective than treating concurrently. There is some evidence to suggest that when one substance is treated individually, use of remaining substances increases.

Table 17.4 outlines the principles of the management of polysubstance use.

Approaches to certain polysubstance use groups

Box 17.2 summarizes the management of sedative abuse in chronic poly-substance treatment. Treatment of coexisting psychiatric co-morbidity is a clinical priority. Psychiatric illness must be considered because of the high rate of chemical dependence amongst the psychiatrically ill. There are multiple potential interactions between substance abuse and prescribed psychiatric medications.

Box 17.2 Sedative abuse management in chronic polysubstance abuse

- Identify and treat co-occurring medical/psychiatric issues
- Stabilize on a long-acting benzodiazepine
- Coordinate treatment providers
- Limit access to benzodiazepines
- Attempt gradual reductions
- Treatment plan identifies and engages in discussion about aberrant drug behaviours
- Arrange regular clinical review, urine testing, and prescription monitoring systems
- Use written treatment agreement
- Document all treatment decisions.

Adapted from *The American Journal on Addictions*, 19(1), Lintzeris N, Nielsen S., Benzodiazepines, methadone and buprenorphine: interactions and clinical management, pp. 59–72, Copyright (2009), with permission from John Wiley and Sons.

Table 17.4 Principles of managing polysubstance presentations

Acute: Stabilize the patient	• Resuscitation: airway/breathing/circulation • Sedated may require airway support/oxygenation/ventilation • Hyper-stimulated or psychotic may require sedation • Risk assessment • Patients often have ingested multiple toxicants • Clinical features may suggest one of several toxidromes (Table 17.2) • Assess: withdrawal risk (alcohol, benzodiazepines, opiates)
Assess primary drug of concern	• Establish primary drug of concern. May not be substance causing presentation, or the most likely to cause target organ damage or exacerbation of mental health problems • Need for detoxification? (out-patient/in-patient) • Assess and prioritize
Assess health and mental health problems	• Coexisting psychiatric disorders: depression, anxiety, bipolar, psychosis, suicidal ideation • A higher proportion of polysubstance users have features of personality (Axis II) disorders • Psychiatric review for more extensive mental health concerns • Establish co morbidities (pre-existing liver or chronic infections, cardiovascular conditions)
Non-acute: Pharmacotherapy	• For opioid dependence (recreational or therapeutic) consider role for opiate replacement therapy • For alcohol dependence consider pharmacotherapy (naltrexone/acamprosate) • Monitor benzodiazepine abuse (see Box 17.1) • Consider SSRIs as first-line treatment of anxiety/depression • Consider mood stabilizers for bipolar disorder (BPAD) • Consider antipsychotics for persisting psychosis
Psychosocial interventions	• Psychosocial interventions (e.g. CBT, motivational interviewing (MI)) for alcohol, cannabis, and tobacco use are effective. Evidence for psychosocial approaches for other substances is less established • Good evidence for effective psychosocial interventions for common psychiatric comorbidities

Box 17.3 Polysubstance use may affect prescribed psychiatric medication by:

- Promoting enzyme induction with altered drug metabolism
- Altering drug clearance and excretion
- Altering CNS neurotransmitters or receptors targeted by medication
- Provoking psychiatric or medical states
- Contributing to poor medical compliance
- Impeding accurate psychiatric diagnosis and impair evaluation of treatment response.

Box 17.3 considers the mechanisms in which polysubstance use affects prescribed psychiatric medication.

Further reading

Connor JP, Gullo MJ, White A, et al. (2014). Polysubstance use: diagnostic challenges, patterns of use and health. *Curr Opin Psychiatry* 27(4):269–75.

Dutra L, Stathopoulou G, Basden SL, et al. (2008). A meta-analytic review of psychosocial interventions for substance use disorders. *Am J Psychiatry* 165:179–87.

Lintzeris N, Nielsen S. (2010). Benzodiazepines, methadone and buprenorphine: interactions and clinical management. *Am J Addict* 19:59–72.

Volkow ND, Frieden TR, Hyde PS, et al. (2014). Medication-assisted therapies – tackling the opioid overdose epidemic. *N Engl J Med* 370: 2063–6.

Injecting drug use

Overdose and overdose deaths 408
Blood-borne virus infections 412
Other medical complications of injecting drug use and their
    management 418
Psychosocial complications of injecting drug use 424

Overdose and overdose deaths

Opioid overdose

People generally do not die during their early adulthood and middle years. Drug overdose deaths are one of the leading causes of death for individuals in these age groups—in many countries, *the* leading cause of death.

Despite their much lower prevalence of use in the general population, heroin and the opioids are implicated in the majority of drug-related deaths (i.e. deaths in which the use of illicit drugs has been listed as the sole cause or as a contributory cause to the death). This is illustrated in Table 18.1.

The term overdose most often applies to the depressant effects of illicit opioids, particularly when taken by injection. Toxicity related to other illicit or prescribed drugs, and of alcohol excess, is covered in the chapters on those substances.

Causes and types of overdose

With regard to suicidal ideation, we can regard drug overdoses as being either:

- accidental drug overdose, or
- drug overdose with clear suicidal intent.

The vast majority of overdoses in this population (more than 80%) are accidental. However, there will also be some in an overlap zone where there was no explicit suicidal intent although there was a recklessness and lack of regard to safety as a result of personal circumstances.

From a pharmacological and physiological perspective, drug overdose may be:

- sudden-onset catastrophic overdose, in which the overdose victim may go unconscious rapidly, e.g. with needle still *in situ*; or
- slow-onset insidious overdose which may go undetected, with risk that the victim may go to sleep and drift into coma without friends or family realizing the danger.

Table 18.1 Mortality associated with illicit drug use compared with prevalence of a drug's use in England and Wales

Drug	Prevalence of use in general population (use in last year, age 16-59)	Number of deaths associated with that drug in 2011
Cannabis	6.9%	7
Cocaine	2.2%	112
Amphetamine	0.8%	62
Ecstasy	1.4%	13
Opioids (incl. heroin & methadone)	0.3%	1082

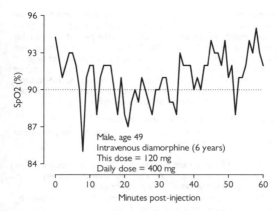

Fig. 18.1 Oxygen saturation after diamorphine injection.

Overdose after intravenous heroin is typically in the sudden-onset cata-strophic category, whilst overdose with oral methadone or oral pharma-ceutical opioids is typically a slow-onset insidious overdose.

The particular risk associated with opioids is not surprising. Opioids are powerful respiratory depressants, and this can be seen with the sharp drop in oxygen saturation levels after opioid injection (Fig. 18.1). Risk of heroin/opioid overdose is increased if there is also consumption of alcohol or other sedative drugs such as benzodiazepines, and this con-coction contributes to many cases of drug overdose death.

Risk of overdose is markedly reduced amongst those in treatment. On commencement of opioid substitution treatment (OST; such as metha-done or buprenorphine maintenance), there is a brief period for a few weeks of increased risk of overdose death (perhaps whilst the patient stabilizes and gets accustomed to the new medication), followed by a period of marked reduction in risk of overdose death for the duration of the OST.

Clusterings of mortality in time and context

The mortality rate from opioid overdose is greater amongst older opioid users, and amongst men (even after allowing for unevenness of distribu-tion of drug use by age and gender), and it is particularly a feature of intravenous heroin use (being rare amongst heroin smokers/chasers).

Treatment is protective against risk of overdose death (see ear-lier in topic)—not only in those treatments requiring total abstinence (such as drug-free residential rehabilitation, and naltrexone antagonist treatments) but also in ambulatory OST treatments (methadone or buprenorphine maintenance). Indeed cessation of OST treatment actually leads to increased risk of overdose death and the period after leaving inpatient treatment or residential rehabilitation is also associated with a rebound increased mortality rate for at least a short period of time.

Heroin users already have a marked excess mortality rate compared with the age-matched population, but this increases approximately eightfold in the weeks following release from prison. This has led to special initiatives to address this period of increased risk.

Preventing heroin/opioid overdose deaths

In the emergency medical situation, the three key specific components of managing the opioid overdose are:
- maintaining the airway
- ensuring sufficient breathing and oxygenation (since opioids are respiratory depressants, a patent airway is not sufficient alone)
- the emergency administration of intramuscular or intravenous naloxone (typically from 0.4–0.8 mg initially, repeated if no response in a few minutes up to at least 2 mg if needed).

A new naloxone nasal spray has been approved recently in the US. If the opioid overdose is caused by a long-acting opioid, then there is a danger that the resuscitated opioid user may slowly drift back into overdose over the subsequent few hours. In some cases, repeat naloxone doses or a slow naloxone infusion is required.

In the wider community situation, four components of preventing overdose deaths should be considered:
- *Secondary prevention:* drug users need to be made aware of the particular danger of intravenous use, of injecting alone, and of mixing heroin with sedative drugs. Harm reduction preventative measures need to have the explicit objective of promoting behaviour change away from injecting, and, if not, then away from mixing drugs and from solitary injecting.
- *For dependent heroin/opioid users:* treatments of various types are protective against risk of overdose death. Good access and early referral to OST treatment can be life-saving.
- *Training of family and friends:* most overdoses occur in the presence of others. Training of family and friends is increasingly being recognized as an essential component of urgent interim management including maintenance of breathing and airway whilst awaiting arrival of emergency medical care.
- *Pre-provision of emergency supply of naloxone,* the opioid antidote, has recently been introduced in some jurisdictions and countries, in order to train first-attenders (e.g. hostel staff or carers) as well as family members and friendship networks in the interim management of the overdose situation. Approximately 10% of naloxone prescribed in this way is typically then used in a real-life emergency situation.

While results from orthodox randomized trials are awaited (and these are difficult to design and conduct), there are already reports of lives saved, and many practitioners now regard this pre-provision as part of competent care of their patient and this is now recommended by the WHO which published guidelines in 2014.

Further reading

Bell J. (2014). Pharmacological maintenance treatments of opiate addiction. *Br J Clin Pharmacol* 77:253–63.

Darke S. (2014). Opioid overdose and the power of old myths: what we thought we knew, what we do know and why it matters. *Drug Alcohol Rev* 33:109–14.

Merrall EL, Kariminia A, Binswanger IA, et al. (2010). Meta-analysis of drug-related deaths soon after release from prison. *Addiction* 105:1545–54.

Sporer KA. (2003). Strategies for preventing heroin overdose. *BMJ* 326:442–4.

Strang J, Babor T, Caulkins J, et al. (2012). Drug policy and the public good: evidence for effective interventions. *Lancet* 379:71–83.

Strang J, Bird S, Dietze P, et al. (2014). Take-home emergency naloxone to prevent deaths from heroin overdose. *BMJ* 349:g6580.

Blood-borne virus infections

Injecting drug users (IDUs) are at risk of one or more blood-borne virus (BBV) infections, and in particular hepatitis C, B, D (HCV, HBV, HDV) and HIV.

Epidemiology

Hepatitis C: infection is associated with a huge burden of disease worldwide as it leads to cirrhosis, end-stage liver disease, and hepatocellular carcinoma in a significant minority of infected individuals. HCV infection is a leading indication for liver transplantation in all Western countries.

- Injecting drug use is the single most important risk factor for HCV infection.
- Following exposure, 25–30% of infections will be cleared spontaneously.
- Many patients have no or minimal symptoms until liver disease is quite advanced.
- Progression to cirrhosis is more likely in males, those drinking alcohol >40 g/day, in patients co-infected with HBV or HIV, in heavy THC users, and in those with non-alcoholic fatty liver disease.
- Treatment is now able to clear the virus in 80–100%.

Prevalence in IDU populations varies from 30% to 90% worldwide (Table 18.2). The annual incidence in the IDU population is 10–30%.

Hepatitis B: is less common than hepatitis C in IDUs and may be acquired through unsafe injecting practices or unprotected sex. Among IDUs approximately:

- 5–15% are actively infected
- 30% are anti-HBc positive
- 50% are immune.

Table 18.2 Examples of the prevalence of blood-borne viruses in injecting drug using populations in some recent reports (%)

Country	HCV	HBV	HDV	HIV
Australia	40–70	2.9–5	0–30	1
Israel	35	3.5		0.9
UK	27–54	0–17.8	0–8.5	1.5
Luxembourg	81.3	3.9		2.5
South Korea	48.4	6.6		0
Iran	34.5–65.9	3.7–30.9		5–9
China	60.9–73.1	3.8–15.4		25.5
USA	69–77	3.5–20	6–50	1–20

A majority of adults infected with HBV will clear the virus, usually after a symptomatic acute hepatitis.

HBV is highly infectious and body fluids such as semen, vaginal fluid, as well as blood may readily transmit the disease.

Hepatitis D: a defective viral particle, requiring presence of HBsAg to enter the hepatocyte. May be acquired as a co- or super-infection in HBV-infected individuals. Prevalence in IDUs may reach 50% in some communities. Discovered in the late 1970s, the epidemiology of this virus has never attracted the interest it deserves. Prevalence rates fell in most communities over two to three decades but more recently rates have increased in some communities. Co-infection increases the severity of liver disease.

HIV: HIV prevalence varies widely in IDUs across the world (Table 18.2) reflecting prevention strategies employed, particularly needle syringe programmes.

- Countries such as Australia and Israel have prevalence of around 1–2%, with US prevalence reaching 20% in some regions.
- In some Asian countries, the prevalence among IDUs is 60–70%.
- In Vietnam, 30% of new HIV cases occur in IDUs.

The impact of needle syringe programmes on BBV infection rates Where such programmes have been implemented, HIV prevalence in IDU populations has remained low. The impact on HCV has been less apparent because of the high prevalence in the IDU population before the programmes were implemented, and because HCV is more infectious and all paraphernalia associated with injecting may transmit the disease.

Assessment

All patients should be assessed fully for evidence of acute or chronic liver disease or for HIV infection at some point early in their contact with drug and alcohol clinic staff. Often these patients do not have a primary care doctor and a failure to identify BBV infection can lead to significant illness. This is an unacceptable outcome as these diseases can be treated and chronic sequelae avoided if early diagnosis is made.

Laboratory tests
The investigations that will demonstrate consequences of BBV infection include:

- LFTs
- FBC and CD4 count
- Viral tests as discussed later in this topic.

All staff in drug and alcohol clinics and in primary care should be capable of, and encouraging of, testing at risk populations for BBV infection as these patients will often not attend another specialty facility while they still have problems with injecting drug use.

Offer serological testing for hepatitis C, B, and D, and HIV to all patients with a history of injecting drug use and, where appropriate, tests for STIs. Be able to test to define the nature of the infection (e.g. current or past) if serology indicates exposure to any of the viruses.

Serological investigations

Serology is the simplest screening tool for each of these viruses and provides information on exposure to viruses without documenting current infection.

Initial tests undertaken are:
- hepatitis C: anti-HCV
- hepatitis B: HBsAg, anti-HBs, anti-HBc (see later in topic p. 415)
- hepatitis D: anti-HDV
- HIV: anti-HIV.

Pre test
- Obtain consent for testing
- Provide information on the significance of a positive or negative result.

Post test
- Provide result in person
- Indicate what further testing is now required
- Arrange appropriate testing and follow-up
- Always ensure patient understands the significance of results.
- Use interpreter services for patients from other countries.

Hepatitis C: serology interpretation and management

Interpretation of hepatitis C serology
- *HCV Ab positive:* current or past infection (40–70% of injecting drug users are anti-HCV positive)
- *HCV Ab negative:* no previous exposure *or* exposure within past 3 months (window period)

Further testing:
- HCV RNA:
  - Negative RNA—no current infection (becomes positive within 2 weeks of exposure)
  - Positive RNA—active viral replication, infectious: order HCV genotype and viral load to direct treatment decisions.

Management of HCV: for many patients focuses on modifying lifestyle factors that may aggravate the liver inflammation.
- Reduce alcohol intake
- Cease cannabis use
- Reduce weight and increase exercise
- Avoid intravenous use of drugs that may cause super-infections with other HCV genotypes, HBV, HIV
- Consider antiviral treatment, once it is established that the patient is willing and able to adhere to treatment requirements.

Treatments for HCV infection continue to evolve rapidly and new drugs offer better control of all genotypes of the disease. The need for pegylated interform and up to 12 months of therapy will no longer be needed for the great majority of patients. Treatments will be based on oral agents, most being directly acting antivirals (DAAs).

New agents include sofosbuvir, simeprevir, daclatasvir, ledipasvir, faldaprevir, ombitasvir, and paritaprevir plus many other agents still in trial. One or other of these is prescribed usually in combination with at least one other drug.

Many opioid substitution clinics now offer HCV treatment on site, having specialists visit the unit regularly or training staff to become competent in HCV treatment. Outcomes equal those in any specialist liver unit.

In future, HCV may be cured in all patients using a primary care-based treatment programme.

Hepatitis B: serology interpretation and management

Interpretation of hepatitis B serology
- HBsAg positive: acute or chronic infection with hepatitis B
- Anti-HBc positive:
  - Where HBsAg is negative, core antibody (IgG) represents past exposure to hepatitis B
  - Where HBsAg is positive, core antibody (IgM) may reflect acute infection or recent flare in chronic infection
- Anti-HBs positive: reflects immune state secondary to either vaccination or past infection
- Anti-HBs and anti-HBc positive: immunity from past exposure to HBV.

Further testing for HBV
If HBs Ag positive:
- Check HBeAg and anti-HBe to define the phase of infection
- Check HBV DNA to direct treatment decisions.

HBV infection is now described in four phases:
- *Immune tolerance phase*: HbsAg positive, HBeAg positive, high HBV DNA, normal ALT
- *Immune clearance phase*: HBsAg positive, falling HBV DNA, raised ALT, seroconversion from HBeAg to anti-HBe (treatment indicated)
- *Immune control phase*: HbsAg positive, anti-HBe positive, HBV DNA positive but lower than immune tolerance phase, normal ALT
- *Immune escape phase*: HBsAg positive, antiHBe positive, HBV DNA rising and ALT elevated (treatment indicated).

Treatment for HBV
- As with HCV, modify those lifestyle factors that may contribute to ongoing liver inflammation.
- While pegylated interferon does have a limited role in treating HBV, the advent of potent oral antiviral agents with very low 5-year resistance rates has changed management markedly.

- The use of a single agent (tenofovir, entecavir, or telbivudine) can control but not cure HBV in the immune clearance or escape phases with a high degree of efficacy. Some countries are training primary care physicians in the assessment and treatment of HBV.

Test all patients to determine their phase and refer on to a specialist unit if:
- the phase of the disease indicates need for treatment *or*
- the stage of the liver disease demands specialist management with regular 6-monthly screening for HCC.

Injecting drug users who are not immune to hepatitis B should be offered vaccination.

HBV genotyping is not currently routine, but may be used in future to provide information on disease severity and treatment responsiveness.

Hepatitis D: serology interpretation and management
- Anti-HDV positive: exposure to HDV and probable ongoing coinfection
- Check HDV RNA: if positive, refer for management of HBV/HDV coinfection.

Management of HDV
- Address lifestyle issues as with HCV and HBV infection
- Consider antiviral therapy for HBV as indicated earlier in this topic.

HIV: serology interpretation and management
Anti-HIV positive: probable HIV infection, confirm with HIV RNA. If positive, refer for specialist care.
   All persons testing positive for HIV Ab should be:
- tested for hepatitis exposure as co-infection is common where needle syringe programmes are not well established and utilized
- referred to the appropriate HIV specialist, e.g. immunologist or infectious diseases specialist to assess the need for treatment and for monitoring.

While treatment of HIV is typically provided in specialty units, some special programmes to increase access have extended HIV management to primary care settings or drug treatment services.

Monitoring for hepatocellular carcinoma (HCC)
All patients with cirrhosis should be screened 6-monthly with abdominal ultrasound and serum α-feto-protein to detect early HCC development.
   Patients with HBV and no cirrhosis are also at increased risk and should also be screened.

Prevention and treatment of blood-borne viral infections

All injecting drug users should be advised of the risk of exposure to hepatitis C, B, and D, and HIV, and should be well educated about the value of monitoring viral status, liver and immune system status, and clinical signs to detect any evidence of disease progression, which may require changed management plans. Patients should be educated on avoiding spread of these BBVs:

- Care with blood spills or open wounds
- Avoid sharing of toothbrushes, nail scissors, or razors
- Safe disposal of sanitary pads
- Washing hands
- Avoiding sexual spread of HBV and HIV. Use of condoms and practising safe sex at all times
- Vaccination against HBV for all at-risk individuals in those countries where universal vaccination is not practised
- Use of post-exposure prophylaxis (PEP) in situations where HIV risk is high.

Further reading

Gidding HF, Amin J, Dore GJ, et al. (2011). Hospitalization rates associated with hepatitis B and HIV co-infection, age and sex in a population-based cohort of people diagnosed with hepatitis C. *Epidemiol Infect* 139:1151–8.

Grebely J, Pham ST, Matthews GV, et al. (2012). Hepatitis C virus reinfection and superinfection among treated and untreated participants with recent infection. *Hepatology* 55:1058–69.

Nelson PK, Mathers BM, Cowie B, et al. (2011). Global epidemiology of hepatitis B and hepatitis C in people who inject drugs: results of systematic reviews. *Lancet* 378:571–83.

Other medical complications of injecting drug use and their management

Causes of complications

Complications may be due to:
- the pharmacology of the drug
- unsafe injecting practices
- contaminants and adulterants
- the associated lifestyle.

Pharmacology of the drug

Opioid effects:
- Drowsiness and hypoventilation are critical issues
- Hypercapnic respiratory failure that may complicate other respiratory disease
- Overdose may present with muscle necrosis, rhabdomyolysis, pressure neuropathy, compartment syndrome(s), and acute kidney injury
- Constipation ranging from mild to narcotic bowel syndrome (pseudo-obstruction related to opioids with abdominal pain)

Stimulant effects:
- Cardiovascular toxicity (tachyarrhythmia, myocardial ischaemia)
- Cerebrovascular accident
- Agitation, psychosis.

Unsafe injecting practices

- Infections: injecting illicit drugs and sharing of injecting equipment places individuals at risk of infections including BBVs (see pp. 412–13) as well as bacteria and fungi
- Vascular and tissue damage: the vasculature and surrounding tissues are also exposed to repeated trauma and sometimes chemical irritation
- Aseptic thrombophlebitis and thrombosis leading to venous scarring (causing 'track marks')
- Lymphoedema
- Indurated, thickened skin, and soft tissue
- Intra-arterial injection may cause limb ischaemia or gangrene. This was a particular hazard with injection of temazepam gel caps while these were available; it may become a problem with new tamper-resistant medications that form gels rather than dissolve in water.

Contaminants and adulterants

Illicit heroin and other injected substances are typically non-sterile and the potency is undefined. The drug may be contaminated or 'cut' with a variety of substances, e.g. starch, talc. The user may experience unexpected allergic reactions, pharmacological effects, or toxic effects. Injection of particulate matter may result in microemboli or granulomas particularly in the liver or lungs.

Associated lifestyle

- Chaotic lifestyle (prioritization of drug use, involvement in the criminal scene, efforts to obtain money for illicit drugs; social disintegration) may undermine efforts to comply with treatment.
- Stigmatization of drug users leads to marginalization, poor interactions with healthcare systems and a lack of trust.
- Nutrition and self-care may be poor leading to wasting and nutritional deficiencies.
- Increased risk of STIs. Chlamydia, syphilis, gonorrhoea, and/or HIV may be acquired through unprotected sex, either as part of sex work to pay for drugs, or unplanned sex while intoxicated.

Bacterial and fungal Infections

Bacterial infections

Most commonly caused by *Staphylococcus aureus*; also *Streptococcus viridans, Pseudomonas*, aerobic Gram-negative rods, anaerobic cocci, *Clostridium*, and rarely, community-acquired MRSA (methicillin-resistant *Staphylococcus aureus*).

Local infections

Infections at the site of injection and surrounding soft tissue—septic thrombophlebitis, abscess (see p. 71, Fig. 5.1) cellulitis, necrotizing fasciitis (mainly with clostridium following subcutaneous injection), necrotizing ulcers, gas gangrene, and pulsatile pseudo-aneurysms, e.g. in the neck or groin.

Systemic or distant infections

Bacterial infections may become systemic and life-threatening. In cases of high unexplained or chronic fever in an injecting drug user, always consider endocarditis, septicaemia, or another hidden focus of serious infection.

Bacterial endocarditis

An important problem with injecting drug use. *Staphylococcus aureus* is the most common organism accounting for 90% of cases. Other causes include *Streptococcus viridans, Pseudomonas aeruginosa*, and rarely *Candida* and other fungal infections.

Although endocarditis classically affects the tricuspid valves it may also affect the mitral or aortic valves, particularly if there is pre-existing valvular disease. In left-sided endocarditis, septic embolization may lead to abscesses in other organs such as the brain or spleen. Mycotic aneurysms may also result from systemic emboli.

Endocarditis may be a cause of unexplained fever and weight loss, with or without a murmur or other the typical features of endocarditis. If there is any suspicion of endocarditis the person should be referred urgently to hospital for investigation.

Do blood cultures in all febrile injecting drug users.

Emboli: thromboembolism, metastatic abscesses (including epidural abscess presenting with back pain and fever), mycotic aneurysms.

Fungal infections
- Mainly due to *Candida, Aspergillus,*and *Penicillium*. Distant or systemic infection including fungal endocarditis, fungal ophthalmitis.
- *Candida albicans:* oral, vaginal, or systemic candidiasis, particularly in patients with HIV (lemon juice used to dissolve substances may be a source of *Candida albicans*).
- Illicit injection of diverted sublingual buprenorphine tablets increases the risk of blood-borne mouth organisms, including *Candida*.

Complications by body system
Cardiovascular complications
- Cardiomyopathy
- Arrhythmias (stimulants)
- Hypertension (stimulants)
- Myocardial infarction (cocaine)
- Endocarditis (see p. 419)
- Vasculitis, vascular damage
- Vascular spasm due to local trauma of injecting, or injecting of cocaine
- Angiitis (amphetamines)
- Intra-arterial injection with distal ischaemia, gangrene
- Embolism
- Arteriovenous aneurysm
- Mycotic aneurysms.

Pulmonary complications
- Most IDUs smoke tobacco which contributes to lung problems
- Pneumonia—bacterial pneumonia, e.g. as a result of septic embolism from endocarditis, pneumocystis (in HIV patients)
- Aspiration pneumonia
- Tuberculosis—consider in patients presenting with pneumonia and HIV infection
- Lung abscess
- Atelectasis
- Pulmonary haemorrhage, pulmonary emboli, pulmonary infarction (from septic thrombophlebitis or coincident cocaine use)
- Non-cardiogenic pulmonary oedema (heroin, particularly if smoked)
- Pulmonary granulomas (from insoluble additives and/or injection of crushed tablets).

Gastrointestinal complications
- Constipation (opioids)
- Bowel infarction (cocaine)
- Acute liver injury, potentially fulminant liver failure (cocaine)
- Hepatitis A, B, C, D.

Musculoskeletal complications
- Osteomyelitis
- Septic arthritis
- Epidural abscess
- Rhabdomyolysis: may result from pressure following prolonged unconsciousness with heroin (and/or benzodiazepines, alcohol); also reported with cocaine or amphetamine use. May lead to acute kidney injury.

Renal complications
- Renal failure
- Glomerulonephritis, interstitial nephritis, or immune mediated in viral hepatitis
- Nephropathy (including HIV-associated).

Dental complications
As opioids (illicit or prescribed) dry the mouth, bacteria can reproduce more readily that cause dental decay. If combined with poor dental hygiene, dental decay is common. This can result in acute or chronic pain, and dental infections (pp. 484–8).

CNS complications
- Overdose/coma or death or cerebral hypoxic injury from respiratory depression (heroin and other CNS depressants)
- Seizures (psychostimulants)
- Cerebrovascular accidents, cerebral infarct, cerebral haemorrhage (psychostimulants).
- Toxic leucoencephalopathy (heroin smoking).

Neuropsychiatric complications
- Anxiety
- Depression
- Agitation, psychosis (stimulants)
- Altered consciousness, organic brain syndrome.

Physical examination
A complete and systematic physical examination is required (see pp. 71–72). In particular, look for relevant complications of injecting drug use:
- General appearance of illness or distress
- Nutritional status (weight, muscle bulk, skin, subcutaneous fat)
- Fever, evidence of sepsis
- Vein damage ('track marks')
- Mental state examination
- Stigmata of liver disease
- Cardiac murmurs, and peripheral signs of endocarditis
- Respiratory failure and localizing respiratory signs.

Laboratory tests

Pregnancy test: in women of child-bearing age.

Blood tests
- FBC
- EUC
- LFTs; isolated elevation of ALT suggests chronic hepatitis C infection; levels may fluctuate
- Coagulation tests (INR, APTT).

Tests for blood-borne viruses
- Hep B surface antigen and antibody, Hep B core antibody
- Hep C antibody and if positive Hep C RNA.
- HIV.

(Also see p. 414.)

Tests for sexually transmitted infections (if at risk or if uncertain)
In addition to tests for BBVs:
- First void urine for *Chlamydia* nucleic acid amplification testing (NAAT)
- If relevant, swab pharynx, anus, genitals for gonorrhoea NAAT and culture
- Hepatitis A IgG and/or IgM.

Other investigations as indicated
- Blood cultures (if febrile, three sets to be taken before commencing treatment with antibiotics)
- Creatine phosphokinase (CK, for rhabdomyolysis; CK-MB for chest pain after cocaine use)
- Urine drug screen (noting any prescribed medication including ambulance given)
- Chest X-ray
- Cardiac ECHO (transoesophageal is more sensitive than transthoracic for vegetations)
- CT head/MRI when indicated (e.g. suspected cerebral abscess).

Treatment of complications

General management of the hospitalized injecting drug user
- Maintain professional, non-judgemental approach, respectful of patient request for healthcare.
- Develop a comprehensive management plan that addresses physical health, mental health, drug health, and psychosocial problems.
- Look for and treat any drug intoxication or withdrawal. Offer nicotine patches for tobacco withdrawal.
- Consult Addiction Medicine service where available for advice.
- Consider commencing or continuing opioid maintenance treatment if opioid dependent.
- Offer analgesia. Pain is a common feature of most of the above-mentioned complications and IDU patients typically are sensitive to pain (may reflect reduced pain threshold in chronic opioid users).
- Assess and manage any comorbid mental health disorder.

- Most IDUs will need social work assistance for housing, welfare support, and support with any legal issues.
- Hospitalized patients should be instructed to cease and discard any drugs or paraphernalia and if not, consider discharge if safe to do so. Non-prescribed drug use complicates delivery of care and may place the patient or staff at risk. Consult senior hospital management for advice.
- If necessary, negotiate limits with the patient regarding absence from the ward, drug use on the ward or requests for analgesia.
- Discharge planning is typically complex and should be planned early. Consider housing, transportation for ongoing treatment, analgesia (access, adequacy, prescribing, and control of dispensing), funding for treatment, integration with addiction care (referral to opioid treatment programme, rehabilitation, or other), access to primary care, and availability of specialist follow-up.

Management of specific complications

Overdose
(Also see pp. 410–11.)
- Assess 'ABC' and if safe, monitor for recovery.
- Oxygen is essential to maintain saturation.
- Antagonists such as naloxone and flumazenil may stave off intubation. Two chief concerns about their use are increased risk of withdrawal if too much is given and potential re-intoxication after these short acting antagonists wear off. Deaths have occurred in patients who disregard advice and leave hospital too soon. Therefore these drugs are used sparingly. Naloxone infusion may be needed for overdose of long-acting drugs like methadone and slow-release oxycodone preparations.

Bacterial endocarditis
- Do three sets of blood cultures in all febrile IDUs before commencing treatment.
- Treat with intravenous antibiotics for at least 6 weeks.
- The team should involve cardiologists, microbiologists, infectious disease specialists, and addiction specialists. A cardiothoracic surgeon should be involved if infection persists, there are repeated emboli or other complications. Uncontrolled drug use is a contraindication for surgery.

Psychosocial complications of injecting drug use

Some individuals inject illicit drugs occasionally and suffer few if any psychological or social consequences. However those who are dependent on an injected drug may find life stressful and very difficult. The illicit status of such drugs greatly increases the financial, legal, and relationship problems that dependent users experience. For some specific drugs (e.g. stimulants), psychological effects can also be directly caused by the drug itself (e.g. stimulant-induced psychosis).

Causes of stress for those who are dependent on injected drugs include:

- financial strain due to the typically high cost of illicit drugs, and the individuals' impaired ability to earn an income; a criminal record can make it a life-long challenge to find employment
- pressures involved in acquiring the money for drugs or in acquiring the drugs themselves, which may include sex work, theft. or dealing
- pressures from being under police scrutiny: if the individual has a criminal record or has come to police attention, even after prolonged abstinence from drug use they may report ongoing police scrutiny, which when delivered inappropriately, can border on harassment
- homelessness
- relationship strain, due to preoccupation with drugs and financial stress
- fights and violence (see following discussion).

Many IDUs have been a victim of violence or abuse as a consequence of their substance use. In addition some (also or instead) have started illicit drug use as a way of reducing the distress of being a victim of past violence or abuse. IDUs are more at risk of involvement in violence because of:

- vulnerability while intoxicated, particularly if using the substance in a public place or if homeless
- violence from unscrupulous drug dealers, or dealers to whom they owe a debt
- increased tendency to become involved in arguments while disinhibited (e.g. injected benzodiazepines) or intoxicated with stimulants.

Intravenous drug use also can be associated with dysphoria or depression, because of:

- shame and guilt, due to internalized stigma, and inability to fulfil obligations that are important to the individual
- a sense of loss of control because of the daunting social circumstances, and inability to control dependent substance use
- social marginalization.

The nature of the drug influences the risk of acute or chronic psychological effects:

- ATS (and some novel illicit drugs) can cause acute aggression, and risk of substance-induced psychosis, or triggering a relapse to an existing psychotic disorder. Depressed mood is common on cessation of dependent stimulant use (see p. 351).
- Lack of sleep (e.g. due to withdrawal from opioids) can contribute to low mood.
- Smoking cessation can contribute to low mood (e.g. on entering a treatment facility if nicotine replacement is not provided).

Addressing the psychosocial complications of injecting drug use

Compassionate and respectful healthcare is key to effective and ethical treatment delivery.

The stress and dysphoria associated with external circumstances typically improves with:

- *commencement of treatment:* and when substance use reduces or ceases, e.g. when a heroin-dependent individual commences opioid maintenance treatment. Once the individual is freed from the cycle of having to spend all of the day acquiring the drug, using, or recovering from use or withdrawing and as health improves, that individual is more able to effectively solve social problems
- *referral to a social worker or skilled case worker:* some individuals require significant support, particularly if they have been removed from mainstream society for some time because of imprisonment or severe drug dependence. Stable housing in particular, can be a key ingredient to improving psychological and physical health and to addressing substance use
- *supportive advocacy:* the treating clinician can often assist with referral or advocacy, e.g. to assist with legal or housing agencies
- *referral to a skilled counsellor:* if psychological symptoms are severe, or remain problematic after substance use is addressed, referral to a skilled counsellor may assist. For those with potential post-traumatic stress disorder (see pp. 467–8 and p. 479) specialist trauma counselling skills are highly desirable
- *psychiatric review and specific treatment if necessary:* will be indicated if diagnosis is in doubt, or the potential role of psychiatric medications needs review.

Assisting particularly complex clients

In individuals with complex psychological or psychiatric comorbidity, or with cognitive impairment, more intensive support can be beneficial. This may involve:

- the support of a community-based case worker
- supported housing
- good communication between health and social agencies (with the individual's consent), to help coordinate efforts.

- regulatory or legal options:
  - where an individuals' substance use puts others at risk, it is important to consider protection of child safety or of public safety (see pp. 575–9 for child protection, pp. 564–9 and pp. 570–2 for driving)
  - in individuals with severe dependence who have been unable to engage with treatment and who face particularly severe social or physical consequences, in some regions compulsory treatment options are available (see pp. 586–7). While evidence for the effectiveness of compulsory treatment varies, occasionally it can provide a 'circuit breaker' and allow the person an opportunity to step back and review their direction and next steps
  - in those with significant cognitive impairment (e.g. brain damage secondary to past overdoses) guardianship arrangements can be helpful (p. 587).

However, for the vast majority of patients, respectful, supportive, and quality voluntary healthcare are the key treatment ingredients. The responsiveness of the treating team to the patient's personal and social priorities contributes to good treatment engagement.

Gambling

Introduction and epidemiology *428*
Pathophysiology *430*
Clinical syndromes and typology *431*
Antecedents *433*
Psychiatric and social comorbidity *434*
Assessment *435*
Management *438*

Introduction and epidemiology

Gambling is betting anything of value, most commonly money, on an event whose outcome is determined largely by chance and hence cannot be correctly predicted.

Gambling in one form or another is engaged in by people from most cultures and countries. For the vast majority of those who gamble, it is merely a social leisure activity; for a small but significant minority it is a problem.

Various terms are used to denote gambling that is causing problems. These include terms such as problem gambling, gambling addiction, and pathological gambling, which are often used interchangeably so there exists some terminological confusion in this field. This also makes comparing studies from around the world difficult and methodologically challenging.

- Problem gambling, is defined as gambling to a degree that disrupts or damages personal, family, or recreational pursuits
- Pathological gambling, an ICD 10 term, is defined as 'frequent, repeated episodes of gambling which dominate the individual's life to the detriment of social, occupational, material, and family values and commitments'
- Disordered gambling is a term introduced by the American Psychiatric Association's DSM-5 classification system, which defines it as 'persistent and recurrent problematic gambling behaviour leading to clinically significant impairment or distress', and which is included in the section on addictive disorders for the first time.

Prevalence and types of gambling

Although gambling is a worldwide pursuit, and thousands of forms of gambling exist, the form it takes differs from country to country, reflecting their historical roots and cultures. There is a trend for certain forms of gambling, especially electronic ones, to become popularized through global economic and other influences.

- In the UK, the British Gambling Prevalence Survey (2010) found that nearly 75% of the population gamble recreationally; 0.9% gamble problematically (about 0.5 million people), and an estimated 6.5% are at risk of developing problem gambling in the future. In the UK, the most popular gambling activities are the National Lottery (57%), scratch cards (20%), betting on horse races (17%), and fruit (slot) machines (14%).
- In continental Europe, the prevalence rates are similar: in Germany the rate of problematic gambling is 0.2–0.6% and in Finland it is 1.1%.
- In the US, prevalence rates vary significantly between states but the average across the country is 2.2%.
- In Japan, gambling opportunities are abundant. An estimated 5.5% of adults are pathological gamblers (defined by a score ≥5 on the South Oaks Gambling Screen). Non-strategic gambling activities, such as pachinko and slot machines, are most popular. Suicide attempts and personal bankruptcy are the most severe consequences of pathological gambling.

- In Australia and New Zealand, although many forms of gambling are popular, poker (slot) machines are overwhelmingly the form of gambling preferred by problem gamblers.

Influences on gambling

- Although problem gambling cuts across age, gender, class, and race, young people and particular ethnic minorities are generally more vulnerable.
- An increase in gambling opportunities will lead to an increase in gambling-related problems.
- Certain forms of gambling, such as poker (slot) machine playing and keno take place commonly in pubs, clubs, and other licensed venues; alcohol consumption may result in the person becoming disinhibited and more likely to gamble and do so excessively.
- Remote (electronic) forms of gambling (Box 19.1) offer anonymity, ease of access, 24-hour availability, and interactivity.
- These features could make them more addictive than traditional gambling activities.
- Perhaps the greatest change in the gambling field currently is the proliferation of remote gambling opportunities.

Box 19.1 Major types of remote gambling

- Internet gambling
- Mobile phone gambling
- Interactive television gambling.

Pathophysiology

Neurotransmitters thought to be relevant in the pathophysiology of excessive gambling are dopamine and noradrenaline plus endogenous opioids. All these have been implicated in other forms of addictive behaviours and so by interpolation may be involved in gambling. There is some evidence for altered dopamine activity in pathological gamblers as well as dysregulated endorphin function. PET scanning has shown that low dopamine D_2 receptor number is associated with negative urges in gamblers, and that dopamine release in increased in pathological gamblers. Endorphin release in response to amphetamine is decreased in pathological gamblers. The insula may be a vital brain region regulating gambling behaviour as lesions here can inhibit the distorted perceptions of near wins that perpetuate gambling in many with gambling addiction.

Further reading

Clark L, Stokes PR, Wu K, Michalczuk R, Benecke A, Watson BJ, Egerton A, Piccini P, Nutt DJ, Bowden-Jones H, Lingford-Hughes AR (2012). Striatal dopamine D2/D3 receptor binding in pathological gambling is correlated with mood-related impulsivity. *NeuroImage* 63: 40–46.

Clinical syndromes and typology

The experience of gambling

For most people who gamble, it is an occasional leisure activity, but in time some people become unable to enjoy and limit gambling as a recreational activity. In some cases, the problem is episodic, but in an important minority of cases, the person's condition persistently deteriorates. They experience a progression that is closely akin to the addictive process:

- The person simply gambles to recover the money lost.
- With repeated gambling, the person loses time and money that should be spent on him/herself, friends, and family.
- He/she becomes unable to focus on studies or work.
- Human relationships become fragmented.
- In order to recover the money, the person begins to bet larger sums and turns to even riskier forms of gambling.
- Losing sight of his/her initial gambling strategy, the person becomes a long-term failed gambler who desperately tries to 'win it all back in one go'.
- The person starts telling lies throughout his/her daily life in order to make his/her story plausible.
- To continue gambling, the person starts borrowing money. When he or she becomes unable to pay the money back, the person asks family and friends for money.
- The person borrows ever more money.
- The person's interpersonal relations deteriorate, resulting in the person spending even more time gambling.
- The person commits criminal acts to fund the gambling (fraud, theft, embezzlement, etc.).

Clinical syndromes

- As terms such as problem gambling, gambling addiction, pathological gambling, and the new term disordered gambling are often used interchangeably, there exists terminological confusion in this field.
- In the ICD 10, pathological gambling sits within the category of 'Impulse control disorders'. It is defined as 'frequent, repeated episodes of gambling which dominate the individual's life to the detriment of social, occupational, material, and family values and commitments'.
- DSM-5's term 'Disordered Gambling' has been placed in the section on addictive disorders. It is defined as 'persistent and recurrent problematic gambling behaviour leading to clinically significant impairment or distress'.
- DSM-5 lists nine diagnostic criteria, of which at least four should be met in the 12-month period to make a diagnosis of gambling disorder (Box 19.2).

Box 19.2 DSM-5 diagnostic criteria for Disordered Gambling

1. Preoccupied with gambling (obsessive thoughts)
2. Increasing bets to achieve the desired excitement
3. Repeated failed attempts to control or stop gambling
4. Restless and/or irritable when trying to control/stop gambling
5. Gambles as an 'escape' from problems or counter dysphoric mood
6. Chases losses: trying to win back losses all at once
7. Lies to others about gambling or its extent
8. Significant negative impact on job or family, or loses opportunities
9. Borrows money to fund gambling.

Grading severity of a gambling disorder
- Mild = if four to five criteria are met
- Moderate = if six to seven criteria are met
- Severe = if eight to nine criteria are met.

Grading the course of a gambling disorder
- Episodic: subsiding for at least several months
- Persistent: continuing for multiple years.

Similar to substance use, gambling behaviours also exist on a scale of escalating severity and adverse consequences, ranging from normal/recreational gambling, through problem gambling, to gambling disorder/addiction.

Antecedents

- Although problem gambling is seen in both men and women and in all adult age groups, young people are more vulnerable to progression.
- In some countries, Indigenous people (first nations) have a higher prevalence of gambling and seem at greater risk of progression.
- In some cases the person has a comorbid mental health disorder; sometimes this is the result of a gambling disorder, but in others the mental health disorder appears to have predisposed to disordered gambling.
- A psychiatric disorder or a developmental disorder may make the person less able to control his/her gambling.
- Alternatively, the person may experience relief of mental symptoms through gambling.
- Certain forms of gambling, such as poker (slot) machine playing and keno take place commonly in pubs, clubs, and other licensed venues; alcohol consumption may result in the person becoming disinhibited and more likely to gamble and do so excessively.

Psychiatric and social comorbidity

Mood disorders and anxiety disorders
- Disordered gambling causes a number of problems and destroys interpersonal relationships, especially with family members and others close to the person.
- As a result, the person can become depressed and suffer a range of anxiety disorders.
- If the person's condition worsens, he/she may have suicidal ideation and may attempt to end his/her life.
- In some cases, the person continues gambling in an attempt to mitigate his/her depression and anxiety.

Alcohol use disorder
- An underlying or comorbid alcohol use disorder is seen commonly in a person with disordered gambling.
- If the person has a comorbid drinking problem, in the course of treatment and recovery, the person's gambling problem may switch to an alcohol use disorder or, conversely, the person's drinking problem may be replaced with a gambling problem.

Drug use disorder
- A drug use disorder sometimes accompanies disordered gambling.
- In particular, illicit drug use is related to illegal forms of gambling.
- Stimulant use is more likely to be associated with gambling
- The presence of illicit substance use worsens the prognosis and makes both problems more difficult to treat and provide recovery support for.

Antisocial personality disorder
- Antisocial personality disorder may underlie a gambling problem.
- In general, this makes for a worse prognosis.

Box 19.3 lists the negative consequences of excessive gambling.

Box 19.3 Negative consequences of excessive gambling
- Stress-related symptoms/conditions
- Psychiatric co-morbidity such as depression, anxiety-spectrum disorders, substance misuse, and personality disorders
- Financial problems such as debts and bankruptcy
- Crime
- Families/friends feel under stress and suffer from anxiety and depression themselves
- Interpersonal violence
- Impact on children—behavioural and emotional problems, and substance abuse
- Loss of productivity and absenteeism at work.

Assessment

Overview

- Many different individuals experience gambling problems. Do not dismiss the possibility because they do not conform to a particular stereotype.
- Most people with a gambling disorder claim they are not addicted to gambling, often because of shame and/or ignorance.
- Outside a specialist clinic, symptoms expressed are usually vague and include commonly seen problems, such as insomnia, stress, depression, anxiety, or interpersonal problems and conflicts.
- Be sensitive and non-judgemental in the assessment of gamblers, given the negative perceptions they are likely to have about themselves.
- Wherever possible, corroborative information should be sought from the gambler's spouse/partner or others in his/her close social network.
- Assessing the individual's daily life may be a useful step towards effective support.

Key points in the assessment of a gambler

- Undertake a detailed assessment of gambling behaviour including:
    - types of games played
    - initiation into gambling
    - progression
    - current frequency (days per week or hours per day)
    - current severity (money spent on gambling proportionate to income)
    - maintaining factors
    - features of dependence
- Take a psychiatric history, including history of presenting complaints, and psychiatric, family, treatment, past and personal histories
- Examine the consequences: financial, interpersonal, vocational, social and legal impact on the person, family, and friends
- Reasons for presentation, motivation to change, and expectations of treatment
- Assessment of suicide risk
- Assessment of psychiatric comorbidity, particularly depression and substance use disorders
- Comprehensive mental state examination.

Making the diagnosis

Information obtained from the assessment should be compared with the criteria for disordered gambling (DSM-5) or pathological gambling (ICD 10). The DSM-5 criteria are likely to predominate over other diagnostic systems.

A diagnosis of disordered gambling is made if four or more criteria are fulfilled:
1. Preoccupied with gambling
2. Increasing bets
3. Repeated failed attempts to control or stop gambling
4. Restless and/or irritable when trying to control/stop gambling
5. Escape from problems or to counter dysphoric mood
6. Trying to win back losses all at once
7. Lying about gambling or its extent
8. Negative impact on job or family, or loses opportunities
9. Borrowing money to fund gambling.

A clinically significant gambling disorder is characterized by continued gambling despite harmful consequences.

Screening tools

Screening tools are available to aid identification of a gambling disorder.

The South Oaks Gambling Screen (SOGS)

This is widely used in epidemiological studies. However, it has many items (20) and poor specificity (0.75), despite excellent sensitivity (0.99).

A one-item screening tool

'Have you ever had an issue with your gambling?'
This has low sensitivity (0.79) though good specificity (0.96). Further investigation should be done if this question is answered positively.

Lie–Bet Questionnaire

This is a two-item screen, which includes the following:
1. 'Have you ever lied to anyone about your gambling?'
2. 'Have you ever increased your bet to get the same sense of thrill or action?'

This has excellent sensitivity (0.99) and good specificity (0.91). Further assessment is needed if an individual answers yes to one or both questions. This tool is useful for frequent screening of high-risk groups, such as clients with substance use disorder.

Brief Biosocial Gambling Screen (BBGS)

In this three-item screen, the questions apply to the previous 12 months.
1. 'Have you become restless, irritable, or anxious when trying to stop and/or cut down on gambling?' (withdrawal)
2. 'Have you tried to keep your family or friends from knowing how much you gamble?' (lying)
3. 'Have you had such financial trouble as a result gambling that you had to get help with living expenses from family, friends, or welfare?' (borrowing money).

This has excellent sensitivity (0.96) and specificity (0.99); follow-up is required for a client who answers yes to one or more questions.

Further assessment of the consequences

- When rapport has been established, more sensitive areas of the history can be explored.
- Enquiry should be made of bankruptcy, domestic violence, divorce, substance abuse, lost productivity; suicidal ideation and illegal activity are often observed.
- Medical consequences include insomnia, lack of exercise, and decreased attention to self-care.

Psychological assessment

Enquire about common traits found in problem gamblers:
- preference for risk-taking
- absence of loss aversion
- sensitivity to immediate rewards.

The Temperament and Character Inventory (TCI) and the Barratt Impulsivity Scale (BIS) are useful assessment tools.

Predictors for prognosis

Almost one-third of pathological gamblers experience natural recovery. Therefore, it is necessary to identify clients with a bad prognosis at an early stage; vulnerable groups include females, adolescents, and people with low socioeconomic status or psychiatric complications, such as substance abuse, attention-deficit/hyperactivity disorder (ADHD), and antisocial personality disorder. Additionally, a family history of addiction is strongly associated with a bad prognosis because of a poor ability to help-seeking behaviour.

Changes in gambling urges and frequency after intervention can be identified using the clinician-administered Pathological Gambling Modification of the Yale-Brown Obsessive Compulsive Scale (PG-YBOCS).

Management

Psychological treatment

- Psychological therapies are the mainstay of treatment, and CBT is perhaps the most commonly used. Self-help interventions such as Gamblers Anonymous (GA) are also very popular.
- CBT consists of a combination of cognitive and behavioural strategies. Problematic gamblers have various cognitive distortions such as illusions of control, overestimates of one's chances of winning, biased memories, etc. And as gambling is about judging the probability of outcomes and decision-making, it follows that cognitive distortions will lead to impaired judgement and poor decision-making. CBT works by identifying these cognitive errors and then working to address them.
- During therapy, consider options such as assessment and treatment of comorbid psychiatric disorders, especially if the patient is not responding.

Gamblers Anonymous

'GA is a fellowship of men and women who share their experience, strength and hope with each other that they may solve their common problem and help others to recover from a gambling problem.' Its under-lying ethos and operating principles are very similar to other 12-step peer fellowships such as Alcoholics Anonymous (Box 19.4).

Secure the remaining assets

- Encourage patients to deny themselves access to ready money, e.g. by prohibiting access to bank accounts, ceasing credit card accounts, and not being paid in cash but by direct money transfer to a bank account, where possible.
- Consider whether the financial affairs of the person should be managed by a guardian, and discuss this explicitly with the patient.

Box 19.4 Guiding principles of Gamblers Anonymous

- Is a fellowship programme
- Believes that no cure, only recovery/control is possible
- Recommends total abstinence
- Is not religious but spiritual
- Considers belief in a higher power is essential
- Is a lifelong commitment
- Anonymity is key
- The essence is repeatedly working through the 12 steps
- There are no fees for GA membership.

Pharmacological treatment

Pharmacological treatments are available but are used in a minority of problem gamblers at the present time. Many medications have been trialled and include those targeting the neurotransmitters concerned with the euphoric and reinforcing effects of gambling, or with mood and mood stability. They include opioid antagonists (naltrexone and nalmefene), selective serotonin re-uptake inhibitors (SSRIs), mood stabilizers, and antipsychotics respectively. Although there have been encouraging results for some agents, methodological weaknesses of pharmacological studies (small sample sizes, inadequate blinding and randomization techniques, high dropout rates, etc.) limit the validity and generalizability of their findings.

- Of the pharmacotherapies trialled to date, naltrexone and nalmefene show the greatest promise. Some gambling and addiction specialists incorporate one of these in the treatment programme. Typically, they are offered for 3–6 months.
- Overall, drug treatment cannot be regarded as first-line treatment for a gambling disorder. No drug is licensed for use in the UK or US.
- Where there is a comorbid psychiatric disorder, suitable pharmacotherapy can be very useful in treating that disorder and allowing the patient to engage in therapy more effectively.
- Dopamine agonists (as used in Parkinson's disease) have been reported to *induce* pathological gambling. Clinicians should monitor this carefully.

Social and welfare support

- Consider necessary forms of social and welfare support.
- Is gambling a way of dealing with the stress faced in daily life?
- Making use of local social resources and providing support that stops a deepening of social isolation helps reduce the damage of a gambling problem in addition to therapy focused on the gambling.

Further reading

American Psychiatric Association (2013). Gambling disorder. In *Diagnostic and Statistical Manual of Mental Disorders* (5th ed), pp. 585–9. Washington, DC: American Psychiatric Publishing.

George S, Bowden-Jones H, Orford J, et al. (2013). Problem gambling: what can psychiatrists do? *Psychiatrist*, 37:1–3.

George S, Murali V. (2005). Pathological gambling: an overview of assessment and treatment *Adv Psychiatr Treat* 11:450–6.

Petry NM. (2005). *Pathological Gambling: Etiology, Comorbidity and Treatments*. Washington, DC: American Psychological Association Press.

Wardle H, Moody A, Spence S, et al. (2010). *British Gambling Prevalence Survey. National Centre for Social Research*. London: The Stationery Office.

Gaming

Types of games and epidemiology 442
Pathophysiology of gaming addiction 444
Clinical syndromes 445
Psychopathology, antecedent, and comorbid psychiatric
    disorders 446
Assessment 447
Treatment 448

Types of games and epidemiology

Games are activities performed for pleasure and based on rules with the outcome deciding victory or defeat. Games have various classifications, but mainly they are classified by the materials associated with playing the game (e.g. board games, sports tools, computers, cards, papers) and the rules (e.g. soccer, poker, chess).

Computer games are those played against specialized computer programs (artificial intelligence) and/or other people using computers. Recently, excessive use of computer games has become associated with health and social problems. Addiction to gaming is becoming a large problem all over the world, with the rapid spread of computer games.

Types of games

Computer games are classified as *on-line games* where an Internet connection is required for their use, and *off-line games* which do not require an Internet connection.

In many online games, players can play with an unspecified number of players (massive multi-player online (MMO) games) and enjoy new elements and stages which can be added to the game scenario at any time. These characteristics of online games can encourage players to continue playing with pleasure for a very long time, and be strongly related to the formation of addiction.

Computer games are also classified by genre.

Main computer game genres
- Action games
- Adventure games
- Role playing games
- Puzzle games
- Simulation games
- Shooting games
- Sports games
- Others.

It is, however, difficult to classify computer games precisely, because the new subgenres are developed rapidly especially in the case of the massive multiplayer online role playing games (MMORPG), and addiction often becomes an important aspect.

Epidemiology of game players and game addiction

- In a 2007 survey, 55–65% of Dutch adolescents played computer games. Male gamers spent an average of 10.5 hours per week on games. Female gamers spent an average of 4.3 hours per week.
- In a 2010 survey, 73% of Korean adolescents played the games with personal computers or smartphones on holidays. The average amount of time Korean high school students spent playing games each day was about 68 minutes (boys 75 minutes, girls 59 minutes).
- In a 2011 survey, 56% of US teenagers spent 30 minutes or more on average playing video or online games each day, and 18% spent over 2 hours playing them.

- In a 2013 survey, 63% of Japanese adolescents use game consoles, and about 40% of them play the online games with personal computers or cell phones.
- A 2014 report suggested that 59% of Americans were playing games.

From this data, it is clear that playing computer games has spread rapidly in many countries over the past few years, and playing them takes up an ever-increasing amount of the time of the young persons involved.

Because the global diagnostic criteria for gaming addiction was not defined until recent years, many of the large-scale surveys used self-recording screening tests.

In a survey using the Video Game Dependency Scale:
- 2.8% (boys 4.7%, girls 0.5%) of German adolescents were classified as 'at-risk' players.
- 1.7% (boys 3%, girls 0.3%) were classified as addicted players on video games.
- 3.8–8.5% of boy's online game players and 1.2–2.8% of boy's offline game players were classified as addicted.

In a survey using the Game Addiction Scale (GAS):
- 1.4–2.3% of Dutch adolescents were classified as addicted.
- 7.6% of Germany adolescents (14–18 years), 3.3% of young adults (19–39 years), and 3.0% of older adults (40 years or older) were classified as problematic users.
- 0.2% of all generation groups were classified as addicted.

In the survey using the Online Games Addiction Scale for Adolescents in Taiwan (OAST), 46% of young Taiwanese frequent MMORPG players were classified as addicted players.

The prevalence of game addiction varies according to the survey methods or subjects, but clearly there are many gamers who have become addicted. Generally, the prevalence of game addiction is higher in youths, men, and online gamers.

Pathophysiology of gaming addiction

Many people can enjoy computer games easily, cheaply, safely, and legally. The games can satisfy various (e.g. conquest, sexual, approval) desires of people. Many gamers can easily achieve the various magnificent aims (e.g. world conquest, excellent soldier) in the virtual rather than in the real world. These characteristics of the games are strongly related to addiction.

Mechanisms to explain how excessive computer game playing comes about have been proposed. It has been suggested that in-game reinforcement and skills induce various affective responses, most notably excitement and frustration. Excessive computer game playing may be maintained by stimulatory effects on reward and sensitization, similar to the long-term changes in the brain reward circuitry believed to maintain substance dependence.

There is evidence supporting the hypothesis that the computer-game playing activates the dopamine reward circuitry in the brain. Compared with healthy controls, subjects with online gaming addiction presented with gaming pictures (and mosaic control pictures) showed heightened activation of the right orbitofrontal cortex, right nucleus accumbens, bilateral anterior cingulate and medial frontal cortex, right dorsolateral prefrontal cortex, and right caudate nucleus, as gauged by fMRI scanning. Craving in online gaming addiction and craving in substance dependence might share the same neurobiological mechanisms.

Clinical syndromes

Computer game addiction and computer use disorder patients demonstrate various clinical syndromes. Several authorities argue that all addictions, including playing computer games, consist of a number of core components:
- Salience
- Mood modification
- Tolerance
- Withdrawal
- Conflict
- Relapse.

Many of the screening tests associated with game addiction consist of similar components. The DSM-5 provisional diagnostic criteria for Internet gaming disorder comprise nine clinical features:
- Preoccupation
- Withdrawal
- Tolerance
- Loss of control
- Loss of other interests
- Excessive use despite adverse effects
- Lies
- Use when feeling distressed
- Social crises.

Game addiction results in various serious adverse effects in addition to the central features listed above (Table 20.1).

Table 20.1 Main clinical syndromes and adverse effects of game addiction

School, work, economic	Psychiatric	Physical	Human relationships
Tardiness	Irritability	Weight loss	Conflicts with parents, wife, husband, brothers, children, friends
Absences	Depression	Obesity	
Dropping out of school	Anxiety	Under-eating	
Repeating the same grade	Staying indoors	Over-eating	Loss of friends
School transfer	Night and day reversal	Reduced ability to exercise	Isolation
Poor grades	Daytime sleepiness	Nutrition disorder	Family depression
Unemployment			Family stress
Reduced income		Metabolic disorders	Family sleepiness
Reduced ability to work			Leaving home
Wasting money			Violent language
Reduced ability to manage housework			Police case
Reduced ability to care for children			

Psychopathology, antecedent, and comorbid psychiatric disorders

Gaming addiction patients commonly have psychological or social difficulties in their backgrounds. Most of them suffer from problems in their social life and in interpersonal relationships, or from comorbid psychiatric disorders. Both personal characteristics and environmental factors contribute to the gaming addiction onset. In general, people who have difficulties in communication in real life also have a predisposition for gaming addiction.

Antecedents to gaming addiction

Personal factors
- Low self-esteem
- Sensitivity or low tolerance to frustration
- Younger age (teenager or young adult), secondary or post-secondary education, and unmarried
- Prior history of depressive disorder or anxiety disorder
- Prior history of substance use disorder or non-substance dependence
- Attraction to novelty
- Unafraid, fearless, or reckless personality
- Suffers from extreme stress
- Poor interpersonal relationships.

Environmental factors/social situations
- Availability of computers
- High level of access to the Internet
- Raised in a neglectful or dysfunctional family; family conflict
- Lack of concern for child's behaviour or activity
- Friend or close acquaintance who also has high skills or knowledge of Internet games
- Has owned a personal computer since a young age
- Tendency to withdrawal socially
- Forced excessive competitive environments (e.g. study for an entrance examination)
- Lack of leisure time or leisure activities.

Comorbid psychiatric disorders

There is an association between various developmental disorders and gaming addiction. Disorders such as Asperger's syndrome and attention deficit hyperactivity disorder (ADHD) are exhibited by many gaming addiction patients (Table 20.2). These disorders may contribute to the causes of the gaming addiction.

Table 20.2 Common associated psychiatric disorders

Nature of disorder	Examples	
Developmental disorders	Asperger's syndrome	ADHD
Neurotic/mood disorders	Social anxiety disorder	Depressive disorder

Assessment

Specific criteria for describing gaming addiction have not been developed yet. Provisional criteria have been developed for DSM-5 and are presented in the section 'Conditions for Further Study.'

For measurement, Young's Internet Addiction Test (IAT) is useful. The IAT identifies and evaluates the severity of Internet addiction. Since most of Internet addiction is Internet gaming, IAT could be used for gaming addiction. IAT is a five-point scale test. The proposed criteria conclude that the key to assessing gaming addiction is to assess its impact on real-life activities and interpersonal relationships, and to examine whether there is a significant loss of individual control or obsession with gaming.

Treatment

The Internet is essential to our daily lives, especially in facilitating electronic correspondence for business or school. *Learning how to use it appropriately* should be the goal of gaming addiction treatment. This is in contrast to the approach for substance dependence, which emphasizes cessation of use of the substance of addiction. Furthermore, the boundary between appropriate and inappropriate use is unclear. This must be established on an individual basis.

In most cases, gaming is not necessary to daily living. Deleting gaming accounts should be part of gaming addiction treatment. Since many patients have a keen attachment to their avatars, they tend to show a strong resistance to account deletion. Patients must have a thorough understanding of, and a strong motivation for achieving, this goal. Motivational interviewing is highly useful in this type of treatment, and a good therapeutic relationship is the key component in patient motivation.

The focus of treatment should consist of motivation and insight. Cognitive behavioural therapy (CBT), psychoeducation, and self-help groups are also useful. Through these therapeutic approaches, patients will deepen understanding of their gaming addictions.

Cognitive behavioural therapy

CBT focuses on changing inappropriate gaming behaviours and reducing their harmful influences on daily life.

CBT:
- enhances the ambivalence between the gaming life's merits and demerits
- focuses on the automatic thoughts connected with obsessive gaming
- imagines positive self-image in the future without gaming
- increases healthy daily activity
- provides coping skills against the gaming obsession
- recognizes re-gaming triggers.

Support groups

The positive effects of support groups are still unclear. Certainly, 12-step therapy self-help groups are active online. For example, On-Line Gamers Anonymous (OLGA) has regular meetings and chat platforms.

Other treatments

- Logging the gaming/Internet use/time, situation, feeling, and whether the patient adheres to the limitations
- Using timers or reminders to set gaming time limits.

Pharmacotherapy

The effect of pharmacotherapy on gaming addiction is unknown because of insufficient data, but antidepressants, mood stabilizers, and naltrexone have been proposed to ease patients' symptoms. For ADHD comorbidity, methylphenidate may be useful, but a definite diagnosis of ADHD should be obtained first.

Other addictive disorders

Social media and social networking *450*
Applications ('apps') *452*
Pornography (Internet and other) *453*
Sexual addictions *454*
Exercise addiction *456*
Food addiction *457*
Other behavioural addictions *458*
The relationship between the behavioural addictions
    and impulse control disorders *459*

Social media and social networking

Social media and social networking services (SNSs) are electronic (Internet-based) ways of transmitting or sharing information with a broad audience. The distinction between the two is that social media are essentially ways of *transmitting* information and images to others, whereas social networking involves *engagement* with others. Groups of people with common interests or similar persuasions associate together on social networking sites, and converse and build relationships with each other. Although research on the addictive effects of social media and SNSs is sparse at present, it appears that engagement is crucial to the potential development of addiction, and this section will therefore focus on SNSs.

Nature of social networking and addictive potential

SNSs are virtual communities where users can create individual public profiles, interact with real-life friends, and meet other people with shared interests. In line with the rapid increase in the use of social networking sites and services, SNS addiction has recently been proposed as a new behavioural addiction.

Although a globally approved definition and diagnostic guidelines of SNS addiction has yet to be developed, it might encompass symptoms such as:

- being overly concerned with SNSs
- being driven by a strong motivation to log on to or use SNSs
- devoting so much time and efforts to SNSs that it causes negative social and health consequences.

Prevalence

As SNS addiction is still an emerging phenomenon, there has been a limited number of epidemiological studies, which have incorporated sound methodologies evaluating the prevalence of this type of addiction. The number of instruments with well-defined cut-offs is sparse, which has limited attempts to estimate the prevalence of SNS addiction. The studies that have been conducted—notwithstanding their limited number—suggest firstly that younger users are more prone to develop SNS addiction than older users, and secondly that there is a female preponderance.

Clinical manifestations

- Spending a great amount of time on SNS activities
- Sleep disturbance and resulting lateness or absence from school or work
- Reduced physical strength and retarded physical development due to physical inactivity and malnutrition
- Lower average grade points and academic achievement
- Reduced productivity and greater economic loss
- Intrafamilial/interpersonal conflicts, such as conflicts between parents and children and relationship dissatisfaction with partners.
- Negative impact on self-esteem and well-being.

Assessment tools

Several self-report measures assessing SNS addiction have been developed. Cross-validation of these scales against each other has not been conducted and there is a lack of certainty regarding the superiority in efficacy of these scales and whether they even assess the same construct.

Treatment

No well-documented treatment specifically for SNS addiction currently exists. More broadly, the assessment of efficacy of various treatment modalities for Internet addiction is still in the early stages.

A meta-analysis of 16 treatment studies of Internet addiction showed that psychological and pharmacological interventions were highly effective in improving Internet addiction, amount of time spent online, and levels of depression and anxiety. The results also revealed that there were no differential effects between pharmacological and psychological interventions on the status of Internet addiction. To what extent these findings apply to SNS addiction remains to be established.

Applications ('apps')

Apps are simple, focused programs which allow the user to contact someone, play a game, or in general terms access information directly from an organization's electronic storage systems. Using an app is an alternative to accessing the material via a website. The advantage of an app is that it can be optimized for viewing on a small screen such as a smartphone. Some apps can be tailored to suit the viewer's personal interests and preferences. There are approximately 3 million apps available.

Apps are attractive and accessible to children from the age of 7–8 years. For this age group they include building games, and for slightly older children social media apps are popular. Apps for teenage boys include 'first-person shooter' games. Many are endless and become addictive.

Apps can be used for dating and to initiate sexual contacts, and for predatory people to find their prey.

Pornography (Internet and other)

Definition and prevalence

Pornography refers to sexually explicit materials intended for stimulating sexual arousal. It may be accessed through magazines, videos, CDs, DVDs, multimedia devices, and the Internet. In recent years Internet pornography use has increased significantly because of its accessibility, affordability (often without any direct charge), and anonymity. Surveys of young adults find that up to 75% of men and 40% of women view online pornography at least occasionally.

Impact on behaviour

Some use of pornography may be considered within the bounds of normal sexual behaviour for adults. Pornography ranges from mild material such as photographs in sales catalogues, through sexual images and photographs in magazines, filmed material produced for primarily educational purposes, material designed for couples and women, to commercial male-oriented pornography, more extreme material, and through to child pornography, bestiality, and other paraphilias. Much pornography is exploitative and degrading, and there is a concern about its impact on human behaviour and development. Some individuals develop problems associated with pornography use including relationship, financial and occupational problems, preoccupation with sexuality, sexual addictions, and sexual offending. However, the distinction between recreational pornography use and problematic/harmful use is not clear.

The influence of exposure to pornography on aggression has been debated for many years. It is speculated that when individuals with high levels of predisposition to violence expose themselves to sexually violent materials, they develop attitudes supportive of sexual violence and aggression against women. However, research findings are mixed concerning the relationship between pornography use and aggression.

Child pornography

Child pornography is illegal in most countries in the world. The consumers of child pornography are predominantly male with relatively high education and socioeconomic status. The association between child pornography use and hands-on sex offences especially involving children is of particular concern. In one study, 24% of the child pornography users had a previous criminal record for a sex offence against a minor, but other studies have reported lower rates. Child pornography use seems to be associated with child sexual abuse recidivism.

Sexual addictions

The nature of sexual addictions

Numerous terms are applied to behaviours where there is excessive preoccupation with and/or involvement with sexual activities. These include:
- hypersexual disorder
- compulsive sexual behaviour
- satyriasis and nymphomania
- sexual addiction.

The excessive desire and involvement is usually directed to unremarkable sexual activities, but may reflect the existence of a paraphilia. These disorders cause many psychosocial problems, however there is no consensus on how to name the conditions. Sexual addictive disorders can occur with a wide range of sexual behaviours including compulsive masturbation, excessive use of pornography, commercial sex involvement such as use of prostitutes, extramarital affairs, paraphilic pursuits, and various forms of risk-taking behaviour.

Prevalence

Epidemiological studies estimate that the prevalence of hypersexuality and sexual addiction ranges from 2% to 10% of the general adult population. Onset is usually prior to age 18 and it peaks between ages 20 and 30. The male to female ratio ranges between 4:1 and 3:1.

Diagnostic criteria

Currently, there are no established diagnostic criteria. However, the common features include:
- persistent and intensive sexual preoccupation, involving arousal, fantasies, urges, and behaviours
- the sexual focus is predominantly non-paraphilic
- much time is spent in preparing for the sexual behaviour, engaging in sexual activity, and recovering from sexual experiences
- individuals show impaired (or essentially no) control over their sexual urges and behaviours
- these behaviours cause clinically significant distress or impairment
- the behaviours persist despite negative consequences.

Often with the development of an addiction there is an increase in the level of pornography or abnormality of behaviour, leading to desensitization to previous types of sexual activity.

Psychiatric comorbidity

Sexual addictions show high levels of co-occurrence with other addictive disorders, and a range of psychiatric disorders such as mood disorders, anxiety disorders, personality disorders, and sexual dysfunctions. Approximately 40% of individuals with sexual addictions have other addictions.

Aetiology and mechanisms

There is a high frequency of childhood physical and sexual abuse in people with sexual addictions. Other psychological factors that seem to play a role in the development and maintenance of sexual addictions include:

- personality characteristic: antisocial traits, low self-esteem, impulsivity, sensation-seeking, nonconformity and alienation
- poor coping mechanisms
- social influences: including the advent of a 'sexualized society' where access to sexual information and opportunities to pursuit one's own sexual desires are abundant.

Neurobiological mechanisms

It is speculated that sexual addictions develop through similar neurobiological mechanisms which occur with other addictive disorders. Thus, repeated exposure to sexual stimulation leads to a sensitization of the incentive-motivational properties of that stimulation. It is associated with elevated intrasynaptic levels of dopamine in the nucleus accumbens.

Treatment

Pharmacological treatment

There are currently no randomized controlled trials (RCTs) of pharmacotherapy for sexual addictions. However, two types of pharmacotherapies are commonly employed: antiandrogen agents and antidepressants. The most commonly used antiandrogens are medroxyprogesterone acetate (MPA) and cyproterone acetate (CPA). However, compliance with these medications poses a serious problem. Of the antidepressants, the SSRIs, especially fluoxetine and sertraline, are most frequently used. These drugs, which are also prescribed for premature ejaculation, may lead to physical desensitization. It is recommended that these medications are used in conjunction with psychological therapies.

Psychological therapies

As for the treatment of other addictive disorders, long-lasting, multi-faceted treatment appears to be the most promising. Therapies include motivational enhancement therapy, cognitive behavioural approaches aimed at relapse-prevention, family/couple therapy, psychoeducation, mindfulness, and peer support groups.

Exercise addiction

Introduction and definitions

Regular physical activity plays a crucial role in health maintenance and disease prevention. However, some individuals engage in excessive physical exercise to the extent that is causes physical and psychological damage. This state can be described as exercise addiction. Some studies have shown that exercise addiction shares similarities with other forms of behavioural addiction, while others have suggested a closer association with obsessive–compulsive disorders. In light of this lack of consensus, it is unsurprising that we have yet to see the establishment of a definition or set of diagnostic guidelines for exercise addiction.

Prevalence

Estimates of the prevalence of exercise addiction have shown significant variance, which reflects the different definitions employed, the type of assessment tools used, and the characteristics of study subjects. Notably, the prevalence in the general population is lower than that of athletes.

Clinical features

- Excessive exercise patterns
- Tolerance, e.g. running increasing distances as the severity of addiction increases
- Presence of withdrawal symptoms, e.g. depression, irritability, and anxiety
- Detrimental social and physical consequences
- Interference with relationships or work.

There is a very high rate of comorbidity with eating disorders, especially anorexia nervosa, and also with body image disorders.

Assessment

Several questionnaire and diagnostic tools have been developed and validated. Some are listed in Chapter 27.

Treatment

Treatment approaches for exercise addiction are based on the cognitive behavioural approach but there is little evidence of the effectiveness of treatments. There are also few studies of pharmacological treatment available although one case study showed that quetiapine produces a moderate improvement in exercise addiction. The course of this form of addiction is unknown however, due to the dearth of longitudinal studies.

Food addiction

Introduction and definitions

Palatable foods, salt, and additives have been shown to be potentially addictive. Indeed, many parallels have been drawn between substance dependence and excessive consumption of such hyper-palatable foods that are known to produce food addiction. Neurobiological studies have shown that certain foods produce responses in the brain neurocircuits resembling those affected by substance abuse. However, thus far globally recognized definitions and diagnostic guidelines in relation to food addiction have yet to be developed.

Prevalence

Studies using the Yale Food Addiction Scale (YFAS) assessment tool have shown that 5–11% of the general population is affected by food addiction. The prevalence increases with obesity status and obesity measurements are also higher in food addicts compared to those of control subjects.

Clinical features

- Compulsive eating and craving for food
- Persistent desire for food or repeated, unsuccessful attempts to cut down
- Continued use despite problems
- Much time spent on obtaining food, eating, or recovering from eating.

There may be particularly strong urges for sugary foods. There is a strong relationship between food addiction and binge eating disorder. In one study, 57% of obese patients with binge eating disorder were classified as food addicted. Food addiction may be a compensatory behaviour in the early weeks of recovery from other addictive disorders.

Assessment

The YFAS with its 25-item questionnaire has been most widely used and validated in several languages.

Treatment

Treatment options for food addiction include behavioural and pharmacological interventions. RCTs using CBT and brief psychoeducation showed improved outcomes in relation to binge eating symptoms. In addition, antidepressants such as serotonin and noradrenaline and reuptake inhibitors (SNRIs), and anticonvulsants like topiramate have shown promise in terms of efficacy and tolerability.

Other behavioural addictions

Introduction

There are many other behaviours that potentially have addictive properties. These include compulsive buying, work addiction, and love addiction, but there are little published data, especially on the last two conditions. Compulsive buying is listed in DSM-5 under 'Other specified disruptive, impulse-control and conduct disorders'.

Compulsive buying disorder

- Globally recognized definitions and diagnostic guidelines have yet to be developed.
- Lifetime prevalence calculated to be 6–7% in adults (in US and Germany) and 11% in high school students in Italy.
- Clinical manifestations include:
  - preoccupation with shopping and spending
  - spending many hours engaged in these behaviours
  - increasing anxiety relieved only when a purchase is made.
- Assessment tools include the Compulsive Buying Scale (CBS).
- Treatments are based on CBT and motivational interviewing. RCTs suggest the effectiveness of citalopram.

The relationship between the behavioural addictions and impulse control disorders

The essential feature of impulse control disorders is the failure to resist an impulse to perform an act that is harmful to the person or to others. The repetitive engagement in these behaviours ultimately interferes with functioning in one or multiple domains.

Whether to group disorders, which are termed in this text 'behavioural addictions,' within addictive disorders or under impulse control disorders is a matter of controversy, only partly influenced by the available data.

In ICD 10, the majority of behavioural addictions, including pathological gambling, together with kleptomania, pyromania, and trichotillomania, are classified under the 'habit and impulse disorder'. Other behavioural addictions such as Internet addiction, exercise addiction, hypersexual disorder, and compulsive buying disorder are coded as the 'other habit and impulse disorders'. Their location in the forthcoming ICD 11 is presently unknown.

In DSM-5, gambling disorder is included in the 'substance-related and addictive behaviours.' The other disorders mentioned earlier are classified under 'disruptive, impulse-control and conduct disorders'.

Reasons for classifying these disorders as addictive disorders include:
* similarities with substance use disorders (SUDs) in their natural histories: exhibiting chronic and relapsing patterns, together with an urge or craving state prior to initiating the behaviours
* similarities with those affected by drug dependence in activated brain regions, including the mesocorticolimbic system and extended amygdala, especially when elicited by behavioural cues
* often a positive response to the same psychosocial and pharmacological treatments of these disorders and SUDs.

Critics have argued that the inclusion of these disorders as behavioural addictions may medicalize bad behaviours when they are simply symptoms of other disorders.

More research is necessary in order to:
* establish the basis of the disease concept of these disorders
* provide more evidence to support their inclusion as behavioural addictions
* promote the development of more effective treatments.

Psychiatric co-morbidity

Introduction and epidemiology 462
Inter-relationships between substance use and mental
   health disorders 464
Synopsis of psychiatric disorders 465
Assessing and managing patients with possible psychiatric
   comorbidity 470
Synopsis of psychiatric management 474
Management of specific comorbidities 480

Introduction and epidemiology

The term *co-morbidity* typically refers to the coexistence or co-occurrence in the same person of a psychiatric (mental health) disorder and a substance use disorder (due to alcohol, medications, or drugs). Patients with comorbid substance use and mental health disorders are often described as having *dual diagnosis* or dual diagnoses. The more specific term *psychiatric co-morbidity* means the co-occurrence of a psychiatric disorder in someone with a substance use disorder.

- Substance use disorders and mental health disorders commonly co-exist in the general population and even more so in clinical populations.
- In the general population, approximately 30% of people with a substance use disorder have a coexisting mental health disorder (Table 22.1), with those with a drug use disorder more likely to have a co-existing mental disorder than those with an alcohol use disorder.
- In clinical populations with substance use disorders, psychiatric co-morbidity may range up to 80%, though in half of these, the psychiatric syndrome is secondary to substance use.
- The mental health disorders which occur most commonly in people with substance disorders are anxiety disorders, mood disorders (depression), and antisocial personality disorder.
- In the general population, approximately 30% of persons diagnosed with a psychiatric disorder have a comorbid substance use disorder ('substance disorder co-morbidity').
- The frequency varies widely, with 30% of those with anxiety and mood disorders having a substance use disorder, but with much higher prevalences in people with schizophrenia, bipolar disorder, and antisocial personality disorder (Table 22.2).
- In general, the *strongest associations* between mental health disorders and substance use disorders are with the less common conditions of bipolar disorder and schizophrenia.

Table 22.1 Occurrence of mental health disorders in people who have a substance use disorder: findings in the general population

Nature of the mental health disorder	% with alcohol use disorder who have a coexisting mental health disorder	% with drug use disorder who have a coexisting mental health disorder
Anxiety disorders	19%	28%
Mood (affective) Disorders	13%	26%
Schizophrenia	4%	7%
Antisocial personality disorder	14%	18%

Table 22.2 Occurrence of substance use disorders in those with a mental health disorder

Nature of psychiatric disorder	% who have a substance use disorder
Anxiety disorder	30%
Phobic disorder	25%
Mood (affective) disorder	30%
Bipolar disorder	50%
Schizophrenia	50%
Antisocial personality disorder	80%

Co-occurrence of a psychiatric disorder with a substance use disorder is particularly common in specialist settings (e.g. psychiatric units and addiction medicine clinics) but the 'other' disorder is often not recognized.

- Only a minority of persons with co-occurring mental health disorders will have that disorder recognized and treated.
- Treatment is more likely to be offered to people who have substance use disorders and (1) particularly severe mental health disorders, (2) multiple co-morbid disorders, and (3) high levels of distress.
- Co-occurring substance use and mental health disorders provide considerable diagnostic and treatment challenges to health professionals involved in the care of these patients.
- It is increasingly expected of both generalist and specialist clinicians that they will be able to provide practical advice to patients who have such combinations of disorders.

Inter-relationships between substance use and mental health disorders

The term psychiatric co-morbidity is purely a descriptive one; it does not imply any particular causal relationship between the substance use disorder and the mental health disorder. Many clinicians find it helpful to subdivide comorbid substance and mental health disorders as follows:

1. The substance use occurs first in the person's life, develops into a disorder, and then the mental health disorder develops secondarily.
2. The mental health disorder develops first and is followed by the development of a pattern of repeated substance use, leading to a substance use disorder (in this case the substance use disorder is regarded as secondary to the mental health disorder).
3. No clear temporal distinction can be made between the onset of the substance use and mental health disorders.
4. The substance use disorder and the mental health disorder occur secondarily to a third disorder (e.g. acquired brain injury).

Others regard this classification as rather simplistic—and it is. Cohort studies show that some symptoms of mental distress may often occur before a repetitive pattern of substance use but the mental symptoms are below the threshold for diagnosis; repetitive substance use often exacerbates the mental symptoms, particularly when dependence develops and a diagnosable mental health disorder may ensue. Typically when a combination of mental symptoms and substance use continues, there is an increase in severity of both the substance use disorder and the mental health disorder. This can result in the symptoms of each becoming intermingled and entrenched.

With regard to management, clarity of diagnosis is important. Some mental symptoms are short-lived and resolve during or in the 2–3 weeks following detoxification. When a substance use disorder coexists with a diagnosed mental disorder *both* should be treated, instead of focusing on one and relying on improvement in that disorder to improve the other one. Some improvement in the mental health disorder may occur with treatment of (and recovery from) the substance use disorder, but it is often incomplete or subject to recurrence, or has a protracted course. Improvement in a substance use disorder is rare when only the mental health disorder is addressed.

Synopsis of psychiatric disorders

Mood (affective) disorders

Major depression

- The diagnosis of major depressive episode requires the presence of *depressed mood and loss of interest or pleasure* for at least 2 weeks associated with at least three of the following symptoms:
    - Significant appetite or weight loss or gain
    - Insomnia or hypersomnia
    - Psychomotor retardation or agitation
    - Fatigue or loss of energy
    - Feelings of worthlessness or excessive guilt
    - Impaired thinking or concentration: indecisiveness
    - Suicidal thoughts/thoughts of death.
- A major depressive episode is different in quality and duration from brief periods of unhappiness related to difficult life circumstances.
- The mood disturbance of a major depression is pervasive in nature, so that the person feels down, flat, depressed (and often irritable) most of the day every day for 2 weeks or more.
- The mood disturbance is associated with a range of biological (or neuro-vegetative symptoms) including:
    - a change in sleep and appetite (either increased or decreased)
    - impaired concentration and memory
    - impaired energy levels and motivation
    - impaired libido.
- Psychomotor agitation or retardation may be present in more severe cases.
- Depressed mood may be associated with depressive thought content, including thoughts that life is no longer worth living and thoughts of suicide.
- There may be thoughts of hopelessness (there is no way out and no future ahead); worthlessness, excessive guilt, and helplessness (there is nothing anyone can do to improve the situation).
- More severe forms of major depression result in significant impairment in functioning, so that the patient struggles to manage the everyday tasks they need to complete.
- Suicidal thoughts may occur with severe major depression and may result in the formation of a suicide plan, with suicide attempts.

Anxiety disorders

Anxiety disorders encompass several common conditions. The lifetime prevalence is around 25% (when not due to substance use or physical illness), with rates for generalized anxiety disorder (GAD) of 5%, phobias (excluding social anxiety) 5%, social anxiety disorder 10%, agoraphobia 5%, post-traumatic stress disorder (PTSD) 8%, and obsessive–compulsive disorder (OCD) 2%.

Generalized anxiety disorder

This is characterized by *excessive anxiety and worry that is difficult to control* and occurs more days than not for at least 6 months.

The anxiety is pervasive, unreasonable, and involves worrying excessively about many situations (not just specific events), and causes significant distress or impairment for the individual.

It involves three or more associated symptoms:
- Restlessness/feeling keyed up/on edge
- Easily fatigued
- Difficulty concentrating/mind going blank
- Irritability
- Muscle tension
- Insomnia.

Panic disorder

With panic disorder, the individual experiences *recurrent, unexpected panic attacks* for a period of a month or more, often associated with the fear of having further attacks.

A panic attack is a discrete period of intense fear or discomfort, accompanied by physical symptoms, which develop abruptly and peak within 10 minutes.

At least four of the following are required for the diagnosis:
- Palpitations, pounding heart
- Sweating
- Shortness of breath
- Chest pain or discomfort
- Feeling dizzy, unsteady, light-headed, or faint
- Numbness or tingling sensations
- Derealization or depersonalization
- Fear of dying
- Trembling or shaking
- Sensation of choking
- Nausea or abdominal pain
- Chills or hot flushes
- Fear of losing control or going crazy.

Agoraphobia

Agoraphobia may develop in which the individual avoids places or situations from which escape may be difficult or help unavailable in the event of a panic attack (e.g. wide open spaces, crowded public places).

Social anxiety disorder (social phobia)

Social anxiety disorder involves an *excessive or unreasonable fear of social situations*, the individual being afraid they will embarrass or humiliate themselves. The individual is aware the fear is excessive or unreasonable, but feels unable to control it, and may experience high levels of anxiety or panic attacks in certain social situations.

Symptoms include:
- blushing
- tremor
- sweating
- difficulty in speaking.

These can lead to significant distress or impairment and the individual may avoid social situations or endure them with intense anxiety.

Commonly feared social phobia situations include:
- parties
- conversations
- meeting new people, especially those of higher social standing
- using public bathrooms
- eating or drinking in front of others
- meetings
- dating
- performing: music, sports, public speaking
- writing in front of others.

Obsessive–compulsive disorder
Obsessions are intrusive, *distressing thoughts, impulses, or images which the individual recognizes as irrational* and tries to manage by suppressing them or neutralizing them with some other thought or action.

Compulsions are associated with obsessions and are *repetitive behaviours* used to try to reduce and manage anxiety related to obsessions (e.g. compulsive hand washing to try to cope with fearful thoughts of contamination in the environment).

Post-traumatic stress disorder
The key features of PTSD are:
1. The *experience of trauma*, which involves exposure to a traumatic event in which:
   a. the person experienced or witnessed events involving death or threatened death, serious injury, or threat to the physical integrity of self or others; and
   b. the response involved intense fear, helplessness, or horror.
2. Current symptoms, which may include:
   a. *persistent re-experiencing* of the traumatic event in one (or more) of the following ways:
      - recurrent, intrusive distressing recollections
      - flashbacks, nightmares
      - acting or feeling as if the traumatic event were occurring again
   b. the *avoidance of any stimuli* associated with the trauma (and numbing of general responsiveness), which may include:
      - avoidance of thoughts, feelings, conversations associated with the trauma
      - avoidance of activities, places, or people that arouse memories of the trauma
      - avoidance of recollections of the trauma, or inability to recall an important aspect of the trauma
      - markedly reduced interest or participation in activities

c. state of *high physiological arousal*, which can include:
   • difficulty falling or staying asleep
   • irritability or outbursts of anger
   • difficulty concentrating
   • hypervigilance (e.g. scanning the environment to ensure there is no threat close by)
   • an exaggerated startle response (e.g. jumping with fright at minor noises in the environment).

Jack's truck crashed into two vehicles, setting one of them alight. A child was trapped in one of the cars and burned to death. For months after the accident, Jack could not get into a vehicle without having an anxiety attack. He avoided using any form of transport and walked everywhere. Seeing trucks on the road or on television would trigger terrifying images of the accident, which were so vivid that he felt as if he was back at the scene of the accident. Whenever he heard a loud bang he would jump and become tremulous.

Exposure to cues that symbolize or resemble an aspect of the event can trigger flashbacks and intense psychological distress.

Because any re-experiencing of the trauma can cause intense fear and distress, there is often:
• feeling of detachment or estrangement from others
• restricted range of affect (e.g. unable to have loving feelings)
• sense of foreshortened future (e.g. does not expect to have a career, marriage, children, or normal life span).

The key features of PTSD can be remembered using the mnemonic TRAP:
• Trauma
• Re-experiencing
• Avoidance
• Physiological arousal.

Adjustment disorder
This is a state of anxiety or depression which occurs in relation to a specific stressful situation, but the anxiety or depression is excessive in nature or causes significant impairment in functioning. The disorder often abates as the stressful event resolves.

Psychotic disorders

Psychotic disorders are characterized by the type of symptoms experienced and their duration. They may last for short periods of time (such as a brief psychotic disorder) or for longer periods of time (such as schizophrenia). Psychotic symptoms can occur in the context of a medical condition, and as part of a depressive disorder or bipolar disorder.

Substance-induced psychosis occurs when psychotic symptoms occur during a period of intoxication or withdrawal from alcohol or other drugs, with resolution of symptoms during abstinence. Types of psychotic disorders include brief psychotic disorder (lasting less than a month and usually triggered by stressful life events), schizophrenia, schizophreniform disorder (similar to schizophrenia but lasting less than six months), and delusional disorder.

During periods of psychosis, individuals often experience the world in a profoundly confusing and disturbing way. They commonly experience delusions and hallucinations, which have the quality of reality. They often have odd behaviour as well as jumbled, disorganized language and abnormalities of mood and affect (such as irritability and agitation, while blunted affect is common in schizophrenia).

Assessing and managing patients with possible psychiatric comorbidity

The assessment of someone with possible psychiatric comorbidity combines an enquiry into the person's substance use and features of mental disorder (as if they were separate entities), and then explores the overlaps and interconnectedness of symptoms and whether a diagnosis can be made of each type of disorder.

Assessment of substance use

This should cover the three domains of:

1. *Intake*:
   a. type of substance
   b. quantity per occasion or day
   c. frequency of use, pattern or variability of use
   d. mode of administration
   e. duration of use
   f. time of last use
2. *Dependence*:
   a. cognitive
   b. behavioural, and
   c. physiological features
      of this syndrome, to identify whether there is an 'internal driving force' to use the particular substance
3. *Consequences or harms,* which can be:
   a. physical (medical) including trauma
   b. psychiatric (and neurocognitive)
   c. social, including financial, personal, and legal.

Eliciting mental symptoms and signs

Relevant questions should then be posed regarding common mental symptoms.

1. *Depression*:
   a. depressed mood
   b. loss of interest or pleasure
   c. insomnia
   d. weight loss
   e. fatigue or loss of energy
   f. feelings of worthlessness
   g. suicidal thoughts

Look for:
   a. flat, depressed affect (may be irritable)
   b. physical agitation (psychomotor agitation) or slowing down (psychomotor retardation)
   c. poverty of speech and language
   d. signs of weight loss
   e. evidence of self-harm
   f. feelings of hopelessness, suicidal thoughts

2. *Anxiety and panic disorders*
   a. excessive anxiety and worry
   b. restlessness, 'on edge'
   c. irritability
   d. 'mind going blank'
   e. insomnia
   f. physical symptoms of panic attacks
   g. excessive or unreasonable fear of social situations
   h. fear of embarrassment

Look for:
   a. tremulousness
   b. sweating
   c. high blood pressure, tachycardia
   d. hyperventilation, difficulty breathing
   e. physical agitation
   f. vomiting
   g. dizziness
   h. redness of face

3. *Post-traumatic stress disorder*
   a. experience of a traumatic event
   b. feelings of intense fear or helplessness at the time
   c. re-experiencing of the trauma (e.g. flashbacks)
   d. avoidance of trauma-associated stimuli (triggers)
   e. physiological arousal

Look for:
   a. signs of anxiety/panic (as listed above)
   b. being easily startled e.g. by sudden movement or loud noises
   c. features of dissociation, disconnection with reality

4. *Psychosis*
   a. social withdrawal
   b. lack of motivation; becoming lethargic and inactive
   c. confused thinking
   d. loss of interest in usual activities
   e. high levels of fear and agitation in response to unusual beliefs and experiences
   f. difficulty keeping track of conversations

Look for:
   a. presence of delusions
   b. presence of hallucinations
   c. evidence of thought disorder: jumbled, disorganised thoughts
   d. blunting of emotional response
   e. inappropriate responses and behaviour
   f. difficulty managing personal hygiene and activities of daily living
   g. lack of insight.

Pay attention to the following

- Mental symptoms may reflect the direct effects of substance use or be a symptom of an underlying mental health disorder.
- There is a need to accept a certain level of ambiguity and uncertainty as to the exact origin of many symptoms.
- Aim to define the substance disorder first.
- Identify any periods of abstinence from substance use in the past—did mental symptoms persist throughout such periods? Or did they reduce in severity and intensity or disappear?
- The diagnosis of a comorbid psychiatric disorder may be only a provisional one at the time of first assessment.
- Defining a comorbid psychiatric disorder and whether it is primary or secondary requires time and the opportunity for subsequent review of symptoms and the mental state.
- In general, if the person has an established substance dependence it is rather more likely this is the primary or predominant disorder than if the substance use disorder is mild or does not reach diagnostic thresholds.
- Allow time to elapse where possible so that the person has a period of abstinence from the substance which allows short-lived substance-induced mental symptoms to lessen or disappear and to provide greater clarity for diagnosis.
- Typically a month of abstinence is required for this but in practice the available time may only be 1–2 weeks post detoxification.

In clinical practice, it is often necessary to make decisions on treatment before clarity of the respective substance use and mental health disorders can be achieved. Decisions may have to be made sooner than is optimal on prescription of (for example) antidepressants or anti-psychotic medications. It may be that a distinction cannot be made between a primary and secondary psychiatric disorder in the available time. Instead the clinician may have to note that the disorder is persistent post detoxification and commence psychiatric treatment in addition to substance disorder treatment.

Every opportunity should be taken to review the diagnoses made as with the passage of time the definitive diagnosis may become clearer, particularly when abstinence is maintained, thus eliminating progressively the masking effects of substance use.

Some temporary substance-induced psychiatric disorders may persist for up to 6 months before finally resolving with abstinence. Typically some psychiatric intervention (medication or therapy) will have been introduced within this period.

Adapting psychiatric treatment for patients with psychiatric comorbidity

- In all patients with dual disorders, early attention should be paid to the substance use and diagnosis of any substance use disorder.
- Cessation of substance use is essential for clarity of diagnosis, to allow temporary substance-induced mental disorders to resolve.

- Supervised detoxification is required for many patients to enable cessation of substance use without risking a withdrawal state.
- Where possible, psychiatric medication should be withheld until a mental health disorder (primary or persistent) has been identified.
- Cessation of substance use is necessary for treatment of a primary or persistent psychiatric disorder to succeed. Improvement in mental state is rarely possible when the person continues with significant substance use, especially if they have a dependence syndrome.
- Continued use of psychoactive substances may not only compromise treatment of a psychiatric disorder, it is also likely to result in hazardous interactions with psychiatric medications. These interactions may be due to interference with hepatic metabolism or interactions at the CNS level causing inappropriate sedation.
- In general, an appropriate psychiatric medication should not be withheld because the person has a history of a substance use disorder; however, it is essential that the psychiatric medication should be safe in case substance use were to resume. Lithium is not prescribed for most patients with substance dependence because of its low therapeutic ratio and range of serious toxic effects.
- The medication regimes outlined on pp. 474–9 have been developed for patients without substance use disorders but can be used as a basis for patients with substance use disorders and psychiatric comorbidity, subject to the caveats made in this chapter.
- Sometimes a single medication may be indicated for both the substance use disorder and the psychiatric disorder but this is uncommon (a possible example is buspirone, which has been shown in small-scale trials to be beneficial for the combination of alcohol dependence and social anxiety).

Adapting addiction treatments for patients with psychiatric comorbidity

- In general the treatment and therapies for addictive disorders may be offered to with psychiatric comorbidity patients.
- Detailed relapse-prevention therapies may not be feasible in patients with certain psychiatric disorders such as major depression.
- Relapse-prevention therapies may need to be modified substantially in patients with co-morbid psychotic disorders; here there should be an emphasis on engaging the patient, rather than pressing ahead with detailed cognitive and skills development strategies, relapse prevention and other therapies may need to be modified in patients who have acquired brain injury or limited intellectual capacity.
- In general, medications for relapse prevention for substance use disorders may be prescribed in patients who have a co-morbid psychiatric disorder; however, there are exceptions such as caution to be adopted if, for example, naltrexone were to be prescribed in someone with co-morbid depression or disulfiram (Antabuse®) were prescribed in somebody with an impulse control disorder.
- Medication for a substance disorder may need to be simplified in patients who have a co-morbid mental health disorder or other condition such as brain injury.

Synopsis of psychiatric management

Depression

Selective serotonin reuptake inhibitors (SSRIs)

- SSRIs are often used as first-line medication for major depression because they are generally well tolerated, have good compliance rates, and are rarely lethal in overdose.
- Anxiety levels can sometimes increase in the early stages of treatment with an SSRI, because of the side effects of the medication, and the anxiety and apprehension of the patient.
- It is therefore advisable to start with a lower dose if an anxiety state is present, and gradually titrate the dose upwards as tolerated by the patient.
- An adequate therapeutic trial of SSRI medication for depression is usually 8–12 weeks, but often longer and at higher doses for OCD.
- If there is only a partial response to an adequate dose of an SSRI and it is well tolerated by the patient, a trial of a higher dose should be considered.
- If the patient has a poor response to an SSRI (because of problematic side effects or a limited treatment response), try another SSRI or look at switching to another class of antidepressant.
- Doses that are generally effective for depression (± anxiety) are as follows:

- Citalopram 20–40 mg
- Escitalopram 10–20 mg
- Fluoxetine 20–40 mg
- Paroxetine 20–50 mg
- Sertraline 50–200 mg
- Fluvoxamine 100–300 mg.

Box 22.1 describes the adverse effects of SSRIs.

Box 22.1 Adverse effects of SSRIs

- Gastrointestinal disturbance: nausea, diarrhoea, constipation, dry mouth, reduced appetite
- CNS side effects: insomnia, agitation, tremors, dizziness, headache
- Sedation can also occur and generally follows this order: fluvoxamine > paroxetine > citalopram > sertraline > fluoxetine
- Sexual dysfunction occurs in up to 30% (in men: delayed ejaculation; erectile dysfunction; in men and women: anorgasmia, reduced sexual desire)
- May trigger mania in bipolar patients; caution advised when not on a mood stabilizer
- Activation of suicidal ideation: patients who are already suicidal and develop agitation as a side effect of an SSRI may be more at risk of an increase in suicidal ideation
- Monitor any suicidal patient closely with SSRI treatment.

Serotonin and noradrenaline reuptake inhibitors (SNRIs)
- SNRIs are comparable with SSRIs for the treatment of depression.
- They act like SSRIs at lower doses (e.g. <150 mg daily for venlafaxine) and may be used for anxiety as well.
- They have more noradrenergic properties at higher doses. They are useful for 'more difficult-to-treat' depression, and may accentuate anxiety at these doses.
- Doses that are generally effective for depression (± anxiety) are as follows:

> - Venlafaxine 75–225 mg
> - Desvenlafaxine 50–100 mg
> - Duloxetine 60–120 mg.

- As with SSRIs, anxiety levels may increase in the early stages of treatment. It is therefore highly advisable to start at a low dose if there is significant anxiety and gradually titrate the dose upwards as tolerated by the patient.
- Side effects are similar to SSRIs at low–medium doses. SNRIs are generally not sedating.
- Blood pressure needs to be monitored at higher doses, with around 5% of patients getting hypertension at doses of venlafaxine >225 mg daily.
- There is an increased risk of seizures in patients with a history of them.
- Discontinuation syndromes are often problematic with SNRIs. Patients should be warned not to stop them suddenly. As for SSRIs, gradually tapering the dose can help minimize the risk of a significant discontinuation syndrome.

Tricyclic antidepressants (TCAs)
- TCAs are effective for the treatment of depression but are generally not used as first-line medications because of side effects, significant drug interactions, and high lethality in overdose.
- Common side effects include sedation, together with blurred vision, dry mouth and constipation (due to their anticholinergic effects), weight gain, and hypertension.
- Because of their sedative properties, TCAs potentiate other CNS depressants such as alcohol, benzodiazepines and opioids.
- They cause cardiotoxicity in overdose.
- There is an increased risk of seizures in patients with a history of them.
- It is inadvisable to give TCAs to patients who are prone to take excessive doses of any prescribed medication with a sedative effect or those with suicidal ideation.
- A discontinuation syndrome can occur if TCAs are stopped abruptly. The symptoms are mainly of cholinergic rebound, and they include GI distress, headache, malaise, chills, muscle aches, insomnia and agitation.
- Starting doses should be low and the dose gradually titrated upwards. The usual dosage range for amitriptyline is 75–150 mg at night (taken then because of sedation).

Noradrenaline and specific serotonergic agents (NaSSAs)
- The commonest drug of this type is mirtazapine.
- May act more quickly than SSRIs
- Good safety profile: minimal anticholinergic effects, no adverse cardiac effects and rarely lethal in overdose.
- Side effects include increased appetite, weight gain, and sedation.
- Sedation is useful for insomnia and relief of anxiety. Any residual day time sedation is often short term.
- Patients should have their weight and BMI monitored during treatment. Monitoring for diabetes should occur in any overweight patients pre-treatment, and in those who gain >5% of their initial weight during treatment.
- Usual therapeutic dose for mirtazapine is 30–45 mg daily, but it is not uncommon to increase the dose to 60 mg daily.
- Mirtazapine can be added safely to SSRIs and venlafaxine to reduce insomnia related to using either of these medications.

Reboxetine
- Reboxetine is a selective noradrenaline reuptake inhibitor.
- Reasonably effective antidepressant, with reported benefits including especially improved energy, social interaction and motivation.
- Side effects include dry mouth, constipation, and urinary hesitancy.
- Typical daily dose is 8 mg/day in divided doses.
- Appears to have lower rates (about 2%) of sexual dysfunction.

Monoamine oxidase inhibitors (MAOIs)
These include tranylcypromine and phenelzine. Tranylcypromine and phenelzine irreversibly block monoamine oxidase (MAO) from breaking down noradrenaline, serotonin, and dopamine, increasing the levels of transmission of these monoamines.
- Complex and potentially dangerous medications to use because of the dietary and medication restrictions involved.
- Limited place in treatment when other medication options have failed, and should be prescribed by psychiatrists. Hypertensive crisis with intracranial bleeding, headache, and death can occur if these medications are combined with tyramine-rich foods or some contraindicated medications.
- Foods rich in tyramine need to be avoided, particularly high-protein food. A detailed list of possible food interactions needs to be provided to patients.
- Hypertensive crisis can occur when used in combination with opioid drugs and drugs with psychostimulant properties (including over-the-counter cough and cold medications).

Moclobemide
- Moclobemide is a reversible inhibitor of monoamine oxidase A (RIMA), reversibly blocking the effects of MAO-A so that if tyramine is taken this can displace the moclobemide from the active site of the enzyme and become metabolized.

- A well-tolerated medication, which is relatively non-toxic in overdose and less likely to cause sexual dysfunction than SSRIs.
- Start with a low dose and gradually titrate the dose upwards. Should be taken with food to minimize side effects. The usual therapeutic dose range is 450–600 mg daily, usually in two divided doses.

Main modalities of psychological therapy for depression

- CBT is commonly used in the treatment of depression and has the best evidence for effectiveness. Cognitive therapy is usually focused on improving distorted patterns of thinking which lead to depression, while behaviour therapy is aimed at changing specific, circumscribed problematic behaviours.
- Interpersonal therapy (IPT) may be helpful for depressed patients in addressing current interpersonal issues.
- Psychodynamic psychotherapy is insight oriented and may be helpful for understanding underlying conflicts and motivations within relationships that contribute to depressive symptoms.
- Supportive psychotherapy aims to provide emotional support during acute periods of crisis and when the patient is too depressed to engage in more interactive and demanding forms of therapy.
- Family therapy may be helpful when the patient's depression is related to family events and is having a negative impact on family relationships.

Anxiety and panic disorders

Antidepressants

- Antidepressants are often used for the treatment of anxiety disorders, typically in the lower dosage range.
- Of these the main ones employed for anxiety are the SSRIs, especially fluvoxamine (lowest risk of cognitive impairment) and mirtazapine.
- SNRIs may be prescribed in low dose.
- Reboxetine can be used in anxiety disorders that are refractory to other treatment. The starting dose should be low: start on 2 mg daily and increase by 2mg every few days as tolerated, aiming for 4 mg twice daily.

Sedating antipsychotic agents

- Newer-generation ('atypical') antipsychotics such as quetiapine, olanzapine, risperidone, and aripiprazole are used in the treatment of anxiety, being approved for this indication in certain countries.
- Doses are much lower than those used to treat psychosis, e.g. quetiapine 25–50 mg two or three times daily.
- They can also be effective in treating insomnia associated with anxiety.
- Although not conventionally regarded as addictive and not activating dopamine reward pathways, abuse can occur, a discontinuation syndrome is recognized, and metabolic effects including marked weight gain can be a serious problem.

Avoid benzodiazepines

While benzodiazepines are highly efficacious for the short-term treatment of anxiety and agitation, there are substantial risks in using benzodiazepines in individuals with a substance use disorder. These include:

- dose escalation
- inducing depression
- impaired cognition
- diversion
- doctor shopping
- drug-affected presentations
- interaction with other CNS depressants.

Drugs with short half-lives have a higher risk of dependence and problematic withdrawal symptoms (inter-dose and early morning anxiety). Drugs with long half-lives cause more residual drowsiness and cognitive impairment.

Because of these risks, benzodiazepines should be avoided in patients with a history of substance misuse unless:

- a compelling indication exists to use them
- there is no good alternative (e.g. failed treatment with CBT and other medication options)
- close follow-up and supervision is provided
- monitoring for misuse is in place.

If benzodiazepines are used, the following guidelines should apply:

- Short-term use only: 2–4 weeks
- Use lowest possible dose
- Give limited supplies
- Intermittent rather than daily use if possible
- Provide supervised administration
- Ensure close monitoring and follow-up
- Explore alternative treatment options: non-benzodiazepine medications and CBT.

Beta blockers

Beta blockers may be useful for performance anxiety (e.g. giving speeches, playing music in front of an audience), by reducing tremor and tachycardia. They can be trialled for other forms of anxiety but the benefit is variable. Usual doses are propranolol 20–40 mg three times daily or 30–60 minutes before performances, or atenolol 25–50 mg. They should be avoided in persons with bronchospasm.

Other agents

Buspirone is non-sedating, non-benzodiazepine antianxiety medication useful for the treatment of GAD. It is not dependence inducing and there is no discontinuation syndrome. The starting dose is 5 mg three times daily and the maintenance dose is 10–15mg three times daily.

Gabapentin shows some promise as a treatment for social anxiety disorder and as an adjunct to other antianxiety medication.

Post-traumatic stress disorder

- Psychological treatments include education about the symptoms of PTSD as well as stress management techniques. These include controlled breathing exercises, progressive muscular relaxation, grounding techniques, and mindfulness.
- Trauma-focused therapy (including exposure therapy and cognitive therapy) helps the person face feared situations, distressing memories, and distressing thoughts about the trauma.
- Where possible, treatment for substance misuse and trauma-focused therapy should be integrated and should occur alongside each other.
- Medication (particularly some of the antidepressant drugs) may be helpful in combination with trauma-focused therapy.

Psychotic disorders

- Both psychological treatments and medication can be helpful in managing psychosis.
- Psychological treatments include psychoeducation about symptoms and early warning signs. Anxiety and stress management techniques are helpful including relaxation techniques.
- Social and living skills training including rehabilitation should be considered.
- Cognitive remediation is helpful for those who have cognitive symptoms related to psychosis.
- Family education is important to provide information about psychosis symptoms and their management.
- Antipsychotic medications reduce the severity and frequency of psychotic symptoms. It is important that the prescribing doctor is aware of any alcohol, tobacco, or other drug use (including any reduction in substance use) because these substances can interact with antipsychotic medication, potentially affecting the blood levels of these drugs.

Management of specific co-morbidities

Management of anxiety disorder with substance use disorder
- CBT is indicated for patients with a combination of alcohol dependence and social anxiety.
- Alcohol-focused CBT is preferred as there are greater improvements in alcohol intake and comparable changes in anxiety levels compared with CBT which addresses both alcohol dependence and social anxiety.
- Caution must be observed when trying to integrate psychological therapies as there may be dilution of the treatment effect if the aim of treatment is too broad.
- Buspirone has been shown to improve outcomes in patients with co-morbid alcohol dependence and social anxiety on measures of both intake and anxiety levels.

Management of comorbid depression with substance use disorder
- TCAs are not first-line treatment due to potentially serious interactions between TCAs and alcohol and various other substances (including cardiotoxicity and death in overdose).
- Evidence for the value of SSRIs for depression in persons with current alcohol dependence is inconsistent; they are indicated post-detoxification for severe, persistent depression.
- Overall, effect on drinking behaviour and abstinence rates appears slight.
- Alcohol dependent patients with early-onset dependence, especially males, may drink more alcohol if prescribed SSRIs compared with placebo.
- In patients with alcohol and other substance use disorders, consider using an antidepressant with mixed serotonergic and noradrenergic actions (an SNRI), given the evidence (albeit limited) of improved mood with these medications.

Management of bipolar disorder with substance use disorder
- For patients with alcohol dependence and bipolar disorder valproate remains the treatment of choice as a single agent. This is largely because of the lack of studies of other mood stabilizers in patients with alcohol dependence and bipolar disorder.
- Lithium has been shown to reduce overall alcohol consumption in patients with alcohol dependence; however, it is a toxic drug with significant risk in this population.
- Quetiapine has been reported to ease depression in patients with alcohol dependence and bipolar disorder but does not affect alcohol intake.
- When naltrexone is added to mood stabilizers, there is a trend to reduce alcohol consumption.

Management of psychosis with substance use disorder

- Among patients with alcohol dependence and co-morbid schizophrenia, clozapine, quetiapine, and olanzapine reduce craving for alcohol.
- Clozapine may reduce alcohol consumption in patients with schizophrenia.
- There is limited evidence for alcohol pharmacotherapies in patients with co-morbid schizophrenia; disulfiram may precipitate psychosis.
- Psychological therapy for alcohol dependence with co-morbid schizophrenia shows mixed results: CBT (in a group format) has been shown to be helpful in some studies but not in others.

Management of trauma syndromes with a substance use disorder

- Consider prescribing a noradrenergic antidepressant (rather than an SSRI) together with alcohol relapse-prevention medication such as naltrexone or disulfiram.

ADHD and substance use disorders

- The key issue is whether there is a legitimate diagnosis of ADHD, with onset in childhood.
- Although the characteristic features of ADHD and the response to stimulant medication should provide useful information, the facts are easily learnt by patients seeking a medical supply of psychostimulants.
- With confirmed ADHD in a patient with psychostimulant dependence, a decision has to be made as to whether to commit to stimulant medication – with dexamphetamine or methylphenidate, or whether this is too risky a proposition. Consider non-stimulant medications and psychological treatments if there are concerns about the risks of prescribing stimulants.
- When stimulant medication is prescribed, it is recommended that each dose is supervised in a pharmacy to prevent misuse and diversion.
- Modafinil is useful as a treatment both for ADHD and relapse prevention in psychostimulant dependence.

Eating disorders and substance use disorders

- Of the eating disorders, bulimia nervosa has the strongest association with substance use disorders.
- But in contrast, anorexia nervosa is negatively correlated with substance use.
- There is little information on medications to reduce substance use and improve psychiatric morbidity in patients with eating disorders.

Autistic spectrum disorders and substance use disorders

- No information is available about the comparative prevalence of substance use disorders in persons with autistic spectrum disorders.
- There is little information about the value of psychiatric medications on substance use.

Further reading

Andrews G, Oakley-Browne M, Castle D, et al. (2003). Summary of guideline for the treatment of panic disorder and agoraphobia. RNAZCP Clinical Practice Guidelines. *Australasian Psychiatry* 11:29–33.

Baker A, Lee NK, Jenner L. (2004). *Models of Intervention and Care for Psychostimulant Users* (2nd ed). National Drug Strategy Monograph series, No. 51. Canberra: Commonwealth of Australia.

Baldwin DS, Anderson IM, Nutt DJ, et al. (2014). Evidence-based pharmacological treatment of anxiety disorders, post-traumatic stress disorder and obsessive-compulsive disorder: A revision of the 2005 guidelines from the British Association for Psychopharmacology. *J Psychopharmacology*, 28: 403–439.

Lingford-Hughes AR, Welch S, Peters L, et al. (2012). Evidence based guidelines for the pharmacological management of substance abuse, harmful use, addiction and comorbidity: recommendations from the British Association for Psychopharmacology. *J Psychopharmacol* 26:899–952. Available at http://www.bap.org.uk

McIntosh C, Ritson B. (2001). Treating depression complicated by substance misuse. *Adv Psychiatric Treat* 7:357–64.

Nutt DJ. (2003). Death and dependence: current controversies over the selective serotonin reuptake inhibitors. *J Psychopharmacol* 17:355–64.

Specific clinical situations

Oral complications of substance use 484
The sleep-disturbed patient 489
The patient who lies 491

Oral complications of substance use

Introduction and overview

Oral and dental diseases are common complications of alcohol and substance use disorders. Often, because of the immediacy of the presenting problem, they are accorded a low priority in the plan of management. However, significant ill health can occur if these disorders are neglected. Certain forms of substance use disorders are associated with a particularly high incidence of oral and dental disease to the extent that some specialist addictions clinics have integrated dental services. In relation to substance use, oral and dental diseases may arise from:

- poor dental and oral hygiene consequent on neglect by the patient
- vitamin and other nutritional deficiency
- the direct toxic effects of the psychoactive substance
- the physical effects of the drug, such as grinding of the teeth (bruxism)
- recurrent vomiting, with reflux of acidic gastric contents into the mouth
- the effects of sugar and other sweeteners in medication, e.g. methadone syrup
- suppression of immune function with predisposition to gingivitis and dental abscesses
- the carcinogenic properties of certain substances, specifically alcohol and tobacco constituents.

The commonest from of dental pathology is accelerated dental caries and gingivitis arising from inadequate dental hygiene compounded by absence of regular dental inspections (Box 23.1).

Dental caries

- Dental caries starts on the tooth surface where dental plaque stagnates leading to decay of the enamel and dentine of the teeth.
- Predisposing factors include xerostomia, poor oral hygiene and sugar-containing drinks and drugs such as methadone syrup.
- May be painless but dentine exposure typically results in hot/cold sensitivity.
- Bacterial plaques (e.g. from *Streptococcus*, *Actinomyces*) are implicated in the occurrence of caries.
- Prevalence of caries has been reduced considerably by fluoridation of water, the removal of sorbitol from methadone syrup, and better oral care with the use of fluoride-containing toothpaste
- Rampant caries is a complication of methamphetamine use due to a combination of poor oral hygiene, xerostomia, bruxism, and high intake of sugar and carbonate drinks; it is known colloquially as 'meth mouth'.

Box 23.1 Dental complications of substance use

Alcohol

- Cheilosis
- Glossitis
- Gingivitis, ulcerative gingivitis
- Xerostomia
- Oropharyngeal cancers, particularly if person is also a smoker
- Dental erosion
- Dental caries
- Signs of trauma, recent or old.

Tobacco

- Stained teeth
- Halitosis
- 'Smokeless tobacco keratosis'
- Pigmentation
- Xerostomia
- Leucoplakia
- Gingivitis, ulcerative gingivitis, gingival recession
- Candidiasis
- Impaired wound healing
- Oral cancers, mainly squamous cell carcinomas. Risk is increased if there is concurrent alcohol abuse
- Increased plaque and calculus
- Caries
- Periodontal disease.

Cannabis

- Tooth loss
- Xerostomia
- Gingival hyperplasia,
- Gingivitis, painful and red associated with white patches
- Leucoplakia
- Erythroplakia
- Increased incidence of carcinoma
- Caries
- Periodontal disease.

Opioids

- Xerostomia
- Caries (particularly patients on methadone syrup)
- Oral complications of injecting drug use.

Psychostimulants

- Xerostomia
- Bruxism
- Tense or painful jaw muscles
- Gingival and periodontal disease
- Rampant dental caries 'meth mouth'
- Nasal septal and palatal perforation (a complication of intranasal cocaine).

Gingivitis/periodontal disease

- Gingivitis is the commonest cause of tooth loss. It arises from accumulation of bacterial plaque, which can become mineralized, with the formation of calculus.
- Gingivitis is usually painless.
- Often results in bleeding when teeth are brushed.
- In time can result in absorption of alveolar bone, loosening of the teeth, and loss of teeth.

Acute pulpitis

Persistent and throbbing dental pain should raise the possibility of extension of the infection and inflammation of the pulp or pulpitis.

Complications of specific substances

(See also Box 23.1.)

Alcohol

Alcohol use disorders cause a multiplicity of oral and dental diseases. Particularly in malnourished alcohol-dependent men, dental pathology can advance to the stage that an entire dental clearance is required. Among the recognized complications are:

- advanced dental caries and gingivitis—due to poor self-care and regurgitation of gastric contents
- fracture of teeth—during alcohol withdrawal, especially with seizures
- vitamin B-complex deficiency syndromes—angular stomatitis and glossitis
- vitamin C deficiency (scurvy)—presents as loosening and dislodgement of teeth, bleeding gums and tooth sockets, regression of the gum line due to gingivitis
- discoloration of the teeth due to acid reflux
- bilateral parotid enlargement—due to recurrent vomiting and reflux of contents into the salivary ducts
- oral cancer.

An alcohol-dependent patient on disulfiram should not be exposed to an alcohol-containing mouth wash.

Tobacco (nicotine)

The main consequences are:
- nicotine staining of the teeth
- dryness of the mouth (xerostomia)
- oral cancer.

Injecting drug use

Injecting drug use is the most important risk factor for spread of hepatitis C and, to a lesser extent, HIV and hepatitis B. It is prudent for dentists to practise universal precautions.

Complications of injecting drug use include:

- bacterial infections of the mouth, gums and pharynx, mouth ulcers
- fungal infections of the mouth, gums, and pharynx, e.g. candidiasis
- oral lesions suggestive of a compromised immune system (HIV/AIDS)
- infective endocarditis may result from *Streptococcus* or *Staphylococcus* infections at times of dental procedures.

Opioids

Oral and dental pathology can be very marked in illicit opioid users, particularly injecting heroin users, whose dependence is such that they typically neglect most aspects of their self-care.

Commonly seen in this population are:
- advanced dental caries due to neglect of dental hygiene
- dental abscesses
- dental caries and wearing of the teeth with exposure of dentine due to diet with high sugar content and also medications such as cough syrup and methadone which contain sugar or other sweeteners
- oral thrush (candidiasis).

Psychostimulants

Dental problems can be severe in users of psychostimulants because of teeth grinding (bruxism), a recognized toxic effect of these drugs.

The most characteristic complications are:
- broken teeth with vertical or diagonal fractures, often resulting in sharp pointed teeth
- trauma to the gums, cheeks, and tongue, with secondary infection and blood loss
- dryness of the mouth (xerostomia).

Prevention of oral and dental disease

A proactive approach is valuable as part of the overall management plan in all patients with substance use disorders. Often patients have not visited a dentist for many years and an appointment for dental examination can be usefully suggested during the patient's initial management.

With detoxification or maintenance on agonist medication the substance dependence should become less symptomatic, thus allowing the patient to attend for dental appointments. Costs may be substantial in many countries, depending on the healthcare system and whether dentistry is provided free of charge or at a subsidized rate.

Accordingly, some addiction services, including opioid maintenance clinics, have integrated dental services or provide referral to a free (or inexpensive) clinic.

Reintroduction to regular dental hygiene will reduce the risk of further complications. The patient should be placed on a multivitamin preparation containing the B complex vitamins and vitamin C. Many patients are also vitamin D deficient and should be placed on appropriate supplements.

Referral for dental examination

In most cases the referral for dental assessment can be an elective one but the following are indications for urgent attention:
- Tooth pain, especially if persistent or throbbing (possibility of acute pulpitis)
- Recent fracture of a tooth, especially with persistent pain
- Sudden displacement of a filling, with persistent pain, which may be due to exposed dentine or to exposed nerve endings
- Acute inflammation of the gums (gingivitis)
- Suspected dental abscess.

Diagnostic pointers

Abnormalities of the teeth can also point to hitherto undetected systemic disease. An example is crowding of the teeth due to maldevelopment of the maxilla in fetal alcohol syndrome.

Further reading

Kidd E. (2009). Oral complications of drug and alcohol misuse. In Latt N, Conigrave K, Saungers JB, et al. (eds) Addiction Medicine (1st ed), pp. 375–8. Oxford: Oxford University Press.
Rees TD. (1992). Oral effects of drug abuse. Crit Rev Oral Biol Med 3(3):163–84.

The sleep-disturbed patient

Introduction and overview

The two most common sleep disorders seen in people who have substance use disorders are insomnia and circadian rhythm disorder. These may occur both while the substance dependence is active and in the early weeks (sometimes longer) of abstinence.

Insomnia

- Symptoms of insomnia include difficulty getting to sleep, frequent and prolonged awakenings during the night, and early morning wakening.
- These are likely to have an impact on next-day functioning and patients may experience fatigue, lethargy, or low mood.
- These symptoms are very common in substance-abusing patients who are abstinent.
- Co-morbidity of substance abuse and depression is common, and the effects of both conditions on sleep are additive.
- Problems with sleeping often continue for weeks after detoxification and can persist for months in some patients.

Circadian rhythm disorder

Symptoms of this disorder include:

- not being able to fall asleep for a long time at night
- difficulty in waking in the morning.

Disturbance of circadian rhythm has often been established for months or years. People who have substance use disorders (be it alcohol, opioids, or stimulant drugs) often have a chaotic lifestyle without routine. They may not suffer from insomnia as such, but their sleeping patterns are irregular and out of synchronization with normal society. They may have a habit of staying up late at night and sleeping late the next morning. Accordingly, their body clock sleep–wake rhythm is shifted through the day, so that morning appointments are missed and they are awake all night.

Overall impact

- Sleep disturbance has a great impact on quality of life in general.
- It can lead to tiredness, difficulties in concentrating, irritability, and sometimes low mood.
- Sleep problems predict relapse in abstinent alcohol-dependent patients, and often in opioid addiction too.

Management of sleep disorders

Treating sleep problems in patients with substance use disorders is a key element in primary goal of preventing relapse. Delayed sleep times are very important to work on because this problem may prevent patients from engaging with therapies.

Maximizing the chances of good sleep involves focusing on the three main drives for sleep in the brain:

1. The homeostatic or recovery drive to sleep

The longer the time without sleep the higher this drive to sleep becomes, and during sleep it declines. The ideal time from one period of sleep to the next is about 16 hours, so if someone is used to getting up at noon, then the maximum sleep drive on this process will be at about 4 am. Taking naps will delay the sleep drive further.

2. The circadian process (body clock)

This clock is reset by light and other stimuli each day, thus making the circadian rhythm stronger. Exposure to daylight in the morning (even on overcast days) resets the body clock via a neural pathway directly from the eyes to the hypothalamus. Other influences on the clock are regular routines such as relatively high levels activity in the day and eating and drinking.

3. Arousal level—influence on sleep

Although it seems obvious, this aspect of sleep propensity is extremely important, particularly when insomnia is a problem. High arousal at bedtime leaves people lying in bed with the mind racing, unable to get to sleep. A very important influence on arousal at bedtime is the availability of games, social networking, and other entertainment on electronic devices such as smartphones and tablets which are often in the bedroom. Use of these before bed or during the night increases arousal (Box 23.2).

Prescription of hypnotic medication is usually not appropriate in this group because of concerns about misuse. Other drugs such as antidepressants are also known to improve sleep, particularly those blocking $5HT_2$ receptors, such as mirtazapine and trazodone, and may be considered in those patients with depression.

Box 23.2 Maximizing good sleep—what we should encourage

- Decide on a rising time and stick to it, even on weekends.
- Stay awake for about 16 hours during the day—no naps.
- Go to bed when tired, but always stick to the rising time.
- Get some daylight in the morning and exercise in the day.
- Keep the bedroom for sleeping, no phone/tablet in the bedroom.
- Wind down towards bedtime, deal with problems early in the evening, no worrying about bills in bed.

Further reading

Wilson SJ, Nutt DJ, Alford C, Argyropoulos SV, Baldwin DS, Bateson AN, Britton TC, Crowe C, Dijk DJ, Espie CA, Gringras P, Hajak G, Idzikowski C, Krystal AD, Nash JR, Selsick H, Sharpley AL, Wade AG. (2010) British Association for Psychopharmacology consensus statement on evidence-based treatment of insomnia, parasomnias and circadian rhythm disorders. *J Psychopharmacology*. 24(11):1577–601.

The patient who lies

Denial is a common feature among patients with substance use disorders. It represents one of the more primitive defence mechanisms, and patients may avoid, cover up, distort, misattribute, underestimate, or simply lie (dissemble) about their alcohol and substance use. The US Centers for Disease Control and Prevention reported that only one in six of 38 million Americans who drink excessively tell the truth about the extent of their drinking (http://www.cdc.gov/vitalsigns/alcohol-screening-counseling/).

The degree of dissembling depends on the severity of the problem. Drug-seeking patients, who complain of pain and/or of insomnia, pose a particular challenge to addiction specialists. Here, a high index of suspicion and attempt to understand reasons behind any untruths is essential.

- Is it to obtain prescriptions for narcotic analgesics or sedative-hypnotics?
- Is it to save face?
- Is it for some gain such as a medical leave certificate, regaining a driver's licence, or for acquiring disability insurance?

Taking into account confidentiality issues, seek collaborative information from the GP, past medical records, family, and friends.

A good systematic history taking, screening for alcohol and substance use, and clarification of inconsistencies is the first step towards a correct diagnosis.

- Introduce alcohol and substance use as part of normal part of a normal health and lifestyle assessment.
- Establish a good therapeutic relationship by being non-judgemental and showing empathy and understanding.
- Use the 'top high' technique (pp. 69–70; p. 78).

In the clinical examination look for clues. For patients with a suspected alcohol use disorder, check for the smell of alcohol on the breath. Look for a puffy bloated face with telangiectasia, conjunctival injection, tremulousness, moist skin, sweating, signs of injury (old or new), tachycardia, hypertension, peripheral neuropathy, truncal obesity or stigmata of chronic liver disease such as spider naevi, palmar erythema, parotid enlargement, bruising, and hepatomegaly (pp. 71–72).

For injecting drug users, look at the general appearance for signs of malnourishment, drowsiness, needle track marks, pupillary size, poor dentition, and heart murmurs (pp. 71–72; p. 421)

Laboratory tests can be helpful in alerting the clinician to undeclared or minimized substance use. These include a urine drug screen or a saliva sample for prescribed medications and illicit drugs.

For alcohol, the options are several:

- blood or breath alcohol concentration
- FBC (macrocytosis)
- LFTs: disproportionately raised GGT and AST/ALT ratio >2 indicates likely alcoholic liver disease
- carbohydrate-deficient transferrin
- ethyl glucuronide.

In the hospital or clinic, ask the nursing staff how the patient behaves (e.g. drug-seeking, demands for psychotropic medication exactly on time, mobility when there is a complaint of acute or chronic pain).

To identify the drug-seeking ('doctor shopping') patient, especially for narcotic opioids or sedative hypnotics, the clinician may have access to telephone enquiry lines or electronic information. For example, in Australia there is a prescription shopping information service. For such patients, regulated, supervised dispensing can be provided either at a specialist clinic or an approved pharmacy.

Special populations

Children 494
Adolescents 496
Young adults 503
Pregnancy and the neonate 505
Fetal alcohol spectrum disorders 514
The elderly 518
Marginalized populations 522
Substance use in different cultural contexts 525
Indigenous peoples 529
Immigrants and refugees 534
Prison inmates 538
The impaired health professional 541
Safety-critical occupations 543

Children

Introduction

When meeting children and families, health professionals should ask about alcohol and drug use as early as the first visit. This provides an opportunity not only to assess but also to educate individuals about the health effects of alcohol and drugs. The extent of alcohol or drug use may not be completely apparent at the first visit and it may take several consultations to get a clear picture. Careful observation of as much of the parent–child interaction (e.g. the parent's manner towards the child and how the child responds) can yield useful information about possible problems that need further investigation.

It is helpful to have a basic understanding of the medical, psychiatric, and behavioural symptoms of children affected by substance misuse and to be familiar with local services and how to refer to them.

Developmental perspective

Children of substance-using parents

The majority of women who misuse substances are of child-bearing age and this has implications for child health and parenting.

Children born to women who used substances in pregnancy are at greater risk of prematurity, low birth weight, impaired physical growth and development, behavioural problems, and learning disabilities.

Some women continue to use substances after childbirth. Most drugs cross the placenta, but even if children are not exposed *in utero* they are at greater risk for childhood problems if their parents are involved in substance use. They grow up in an environment where there may be increased prevalence of mental health disorders, histories of physical or sexual abuse, serious medical problems, poor nutrition, relationship difficulties (including domestic violence), and limited social supports. This may manifest in the child as delays in language development, learning problems, behavioural disturbances or adjustment problems in home, health, social, and emotional domains (see Box 24.1).

Children who become substance users

There is a relationship between parental substance use and substance use in children. These children are found to be at increased biological, psychological, and environmental risk through many factors including genetic predisposition to substance use and mental health disorders, decreased parental monitoring, increased availability of substances in the child's environment (sometimes being almost 'normative'), permissive attitudes to substance use, social isolation including lack of encouragement to attend school or opportunity to pursue other constructive activities (e.g. sport, hobbies), stress, negative affect or other mental health conditions. Often a combination of risk factors exists.

Box 24.1 Warning signs that may suggest substance use in a child's environment

- Developmental delay
- School difficulties
- Behavioural problems
- Psychosomatic symptoms
- Emotional difficulties and mental health problems (e.g. depression, anxiety).

Management of children from alcohol or other drug backgrounds

Linking with support services

Early detection of families where substance use is occurring enables monitoring of the child's development and provision of assistance for families. While women may be reticent to disclose substance use, fearing the involvement of authorities such as Child Protection, a non-judgemental discussion about the supports available can help ameliorate some of this concern. Support can occur as early as antenatal classes in preparing for childbirth and childcare or parenting support in early childhood.

In some cases, assistance is required to deal with domestic violence, risk of homelessness, legal, or other complications. Referral to government-funded community health services or non-governmental agencies and social services is required in these situations.

Importance of intervention for parental substance use

A non-judgemental discussion with the parents about the importance of addressing substance use for the benefit of the child as well as for themselves is important. This can include treatment options and detail about services available.

In certain cases, child protection authorities do need to be notified because of the severity of psychosocial risk. In most cases, this management plan should be communicated openly and transparently to reduce the risk of further complications or negative outcomes.

Monitoring the growth and development of the child(ren)

The growth and development of children of substance-using parents should be monitored regularly if possible; otherwise opportunistically so that where problems (e.g. developmental delay, learning difficulties) are identified, early intervention can occur.

Adolescents

The nature of adolescence

Adolescence is an important developmental period during which the transition from childhood to adulthood occurs. Adolescent development is more than the physical phenomenon of puberty. Cognitive maturation and psychosocial development are also important aspects of adolescence. (See Table 24.1.)

Physical development commences with the onset of puberty, and is characterized by physical growth and the development of secondary sexual characteristics and reproductive capability.

Cognitive development progresses into the young adult years (around 20 years of age). During this time, cognitive capabilities move from concrete thinking in early adolescence to abstract thinking by late adolescence. For instance, talking about the long-term effects of alcohol, such as liver disease, rarely has impact on the early adolescent. It is better to talk with the young adolescent about how heavy drinking contributes to difficulties in their relationships with peers or family, or difficulties performing at school.

Psychosocial development includes the development of a stable and independent identity, relationships beyond family to peers, a moral and value system, an understanding of sexuality, and acquisition of skills for a future vocation.

Substance use and adolescent development

Regular or heavy substance use frequently inhibits adolescent development by delaying the time that psychosocial milestones are reached, impairing cognitive maturation, reducing educational achievements, impairing the development of healthy relationships, and increasing the likelihood of mental health problems in adolescence and adulthood.

Alcohol and drug use impacts on the developing brain in adolescence. It manifests as structural changes especially in the hippocampus and prefrontal cortex. Neurocognitive impairments particularly in relation to memory and learning have also been identified. Depending on the severity of the substance use, some changes do not reverse with prolonged abstinence.

Differentiating significant problems from occasional use

Adolescent substance use fits a spectrum. When consulting with an adolescent, it is important for the health professional to discern where the adolescent is in the spectrum of adolescent substance use.

Experimentation with substances by young people is much more common than progression to regular use. Sometimes adolescents use drugs only in specific situations, for instance, only when attending parties or when socializing with certain peers. This is sometimes referred to as 'situational' or 'recreational' use. Other adolescents use drugs to self-medicate difficulties with sleep or emotional difficulties.

Table 24.1 Developmental stages of early, middle, and late adolescence

Early adolescence (~11–13 years)	Characterized by the physical and physiological changes of puberty
	Frequently concerned about whether their development is 'normal' and in keeping with their peers
	Usually still dependent on family, but peers (usually of the same sex) become increasingly important
	Characterized by concrete thinking
Middle adolescence (~14–16 years)	Characterized by the increasing development of autonomy
	Identity becomes very important to the young person. Attachment to peer groups takes place and being attractive, accepted, and popular are often a focus
	Experimentation and risk taking are very common. This may include with alcohol and other substances
Late adolescence (~17–20 years)	More mature intellectual abilities have developed
	Independence and a sense of identity and self-worth are usually evident, plus plans and aspirations for the future, including employment and relationships

Abuse or harmful use: here alcohol or drug use is repeated and is resulting in problems. Examples of problems include difficulties with family or friends, failure to fulfil study requirements, or even attend school because of substance use.

Dependence on a substance refers to an internal drive to use psychoactive substances (sometimes termed compulsive drug-seeking behaviour despite negative consequences).

Risk factors for substance use and its progression

Research continues to explore what the determinants are of progression from experimentation to abuse or dependence. The role of environment in the expression of genetic risk for heavy alcohol or drug use is becoming evident.

Patterns of substance use that influence progression to problems include:

- onset of alcohol or other drug use in early adolescence
- heavy use, in terms of dose and/or frequency.

Risk factors and protective factors

Understanding how adolescent drug use comes about is often explained in terms of a risk factor and protective factor framework. This framework helps to understand why some adolescents follow trajectories that lead to substance use problems while others, even in the face of severe psychosocial stressors and substantial adversity, do not develop drug or alcohol, or other problems. Resilience refers to the ability to be well adjusted and interpersonally effective despite an adverse environment. Factors that counter risk factors and help people deal positively with life

Table 24.2 Some risk and protective factors for substance misuse in adolescents

Biological factors	Genetic, physiological factors
Temperament and personality traits	Antisocial personality disorder, sensation seeking trait, impulsivity
Familial factors	Familial attitudes that are favourable to substance use, parental modelling of substance use, poor or inconsistent parenting practices
Early onset of substance use	Alcohol or drug use before age 15 years
Emotional and behavioural problems	Depression, anxiety, conduct disorder, attention deficit/hyperactivity disorder
Poor social connections	To school and community groups
Peer use of substances	Attitudes and behaviour favourable to substance use

changes are referred to as protective factors. Protective factors may be events, circumstances, or life experiences (see Table 24.2).

Approaches to managing adolescent substance use aim to reduce risk factors and strengthen protective factors where possible.

There is no one single risk factor that can be attributed to adolescent drug use. Psychosocial risk factors tend to 'cluster'. That is, individuals tend to have several risk factors that impact on their development. This explains why many health-risk behaviours (alcohol misuse, heavy tobacco use, other substance use, unprotected sex, delinquency) often co-occur.

Specific aspects of the substance use history

Polysubstance use

Polysubstance use is common among adolescents. When obtaining a drug use history from young people, it is important to specifically ask about each substance, including alcohol and tobacco. Good communication skills are important (Table 24.3).

For any given substance, gather information on:
- how often they take that substance
- the dose used (i.e. how many drinks on a given occasion, how many cigarettes a day, how many times they use marijuana in a given week or on a given day)
- whether episodic heavy use occurs and if so, how often.

Differentiating problematic from experimental use

In addition to the extent of use, it is helpful to find out whether the young person has experienced problems (physical, emotional, social, or legal) with their substance use (see Box 24.2). A sample question is 'Do things happen when you use drugs/drink heavily that you later regret/wish didn't happen?'.

Table 24.3 Principles of engaging adolescents

Confidentiality	Confidentiality is extremely important in the relationship between a young person and a health professional Adolescents frequently will not disclose the details of their substance use if they are concerned that confidentiality will not be maintained by the health professional
Take a broad psychosocial history	Adolescents respond well to a holistic approach, rather than a focus on their substance use
Screen for mental health problems	Mental health problems often emerge in adolescence and should be screened for regularly
Avoid judgement	Any perception of judgement about the adolescent's substance use on the part of the health professional impedes engagement with the young person

---

Box 24.2 Warning signs of substance use in adolescents

- Drop in school grades
- Behavioural changes—change of friends, lack of interaction with family, increasing isolation
- Changes in appearance—red eyes (cannabis), loss of weight, skin sores (amphetamines)
- Loss of interest in hobbies, sport, activities
- Changes in eating pattern (cannabis increases appetite, amphetamines reduce it)
- Changes in sleeping pattern
- Lethargy, loss of motivation
- Mood swings ('uppers and downers')
- Financial concerns (increased need for money but on what spent not apparent)
- Problems with the law (drink driving, assault, break enter and steal, criminal activity).

Where there is a history of heavy substance use obtained, ask the young person whether they experience:

- difficulty controlling use of the substance
- withdrawal symptoms when they do not use a substance (e.g. 'if you don't' use marijuana, how do you feel?').

These features of physical drug dependence may commence in adolescence, rather than later in adulthood.

Management of substance disorders in adolescents

- Management of substance use disorders in adolescents requires a multipronged approach, which takes into account the adolescent's stage of development.
- Management includes behavioural strategies, intervention for mental health and well-being, and in some cases, medication.

- Open, non-judgemental discussion with young people about substance use is best.
- Risks need to be communicated. For instance, with alcohol discussions can occur around loss of consciousness ('coma drinking'), accidents and injuries, assaults and trauma (including road trauma), and sexual risk-taking (sexual assault, unprotected intercourse).
- Discussing with the young person the pros and cons of potential strategies to reduce consumption is helpful.
- In severe cases, alcohol withdrawal management ('detox') may be required.
- Concomitant mental health problems need attention.
- The use of pharmacotherapies for alcohol and for tobacco dependence in young people is under evaluation.

Cannabis

Cannabis use is particularly common among young people.
- Advise that cessation of cannabis often leads to significant irritability, anxiety and/or insomnia and these symptoms can precipitate relapses if not anticipated and managed.
- There is now sufficient evidence that in certain vulnerable individuals with a genetic predisposition, cannabis can increase their risk of developing a psychotic illness later in life.
- Previous exposure to cannabis without apparent ill effect does not mean that subsequent exposure will be equally harmless.

Opioids

In most cases, pharmacological management of opioid dependence in the adolescent is with opioid substitution therapy. Careful diagnosis of dependence is required before commencing this treatment.

The family

Depression and anxiety often occur in parents of substance abusing adolescents, sometimes reaching clinical levels of severity. Parents frequently describe feelings of helplessness and a lack of confidence about having the appropriate parenting skills to deal with their teenager's drug use.

The health professional can help empower parents through:
- education about substance use
- advice and/or referral for assistance with parenting strategies
- management of depression of anxiety.

With more entrenched substance misuse, disengagement with the family may have occurred. Families are an integral part of the adolescent's world and it is therefore important to try to assist the young person to rebuild connection. Depending on the individual circumstance this connection may be achieved through mediation by the health professional or more formally with family counsellors.

Increasing access to treatment

Outreach

Adolescents often do not engage with alcohol and drug services for adults. They sometimes need specific outreach and proactive services that cater appropriately for their developmental stage and incorporate a consideration of their cultural background, lifestyle, and in many cases their family.

Opportunistic healthcare

This is very important in young people, particularly the homeless, and can be a useful means of encouraging the young person to engage with healthcare services. In attending to screening and management of blood-borne viruses and STIs, addressing intercurrent health problems (chest infections, skin rashes, etc.), a rapport can be developed with the young person which encourages them to continue to attend to their healthcare.

Mental health problems should always be monitored in young people. Substance use may complicate depression and anxiety that are common in adolescence, but these conditions may not be articulated as such by the young person. Suicidal risk in the young person needs to be assessed frequently. Psychosis (drug induced or otherwise) can also occur with heavy substance use.

Transition from adolescent to adult drug treatment services

The transition from developmentally focused youth drug treatment services to more independently orientated adult services can be challenging for young people. The aims of successful transition of young people to adult-orientated health services are to optimize both their health and their ability to adapt to adult roles. The transition process needs to include the coordination of primary and specialty health services, as well as the development of up-to-date detailed written transition plans, in collaboration with young people and their families. Confidentiality and informed consent must be maintained for the adolescent or young person as they traverse systems and engage with different health professionals. This usually means discussing with the young person what information is clinically relevant for the adult health service to be aware of.

Harm reduction in the adolescent context

As for adults, principles of harm reduction apply to the adolescents, although they need to be appropriately modified for young people of differing developmental stages and they need to take into account the adolescent's context. For example, specific advice on the less harmful methods of using drugs may be appropriate in adolescents whose substance misuse is unlikely to cease for some time.

Prevention of substance use disorders in adolescence

Resilience in adolescence can help protect against substance use. There is evidence that resilience can be promoted by increasing a sense of connectedness of the adolescent, e.g. to family, school, or to sporting, religious, or cultural groups (see Box 24.3).

Box 24.3 Tips for parents in preventing adolescent substance use problems

- Spend time with young people, communicate with them, be involved in their lives
- Get to know their friends, and their friend's parents
- Set a good example—good role modelling is important
- Be alert to early warning signs of drug use
- Do not over react, be calm, avoid conflict
- Do not nag or lecture—reason honestly with them
- Set sensible ground rules and boundaries
- Ensure adult supervision at parties, plan how they and their friends get home
- Seek professional help—from GPs, psychologists, addiction specialists, psychiatrists—if problems arise.

Young adults

Cognitive development

Managing young adults differs from adolescents. Being more mature, young adults understand the broad impact of their substance misuse. It is important to note that in cases of severe substance misuse, there may be substantial cognitive impairment or acquired brain injury. If not excessive, this may improve with abstinence and cognitive rehabilitation, although research to date suggests that some degree of impairment will remain indefinitely.

Psychosocial development

When compared to adolescents, young adults tend to be more focused on their future and there is greater motivation to address substance misuse, mental health, education and employment. Intimate relationships are very important to the young adult and in many cases can be a strong motivating factor to address substance misuse and mental health.

Management of substance use disorders in young adults

Pharmacotherapy

Pharmacological management of substance dependence in young adults is similar to older adults. Concomitant treatment of mental health disorders such as depression, anxiety, or other disorders such as attention deficit disorder may also need pharmacological intervention in addition to psychological interventions

Psychosocial rehabilitation

Psychosocial rehabilitation is a significant aspect of management of young adults. Engaging the young adult in appropriate educational endeavours or in suitable employment, sometimes starting with minimal contact hours with gradual increases is recommended. It is important for the medical practitioner to have an awareness of local resources that can assist with this.

Adult drug treatment services

Adult drug treatment services differ from youth services in that there is greater onus on the young adult to drive their healthcare. Compared to youth workers, there is less capacity for adult treatment services to arrange and coordinate appointments or perform outreach for adults, although some services will provide this in the early stages of transition from youth to adult treatment services. It is best to advise individuals of the differences between treatment systems to avoid unnecessary distress about the change in paradigm. (See earlier section on 'Transition from adolescent to adult drug treatment services', p. 501).

Relapses

Addiction is a chronic relapsing disorder. Young adults need to be aware that relapses will occur and therefore not to 'lose heart'. Important messages include that they (1) can learn what the triggers for relapse tend to be for them and what works best to minimize their frequency and (2) rather than avoiding treatment (e.g. because of shame or despondency), it is easier to attend to relapses promptly to curtail their duration.

Further reading

Hermens DF, Lagopoulos J, Tobias-Webb J, *et al*. (2013). Pathways to alcohol-induced brain impairment in young people: a review. *Cortex* 49:3–17.

Kang MS, Skinner R, Sanci LA, *et al*. (2013). *Youth Health and Adolescent Medicine*. East Hawthorn: IP Communications.

Saunders J, Rey J. (eds) (2011). *Young People & Alcohol: Impact, Policy, Prevention, Treatment*. Chichester: Wiley Blackwell Press.

Spear L. (2000). The adolescent brain and age-related behavioral manifestations. *Neurosci Biobehav Rev* 24:417–63.

Pregnancy and the neonate

The number of women misusing drugs has increased considerably and a significant number of women presenting to drug misuse services for treatment are of child-bearing age. Every woman thought to have a possibility of pregnancy requires appropriate history-taking, assessment, and screening for alcohol and other drug use. Drug and alcohol use during pregnancy is associated with both maternal and fetal/neonatal outcomes. Maternal outcomes include not receiving adequate prenatal adverse care and fetal outcomes relate to a failure to thrive. Women of child-bearing age who smoke, consume more than two standard drinks a day, or use other psychoactive drugs, should be informed of the potential risks to both themselves and the fetus, and offered advice and if necessary told where to get help.

Pregnancy offers healthcare professionals a window of opportunity to help reduce the harm associated with problematic alcohol, nicotine, and other drug use. Although pregnancy may act as a catalyst for change, drug misusers often fail to use general health services and are, therefore, more vulnerable to mental health, medical, and obstetrical complications. It is important that obstetric care is organized once pregnancy is confirmed. Where harmful, hazardous or dependent use of psychoactive substances is suspected or confirmed, a specialist healthcare professional with expertise in drug and alcohol misuse should be involved. In collaboration with the antenatal team, the drug and alcohol specialist(s) can provide specific guidance on treatment and will monitor the patient's alcohol and other drug use during pregnancy. This is particularly important at 12, 18–20, 25 and 26 weeks.

Following the birth of the baby, monitoring is continued by the neonatal team and the drug and alcohol expert(s). A risk assessment should be conducted and if the infant is considered to be at risk, involvement with child protection agencies or departments is mandatory.

Effects on the fetus/infant

The development of the fetus will be affected by factors such as quantity and frequency of substance use, and depending on the gestational stage, drug or alcohol use may lead to:

- prematurity
- low birth weight
- perinatal mortality
- respiratory distress
- withdrawal syndromes
- convulsions
- sudden infant death syndrome: increased four- to fivefold in infants born to pregnant drug users
- teratogenic effects.

Effects on the mother

Pharmacological effects of the drug

Chaotic use may lead to:
- overdose/intoxication
- withdrawal syndromes (alcohol, nicotine, benzodiazepines, stimulants, cannabis).

If injecting drugs, *complications of injecting*:
- Bacterial infections:
  - Septicaemia
  - Subacute bacterial endocarditis, septic thrombophlebitis
- Viral infections: hepatitis B, C, HIV (see Box 24.4)
- Fungal infections: candidiasis.

Other medical complications
- STIs such as chlamydia and herpes
- Poor nutrition
- Vitamin deficiencies
- Anorexia (especially stimulants)
- Anaemia.

Emotional/psychiatric complications
- Anxiety
- Depression
- Insomnia.

Obstetric complications
- Placental insufficiency, abruptio placentae, placenta praevia
- Intrauterine growth retardation (IUGR)/death
- Premature rupture of membranes/premature labour
- Pre-eclampsia/eclampsia
- Chorioamnionitis
- Premature delivery
- Postpartum haemorrhage.

Psychosocial issues
- Domestic violence
- Housing problems
- Financial problems
- Prostitution
- Criminal activity.

General complications of alcohol and other drug use during pregnancy

In general, risk of damage is greatest in the first trimester of pregnancy (especially the first 8 weeks) but caution should be exercised during the second and third trimesters. Transport of drugs across the placenta is greatest in late gestation when placental blood flow is greatest.

Box 24.4 Blood-borne viruses: hepatitis C, B, and HIV in pregnant injecting drug users

All pregnant mothers should be offered screening for hepatitis B, C, and in selected cases HIV.

Hepatitis C: up to 10% of mothers with chronic hepatitis C infection who are HCV RNA (PCR) positive can transmit hepatitis C virus to the fetus. Caesarean section has not been shown to reduce the risk of vertical transmission. Ideally, the infant should be tested for HCV RNA PCR at 4–6 months and after 18 months when transplacental antibodies have disappeared. However, follow-up is often difficult and infants are not tested.

If HCV RNA PCR is positive after 6–18 months—refer to Paediatric Hepatologist or Infectious Disease Specialist.

Hepatitis B: women who are HBsAb negative should be offered hepatitis B vaccination after birth. All newborn infants in Australia receive hepatitis B immunization. In addition, babies of HBsAg-positive mothers are given immunoglobulin within 12 hours and a total of four doses of hepatitis B vaccination—at birth, 2, 4, and 6 months. Caesarean section is not justified.

HIV: the risk of vertical transmission of HIV is greatest during the last week of pregnancy and during birth. The risk can be reduced by elective caesarean section and intravenous antiretroviral therapy before birth. Zidovudine therapy reduces the risk of vertical transmission from 25% to 8%. It is further reduced by combination therapy. Refer to appropriate Infectious Diseases Specialist and Obstetrician for appropriate advice and treatment.

Women who misuse drugs and alcohol during pregnancy should receive education and advice about safe sex and risk reduction strategies, and be screened for blood-borne viruses that are spread by vertical transmission. It is advisable that tests are conducted for blood-borne viruses (hepatitis C, B, and HIV) early in pregnancy (see Box 24.4). All testing should be conducted in conjunction with pre- and post-test counselling (see sections p. 414). Patient confidentiality must be maintained at all times.

The significance of maternal infections is evident but has not been well documented in substance misusers. Women who misuse drugs and alcohol may be at greater risk because of promiscuous sexual behaviour and involvement in the sex industry is not unusual. Vertically transmitted infections such as syphilis may lead to malformations and neurodevelopmental delay. Maternal genital infections may increase neonatal infection by intrapartum transmission (genital herpes). For other infections such as *Neisseria gonorrhoea* and *Chlamydia trachomatis* infection, alcohol intoxication, substance misuse, and hazardous drinking levels were factors significantly associated with transmission (see Box 24.5). Education during pregnancy should include advice about safe sex and risk reduction

Box 24.5 Sexually transmitted infections in pregnant drug users

Pregnant mothers known to be sexually promiscuous and/or involved in the sex industry should be offered screening for STIs.

Syphilis: syphilis in pregnancy poses major health risks for the mother and the fetus through vertical transmission. Injecting drug use was observed in female sex workers in Iran where the prevalence of syphilis was 7.2% and herpes simplex type 2 (HSV2) was 18%. Ideally, infected individuals should be treated with a weekly injection of benzylpenicillin for 3 weeks. The infant should be followed up until 18 months old to diagnose congenital syphilis. However, follow-up is often difficult and infants are not tested.

Genital herpes: women who experience their first genital herpes simplex virus (HSV) infection in pregnancy are at highest risk of transmitting the virus to their neonate. Oral aciclovir and valaciclovir given prophylactically in late pregnancy can limit clinical reoccurrence of genital herpes, shedding of HSV at delivery and the rate of caesarean delivery for past HSV disease.

Chlamydia trachomatis genital infection (CTGI): in adolescent girls in Quebec (28% with a history of pregnancy) prevalence of CTGI was 9.3%. In pregnant women it can cause premature delivery and in newborns the clinical manifestations are pneumonia and conjunctivitis.

Refer to appropriate Infectious Diseases Specialist and Obstetrician for appropriate advice and treatment.

strategies. In collaboration with Genitourinary Medicine Services, sexual health should be assessed and screening for STIs should be undertaken if necessary.

Effects of specific drugs

Nicotine

The vasoconstrictor effects of nicotine impair placental blood supply, while carbon monoxide reduces availability of oxygen to the fetus. The risk of harmful effects is greater in older mothers who smoke. Smoking cessation in early pregnancy will give the greatest benefit, although quitting smoking at any time during pregnancy is beneficial for both the mother and fetus and is rarely addressed as a priority in substance misuse populations. (Also see Chapter 8.)

Maternal risks: premature delivery and greater risk of complications

Fetal/infant risks
- Low birth weight (the risk increases in mothers who continue to smoke during pregnancy)
- Increased risk of perinatal mortality
- Sudden Infant Death Syndrome (SIDS).

Nicotine replacement therapy: as yet there is only limited evidence regarding the safety of nicotine replacement therapy or bupropion during pregnancy and lactation.

Alcohol

There are no internationally agreed guidelines regarding safe limits of alcohol consumption during pregnancy. The UK Department of Health recommends not more than 1–2 units of alcohol once or twice a week. Many countries follow similar guidelines as the US which advises total abstinence during pregnancy or in women who are considering pregnancy.

Fetal alcohol syndrome (FAS)

FAS is the result of harmful exposure to alcohol early in pregnancy. It is reported to be the leading preventable cause of mental retardation in Western countries (see Box 24.6 and pp. 514–17). There is a broader range of harmful effects which are termed fetal alcohol effects (FAEs). In North America, estimates for FAEs and alcohol-related neurodevelopment disorder (ARND) are 10-fold those for FAS. The term fetal alcohol spectrum disorders (FASDs) has been used to incorporate less severe fetal effects of drinking.

The detrimental effects of alcohol are greatest during the first trimester of pregnancy, often before the woman knows that she is pregnant. Thus, all women of child-bearing age should also be advised of the risks of drinking and restrict their drinking to a minimum if they are likely to become pregnant. Risks are greater for women older than 30 years of age.

The common pathway of alcohol teratogenesis appears to be its deleterious effects on the developing brain and nervous system. The times of greatest sensitivity of the fetal brain to maternal alcohol consumption are the first and third trimesters.

Sudden cessation of alcohol consumption in pregnant alcohol dependent women is associated with a high risk of seizures. Alcohol detoxification should not be conducted in the community, and needs very careful supervision by obstetricians and alcohol treatment specialists.

Box 24.6 Fetal alcohol syndrome

The teratogenic effects of alcohol cause developmental delay and birth defects

- Characteristic facial abnormalities with underdevelopment of the middle of the face—depressed bridge of nose, thin upper lip, absent philtrum, flattened maxilla; also 'bulls eyes' and low set ears
- Growth retardation (prenatal or postnatal)
- Cardiac abnormalities
- Behavioural disturbances
- Learning disability
- Prematurity, low birth weight; small for gestational age
- Fetal or neonatal death.

Heroin

The incidence of opioid misuse is still increasing in many European countries, with most addicts seeking treatment for the first time between the ages of 20 and 30 years. An estimated 30,000 pregnant women use illicit opioids each year in the European Union. Despite some efforts to address the lack of guidance on managing the pregnant opioid user, an optimal methadone-dosing strategy has yet to be established.

It is clinically agreed that opioid-dependent women fare better if they are maintained on opioids while pregnant rather than attempt abstinence. Conversion of heroin to methadone has been found to be the most effective treatment for opioid-dependent pregnant women, although in some countries buprenorphine may be preferred.

Enrolment of the opiate-addicted woman in a methadone maintenance programme gives the medical community an opportunity to intervene and optimize neonatal outcome in these high-risk pregnancies. It has been demonstrated that methadone improves prenatal care, neonatal outcome, reduced illicit substance use, and improves the overall health of pregnant women. However, the benefits can be negated if inadequate methadone dose is prescribed and heroin is used 'on top'. The dose of methadone may need to be increased in the third trimester of pregnancy.

Pregnant intravenous drug users often have poor antenatal attendance, chaotic lifestyles, and poor nutrition, and detoxification of pregnant heroin-dependent women is risky. Maternal abstinence may result in fetal distress that is more harmful than passive dependence, and may induce abortion or premature labour. The highest risk period is before the 14th week and after the 32nd week of gestation.

Methadone maintenance treatment in conjunction with a comprehensive drug and alcohol and prenatal programme is the treatment of choice to maintain the patient in a comfortable state (average dose of methadone: 30–80 mg daily). Although neonatal opioid dependence as well as neonatal abstinence syndrome (see Box 24.7) may occur, this is not life-threatening and can be managed easily in Special Care Baby Units. Babies born to opioid-dependent mothers should be monitored for the neonatal abstinence syndrome (Box 24.7).

Benzodiazepines

The use of benzodiazepines, particularly during the first trimester of pregnancy, is thought to be associated with decreased fetal growth. There is controversy as to whether fetal abnormalities occur and whether benzodiazepines should be prescribed in pregnancy.

Examination of pooled data from cohort studies found no association between fetal exposure to benzodiazepines during the first trimester and risk of major malformations or malformations of the oral cleft alone (cleft lip and cleft palate), but case–control studies show a small increase in risk for oral cleft palate. Some authorities advise fetal ultrasonography to screen for cleft lip/palate when benzodiazepine abuse or dependence is observed.

A neonatal benzodiazepine withdrawal syndrome is described (Box 24.8)

Box 24.7 Features and management of neonatal abstinence syndrome

Neonatal heroin abstinence syndrome
- Onset following last illicit use: 24–36 hours after delivery
- Duration: >1–2 weeks.

Signs and symptoms
- CNS: high pitched cry, tremor, sleep disturbance, increased muscle tone, myoclonic jerks, convulsions
- Respiratory: sneezing, yawning, nasal flaring and stuffiness, tachypnoea, respiratory distress
- Gastrointestinal tract: poor feeding, excessive sucking, regurgitation, projectile vomiting, diarrhoea.

Neonatal methadone withdrawal syndrome (severity may be reduced if breast-fed)
- Onset: 5–15 days after delivery (i.e. following last dose)
- Duration: >2–3 weeks.

Signs and symptoms
- CNS: high pitched cry, tremor, sleep disturbance, increased muscle tone, myoclonic jerks, convulsions
- Respiratory: sneezing, yawning, nasal flaring and stuffiness, tachypnoea, respiratory distress
- Gastrointestinal tract: poor feeding, excessive sucking, regurgitation, projectile vomiting, diarrhoea.

Treatment
- Monitor severity of symptoms using a neonatal abstinence syndrome scale
- Nurse in a quiet environment and minimize stimuli
- If withdrawal symptoms are severe, administer morphine 0.5 mg/ mL solution (0.5–0.9 mg/kg/day in four divided doses) and reduce slowly by 0.1 mg 6 hourly every 4 days or longer.

NB: administer morphine with caution and only after seeking advice from the specialist neonatologist.
- Discharge planning is important
- Consider the safety of the child. In many regions there is an obligation to notify the Child Protection Services if the child is considered to be at risk.

Box 24.8 Neonatal benzodiazepine withdrawal syndrome

- 'Floppy infant syndrome': hypotonia, sucking difficulties, hypothermia or impaired temperature control
- Tremor
- Irritability
- Hyperactivity
- Cyanosis.

Cocaine/crack cocaine

Cocaine causes vasoconstriction, thus reducing the blood flow to the placenta and increasing the risk of placental abruption. It also increases uterine contractility, thus increasing the risk of spontaneous abortion and premature delivery. The use of cocaine during pregnancy is associated with an increased risk of Sudden Infant Death Syndrome (SIDS) in the baby. See Box 24.9.

Box 24.9 Neonatal stimulant withdrawal syndrome

- Increased muscle tone (stiffness)
- Tremor
- Irritability
- Restlessness
- Itching/scratching
- High pitched crying
- Irregular sleep–wake cycle
- Photosensitivity.

Treatment
- Monitor severity of neonatal abstinence syndrome scale
- Swaddle
- Nurse in a quiet environment and minimize stimuli.

Multiple substance use

Multiple drug use during pregnancy is common and associated with increased rates of prematurity and IUGR, and also with increased rates of problems during labour including premature rupture of the membranes, meconium-stained liquor, and fetal distress. Women using cocaine and multiple substances are at particular risk.

Substance use is not necessarily attenuated during pregnancy. An Irish study showed that 2.8% of urines from a sample of 504 pregnant women screened positive for illicit substances at their first antenatal visit, whereas 5.6% of urines from a separate sample of 515 women screened positive 6 weeks after delivery. The substances identified included benzodiazepines, cannabis, amphetamines, opiates, and cocaine. Less than 2% tested positive for alcohol. Positive screens were associated with women being single, unemployed, and having had a previous pregnancy.

Breastfeeding

Breast milk is generally regarded as the best nutrition for the child. In general, mothers should not be discouraged from breastfeeding but should be given full information of the risks associated with continued use of alcohol and other substances. See Box 24.10.

Box 24.10 Excretion of substances in breast milk

Tobacco

- Minimal amounts are excreted into the breast milk
- Offer the mother nicotine patches to reduce the risks associated with passive smoking.

Alcohol

- Alcohol passes through the breast milk so drinking during breastfeeding is not recommended
- If the mother insists on drinking, consumption should not exceed one standard drink (10 g) per day and then only after breastfeeding.

Opioids

- Mothers who are stable on methadone maintenance treatment may breastfeed, but those who are unstable should not be encouraged to do so
- The safety of buprenorphine has not yet been established but the amount in breast milk is probably clinically insignificant.

Psychostimulants

- Advise regular and unstable users against breastfeeding
- Inform users of the risks associated with breastfeeding.

Cannabis

- Some cannabis is excreted in the breast milk, but the effects on the infant are unknown.

Further reading

Cook J. (2003). Biochemical markers of alcohol use in pregnant women. *Clin Biochem* 36:9–19.

Finnegan LP. (1991). Treatment issues for opioid dependent women during the perinatal period. *J Psychoactive Drugs* 23:191–201.

Floyd R, O'Connor M, Skol RJ, *et al.* (2005). Recognition and prevention of fetal alcohol syndrome. *Obstet Gynaecol* 106:1059–64.

NSW Department of Health (2006). *National Clinical Guidelines for the Management of Drug Use During Pregnancy, Birth and the Early Development Years of the Newborn.* Sydney: NSW Department of Health. Available at: www.health.nsw.gov.au

Perez-Montejano R, Finch E, Wolff K. (2013) A national survey investigating methadone treatment for pregnant opioid dependent women in England and Wales. *Int J Ment Health Addiction*11(6):693–702.

Fetal alcohol spectrum disorders

Causes

Alcohol consumption during pregnancy can result in adverse child outcomes, including miscarriage, premature birth, stillbirth, and birth abnormalities. The severity and type of condition is related to the amount of maternal alcohol consumption and timing of exposure.

Definitions

Prenatal alcohol exposure (PAE) can cause fetal alcohol spectrum disorders (FASDs). The term FASDs is not a clinical diagnosis, but an umbrella term that covers several categories of disorders resulting from fetal alcohol exposure. These disorders include:

- fetal alcohol syndrome (FAS)
- partial fetal alcohol syndrome (pFAS)
- alcohol-related neurodevelopmental disorder (ARND)—this term is being replaced by:
- neurobehavioral disorder associated with prenatal alcohol exposure (ND-PAE)
- alcohol-related birth defects (ARBDs)
- other neurodevelopmental disorder associated with PAE.

Diagnosis

Fetal alcohol syndrome (FAS) diagnosis is based on:

- Facial dysmorphia (Fig. 24.1):
  - Smooth philtrum
  - Thin vermillion border
  - Small palpebral fissures (≤10th percentile)
- Below average height and/or weight
- CNS abnormalities (IQ is typically low (≤70))
- History of PAE.

If information about PAE is unavailable, FAS is diagnosed if the other three criteria are present. *Diagnosing other FASDs requires a history of PAE.*

Partial FAS (pFAS) is considered when a person with a history of PAE does not meet full diagnostic criteria for FAS, but has some facial features and growth deficits or CNS abnormalities.

Alcohol-related birth defects (ARBDs) are structural birth defects associated with PAE, including cardiac, skeletal, renal, ocular, or auditory system malformations.

Neurobehavioral disorder associated with prenatal alcohol exposure (ND-PAE) was introduced in (DSM-5) as a 'Condition for Further Study' (see Box 24.11).

Diagnosis is based on deficits in the following in individuals with a history of more than minimal PAE:

- Neurocognitive functioning
- Self-regulation
- Adaptive functioning.

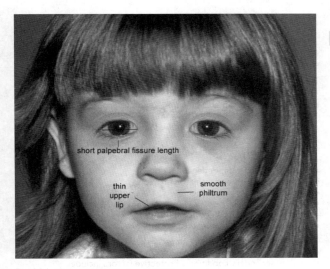

Fig. 24.1 Diagnostic facial features of FAS.

Reproduced from Astley, S.J., *Diagnostic Guide for Fetal Alcohol Spectrum Disorders: The 4-Digit Diagnostic Code*, Third Edition, Copyright (2004), with permission from University of Washington Publication Services.

Box 24.11 Terminology: ND-PAE compared with ARND

The term ND-PAE replaces the term alcohol-related neurodevelopmental disorder (ARND). In the interim, the American Psychiatric Association has recommended the use of the code 315.8 in DSM-5, with the designation of *Neurodevelopmental disorder associated with prenatal alcohol exposure*. This diagnosis applies when a person with a history of PAE has symptoms causing social, occupational, or other impairment that do not meet full criteria for any other disorder in the diagnostic class.

'More than minimal' is defined as maternal alcohol consumption of 1–13 drinks per month, but ≤ 2 drinks per occasion. An ND-PAE diagnosis can be made with or without facial dysmorphia.

Other neurodevelopmental disorders
Patients with other birth defects and genetic conditions, such as Williams' syndrome, may have clinical characteristics similar to FASDs. Careful evaluation is needed to exclude these conditions.

Prevalence

The prevalence of FASDs is estimated to be 2–5% of school-age children in developed countries. Higher rates are reported in populations with high alcohol consumption. FAS is estimated to affect 2–7 per 1000 children in developed countries.

Prognosis and treatment

FASDs are lifelong conditions. The extent of impairment ranges from profound developmental disabilities to subtle problems. Although the impact may be minor in less severe cases, public health significance is magnified by the prevalence of FASDs in the population. Such individuals often develop other conditions:

- Mental health problems
- Conduct disorders
- Alcohol and drug dependence
- Depression or other psychiatric problems
- Disrupted school experience
- Trouble with the law
- Inappropriate sexual behaviour
- Inability to live independently and/or hold a job as adults.

There is no cure for FASDs. With early identification and diagnosis, children can receive services that help maximize their potential and decrease the risk of secondary conditions. Protective factors include:

- diagnosis before age 6
- living in a stable, nurturing home
- not experiencing violence
- receiving special education and social services.

Individuals with FASDs benefit from early interventions, individualized education programmes, preparation for school to work transitions, and continuing services as adults.

Effective prevention depends on knowledgeable physicians and educated women.

Prevention

FASDs are preventable. Any alcohol consumption during pregnancy may increase the risk for FASDs. Women should be educated about the risks of alcohol use during pregnancy and advised to avoid alcohol consumption while pregnant or when conception is possible. Physicians should be trained to implement screening and brief interventions for FASDs prevention.

- There is no safe time to drink during pregnancy.
- There is no known safe amount of alcohol consumption during pregnancy or when trying to conceive.

Further reading

American Academy of Pediatrics. *The Fetal Alcohol Spectrum Disorders (FASD) Toolkit.* Available at: http://www.aap.org/en-us/advocacy-and-policy/aap-health-initiatives/fetal-alcohol-spectrum-disorders-toolkit/

Centers for Disease Control and Prevention (CDC). *National Center on Birth Defects and Developmental Disabilities (NCBDDD).* Available at: http://www.cdc.gov/ncbddd/fasd/index.html

May PA, Gossage JP, Kalberg WO, *et al.* (2009). Prevalence and epidemiologic characteristics of FASD from various research methods with an emphasis on recent in-school studies. *Dev Disabil Res Rev* 15:176–92.

Streissguth AP, Bookstein FL, Barr HM, *et al.* (2004). Risk factors for adverse life outcomes in fetal alcohol syndrome and fetal alcohol effects. *J Dev Behav Pediatr* 25(4):228–38.

The elderly

The subject of substance use in the elderly is important because of the sheer scale of the problem, the morbidity and mortality, and the social impact and costs. By 2020, the prediction is that the proportion of older people (usually defined as over 60 years of age) in the population in the Western world and many Asian countries will reach 25%.

Epidemiology

Since older people are using more substances than in the last two decades, and the numbers of older people are rising, the likelihood is that there will be an increase in the need for treatment.

The 'baby boom' generation (those born between 1946 and 1964), who were the first cohort to use drugs recreationally and dependently, are ageing. This group have had the benefit of improved treatment for substance misuse, but also suffer from a host of medical and psychiatric conditions.

In the UK it is estimated that:
- 13% of men and 12% of women over 60 years of age smoke
- over the last 10 years there has been a 25% increase in the number of older men and a 300% increase in the proportion of older women drinking above recommended daily limits of alcohol
- 25% of care home residents in the US are prescribed a benzodiazepine; 10% are misusing these due to the lack of vigilance about dependence.

'Safe limits'
- There is probably no such thing as a safe limit.
- The recommended limits for adults are very likely not applicable to older people.
- The US NIAAA has recommended that for some older people one US drink (14 g alcohol) a day and no more than seven US drinks per week is sufficient. More than three US drinks a day is considered likely to lead to harm.
- Older people should be advised to eat before drinking, to drink slowly, not to drink and drive, not to use machinery when they have been drinking, and not to swim after drinking.
- For those people with comorbid conditions and on medications, sensible advice might have to be that they do not drink.

Costs
Older people incur greater costs:
- The cost of alcohol-related admissions in England for 55–74-year-olds was more than ten times that for 16–24-year-olds.
- The cost of alcohol-related admission for older men was almost double that for older women.

Distinctive issues in older people

Even if older people continue to use substances in the same way as when they were an adult, the impact may be different. They do not need to use excessive amounts to be affected adversely especially if they are using combinations of substances.

Older people are at greater risk of the impact of substances for the following reasons:

- The development of chronic complex physical and mental health problems.
- As a consequence older people are prescribed medications, often multiple, so that drug interactions are more likely.
- Increased vulnerability due to physiological changes related to the ageing process, e.g. decreased metabolism leads to accumulation and increased brain sensitivity to substances leads to adverse effects.
- Acute confusional states and memory difficulties may lead to consumption.
- Presentation with somatic, mental, and functional impairment not attributable to substance use may lead to worsening of any aspect of health, and even overdose, due to inappropriate prescribing.

The lifespan perspective

Addiction can be a lifelong problem: some people start in their teens and continue relentlessly into older age, for some cessation with resumption is the pattern, whilst others begin when they reach older age.

Risk factors in older age include boredom, isolation, losses associated with retirement, bereavements, disability, comorbid medical conditions, occupation, and ethnic group.

The so-called geriatric giants, i.e. iatrogenesis, immobility, intellectual deterioration, incontinence, and instability, can reflect substance problems.

Assessment

Older people should not be exempt from a thorough physical and psychosocial assessment which should be updated with regularity and this should be recorded.

The details of a substance use assessment have been covered in Chapter 5.

Social factors are central

- Assessment of consent and capacity
- Social vulnerability, e.g. isolation, risk of falls, financial abuse
- Social function: activities of daily living, support from formal and informal carers and family
- Social environment: any change which presents as uncharacteristic behaviour or new symptomatology which is unexplained should be cause for suspicion, e.g. sleep, eating, mood, memory, weight loss, irritability, agitation and escalating doses of prescription drugs
- Evidence of comorbid disorders and their treatment with medication.

Barriers to detection

- Lack of training, stigma, and stereotyping may lead to inability to detect presentations in older people especially if they are atypical.
- Perception of too little time in which to undertake an assessment and lack of confidence in delivering an intervention and knowledge about appropriate referral.

A formal aged care assessment is indicated when:
- further assessment and observation is required
- the patient is deteriorating
- treatment, e.g. withdrawal management or stabilization, cannot take place at home
- needs are complex due to physical, mental, and social problems
- the patient is unable to be cared for at home
- isolation and/or chaotic domestic situation
- the person is unable to function at home
- previous treatment is proving ineffective
- the patient is suicidal.

Pharmacological interventions

Whether to prescribe to a patient who is already on multiple pharmaceuticals

Pharmaceutical interventions should be initiated and prescribed with caution and care. Lower doses are usually appropriate for older people though formularies rarely give specific guidance for older people.

Medications for substance use disorders such as acamprosate, naltrexone, and disulfiram should only be considered if the patient can be monitored by an expert team. A multidisciplinary team comprising an addiction specialist and a geriatrician with their teams should initiate and review treatment. Pharmacological interventions should only be provided if there is a psychosocial package of care in place.

It is a clinical decision requiring experience, expertise, and sometimes even intuition as to whether an additional medication is appropriate for the patient (who may be on a host of other medications). However, it is also imperative that patients should not be denied the benefit of pharmacological agents just on the basis of age. This is sometimes a difficult balance that only those skilled can undertake.

The specific medications should only be prescribed if the patient is dependent and/or in withdrawal, while taking consideration of all other medications they are prescribed and/or have consumed at the same time. Older people may not exhibit the features of dependence as younger people. However, low doses of drug may still impact on them adversely even if they do not present with the symptomatology. Older people and their carers often are not aware of the effects many substances may be having on functioning. Meticulous probing and corroboration with medical professionals and carers and family should be undertaken to ensure that it is safe. Older people are often using analgesics, sedative hypnotics and other substances which may or may not be obtained through legitimate sources (e.g. doctor, pharmacy) or through contacts and the Internet.

Psychological interventions

Most of the research that has been undertaken has been on psychological interventions in older alcohol misusers.

The overall message is positive in that older people achieve comparable outcomes across a variety of domains (social, psychological, physical, legal) as their younger counterparts do: in some cases they may even fare better. Older adults who seek treatment do have the capacity to change, so that there is benefit in proactively seeking and providing treatment.

Implications of substance dependence for retirement facility living

Care home policies should include substance misuse assessment and management in their care plans.

Patients in care homes need to be assessed and regularly monitored. Although alcohol is the most commonly misused drug, there should be a high index of suspicion about ongoing substance use and long-term prescription, e.g. benzodiazepines and opiates.

Residents will be at risk of falls (due to effects of alcohol on muscle tone and balance, and osteoporosis). They will be at risk of interactions with many commonly prescribed medications for older people, e.g. antihistamines, acid-lowering drugs, epilepsy medication, and antibiotics. These interactions with, e.g. alcohol and benzodiazepines, will render them at risk of the development of intoxication whilst withdrawal may manifest as a confusional state or delirium.

Short-term treatment with benzodiazepines can inadvertently merge into long-term dependence as may analgesics. Alcohol may enhance the sedative effects of hypnotics and sedatives as well as antidepressants and antipsychotic medication.

It is the responsibility of the care home staff (both management and professional primary care, physicians and psychiatrists, and their teams) as well as family, friends, and carers to be aware that substance use may have an important bearing on the subsequent stability and treatment of the resident. The collaboration of these professionals is key in monitoring the prescription regimens in the context of the residents' behaviour, symptomatology, and overall management. This might necessitate referral to addiction services so that medication can be safely reduced and lead to positive outcomes.

Further reading

Crome IB, Li TK, Rao R, et al. (2012). Alcohol limits in older people. Addiction 9:1541–3.

Crome IB, Rao T, Tarbuck A, et al. (2011). Our Invisible Addicts: Council. Report 165. London: Royal College of Psychiatrists.

Crome IB Wu L-T Rao T Crome P (eds) (2014). Substance Use and Older People. London: Wiley.

European Monitoring Centre for Drugs and Drug Addiction (2008). Substance use among older adults: a neglected problem. Drugs in Focus 18.

Lingford-Hughes A, Welch S, Peters L, et al. (2012). BAP updated guidelines for the pharmacological management of substance abuse, harmful use, addiction and comorbidity: recommendations from BAP. J Psychopharmacol 26(7):899–952

Moore AA, Blow FC, Hoffing M, et al. (2011). Primary care-based intervention to reduce at-risk drinking in older adults: A randomized controlled trial. Addiction 106(1):111–20.

Moy I, Frisher M, Crome P et al (2011). Systematic review of treatment for older people with substance problems. Eur Geriatr Med 2(4):212–36

Rao T Crome IB. (2011). Substance misuse among care home residents. NRC 13(11):2–4.

US Department of Health and Human Services (1998). Substance Abuse among Older Adults (Treatment Improvement Protocol (TIP) Series No. 26). Washington, DC: US Department of Health and Human Services.

Marginalized populations

The issue of marginalization

People can be marginalized for a variety of reasons—from their sexuality, sexual activity, or drug-taking, to their ethnicity, language, or appearance amongst many things. Being marginalized means a person's perceived social worth is less, and they are often treated accordingly. This matters because marginalized populations face significant barriers in accessing services and receiving good quality treatment and care. They face stigma and discrimination—in some cases their behaviour is classed as illegal, making it harder again to access care. It is harder for them to achieve and to maintain good health, and so unsurprisingly their overall health and well-being is far lower than the general population. This is not because their physiology differs from any other person, but because of the social determinants of their health. According to the WHO, these are the conditions in which people are born, grow, live, work, and age. These circumstances are shaped by the distribution of money, power, and resources at global, national, and local levels. And when working with marginalized clients, these are the things that have often determined the trajectory of their lives.

As a clinical workforce, we must be cognizant of this. We need to consider the early events in someone's life that may have led to their substance use, the high likelihood of previous trauma amongst those who use drugs, and the common coexistence of mental health and substance use issues.

And in understanding this, we must advocate for, and provide, more flexible/appropriate/and non-judgemental health services. We may need to consider outreach services and early or late clinics in alternative locations other than hospitals. We must ensure our services are where they need to be, open during hours that work best for those we seek to see, and have staff that openly welcome all who enter. Consider co-location of services. Consider low literacy resources. We need to design our services to best suit our clients' needs, rather than our own. Include them in the planning if you can.

General considerations when working with marginalized groups

- Be kind, be considerate, and leave your judgement at the door.
- Be honest and open, and acknowledge your own limitations.
- Acknowledge that they will know far more than you about certain details—so ask for their help and advice to improve your understanding.
- Focus on practicalities and on positives. Avoid catastrophizing, no matter how concerned you may be.
- Try and come up with small practical steps, rather than detail how someone might reshape their entire life.
- Take things slowly—trust takes time, and you need trust to develop a therapeutic relationship.

The following sections set out some considerations for special groups.

Sex workers

- Sex workers have *lower* rates of STIs than the general population. It is good to acknowledge this.
- There are many people who undertake sex work voluntarily, as well as those who do so less voluntarily (e.g. in order to fund their drug dependence). We should work respectively and sensitively with both.
- Sex workers may need a certificate for their workplace to state they have been screened for STIs. Work with them to provide them with what they need and acknowledge the positives in what they are doing.
- It is useful to know the context of a person's sex work as risk may vary enormously. A person working from the street, for example, may be at higher risk of personal violence and sexual assault compared to someone working from a well-supported and regulated brothel. A person sex working to support their drug dependence may be more likely to engage in unsafe sex in order to make money more quickly. And a sex worker using drugs with a client together may lead riskier practices and unsafe sex due to disinhibited behaviour.
- It is useful to know that sometimes condom use may be how a sex worker distinguishes between their sexual practices at work and at home. So there are many sex workers who would use condoms 100% for work, but not necessarily with their partner/s. It is important when taking a sexual history to determine risk of STIs to ask about both.
- Don't forget about contraception, as well as STI risk.

At-risk youth

- It is essential to understand mandatory reporting considerations, as legislation may differ in different countries or jurisdictions.
- It can be helpful to acknowledge that you may not know the young people's 'lingo'. Ask them what they mean if you don't understand. Most people like to feel helpful and knowledgeable and will be willing to teach you if you ask respectfully.

Homeless

- On average, people who are homeless and street based die about 20 years earlier, and have a physical 'age' of someone 20 years older.
- It is important to consider practicalities. They may have nowhere to store any medications, no access to refrigeration, and limited or no access to running water. Depending on the situation and their needs, be prepared to think outside the box. Can you see them each day? Can you store medications for them? Can someone else?

Sexual identity and sexual behaviour

- Do not assume that how someone identifies in terms of their sexuality (e.g. homosexual, heterosexual, bisexual) necessarily determines their sexual practices. A man who considers himself heterosexual may still have sex with men. A gay woman may have sex with men in the context of sex work. Be clear when asking about specific behaviour, without judgement and without assumptions.

- With sexual identify, it can be helpful to simply ask 'Do you prefer to have sex with men, women, both, or neither?'
- And when asking about actual sexual practices, it can be helpful to introduce it by saying 'In order to work out any risks, I need to ask about all sexual contact you have had, no matter who it was with, when, where, or how. So that includes regular partners, casual partners, paid sex work, and everything in between. Is it OK if I ask about this?'.
- And to accurately determine clinical risk of STIs and/or HIV/AIDS, you will need to know details. Among men who have sex with men, for example, you need to ask about anal intercourse, and get the details as to insertive/receptive and with/without condoms or any broken condoms. Be open and ask/acknowledge your own limitations if need be.
- If you are embarrassed, they are more likely to be. If you can be matter of fact, they are more likely to be.

People who inject drugs

- Remember that their priorities may not be your own. Ask them what it is that you can help with, and focus on what they want/need.
- Always ask not only what people are using, but where they are using. Ask to inspect injection sites if they consent.
- Are they interested in reducing/stopping? Would they like your help with that? And if they are not ready/willing/able to consider ceasing their drug use, be prepared to offer harm reduction messages instead.
- Avoid scaremongering. Instead of 'You are going to die if you don't get treatment for that' consider reframing and focus on solutions. 'I can hear you're worried about this, despite everything that is going on for you right now, and I know you would like to get some treatment. How can I best help you with that?'
- Know something about filtering, and how/where they may access wheel filters if they are interested.
- Remember other practical interventions—hepatitis B vaccination, for example, or take-home naloxone.

Substance use in different cultural contexts

Cultural issues in clinical practice

In many countries, patients with alcohol or substance use disorders have diverse cultural and linguistic backgrounds with differences in practices and beliefs. Socioeconomic factors, living conditions, physical environments, and access to education and healthcare affect people's use of alcohol and/or other substances and subsequent problems. Effective communication is important in understanding and managing these, and clinicians need to be aware of the specific factors that have an impact on patients and their families.

Types of substance used

Some substances are only used or popular in particular areas; often these are local plants or herbal mixtures, e.g. kratom (*Mitragyna speciosa*—a plant with mild narcotic properties), kava, and coca leaves. Some of these substances were used traditionally by local people long before becoming modern substances of abuse. For instance, kratom was used by rural people in southern Thailand as an energizer for hard work and medicine for several illnesses for over a hundred years. It has now become a substance commonly abused by youths in a mixture with other addictive substances, e.g. benzodiazepines and codeine cough syrup. Kava (*Piper methysticum*) is used in the Pacific in the form of a traditional herbal drink to welcome guests at important sociopolitical events. It has been abused in other places as the kavalactones in it can produce euphoria and relaxation.

The use and misuse of drugs have escalated with newly emerging and re-emerging substances coming on to the market. Some substances are used to cause 'legal highs' in some countries or states but are illegal in others. A wide range of unregulated products can now be developed quickly; these include herbal mixtures and synthetic designer drugs, frequently with concealed ingredients, often aggressively advertised and marketed over the Internet and sold in specialty shops as incense, room odourizers, plant food, bath salts, or research chemicals.

Due to innovative marketing and rapidly changing compositions, suppliers can circumvent regulations. In some jurisdictions these drugs, despite being similar in structure to prohibited drugs, are traded regardless of the drug's legal status; in others they are grey market goods. Examples include 'Spice' (herbal mixtures laced with synthetic cannabinoids) and 'bath salts' (mephedrone, amphetamines, and cathinones). When there is a scarcity of some drug, a new or modified kind of abuse emerges, such as the use of 'krokodil'—a 'flesh-eating' mixture made by cooking crushed codeine pills with household chemicals, which allegedly has effects like those of heroin. It was first produced in Russia when a scarcity of heroin and abundance of over-the-counter codeine fuelled a pandemic peaking in 2011. Various street names of the substances are known only to people from the same community. Clinicians should be knowledgeable about the common types and patterns of alcohol or substance use in their community and use this information in their assessment of patients.

Quantification of alcohol or drug intake

Many cultural influences make the quantification of substance intake difficult. People in many countries are unfamiliar with a standard unit of alcohol and may not use a standard-sized container to drink it. In some situations drinkers share a container when they drink together in a closed group. The use of other substances, such as cannabis and heroin, may also be difficult to quantify as users often report the amount they consume in the unit familiar to their community or share the substance from the same container. Some users mix together two or three different substances.

To obtain the best estimate of the quantity of substance used, the clinician needs to inquire about the method of administration, size of the container used, street names of the substances and 'units', form of the substance—leaf, liquid, pill, or powder—and places or situations where they are used. Asking how many people share the supply (e.g. a bottle of wine), the frequency of drinking (e.g. payday only or daily), how much money the person spends on the substance each day, and number of associates in the drinking group are also helpful in assessing the amount consumed and risk of complications.

Social attitudes and norms

Substance use is a matter of public concern and debate worldwide because of its negative and often tragic associations and there is high-profile media coverage of substance-related issues. Substance use is a part of normal life and support for legalizing some drugs, e.g. cannabis and Ecstasy, and harm reduction varies between countries and shifts over time. In this digital era where online social networking is a key part of everyday life and transportation systems are good, forms of drug trade and epidemic have changed and cross-border drug-related activities are common. The spread of the 'drug culture' and increasingly tolerant attitudes—at least towards cannabis—occur worldwide. They affect how people in a society admit or deny drug use when asked in a clinical or non-clinical setting.

Indigenous people may be at increased risk of substance- and alcohol-related problems because they are marginalized and at a social disadvantage. They may also face barriers when accessing mainstream services for help, as a result of which they present late for treatment. This may occur because most services are designed for and by the majority cultural groups or because of unawareness of services available. Thus, active detection of substance-related problems is important to improve access to indigenous-specific and other treatment services. Increased cultural sensitivity in mainstream services is needed. Partnership between these services and indigenous health professionals, services and communities increases the chance of achieving reduction in substance-related problems both at individual and community levels.

Beliefs about the causes of substance use

The perception of causes or explanatory models of illnesses differ among ethnic groups. In more highly educated societies, people are more likely to understand the bio-psycho-social model of substance use and accept substance dependence as a disorder of the brain. However, some cultures regard alcohol or substance use as a moral issue. Substance dependence is believed to reflect disadvantages associated with people's backgrounds (which include poverty and mental illness) or to result primarily from individual decisions and choice.

Failure to control the use of substances may be viewed as moral inadequacy or weakness of mind and modern treatments may be considered inappropriate. As stigmatization is very strong in some cultures the need for treatment, especially long-term treatment, may be interpreted as an index of severity, leading to poor compliance with treatment. Symptoms such as tremor and sweating due to alcohol withdrawal or stimulant-induced psychosis may be thought due to breaking a taboo or being possessed by a spirit.

It is helpful for the healthcare team to adopt an educational approach, discussing bio-psycho-social aspects in simple terms and explaining pathological patterns of dependence, including the repeated desire to cut down, the prolonged use of substances and taking larger amounts than intended as behavioural symptoms of a disorder and not as a moral weakness. Pharmacotherapy and psychosocial intervention should be explained as means of relieving troublesome symptoms, but responsibility for change should always remain with the patients, with the success of treatment being largely theirs.

Taboo and stigmatization

Alcohol and substance use is taboo in some cultures, families, or religions. In many Muslim countries, alcohol consumption is strictly prohibited. In Buddhism, lay people are taught to conform to the Five Precepts, the fifth of which is to refrain from using distilled or fermented intoxicants, including alcohol, tobacco, and other addictive substances, which often lead to undesirable behaviour. In some countries it is thought that alcohol use is acceptable 'macho' behaviour, while stigma is attached to drinking by women.

Many people believe that substance misuse is a problem of other people or of those from other ethnic communities and cannot accept that it is also their own problem. People may therefore be too embarrassed to report that they or their relatives need help. They may also feel ashamed that they will be judged as a bad person or even a criminal. Responses to questions may depend on social attitudes, and marital or family problems resulting from drinking may be kept secret, with women being taught not to discuss the problems outside the family. Clinicians need to recognize that people from all communities use substances, licit or illicit, and anyone can experience harm due to intoxication, overdose, or dependence. It is important to find the most comfortable way to help people to talk about their alcohol or substance use and related issues.

Communication and treatment issues

- It is important to assess whether patients' symptoms are culturally normal or abnormal. Someone may spend a long time in a drinking group in a community where the alcoholic beverage is consumed from the same container until the supply is depleted, yet an individual within the group drinks little. Therefore, when asking if he/she spends a lot of time drinking, gets intoxicated, or has hangovers, he/she may give an affirmative answer leading to a mistake in diagnosis.
- Clinicians may have difficulty exploring symptoms which are culturally specific when they are unfamiliar with the patterns of behaviour within a particular social group. In small, closed communities, where people know each other's business and are unconfident about assurances of confidentiality, patients may not admit to substance use. In addition, people who find it hard to disappoint or hurt others may give over-obliging, favourable responses to therapists or fail to disclose their lack of adherence to medication.
- In traditional Asian cultures, families are largely close-knit and extended and the family plays a very important part in daily living and a patient's decision to seek and/or take treatment as recommended. Information from family members about a patient's substance use and its consequences may sometimes be more reliable than information from the patient him/herself. Such information may be the sole source, particularly in those intoxicated, having severe withdrawal symptoms, or otherwise disturbed. If clinicians and the treatment team are sensitive to the importance of the family and can communicate with them directly, this will help the patient to remain engaged in treatment and reduce the risk of relapse. However, some may not want their family to know that they use a substance, and their wishes should be ascertained before contacting them.
- It is necessary for a clinician to be sensitive to and acknowledge the cultural factors that determine the patient's disorder, and at the same time understand and respect their right to adhere to their cultural beliefs and practices, in order to assess and treat them effectively.

Further reading

Center for Substance Abuse Treatment (2009). Substance abuse among specific population groups and settings. In *Substance Abuse Treatment: Addressing the Specific Needs of Women*. Treatment Improvement Protocol (TIP) Series, No. 51. Rockville (MD): Substance Abuse and Mental Health Services Administration (US). Available at: http://www.ncbi.nlm.nih.gov/books/NBK83240/

National Institute on Drug Abuse, National Institue of Health (2003). *Drug Use Among Racial/Ethnic Minorities – Revised*. Bethesda, MD: US Department of Health and Human Services, National Institutes of Health, National Institute on Drug Abuse.

Indigenous peoples

Indigenous peoples are those who have inhabited a land for thousands of years as distinct from those who have lived there only a few hundred years. They typically have a strong concept of unification of people with the natural world. Each has a distinct culture, spirituality, and traditions, and many speak a distinct language or languages.

Indigenous peoples include Aboriginal and Torres Strait Islander Australians, Māori (or 'Tangata Whenua'—'people of the land') in New Zealand, First Nations in North America and Canada (including Indian, Métis, and Inuit) among many others.

Risk factors for substance use disorders

In some countries, the indigenous people form the largest population group and hold power (such as in Fiji). However, in many countries indigenous populations have been subject to colonization, and have become economically and socially disadvantaged. In such countries indigenous peoples have typically faced considerable challenges across many generations through loss of individuals' identification with their culture, disempowerment, loss of land, lack of access to quality education, employment, and wealth, as well as challenges to traditional sense of worth, law and identity. All of these factors predispose to increased risk of both substance use disorders and mental health disorders.

Specific factors which contributed to increased risks include:

- The introduction of new, stronger, and readily available psychoactive substances at the time of colonization, in the context of threats to community values and authority.
- Indigenous peoples were encouraged or forced to leave their traditional land in several countries for a time, e.g. Australia, US and Canada. Instead the peoples lived in defined communities, often in mission settlements.
- Enforced removal of children from their parents occurred in some cases, with the intention of hastening assimilation into the mainstream. In some areas this practice occurred as recently as the 1960s.
- Childhood separation, loss of sense of identity, and in some cases exposure to physical or sexual abuse within institutions have often left psychological scars that may include anxiety, depression, and post-traumatic stress disorder. These mental health disorders further predispose to substance use disorders.
- Some Indigenous adults then face major challenges bringing up their own children, having had limited opportunity to observe parenting skills. This can result in transgenerational transmission of substance use and mental health disorders.
- Other historical factors (e.g. payment or rations provided in the form of alcohol or cigarettes) contributed to normalization of episodic heavy drinking or smoking in some communities.
- There has been considerable speculation that genetic influences may explain an increased risk of substance use disorders, however for most indigenous peoples (e.g. Aboriginal and Torres Strait Islander Australians) this theory has never been tested, and there are ample social stressors to explain the increased risk.

Prevalence and impact of substance use disorders

- Data on the prevalence of substance use disorders in Indigenous communities is often limited.
- Available studies generally show higher rates of abstinence from alcohol, but among those who do drink, higher rates of unhealthy drinking. For example, Māori are more likely to be non-drinkers than are other New Zealanders, but drink 40% more on average per drinking occasion.
- Smoking rates in Indigenous communities are typically double that of the non-indigenous population in the same country.
- There may be a higher prevalence of cannabis and other illicit substance use. Some Aboriginal and Torres Strait Islander communities, in Northern Australia, report significant problems from cannabis, including high financial outlays, psychiatric complications, and stress or even violence when cannabis is not available.
- There may be higher prevalence of solvent misuse, including glue and paint sniffing in urban settings, and petrol sniffing, particularly in rural and remote regions.
- Prevalence of injecting drug use and of sharing of injecting equipment can be higher (e.g. among Indigenous Australians), with associated increased risk of blood-borne viruses.

Other health disorders and substance use

In disadvantaged indigenous communities there can be a high prevalence of physical disease. For example, Aboriginal and Torres Strait Islander communities in Australia often have a high prevalence of diabetes, renal failure, and rheumatic heart disease.

- The distress of disease and of recurrent premature deaths in the community may be a trigger to substance use.
- Alcohol or drug use may impact significantly on the ability of the individual to manage their own chronic disease.
- Alcohol use may complicate the course of a comorbid disease. For example, acute alcohol consumption may precipitate hypoglycaemia in a person taking hypoglycaemic medication, while chronic heavy consumption may increase insulin resistance. Unhealthy alcohol use combined with obesity and/or viral hepatitis can greatly increase the risk of liver disease.
- Any experience of alcohol withdrawal may be more severe in persons with multiple medical disorders.
- Any pharmacotherapy suggested for alcohol dependence needs to selected with an understanding of the challenges the individual will face with adherence if they are living in a stressful setting or overcrowded housing. For example, once-a-day naltrexone may be more suitable than a three-times-daily acamprosate regimen. In carefully selected and informed individuals, disulfiram may be possible, though chronic disease may make that medication too risky in others.

Treatment for indigenous persons with substance misuse

The concept of 'cultural competence' describes the set of attitudes, knowledge, and skills that allow the healthcare professional to care effectively for a person from another culture (see p. 526 on cross-cultural care). This typically incorporates not only awareness of and respect for the culture of the patient, but also awareness of the clinician's own culture and how it can affect their approach. The ability to develop relationships that engender trust and respect is critical (see Box 24.12).

Communication with indigenous clients can be assisted by the following:

- Taking ample time for effective communication
- Introducing yourself as a person, and starting to get to know the patient you are talking with as an individual
- Bringing no preconceptions with you
- Willingness to learn about the patient's culture and environment
- An awareness that one's own culture influences one's beliefs and interactions
- Indigenous health professionals or clinical aides can typically enhance the quality of communication and engagement, and help ensure a welcoming and culturally comfortable environment
- Where language differences impair communication, quality translation is essential.
- In a clinical assessment, a less structured conversation which allows the patient to tell their story can be more effective in history taking and engagement than a series of directed questions. This can be followed up by 'filling in the gaps' with more structured questions, linking this in with the story you have already heard.
- A holistic approach to medical, psychological and social needs is recommended.

In providing counselling or support, it is particularly important to consider culturally appropriate forms of communication and the home,

---

Box 24.12 Developing relationships

Some indigenous communities may have fundamental differences from European cultures in basic concepts, such as:

- time
- cause and effect
- individualism
- systems of logic and reasoning
- modes of polite communication—in some cultures, a series of direct questions can be perceived as disrespectful interrogation
- responsibilities: responsibility to family and community are particularly important, and can outweigh commitments to attending a medical appointment

Seeking advice and support from an Indigenous person from that community is of great assistance. Where available, an Indigenous health professional can greatly improve the quality of communication.

family, and community context. Extended family and kinship or community ties, and responsibilities can be particularly strong. These ties can bring both challenges and resources. If close kin are also problem drinkers, it can be challenging for a dependent drinker to avoid cues to drinking. On the other hand, non-drinking relatives may provide great support. The patient may wish to involve family in the treatment process.

Traditional or community-controlled treatment approaches

Indigenous peoples have their own cultural beliefs regarding health and treating sickness, which must be acknowledged and respected. In some indigenous communities, specific traditional approaches to healing have been utilized in treatment of substance use disorders.

Efforts need to be made to ensure that treatment respects the patient's culture, but also includes access to the full range of modern therapies, including relapse prevention medicines for alcohol dependence, or opioid maintenance pharmacotherapies (see Box 24.13). Explaining the role of modern medicines clearly is important.

In many countries health services run by indigenous communities provide a highly accessible alternative to mainstream services or work in collaboration with mainstream services.

The patient in the context of the community

At times, whole communities may be seriously affected by unhealthy alcohol or drug use. This tends to normalize risky substance use, and also provides a traumatic or difficult environment for children and adults alike. In communities such as these, where an individual seeks to stop substance use they can face immense challenges, with constant cue exposure, e.g. to cigarettes or episodic heavy drinking. Considerable leadership and strength has often been shown by communities which have effectively made changes in these circumstances. Support of community-driven efforts to address substance use is likely to increase the chance of success of any one individual who is seeking to address their substance use.

Box 24.13 Principles for improving a treatment service for indigenous peoples

- Consultation with indigenous community representatives—to identify and address any barriers to treatment access
- Partnership and consultation with indigenous-controlled services where available
- Cultural awareness training
- Employment of indigenous staff, including translators where necessary, and their involvement in service planning and delivery
- Particular attention to a friendly, welcoming, flexible atmosphere
- A visually appealing service and printed materials
- Healthcare that integrates services for mental, physical, psychological, and social needs as far as possible
- Keeping in mind the individual as part of the family, extended kinship, and community.

Some remote indigenous communities affected by widespread unhealthy alcohol use have successfully sought out a range of supply controls, including:
- regional alcohol bans
- restrictions to the amount or time, or location of alcohol sales
- restriction of sales to low alcohol beer
- a system of individual permits to buy alcohol, where a permit is lost in the case of alcohol-related violence.

These measures, which are sometimes opposed by the alcohol industry, have had documented success. They are often combined with opportunities for community development.

In efforts to reduce petrol sniffing (volatile substance misuse) in Australia, good results have been obtained by supply control, with the switch of whole regions to non-sniffable fuel. This has been successfully combined with increased opportunities for young people and for general community members.

It is important that services and health professionals work in partnership with indigenous communities to ensure that solutions are relevant, appropriate and likely to be successful.

Further reading

Gray D, Saggers S, Sputore B, et al. (2000). What works? A review of evaluated alcohol misuse interventions among Aboriginal Australians. *Addiction* 95:11–22.

Kirmayer LJ, Brass GM, Tait CL. (2000). The mental health of Aboriginal peoples: transformations of identity and community. *Can J Psychiatry* 45:607–16.

Saggers S, Gray D (eds) (1998). *Dealing with Alcohol: Indigenous Usage in Australia, New Zealand and Canada.* Cambridge: Cambridge University Press.

Immigrants and refugees

The prevalence and patterns of substance use and mental disorders among immigrant and refugee groups is highly variable. Immigrant status, in itself, is not associated with either increased or decreased risk for substance-related or mental health disorders. However, among groups most vulnerable to the development of substance and mental health problems are refugees and asylum seekers.

It is the *specific circumstances* of pre-migration experience, migration, and settlement that are important in influencing risk for mental disorder.

Risk factors among immigrants and refugees

- Traumatic experiences or prolonged stress prior to or during migration
- Being adolescent or elderly at the time of migration
- Separation from family
- Inability to speak the language of the host country
- Prejudice and discrimination in the receiving society
- Low socioeconomic status and, particularly, a drop in personal socioeconomic status following migration
- Non-recognition of occupational qualifications
- Isolation from persons of a similar cultural background
- Extent of acculturation.

The global picture

To longstanding patterns of migration for economic and family reasons have been added mass movements of people because of persecution, civil war, and conflict.

Instability in the Middle East, Africa, and Central America has been a primary reason for the shifting flows of the displaced around the world in recent years. Economic reasons are also still motivating those fleeing parts of Central America and Africa.

The changing pattern of war means that the nature of displacement is very different from previous eras. It has shifted from pitting countries against each other to warring factions vying for control within countries, often with weapons and gunmen and combatants from abroad (e.g. Syria).

This means the likely needs of displaced persons are different.

Origins and destinations for migrants and asylum seekers

- The biggest group of asylum seekers in recent years has come from Afghanistan, followed by those from Pakistan and Iran, which have hosted large numbers of refugees from a succession of wars in Afghanistan in recent decades.
- In 2014, the largest group are Syrians fleeing more than 3 years of civil war (to Egypt, Jordan, and Lebanon mainly).
- Other main sources of asylum seekers are Iraq, Eritrea, Sudan, Gaza, Libya, Ukraine, and Somalia.

- The most sought-after destinations are Europe (Germany, Sweden, France, and Italy), North America parts of the Asia Pacific, and Turkey, Egypt, Jordan, and Lebanon.
- Increasing proportion of asylum seekers applying to the US are from Mexico and Central America, escaping drug cartel and organized crime violence.
- China remains a main country of origin for those seeking asylum in the US—as per previous years.
- The recent surge of migration from Central America (El Salvador, Honduras, Guatemala) to the US, increasing numbers are women and children. More than 50,000 *unaccompanied minors* crossed illegally into the US from October 2013 to June 2014—a record.
- Of the total number of people forcibly displaced from their own countries, about *half are children*.

Internally displaced groups

- There are now many displaced people who live in their own countries.
- Syrians today make up the single largest group of internally displaced persons, with 6.5 million displaced within the country by the end of 2013.
- In Colombia, although rebellion is waning, 5.4 million remain displaced, and another 3 million in the Democratic Republic of the Congo.

Epidemiology

Studies of the epidemiology of substance use disorders in immigrant receiving countries show no overall difference in the prevalence of sub-stance use disorders compared with the 'home' population. However, there is great variation between immigrant groups, which reflects:

- the variation in the demographic, cultural, and migration profiles of the groups being studied
- the wide variation in national health service, social support, and legal systems
- the significant methodological and practical challenges to carrying out high quality research in immigrant and refugee communities.

The patterns of alcohol use tend to reflect patterns in the home coun-tries of immigrants. To a significant extent this is also the situation with injecting drug use, although the rates of drug use in some young immi-grant and second-generation groups is of great concern.

Socioeconomic position and cultural dislocation are important con-tributors. Co-morbidity is very common, with causality operating in both directions. The presence of a mental disorder increases the risk of alcohol and other forms of drug abuse and dependence, and the pres-ence of drug use disorder increases the incidence of mental disorder, particularly mood disorders, most commonly depression and anxiety.

Accessing treatment and prevention services

A consistent finding in English-speaking countries with large immigrant populations is *lower levels of utilization of mental health services* by immigrant communities, although there is wide variation. It is not known whether this is due to lower prevalence of mental disorder among these communities or whether the lower rates of service use may be explained by factors such as:

- conceptions of mental health and illness that do not accord with mainstream views
- higher levels of stigma associated with using mental health services, perceptions of inappropriateness of services
- a lack of awareness of what services are available.

There is little information on whether the quality of treatment outcomes for immigrant and refugee patients is the same or different to that of majority communities. The existence of culturally appropriate treatment and prevention services for mental and substance use disorders is the exception rather than the rule.

Where such services do exist they are almost never rigorously evaluated. In most countries, mental health services and drug and alcohol services are separately administered. Given the very high rates of co-morbidity this is generally an unsatisfactory situation. Mental health services are usually not competent to treat drug and alcohol problems, and drug and alcohol services are generally not competent to treat mental disorders. People with both types of problems bounce around between services and, more often than not, receive poor quality care.

There is increasing recognition of this system-level problem and attempts to integrate mental health and drug and alcohol services are becoming more common, as is the recognition that mental health clinicians require at least basic training in skills relevant to drugs and alcohol, and drug and alcohol clinicians require basic mental health competencies.

All clinicians require additional training in effective cross-cultural clinical practice, and health services require assistance in developing effective models of service delivery to cultural minority groups.

Immigrant diversity: a policy challenge

In some countries with a long history of permanent immigrant settlement, there is generally a policy framework that recognizes the cultural and linguistic diversity of populations, and the responsibility of services (variably, and never fully, discharged) to respond effectively to this reality of diversity.

However, in countries that have become immigrant-receiving countries only in recent decades there is generally both a lack of epidemiological and other necessary information, and little in the way of policy and practical service response to diversity.

There is much to be learnt about:

- the hundreds of millions of internal, rural to urban, migrants in China, India, Indonesia, Brazil, and other countries
- temporary labour migrants, most commonly women and almost entirely from poor countries

- the large numbers of trafficked women
- tens of millions of international students
- huge numbers of illegal migrants living in countries without the benefits of permanent residency or citizenship and in constant danger of imprisonment and deportation.

These less visible and under-researched groups are likely to be most at risk of developing mental and substance use disorders, and are least likely to have access to effective services.

Prison inmates

Introduction and epidemiology

The prison environment is unique and challenging. The dominant culture is one of control, and healthcare services often sit uncomfortably within this. There is, furthermore, a nexus of antisocial behaviour, personality disorder, disadvantage, mental health disorders, physical illness, infectious diseases, risky sexual behaviour, and substance use that poses huge health risks to inmates. Box 24.14 offers a snapshot of a sample prison population in New South Wales (NSW), Australia.

The rate of incarceration throughout the world varies from 29 per 100,000 adults in Liechtenstein to 750 per 100,000 adults in the US. The variability in incarceration is strongly linked to drug-law policies (the so-called War on Drugs), and to health and social welfare indicators linked to poverty, social dislocation, and disrupted relationships. A high proportion of prisoners have a history of alcohol or drug misuse.

Psychiatric comorbidity

Individuals who misuse drugs disproportionately suffer from mental disorders. Either condition can precipitate non-compliance with treatment and this, in turn, strongly predicts interaction with the criminal justice system. Some prisoners also have adult ADHD which is often primary to their addiction. The appropriate treatment of this (e.g. methylphenidate) has been shown to be useful among prisoners.

Drugs and crime

The following crime classification has been developed to provide the criminal justice sector a health paradigm for the interactions between substance misuse and crime:

- Psychopharmacological crimes: crimes committed under the influence of a psychoactive substance, as a consequence of its acute or chronic use
- Economic-compulsive crimes: crimes committed in order to obtain the means to support drug use

---

Box 24.14 A snapshot of substance use in the NSW prison population

- Approximately half of male and female prisoners drank in the harmful range (by AUDIT score) immediately prior to coming into prison.
- In 2009, 84% of prisoners had used at least one illegal drug at some time prior to incarceration.
- Over 40% of prisoners continue to use illicit drugs while in prison.
- One-third of females and one-fifth of males inject drugs while in prison.
- Of those who inject, 70% share injecting equipment.
- An estimated 1 in 30 prisoners inject for the first time while in prison.

(Data from New South Wales Inmate Health Survey, 2009.)

- Systemic crimes: crimes committed within illicit drug markets—drug supply, distribution, and abuse
- Drug law offences: crimes committed in violation of drug and other related legislations.

Avoiding imprisonment

Attempts to re-engage clients with substance use disorders with community health and welfare services, through low-level courts, is the subject of a number of diversion programmes being trialled in different jurisdictions. 'Drug Courts' are just one example.

Prevention of drug and alcohol use in prisons

Alcohol

Controlled in prison reasonably well, as the quantities required make it difficult to conceal, and easy to detect. Also, because of the disinhibitory effects of alcohol, with consequent disruption to a closed and overcrowded community, tolerance by both custodial authorities and inmates is low, and when tolerated, short-lived.

Other drugs

Supply is constrained through regulation and physical barriers, but the success of supply reduction has never been supported with evidence. Random urine testing of prisoners confirms that drugs, licit and illicit, available in the community, are being brought through to prisoners—either through corrupt staff or contractors, or by coercion of families and friends.

Diversion of prescribed medications is minimized through supervision of medications by health service staff. Custodial staff have an important ancillary role to play, but non-compliance and diversion will always be threats to a prescribing service in the prison.

Management of drug and alcohol use in prisoners

Incarceration may result in:
- catastrophic interruption of substance use (transfer to a coercive, non-therapeutic environment)
- continuation of interrupted therapeutic associations
- an opportunity to address substance use in a relatively controlled environment (particularly polydrug misuse).

Prison-based opioid pharmacotherapy programmes are available in some countries and states but not others. The may include:
- maintenance—some systems impose low fixed-dose regimens, while others restrict the particular correctional centres that 'allow' opioid pharmacotherapies through the prison classification system
- reduction—clients from community programmes are withdrawn from their treatment, in a non-consensual manner
- enforced withdrawal—in jurisdictions where no opioid pharmacotherapies are sanctioned.

Harm reduction
- Harm reduction in the prison environment, despite extreme risks of blood-borne virus transmission often receives inadequate attention.
- Undue priority is given to supply reduction (e.g. surveillance, interdiction).
- Demand reduction—psychological approaches are favoured by custodial authorities; therapeutic approaches are constrained; limited number of prison-based therapeutic communities; most experience is with methadone, and little with buprenorphine or naltrexone.
- Harm reduction is limited to immunization programmes and rarely extends to education about bleach and making bleach available for cleaning injecting equipment. Outside of 11 countries worldwide, there is no access to regulated exchange of injecting equipment.

Management of psychiatric comorbidity
Imprisonment may provide an opportunity for management of psychiatric co-morbidity including sometimes undiagnosed primary psychiatric conditions.

Transition to the community
The period immediately after release from prison is a *very dangerous one*. Often tolerance to drugs such as opioids or benzodiazepines is reduced due to enforced abstinence, but the desire to use a substance is high. Australian male prisoners were nearly four times more likely to die soon after release than their non-incarcerated peers, and women on release from prison were nearly eight times more likely to die. Drug-related causes of death were the most common.

Efforts to reduce post-release mortality include education, offering increased doses of opioid maintenance pharmacotherapy just prior to release, and ensuring a smooth transition to community-based treatment and support services.

Summary
Despite some improvements in recent years, there remains an overwhelming need for enhanced responses to mental health and substance use disorders for people who are or have been in prison. The inconsistencies between prison systems, and sometimes even within the system, make the transition from community to prison and back to community difficult for service providers, and dangerous for clients.

Further reading
European Monitoring Centre for Drugs and Drug Addiction (2007). Drugs in Focus: Drugs and Crime—a complex relationship. Lisbon: EMCDDA. Available at: http://www.emcdda.europa.eu/attachements.cfm/att_33064_EN_2007_2721_EN_WEB.pdf

Larney S, Kopinski H, Beckwith CG, *et al.* (2013). Incidence and prevalence of hepatitis C in prisons and other closed settings: results of a systematic review and meta-analysis. *Hepatology* 58:1215–24.

Zlodre J, Fazel S. (2012). All-cause and external mortality in released prisoners: systematic review and meta-analysis. *Am J Public Health* 102:e67–75.

The impaired health professional

Approximately 10–15% of all healthcare professionals will misuse drugs or alcohol at some time during their career. Though recent studies suggest that the prevalence is similar to the general population, given their level of responsibility, any impairment could potentially place patients at risk. Drug-dependent health professionals represent a specific subtype of drug misuser, given their access to licit drugs, particularly opioids, sedatives, and tranquillizers.

While risk factors for substance use disorders are similar to those for the general population, health professionals have additional risk factors related to their chosen profession. These include the relative ease of access to a range of prescription medications, as well as the stressors commonly encountered in clinical practice (Table 24.4).

Dealing with an addicted colleague

Recognition of warning signs is an important step in dealing with an addicted colleague (see Table 24.5). Once a problem is identified, there are many barriers to receiving treatment. The impaired practitioner will often rationalize, deny, and minimize their problem. They may fear being stigmatized, ostracized, and deregistered. Others are often reluctant to confront or deal with warning signs, fearing unpleasant consequences for their colleague (loss of livelihood and reputation) and themselves (time-consuming investigations, legal repercussions, loss of collegiality). Take the following steps:

- Seek advice from senior colleagues/health advisory services
- Arrange a time to meet privately with the colleague of concern
- Inform them that you are concerned and why
- Ask them to consult an appropriate doctor, provide relevant contact information, and follow-up to ensure advice is take.

Table 24.4 Risk factors for substance misuse

Vulnerable individual	Family history of mental illness, substance misuse
	Adverse childhood experiences
	History of mental illness, physical illness, pain
	Marital discord; poor support networks
	Poor coping skills with stress
	Personality factors e.g. perfectionistic, obsessional, self-sacrificing, ambitious, rigid, difficulties with emotional expression
Drug factors	No treating GP; prone to self-medication
	Ready availability e.g. opioids, benzodiazepines, anaesthetic agents, other sedatives
Occupational factors	Overwork, sleep deprivation
	Impaired work–life balance
	Exposure to trauma and death
	Treatment failures; medico-legal concerns
	Inadequate resources and support
	Ethical and diagnostic dilemmas

Table 24.5 Warning signs of substance misuse at work

Clinical performance	Appearance and behaviour
Increased sick days	Dishevelled appearance
Reduced efficiency and decisiveness	Change of mood, personality
Patient complaints, e.g. poor analgesia	Unexplained loss of consciousness
Inappropriate prescribing	Smells of alcohol at work
Overt evidence of drug use—ampoules, syringes, pills	Evidence of drug use—track marks, drowsy, tremulous, ataxic
Filling patient's prescriptions	

Notification to regulatory authorities

Consideration should be given to making a formal notification to the appropriate regulatory authorities where there are concerns that the health professional:

- has practised the profession while intoxicated or otherwise affected by alcohol or drugs
- has placed or may place patients at risk of harm during their practice (a) because of a substantial departure from expected professional standards due to substance use (b) because of impairment from substance use.

Reporting obligations vary across different jurisdictions, and health practitioners should consult their local regulatory authorities to determine if reporting is mandatory or not. Even without mandatory reporting, health professionals often have an ethical and professional responsibility to report behaviour of concern. Impaired colleagues should also be encouraged to self-notify.

Effective health programmes for impaired practitioners have high success rates and provide a combination of structure, treatment, supervision and monitoring (e.g.. thrice weekly urinalysis; urinary EtG; breathalyser testing; testing blood for MCV, LFTs, CDT).

When treating *an impaired health professional,* treat them as you would any other patient. Be aware that over-identification with a colleague and defence mechanisms such as collusion, denial, avoidance, minimization, and rescuing are barriers to treatment.

Preventive strategies include more education in training programmes about risk factors and protective factors for substance misuse, and early access to appropriate treatment and rehabilitation programmes.

Further reading

Baldisseri M. (2007). Impaired healthcare professional. *Crit Care Med* 35:106–16.
Kenna G, Lewis D. (2008). Risk factors for alcohol and other drug use by healthcare professionals. *Subst Abuse Treat Prev Policy* 3:3.

Safety-critical occupations

Introduction and epidemiology

Certain occupations have a special responsibility for public safety because of the nature of the work. These include airline pilots, air traffic controllers, and some other transport personnel, certain medical and other healthcare practitioners, and emergency services personnel.

- Of 1353 US pilots who died in aviation accidents between 2004 and 2008, 507 were found to be taking drugs and 92 had ethanol in excess of 0.04 g/dL.
- Many safety critical industries (e.g. airlines, forestry) run comprehensive alcohol and drug programmes to reduce risk; those who don't, should.

Approaches to policy and prevention

Best practice considers:
- workplace alcohol and drug policies
- detecting and monitoring those with intoxicant use problems
- employee privacy
- staff training
- what local resources and specialists are available?
- when is an affected employee work safe
- management of relapse
- continuous programme improvement.

An enthusiastic senior staff member should lead the programme together with a governance group of managers, unions, staff, and health-care professionals. All should debate and agree common goals for the programme.

Information

Workplace policies may extend to employees' behaviour outside of the workplace, setting a zero tolerance of workplace alcohol or drug use, discussing alcohol use at company functions, and devoting particular attention to risk. Policies should be publicized and include ongoing staff education.

Access

This includes voluntary presentation, referral by unions, peers, management, and health services, and pre-entry or reasonable cause drug and alcohol tests. Staff need assurance that participation and compliance with treatment can enable them to continue in employment.

Intervention

- With trained staff, screening and brief intervention may be possible, but focus should include possible intoxicant-related problems, e.g. antisocial behaviour, accidents and trauma, or apparent intoxication at work.
- Programme staff should discuss concerns with the employee and refer them to alcohol and drug practitioners for assessment, treatment, and advice about ongoing monitoring and support.
- Monitoring can involve blood and urine tests and regular meetings with health services.
- Urine testing can detect drug use. The best biomarker of relapse to heavy drinking is the CDT test. This is not as useful in initial assessment.
- Support may involve counsellors, others in recovery, and recovery group attendance.

Work

After an agreed treatment period an employee who ceases unsafe use of intoxicants and who complies with monitoring and support should return to work. Relapse should trigger re-assessment, decisions about further assistance, and whether the employee remains work safe.

Further reading

Canfield DV, Dubowski KM, Chaturvedi AK, et al. (2012). Drugs and alcohol found in civil aviation accident pilot fatalities from 2004-2008. *Aviat Space Environ Med* 83(8):764–70.

Csiernik R. (2003). Ideas on best practices for employee assistance program policies. *Employee Assistance Quart* 18:15–32.

Flynn CF, Sturges MS, Swarsen RJ, et al. (1993). Alcoholism and treatment in airline aviators: one company's results. *Aviat Space Environ Med* 64(4):314–18.

SAMHSA Advisory (2012). *The Role of Biomarkers in the Treatment of Alcohol Use Disorders, 2012 Revision.* Available at: http://store.samhsa.gov/product/The-Role-of-Biomarkers-in-the-Treatment-of-Alcohol-Use-Disorders-2012-Revision/SMA12-4686

Substance use and specific healthcare settings

Substance use disorders in primary healthcare 546
Substance use disorders in consulting rooms practice 549
Specialist addiction services 551
The emergency department 552
The consultation-liaison service 559
Dance parties and other public venues 561

Substance use disorders in primary healthcare

The vast majority of people with substance (alcohol and other drug) use disorders do not receive treatment in specialty settings. And most of the consequences of substance use accrue to those without a disorder—those with use that risks consequences (sometimes referred to as hazardous or at-risk use). Yet most people, including those with unhealthy substance use, visit community-based general health practice settings for a variety of health concerns, from the simple and acute to the more complex and chronic. Such settings often include preventive care as part of expected services.

General practice settings are well suited for addressing unhealthy substance use. There, patients are accessible both for case identification, and management of disorders. Generalist clinicians (e.g. physicians, nurse practitioners, and physician assistants) can incorporate brief screening questions into other preventive care services. Brief behaviour change counselling is becoming a staple of everyday practice since it is essential for managing risk factors (e.g. diet, physical activity, and sleep habits), and chronic conditions (e.g. medication and visit adherence).

Extending these approaches to alcohol, tobacco, and other drug use fits well. An established longitudinal and continuous care relationship can make asking about substance use for health appear more justified to the patient who recognizes that their clinician is asking for their benefit. The relationship is also likely a key part of the efficacy of brief counselling that can be more sincere, and is repeated over time in the context of a trusting, confidential, comprehensive role. The generalist clinician can take into consideration the medical, social, family, and mental health history when assessing substance use and determining its priority as a health issue for the patient and how to address it best.

A number of approaches have been proven efficacious in primary healthcare settings. These include screening and brief intervention for unhealthy alcohol use, and medication treatment of alcohol and opioid use disorders (with naltrexone and acamprosate for the former, and buprenorphine and methadone (where regulatory structures permit them) for the latter). Outpatient alcohol and opioid detoxification is also feasible in these settings provided staff can be available for the time required (observation and short-term follow-up calls and visits). Psychosocial treatments are important components of any of these approaches and will often not be provided by the physician. Thus to successfully implement this care, the psychosocial components should be provided either by someone in the practice qualified to do so or by referral. Also, since opioid agonist treatment often involves complexity in both prescribing (which may need to be frequent), and in testing (e.g. random urine testing), staff in the practice are needed to support this care (e.g. a nurse care manager).

Unhealthy substance use can be handled in these settings like other risk factors and chronic conditions. Identification on a positive screen is followed by feedback about the risk and discussion of strategies to reduce risk much like might be done for an elevated blood glucose or cholesterol. Brief behavioural or medication treatment, or referral to a specialist, once instituted, can be followed by reassessment of key measures for response, any adverse effects, and adherence. For example, for alcohol use one might reassess the number of heavy drinking days or a measurement of a previously elevated liver enzyme level; for opioid use, a urine toxicology result. This approach is similar to following a haemoglobin A_{1C} level in diabetes or a blood pressure in hypertension. When necessary, the treatment can be changed, intensified, or discontinued based on response.

When too complex or if the condition is not responding (substance use continues, increases, or is complicated by consequences or co-occurring mental health or medical conditions), the clinician can refer. Ideally such referrals should look just like other medical referrals to be successful. Clinicians should know the name of the specialist and what might happen to the patient when they see them. With patient permission, the clinicians (generalist and substance disorder specialist) should communicate about the patient (reason for referral, and result of specialty assessment and intervention) and the patient should return to the generalist for long-term follow-up. Because substance use disorder specialists and treatment programmes are often in physical locations and even care systems distant from primary healthcare, extra efforts should be made for warm handoffs—personal communication between the clinicians and the patient and provision of as much information as possible to the patient. Clinicians can choose to handle levels of severity of unhealthy use with which they are comfortable and competent, just like is done for other conditions (e.g. some clinicians are comfortable handling cardiac dysrhythmias; others would refer to a specialist and then continue to see the patient thereafter).

Because substance use has traditionally not been well addressed and managed in general healthcare settings, however, many challenges and barriers exist for delivery of high-quality care. Patients may not tell the truth in response to screening questions because of a fear the clinician will think less of them. They may also fear having substance use results documented in their medical records since that might affect their insurability or even employment or legal status. While clinicians cannot completely mitigate these consequences, they can address substance use non-judgementally as a health risk factor just like any other, and reassure patients of this purpose. After all, even if the clinician does not manage the substance use itself, it would be impossible to diagnose and treat just about any symptom or disorder appropriately without knowing if substance use was present as a cause (e.g. of sleep disturbance, anxiety, acid reflux) or as a factor that might interfere with high quality care (e.g. medication interactions, non-adherence, chronic pain management).

Another barrier for clinicians is lack of knowledge of substance use disorders and relevant treatment resources, because of lack of training and the separateness of care systems. More resources are becoming available for continuing education in this area, local resources can be investigated, and many clinicians and patients become quite satisfied when it becomes possible to manage substance use disorders alongside other health conditions.

Limited time is a key barrier to addressing unhealthy substance use in general practice. In some ways this is a 'straw man'—time is not cited often as a reason to not address a new diagnosis of diabetes or heart disease, though it is referenced as a reason for lower quality of care of such conditions. Regardless, a number of features of the transformation of healthcare to include patient-centred medical homes and the importance of general practice for coordinating care are relevant to managing unhealthy substance use. For example, electronic records can prompt screening and follow-up reassessment and care and track results. Office staff such as medical assistants can help facilitate screening and follow-up testing. Health educators who are appearing more commonly in such settings can provide brief behaviour change counselling for substance use as well as for other health behaviours. Health behaviour change specialists (e.g. psychologists, social workers, mental health counsellors) can provide counselling for unhealthy substance use as well as for other mental health conditions. Nurse care coordinators (now working often to coordinate care for diabetes and heart failure) can take time to coordinate care for unhealthy substance use. Physicians and other prescribers can work at the 'top of their licences' by prescribing medications, prioritizing among other conditions, by emphasizing the importance of the condition to patients, and by directing the care among the many options available including referral.

In sum, general practice settings make sense for addressing unhealthy substance use. Access is easier and more likely for patients, and there are many things clinicians can do successfully. Patients appreciate getting their care from one clinician when possible—it is more convenient and higher quality, less prone to errors related to unawareness of conditions identified and care provided elsewhere. A patient with anxiety, opioid use disorder, and asthma, with young children at home can have her conditions assessed and medications prescribed during the course of one visit. A clinician frustrated with prescribing opioids to a patient with chronic pain who seems demanding can address both the pain and substance disorder issues simultaneously. Patients with substance use disorders who normally would not have them addressed until they reach their fifth decade are appreciative of earlier access to care when many consequences can be avoided and the condition addressed more easily than a more firmly established disease. Clinician training and adequate staff resources can make this sort of care a reality.

Substance use disorders in consulting rooms practice

The nature of consulting rooms practice

In many healthcare systems, medical consulting rooms represent the first point of contact for persons wanting to access healthcare. General (or family) medical consulting rooms provide comprehensive general care to individuals and families, and they are easily accessible. Depending on the particular health and welfare system, they can provide important connections with social and welfare services, schools, and local authorities. This is important because an intersectoral approach may be necessary for effective interventions to be implemented.

Doctors and health professionals who run these practices are typically very busy. Their attitudes usually depend on (1) time, (2) education, (3) role security, and (4) therapeutic commitment. Whether they have a disease-centred (and often 'reactive') approach or a more proactive, capacity building, and empathic attitude, health professionals should always incorporate strategies for the management of substance use disorders. A holistic approach ensures that the life conditions that are at the base of addictive disorders are addressed and understood.

The patients

From a substance use point of view, patients in consulting rooms can be classified into four groups.

1. Patients already in treatment for addiction within the rooms (office). In this case, the doctor is likely to be an addiction expert. He/she will know how to identifying addiction, how to treat the health consequences and which rehabilitation approaches to recommend.
2. Patients accessing the office for extra prescriptions of benzodiazepines or opioids as pain-cough relievers. These patients are typically well aware of their addiction and how to access their preferred drugs. They hope to take advantage of a busy practice, and wander from one practice to another ('doctor shoppers').
3. People attending the office seeking generic medical consultations. They may or may not be aware of having an addiction and use substances to maintain their lifestyle and/or the addicted state. They may think they have control over their use. These patients represent the majority of patients seen in medical practice who have addictive disorders and should be the principal focus for practitioners managing addiction disorders. They may also access the practice for non-medical purposes, such as applying for a licence to drive or to carry a weapon.
4. People reporting unusual behaviours or health problems of a family member.

What to do

In each of these instances the medical practitioner should try to work collaboratively with other services. Be aware of stigma.

- No matter the approach, effective addictive disorders management entails helping the patient to *live and enjoy life* within the local community. The aim is to prevent losing control over substance use, which for some people (e.g. those with dependence/addiction) may require abstinence from the substance.
- Most of the time, referral to a specialist centre or a self-help group is perceived like telling everyone there is a problem. In some countries, substance users may be compelled to attend these services because of legal mandate or a decision of a court. In these circumstances, substance users usually deny their problem and may prefer to interrelate only with their practitioner.
- Specialists in addiction practice should be aware of this and try to establish contacts with the family, social services, or specialist centres—but only with permission of the client. Specific techniques, such as Brief Intervention and Motivational Interviewing, can be helpful in finding the right approach to the patient.
- In situations (1) and (2) listed earlier, consultants should find ways to cooperate with local community services and check if treatment or rehabilitation can be initiated or improved. Contact with the specialist centres should be made to share responsibilities of therapy.
- The third situation is the most common. The medical practitioner should be alert to signs and symptoms that can help 'raise the issue'. Hypertension, sleep disorders, anxiety/depression, family, and/or socioeconomic problems are only some of the presenting signs. Normal blood tests should not prevent from thinking about and identifying addiction.
- Disease-oriented practitioners can address the importance of ensuring problems do not worsen, while proactive practitioners should stress the importance of a co-shared health with empowerment and health promotion being at the base of their intervention.

In summary

- Think of, and identify possible addictive disorders.
- Check on physical and neurological health.
- Use brief advice and/or motivational interviewing to create an empathic, non-judgemental relationship and increase chances of success.
- Facilitate/activate any possible link and support from local social services.
- Pharmacotherapy can be utilized for abstinence-oriented goals, or for harm reduction ones (e.g. methadone maintenance).
- Referral to specialized services is important for patients with established substance dependence.
- Stigma is an important issue for many patients and the patient's perception of this should be evaluated.
- New technologies can be helpful for busy practices especially with new evidence supporting the effectiveness of specific website interventions (e.g. for alcohol risk reduction).

Specialist addiction services

- Specialist addiction services play an important role in providing outpatient or inpatient treatment for substance use disorders. Their availability is far from universal, even in the developed world.
- The range of specialist services varies considerably, from sole specialist practitioners to complex outpatient or residential services.
- Specialist services may cater for just one disorder, e.g. opioid maintenance programmes; or may provide comprehensive addiction medicine or addiction psychiatry services.

Outpatient services

Specialist outpatient services may provide diagnostic, assessment, withdrawal management, and ongoing care. This may include one or more of:
- ambulatory withdrawal management
- outpatient diazepam reduction regimens
- opioid substitution therapy: with dispensing of the medication onsite or through local pharmacies or clinics
- counselling and relapse prevention approaches, including relapse prevention medicines, individual or group counselling
- provision of facilities (at cost) for mutual support groups
- prevention, diagnosis, or treatment for common comorbidities, e.g. testing and vaccination for viral hepatitis.

Some services provide a still broader range of health and social care including:
- onsite specialist medical or psychiatric care (e.g. for management of viral hepatitis, HIV, STIs, contraception, mental illness)
- holistic primary healthcare
- assistance with housing, legal needs, and government benefits.

Such 'one-stop shops' can greatly increase access to care for marginalized or chaotic patients.

Some specialist clinics also provide outreach services (e.g. from a van) to deliver care to the most vulnerable and marginalized clients.

These services play an important role in supporting family physicians and providing skills development and shared care opportunities.

Residential services

Specialist residential rehabilitation services are available for people with especially severe substance use and addictive disorders. They are often based on a therapeutic community model, where the staff and counsellors are usually in recovery themselves. Residents progress through a series of levels of increasing responsibility for self-care and for the community. This can include preparation of food, maintenance of the facility, enforcing community rules, and support for new residents. Most services require the prospective resident to contact them directly and repeatedly. Most are based on the 12-step model of recovery, but there are often additional focuses such as childhood abuse and comorbidity.

The emergency department

The ED is a busy and often pressured environment which provides treatment for acutely sick people. The emphasis is on rapid assessment, resuscitation, and stabilization, and then transfer (or discharge). However, it also provides an opportunity for detection and mangement of an incidental substance use disorder. For many such patients it is their first contact with the health care system.

Patients with substance use disorders are seen frequently; indeed in some EDs they comprise up to half the patients. They may have a mix of physical and psychiatric problems and often major psychosocial difficulties. Those with trauma are an important subgroup and are characterized as being:

- predominantly younger males
- having combined alcohol use disorders (25–50%), smoking (up to 60%), and other substance use (up to 40%)
- exhibiting high levels of risk-taking behaviour
- sensation-seeking
- poor coping mechanisms.

Social exclusion, violence (as victim or perpetrator), criminal activities, and antisocial behaviour may sometimes complicate the management of substance-using patients.

The impact of substance use

Among the factors that need to be considered when managing patients with substance use disorders in the ED are:

- the wide range of physical and psychiatric morbidity
- the multiplicity of substances used
- the spectrum of severity of substance use disorders (e.g. intoxication/overdose, withdrawal; presence of medical, neuropsychiatric and/or social complications)
- the masking effects of acute intoxication (with or without delirium) on the clinical features of other conditions, e.g.:
  - traumatic brain injury
  - Wernicke's encephalopathy
  - severe infection (in drug-dependent individuals often with multi-resistant strains).

Other examples of the impact of substance use disorders include:

- increased infection rates due to immune impairment often combined with stress axis disturbances
- clotting disturbances due to disturbances in coagulation factors or platelet numbers or function (due to liver impairment or substance-induced)
- impaired wound healing due to malnutrition or alcohol use.

A multidisciplinary approach is crucial to successful determination of the cause of abnormal behaviour as well as ensuing management. Patients with a history of substance misuse are likely to have involvement with a range of hospital and community-based services. Early availability of information from these will support more informed decision-making.

Agitation and aggression

Agitated and aggressive patients (see Boxes 25.1 and 25.2) often require several members of staff to gain a measure of control and calm. At the same time they are often extremely unwell, with a range of complications ranging from acid–base disturbance, hyperthermia, hypoxia, and dehydration as well as brain injuries.

Approaches for dealing with agitated patients

Key principles guiding the management approach are as follows:

- Consider the past history of the patient including past successful approaches to maintain control and calm.
- Keep the clinical needs and reduction of associated risks to the patient as a priority.

Box 25.1 Drug causes of acute agitation

- Intoxication:
  - alcohol
  - sedative hypnotics/anxiolytics, in particular benzodiazepines
  - cannabis
  - cocaine
  - amphetamines and derivatives
  - hallucinogenic agents
- Side effects/interactions/toxicity:
  - antidepressants
  - salicylate toxicity
  - serotonin syndrome
  - neuroleptic malignant syndrome (NMS)
  - anticholinergic syndrome
  - antipsychotic reaction
- Withdrawal syndromes.

Box 25.2 Some non-toxicological causes of agitation

- Hypoxia
- Hypoglycaemia
- Acid–base and electrolyte disturbances
- Sepsis
- CNS disorders such as:
  - trauma (including subdural or subarachnoid haemorrhage)
  - meningoencephalitis
  - cerebrovascular accidents
  - seizures
- Hyperthermia
- Endocrine disturbance
- Autoimmune disease
- Organ failure
- Acute alcohol or drug withdrawal.

- Consider duty of care for other patients and for staff.
- The layout and availability of services and support within the facility will help determine appropriate clinical management.

Specific management steps:
- Early assessment and differential diagnosis of any patient with delirium (differential diagnosis: See Box 25.4).
- Seek collateral history/information from medical records, other services or family.
- Avoid confrontation, ensure adequate assistance, defuse tensions, adopt de-escalation strategies, ensure safety of other patients and staff.
- Establish patient's concerns, reassure patient and any accompanying relatives/friends, encourage reasoning by offering appropriate options and through non-threatening actions.
- If efforts to de-escalate have succeeded, then conduct a medical and mental health assessment. Consider oral sedation to assist in maintaining calm and compliance.
- Consider oral sedation to assist in maintaining calm and compliance.
- If there is increasing urgency or failure of de-escalation, then consider the role of physical restraint with view to acute sedation. Discuss this within the treating team.
- Frequently monitor both the physical and mental state. Use validated scales to monitor, e.g. pain, delirium, sedation, or anxiety.

The situation should be under early control, to allow determination of the underlying physical ± associated psychological causes. A period of observation is important (e.g. within an observation unit) for further investigations or monitoring prior to discharge. If in doubt, patients should not be discharged.

Management will require input of colleagues from internal medicine to rule out severe organ failure, and from psychological medicine, addiction services, and social services. It is important that a suitable psychological risk assessment is made prior to hospital/unit discharge, together with review through community and liaison services as part of a planned discharge.

Reduced level of consciousness

Maintenance of an adequate airway and ensuring sufficient ventilation, adequate cardiocirculatory support and immediate neurological assessment are key initial steps for clinical care. Box 25.3 outlines the immediate steps to be taken.

Patients must be carefully evaluated to seek causes of coma. At the same time preventative steps must be taken to ensure that complications of coma are avoided or minimized.

The ingested drugs are usually unknown in intoxicated ED patients. Care should be supportive, including necessary ventilatory and circulatory support, while excluding other possible causes. If opioid overdose is suspected, careful use of the antagonist naloxone can be considered. Minimize risk of acute withdrawal stress, which may have severe

---

Box 25.3 Immediate steps in managing an emergency

- Consider the need for self-protection—in potentially dangerous situations security or police should be called.
- Is cardiopulmonary resuscitation (CPR) needed?
    - basic life support
    - advanced cardiac life support: ABCDE (airway, breathing, circulation, disability, exposure/elimination).
- Vital signs:
    - pulse rate
    - blood pressure
    - respiratory rate
    - auscultation of lung fields
    - oxygen saturation
    - temperature.
- ECG (QTc prolongation seen with many CNS depressants; tachyarrhythmias, myocardial ischaemia with psychostimulants).
- Establish IV access.
- Ensure continuation of adequate airway and sufficient ventilation
- Consider the need for intubation if GCS is < 9 or respiratory failure occurs.
- On physical examination, check in particular for traumatic or other brain damage (e.g. ischaemia, subarachnoid haemorrhage, intracranial haemorrhage), assault (including rape), and recent injection
- Routine blood tests including glucose, CPK, troponin, coagulation.

---

consequences in addicted and critically ill patients. If a toxicological cause is confirmed, specific therapy can be provided such as the use of an antidote (seek toxicological advice).

A reduced level of consciousness or coma may be:
- a result of direct toxic effect on the CNS
- secondary to the effects of CNS depression, e.g. hypoxia, hypoglycaemia, hyponatraemia, hypotension, seizure
- a non-toxin medical issue, e.g. sepsis, meningoencephalitis, cerebrovascular accident, space-occupying lesion.

Delirium

Delirium may vary in its nature depending on any combination of substances taken (alcohol, sedative-hypnotics, psycho-stimulants and hallucinogens) and other medical conditions (Box 25.4). Other causes are:
- anticholinergic syndrome
- serotonergic syndrome
- neuroleptic malignant syndrome
- increased toxic effects of drugs due to altered metabolism.

The management of delirium is outlined in Box 25.5.

Box 25.4 Differential diagnosis of acute delirium 'I WATCH DEATH' acronym

- Infections
- Withdrawal state
- Acute metabolic disturbance
- Trauma
- CNS disease
- Hypoxia
- Deficiency syndromes
- Endocrine disorders
- Acute vascular event
- Toxins including alcohol, drug overdose, illicit drug use, multiple substance use
- Heavy metal poisoning.

(Also see differential diagnosis of delirium p. 96.)

Box 25.5 Management of delirium

- Consider differential diagnosis, consider additional morbidity, and treat accordingly.
- Evaluate suicidality, protect and intervene as appropriate.
- Treat pain.
- If patient is agitated, talk them down in a calm manner and create a calm environment.
- If patient is severely agitated, consider benzodiazepines unless contraindicated (but beware of potentially delirogenic effects, e.g. in older patients, their use can further cloud consciousness); benzodiazepines are first choice in an alcohol-sedative withdrawal state.
- Consider prescribing neuroleptics—but beware of lowering seizure threshold and exacerbating hyperthermia.
- Other potential medications include antiepileptics, beta blockers, and alpha-2 agonists.
- Consider the place of an antagonist: is there confirmed intake of a single substance?; beware of unexpected interactions; seek toxicological advice.
- Where likelihood of psychostimulant toxicity, consider antihypertensive medication but beware of vasospasm; use alpha blockers before beta blockers; avoid aspirin.
- Does gastric lavage have a place to remove unabsorbed drug?—this is rarely the case unless very recent ingestion (less than 1 hour).
- Consider plasma expansion with crystalloid when patient is hypertensive or there is evidence of rhabdomyolysis.
- IV fluids in rhabdomyolysis ± dialysis; some centres use alkalinization of urine (after hydration) aiming for urinary pH of 7.45–7.55).

Box 25.5 *(Contd.)*

- Severe metabolic acidosis: sodium bicarbonate only if circulatory failure has occurred.
- Management of hyperthermia—physical cooling, hydration consider the place of benzodiazepines, dantrolene, and antipyretics, in case of hyperkalaemia use immediate dialysis.
- Hypothermia—protect, allow gradual warming, avoid shivering or hyperthermia.
- Electrolyte balance.
- Hyperglycaemia and hypoglycaemia: treatment as appropriate.
- Administration of vitamins, especially parenteral thiamine.

Detection and intervention for substance use

Given the impact of substance use disorders on the clinical presentation, all patients should be screened for substance use disorders using appropriate questions, or by means of questionnaires. Those identified with substance use disorders should be further evaluated. Use of alcohol and other drugs is particularly relevant in the patient with acute injury. Measuring breath alcohol concentration and urine drug screening (UDS) are indicated.

The ED plays an important role in providing treatment for patients with substance use disorders including:

- management of acute intoxication
- detoxification and withdrawal management
- use of substitution treatment (e.g. for opioid dependence) in some settings
- opportunistic interventions (screening and brief intervention) particularly for those who are injured or have substance-related disorders (will also facilitate ongoing care for these disorders) (see Box 25.6).

Box 25.6 Intervention for alcohol and other substance use disorders

- Systematic screening, using explicit questions or a questionnaire.
- Biological markers of alcohol (including BAC) and urine drug screen may alert to unexpected substance use.
- Brief intervention (e.g. FRAMES or FLAGS approach), with the provision of tailored information and advice, encouragement to change, and self-management.
- Initiation of withdrawal management.
- Advice on abstinence from the substance if dependent, or if co-morbid mental health problems.
- In opioid dependence, consider the role of substitution treatment.
- Information and referral options for elective withdrawal management (detoxification) and rehabilitation programmes.

Having a drug and alcohol consultation service available within the ED can further improve quality of care. Also, education on substance use should be incorporated into health professional training and post-graduate skills development for all clinicians providing ED care. It is of utmost relevance that clinicians address substance misuse and perform brief motivational interviewing, e.g. according to the FRAMES criteria.

For further details on assessment and management see sections on:

- toxicity and withdrawal states for individual substances
- acute psychotic states (pp. 98–101) and suicidality (p. 94)
- domestic/interpersonal violence (pp. 580–2).

Further reading

European Resuscitation Council website: http://www.erc.edu

Kork F, Neumann T, Spies C. (2010). Perioperative management of patients with alcohol, tobacco and drug dependency. *Curr Opin Anaesthesiol* 23:384–90.

Runge JW, Hargarten S, Velianoff G, *et al.* (2001). Recommended best practices of emergency medical care for the alcohol impaired patient: screening and brief intervention for alcohol problems in the emergency department. Available at: http://www.nhtsa.dot.gov/people/injury/alcohol/EmergCare/tech_doc_page.htm

Spies CD, Rommelspacher H. (1999). Alcohol withdrawal in the surgical patient: prevention and treatment. *Anesth Analg* 88:946–52.

Tønnesen H, Nielsen PR, Lauritzen JB, *et al.* (2009). Smoking and alcohol intervention before surgery: evidence for best practice. *Br J Anesth* 102:297–306.

The consultation-liaison service

There is a high prevalence of substance use disorders among hospital in-patients and those attending hospital-based clinics. In the great majority of cases patients have not presented because of concern about their substance disorder and requesting treatment and help for it. Rather, they present with the variety of physical and psychiatric disorders that arise from psychoactive substance use. Additionally, some patients are admitted for disorders which are unrelated to substance use, but concomitantly have a level or pattern of substance use that is injurious.

Addiction medicine consultation-liaison (C-L) services exist in many hospitals and form an important component of service provision. C-L services in general hospitals contribute to the management of patients with disorders caused by the use of alcohol, tobacco, prescribed medications, and illicit drugs, although some are more restricted in their focus. Some C-L services operate within psychiatric hospitals and prison medical facilities. Variants of C-L services involve outreach to high-risk populations such as homeless and transient people, the mentally ill, and former prisoners.

Aims of C-L services

The principal aims of C-L services are threefold:

1. To provide advice on the clinical management of patients who have a known or suspected alcohol, tobacco, medication, or illicit drug problem, with the goal of optimizing their treatment and avoiding complications (such as an uncontrolled withdrawal syndrome) and extended lengths of stay.
2. To provide referral options for patients with substance disorders— to a suitable addiction specialist, to their general practitioner for ongoing treatment, to a voluntary/non-governmental organization, or to a self-help group.
3. To enhance the overall skills of hospital staff in identifying and managing patients with substance use disorders so that the overall standard of care for these patients is enhanced and contributes to good standards of professional practice throughout the hospital.

The scope of clinical management

C-L services are very diverse in terms of the clinical management that they provide. At a very basic level, the service may be confined to the provision of information material about substance use and its attendant disorders, and on telephone helplines, counselling agencies, self-help groups, and other relevant local services. At a more well-formed level, the service may provide assessment and brief therapy for hazardous substance use or substance dependence, which might include a session of counselling on the ward or arrangements made for the person to attend a self-help group.

More comprehensive C-L services provide specialist assessment of the patient's substance use and related disorders in the context of their presenting condition and psychosocial background. Such C-L services are typically multidisciplinary. The initial assessment may be undertaken by a specialist C-L nurse, with training in addiction, psychiatric or medical nursing, a medical resident, a postgraduate medical trainee in addiction medicine, psychiatry, or general medicine, or a medical addiction specialist. Typically there would be regular meetings of the multidisciplinary team to confer, update team members, and establish a management plan for the patient from a multidisciplinary perspective.

The most common forms of management such a team would provide include:

- assessment of the risk of withdrawal syndrome
- management of detoxification from alcohol, tobacco, prescribed medication, or illicit drugs
- comprehensive assessment of substance use where the history has been difficult to elicit or is inconsistent, to identify the aetiological significance of substance use for the presenting disease
- the management of acute (e.g. postoperative) pain in a person with known or suspected substance (particularly opioid) dependence
- the assessment and management of a person with chronic pain and known or suspected drug (particularly opioid) dependence
- the management of drug-seeking behaviour particularly in a hospital setting
- the differential diagnosis of postoperative delirium in a patient with known or suspected substance dependence
- linking patients to continuing therapy for their substance use disorder following discharge from hospital
- contributing to the discharge planning process from a substance use disorder perspective.

Enhancing the skills of hospital staff

The second and equally important objective of C-L services is to enhance the knowledge, skills, and professional practice of staff who have not been specifically trained in addiction management. The underlying principle is that of a multiplicative effect: the C-L service contributes to the optimal management of patients with substance use disorders to a greater extent than could be achieved by direct patient management alone. The C-L Service would typically provide in-service training sessions for hospital ward staff in the assessment of substance use and related disorders, the assessment of risk of withdrawal, training in monitoring withdrawal states, and in the nursing and pharmacological management of patients in withdrawal states. Other topics might include the recognition and management of drug-seeking behaviour and the development of policies to manage such patients. The in-service sessions may take the form of case presentations or may adopt a more didactic approach in the form of a lecture or tutorial.

Dance parties and other public venues

Substance use in some public venues may be very high. Sometimes it is visible, sometimes not. In some public venues, emergency services personnel (e.g. ambulance officers and paramedics) are in attendance. At others, first-aid facilities are provided and staffed by voluntary organizations (such as St John's Ambulance).

In dance parties and 'raves', rates of drug use can be exceptionally high (up to 80% of attendees). In these settings, the drugs most commonly used are:

- psychostimulants, e.g. MDMA (Ecstasy), cocaine, amphetamine-type substances, and new psychotropic substances
- gamma hydroxyl-butyrate (GHB) and its analogues, which are predominantly sedatives but may have an initial stimulant effect on behaviour
- ketamine.

Those which are stimulants and empathogens/enactogens (such as MDMA) allow people to stay awake for longer and achieve a sense of euphoria.

Clinical

Given the rates of drug use, adverse consequences are relatively uncommon but when they do occur, they can be serious and life-threatening. These include the following:

- Hyperthermia (stimulants): caused by high ambient temperatures, central thermoregulatory changes, and increased heat generation by skeletal muscle. If severe can result in multiorgan failure, DIC, and death.
- Seizures (stimulants, GHB).
- Hyponatraemia (stimulants and MDMA): caused by syndrome of inappropriate secretion of antidiuretic hormone (SIADH) and excessive water intake. Can result in seizures, cerebral oedema, and death.
- Rhabdomyolysis (stimulants): can result in acute kidney injury.
- Vascular complications including myocardial ischaemia, cerebral haemorrhage (stimulants).
- Agitation and behavioural disturbance (all drugs).
- Decreased level of consciousness and respiratory depression (GHB + derivatives); profound and prolonged coma and respiratory depression can occur when consumed with alcohol.
- Trauma related to intoxication (all drugs).

Risks

Partygoers particularly at risk of adverse effects include:

- inexperienced users
- people left alone
- those who take all their drugs at once (dumping) for fear of detection
- those who drive home from the venue.

Harm reduction

Very few strategies have been successful in reducing drug use at dance parties and so harm reduction is the main focus. Approaches include:

- encouraging individuals to research through peer networks and Internet
- encouraging people to stay with friends and not go off alone
- medical cover is often provided at larger dance parties, which allows rapid onsite triage and management
- drug rovers are often volunteers who move around the dance floor and more secluded areas to detect people who may be at risk
- providing transport to and from the venue.

Police presence and sniffer dogs

Evidence shows that this has very little effect in reducing drug use at parties and may in fact increase harm by encouraging people to 'dump' their drugs.

Roadside testing may reduce driving under the influence (DUI) following the event.

Legal and ethical issues

Drinking and driving 564
Drugs and driving 570
Seizures and driving 573
Child protection 575
Interpersonal violence 580
Workplace safety and interventions 583
Involuntary treatment and diversion programmes 586

Drinking and driving

The World Health Organization recommends an upper limit for legal blood alcohol concentration (BAC) for drivers of 0.05 g/100 mL. Eighty-nine countries covering 4.6 billion people (66% of the world population) have a BAC limit of 0.05 g/100 mL or less. With a BAC of 0.05–0.079 g/100 mL, a driver is four times as likely to die in a road crash as one with no alcohol, and twice as likely to be in any crash. Risk rises rapidly with further increases in BAC.

In order to comply with a BAC maximum of 0.05 g/100 mL for driving, a general guideline for an average healthy person is that:
- women drink no more than one standard drink in the first hour, then only one drink per hour thereafter
- men drink no more than two standard drinks in the first hour, then no more than one standard drink per hour thereafter.

NB: some people of small build, or who are ill, or who have concurrent medical problems, or who are on medication (e.g. sedatives), will need to drink less or not at all.

In some countries/regions a medical practitioner is obliged to report to the driver licensing authority a driver who is repeatedly drinking to the extent that their driving ability is impaired or is unfit to drive. Medical practitioners need to weigh the benefits of patient mobility with the increased risk posed to other road users and make themselves aware of local guidelines.

Drinking-driving

'Drinking-driving' is the favoured term for the criminal conviction of driving a vehicle under the influence of alcohol. Drinking-driving accidents are a problem in all countries that make use of motor vehicles for transportation. Drinking-driving countermeasures have been developed and many of these have been evaluated.

In the field of traffic safety, the BAC is expressed as g/100 mL, (e.g. 0.10% or 0.10 g/dL or 100 mL) in the US and Australia. In the UK, it is expressed as mg per 100 mL (e.g. 100 mg/100 mL). The legal driving limit differs in different countries: in the UK and the United States it is 0.08% (expressed as 80 mg/100 mL in the UK). In Australia and in most of continental Europe it is 0.05%.

The risk of a fatal crash for drivers with a positive BAC rises more steeply for drivers under the age of 21 years than for older drivers. Table 26.1 shows that there is a marked deterioration in performance between BACs of 0.05% and 0.09%.

BAC can be measured by taking a blood sample from a driver, but also via analysis of breath alcohol. The invention of the breathalyser test and other portable devices for collecting samples of drivers' breaths has had a major impact on the enforcement of drinking-driving countermeasures.

Table 26.1 Relative risks for a single-vehicle fatal crash for various BACs

BAC level: g/100 mL	Relative risk of a single-vehicle fatal crash
0.02–0.04	3.8
0.05–0.79	12.2
0.08–0.099	31.9
0.10–0.149	122.3
>0.15	4728

Source data from *J Stud Alcohol Drugs*, 73(3), Voas et al., Alcohol-Related Risk of Driver Fatalities: An Update Using 2007 Data, pp. 341–350, Copyright (2012), with permission from Alcohol Research Documentation, Inc.

A number of factors influence alcohol-induced impairment:
- *Alcohol tolerance*: the repeated performance of a particular task in association with alcohol consumption can lead to a form of adaptation known as 'learned' tolerance. This acts to reduce the alcohol-induced impairment under routine circumstances.
- *Age*: the fatality rate for 16–19-year-old drivers is four times higher than that for their 25–69-year-old counterparts. For male drivers under 21 years, an increase in BAC of 0.02% will more than double the relative risk of a fatal single-vehicle crash. The greater risk in younger people can be explained in part by lack of experience and overconfidence. The risk increases if there are other teenagers in the car.
- *Gender*: women metabolize alcohol differently from men and achieve higher BAC levels for the same 'dose' of alcohol.
- *Medication*: combining certain types of medication with alcohol increases crash risk. This applies particularly to sedatives and tranquillizers (e.g. benzodiazepines), which have an increased crash potential when taken on their own. Other drugs implicated include anti-depressants, codeine and other morphine-like analgesics, anti-histamines, also some cardiovascular and antipsychotic medications. The risks of driving after drug use are less than driving with a BAC of 0.08% or higher. But the risks of driving after drinking and using drugs are greater than the additive risk of driving after alcohol or drugs alone.
- *Sleep* deprivation: drowsiness increases crash risk and alcohol consumption increases the adverse effects of sleep deprivation.

Factors influencing blood alcohol concentration levels
Different people metabolize alcohol at different rates. As a rule of thumb, 1 unit of alcohol (10 g) will lead to an increase of 15 mg% (0.15%) in the BAC. The body eliminates about 15 mg% of alcohol per hour.

Listed here are some of the factors that influence the concentration of alcohol in a person's breath or blood (BAC):

- The quantity and concentration of alcohol consumed
- The time since the last drink, and the rate of drinking
- Whether alcohol was consumed on an empty stomach
- The amount of alcohol that remains in the stomach
- The amount of alcohol already metabolized by the liver
- The general condition of the liver
- The person's metabolic rate
- The person's emotional state
- Physical factors, including gender, weight, body size, and lean tissue to body fat ratio
- The volume of water in the tissues of the body, which can be affected by such factors as medication, illness, and the menstrual cycle.

Decline in drinking and driving

Since the early 1980s there has been a general decline in the incidence of drinking-driving in the developed world, where alcohol-related traffic deaths have been cut dramatically as the result of drink-driving legislation. In the US, the institution of preventive measures such as lower legal BAC (*per se*) limits and administrative licence revocation reduced alcohol-impaired driving. In 1982, 48% of people died in crashes involving drivers with BACs of 0.08% or higher. The percentage declined to 31% in 2012. Among 16–20-year-olds, the respective percentages were 36% in 1982 and 18% in 2012, largely as a result of raising the minimum legal age of drinking to 21 years and the passage of zero tolerance laws for drivers under 21.

General deterrence as prevention

Lowering BAC limits: the implementation of strict legal alcohol limits (e.g. 0.08% or 0.05% or above for the whole population and 0.02% for young drivers) have been successful in reducing the level of the problem. However, the impact of these measures is eroded over time, and this has led to countries implementing more stringent BAC levels.

Enforcement: intensification of police enforcement of breath testing reduces accidents in the short term, but the effects are generally temporary. Highly visible, random breath testing is effective at reducing drinking-driving and the associated crashes, injuries, and deaths.

Severity of punishment: punishments include fines, suspension of driving licences, court-mandated treatment for alcohol problems, and imprisonment. Licence loss has been shown to be the most consistently effective deterrent.

Repeat offenders: in a number of jurisdictions repeat offenders are subject to more draconian interventions, such as confiscation and loss of their licences for longer periods, and imprisonment. The impact of routine punishments can be enhanced when combined with alcohol treatment. This can range from short-term educational sessions to longer programmes lasting up to 1 year.

Restrictions on young or inexperienced drivers

A numbers of prevention strategies have been successfully implemented, as follows:

- Lower BAC limits: sometimes called 'zero tolerance laws', set the legal BAC limit for drivers under 21 at 0.00% or 0.02%. They have been successful in reducing the proportion of drinking drivers involved in fatal crashes in the under-21 year age group in the US. They also invoke other penalties, such as automatic confiscation of the driving licence.
- Licensing restrictions: graduated licensing schemes that include delayed access to a full licence and curfews for young drivers have been well accepted where implemented and have shown safety benefits.

Examples of national experiences

United Kingdom

In the UK, 3000 people on average are killed or seriously injured per year in drink-drive collisions (Department for Transport, 2007). Nearly one in six of all road deaths involve drivers who are over the legal limit. Although drinking and driving occurs across all age groups, young men aged 17–29 years are most often involved, as perpetrators and casualties. The legal alcohol limit is 80 mg/per 100 mL of blood, which can also be expressed in terms of levels in the breath (the official measure) or in urine:

- Breath alcohol: 35 mcg/100 mL or
- Urinary alcohol: 107 mg/100 mL.

This is roughly equivalent to 2 pints (4 units) of ordinary strength beer in an average man and less for a woman. Men should therefore consume no more than 4 units and women no more than 3 units if they wish to remain below the legal limit. Just two 175 mL glasses of 12% wine would put the average woman over the legal limit.

Australia

Australian-born single men under the age of 30 years are more likely than any other group to drink and drive. There have been intensive media campaigns and concentrated police efforts, including an increase in random breath testing, to discourage people from drinking and driving.

The legal limit for drivers in all states in Australia is below 0.05%. No alcohol is allowed for drivers on a probationary licence (P plates) or learner drivers (L plates). The laws impose severe penalties for convicted drink drivers, including licence loss, fines, and occasionally imprisonment.

United States

In the US in 2012, 10,322 of the 33,561 (31%) of the people who died in motor vehicle crashes died in a crash involving a driver with a BAC of 0.08 g/100 mL or US. Every state and the District of Columbia define impairment as driving with a BAC at or above this level. In addition, they all have zero tolerance laws prohibiting drivers under the age of 21 from drinking and driving. Generally, the BAC in these cases is 0.02 g/100 mL.

Drink-driving campaigns target drivers under the age of 21, repeat offenders, and 21–34-year-olds, the age group that is responsible for more alcohol-related fatal crashes than any other.

Intervention programmes

In several countries intervention programmes exist with the aim of preventing further drink-driving offences through a combination of:

- education
- ignition interlock devices
- monitoring

Education programmes may be provided in a group format ('driver offender courses'), or may be individualized in the form of a brief alcohol intervention, or for drivers with a more established alcohol use disorder, with pharmacological and psychological treatment.

Multicomponent community intervention programmes

combining the following have further reduced alcohol-impaired driving:

- Community organizing
- Strategic planning
- Heightened police enforcement of drinking and driving and underage drinking laws
- Publicity concerning laws and their enforcement and rationale
- Expansion of screening of brief intervention and treatment
- Monitoring and evaluation.

Ignition interlock devices prevent the driver from starting the car until he/she has passed a breath test. Modern machines allow download of data periodically, so that authorities can monitor if the person is still attempting to drink and drive. Such attempts can trigger additional treatment if needed, or an extended period on the interlock.

Monitoring of response to intervention typically involves periodic analysis of blood markers of alcohol use. These include GGT and other standard liver function tests, carbohydrate-deficient transferrin (CDT) and ethyl glucuronide (EtG).

There is growing evidence for an approach combining treatment including counselling plus licence suspension.

Further reading

Asbridge M, Hayden JA, Cartwright JL. (2012). Acute cannabis consumption and motor vehicle collision risk: systematic review of observational studies and meta-analysis. *BMJ* 344:e536.

Australian Roads (2003). *Assessing Fitness to Drive: For Commercial and Private Vehicle Drivers.* Sydney: Austroads Inc.

Babor T, Caetano R, Casswell S et al. (2003). *Alcohol: No Ordinary Commodity.* Oxford: Oxford University Press.

Blomberg RD, Peck RC, Moskowitz H, et al. (2009). The Long Beach/Fort Lauderdale relative risk study. *J Safety Res* 40(4):285–92.

Driver and Vehicle Licensing Agency (2007). *At a Glance Guide to Medical Aspects of Fitness to Drive.* Swansea: DVLA.

Elvik R. (2013). Risk of road accident associated with the use of drugs: a systematic review and meta-analysis of evidence from epidemiological studies. *Accid Anal Prev* 60:254–67.

Goodwin A, Kirley B, Sandt L, et al. (2013, April). *Countermeasures that Work: A Highway Safety Countermeasures Guide for State Highway Safety Offices* (7th ed.). (Report No. DOT HS 811 727). Washington, DC: National Highway Traffic Safety Administration.

Li MC, Brady JE, DiMaggio CJ, et al. (2012). Marijuana use and motor vehicle crashes. *Epidemiol Rev* 34(1):65–72.

National Highway Traffic Safety Administration (2014). Traffic Safety Facts 2012. DOT HS 812 032. Washington, DC: U.S. Department of Transportation.

National Institute on Alcohol Abuse and Alcoholism (2001). *Alcohol and Transportation Safety.* Alcohol Alert Number 52. Available at: http://pubs.niaaa.nih.gov/publications/aa52.htm

Voas RB, Torres P, Romano E, et al. (2012). Alcohol-related risk of driver fatalities: an update using 2007 data. *J Stud Alcohol Drugs* 73: 341–50.

World Health Organization (2013). *Global Status Report on Road Safety 2013: Supporting a Decade of Action.* Geneva: WHO.

Zador PL. (1991). Alcohol-related relative risk of fatal driver injuries in relation to driver age and sex. *JStud Alcohol* 52(4):302–10.

Drugs and driving

Introduction

- Impairment of driving by drugs is an increasingly recognized problem (Box 26.1); its prevalence is probably higher than has been thought because of logistical difficulties in testing an apprehended driver for the range of drugs that may be involved.
- Besides alcohol, cannabis and benzodiazepines are most often found in impaired drivers, opiates and stimulants less often.
- Drugs may be prescribed (e.g. for pain), purchased in pharmacies ('over the counter'), or illicitly taken.
- Half of all impaired drivers have used multiple drugs.

Effects of individual drugs

Cannabis

- Raised concentrations of THC are associated with increased road traffic crash risk.
- Perception, psychomotor performance, and cognitive and affective function may be affected.
- Odds ratio for a serious or fatal injury whilst driving under the influence of cannabis ranges from 1.22 to 9.50.
- Accident risk is significantly increased when THC concentration in blood is at least 5 mcg/L, whether or not ingestion had occurred recently.
- The effects of drug use setting (e.g. polydrug use, concomitant alcohol use, and sleep deprivation) are intertwined and significantly contribute to unsafe driving.

Cocaine

- Both acute intoxication from cocaine use and the impact of exhaustion and tiredness following use have a negative impact on driver safety.
- Risk taking may be increased.
- Odds ratio for a serious or fatal injury whilst driving under the influence of cocaine ranges from 2 to 22, with the extent and significance of the increase in risk depending upon the population of driver investigated.

Box 26.1 Factors influencing driving impairment

- Sedative drugs cause more impairment especially when taken with alcohol.
- Higher doses cause more impairment.
- Mode of administration influences impairment; drugs taken by injection cause more impairment.
- Time after intake influences the degree of impairment; e.g. cannabis impairs driving skills for 2–4 hours.
- Half-life influences accumulation of the drug, e.g. long-acting benzodiazepines may impair more than short-acting ones.
- Development of tolerance is important when dose changes or a new drug is started.
- Liver disease may increase susceptibility to drug effects.

Amphetamine-type drugs

- Amphetamine and methamphetamine produce stimulatory effects, significantly increasing alertness and confidence, which may increase risk-taking whilst driving.
- Drivers may use amphetamines to keep awake whilst driving long distances.
- The 'come down' or 'crash' that follows 6–24 hours later, which is characterized by irritability, agitation, craving, and sleep disturbance, impairs driving.
- Odds ratio for a serious or fatal injury when driving under the influence of amphetamine/methamphetamine ranges from 2 to 24 in different studies.
- Use of prescribed amphetamines or similar drugs may also impair driving.

MDMA

- The 'come down' from MDMA associated with sleep deprivation is a risk factor for impaired driving.
- Odds ratio for a serious or fatal injury when driving under the influence of MDMA ranges from 5 to 30.

Ketamine
- Drowsiness, perceptual distortions, time disturbance, and feelings of unreality (effects of ketamine at moderate doses) impair driving abilities.

Opioids

- Odds ratio for serious injury or death for drivers testing positive for medicinal opioids is between 4.8 and 9.2.
- Those taking prescription opioids (e.g. codeine, tramadol, oxycodone) for pain may be impaired, although in some cases reduction of pain may reduce their impairment.
- Long-term patients show tolerance to sedative effects which may reduce their impairment over time.
- Illicit heroin users frequently use other drugs which may add to their impairment.
- In many countries, patients prescribed methadone can keep their driving licence; there is evidence that stable doses of methadone do not increase road accidents above the community average.

Benzodiazepines

- Acute intake of benzodiazepines is followed by a concentration-dependent deterioration of performance. Low levels of these drugs taken therapeutically may impair driving.
- Any benzodiazepine use increases twofold the risk of a road accident in a concentration-dependent fashion: risk is significantly higher when blood concentrations are above the normal therapeutic range (OR: 3.75; confidence interval: 1.46–9.63).
- Benzodiazepines are often used in combination with other drugs and then substantially impair driving.

Testing for drugs

In several countries, driving impairment is tested by roadside tests of function supported by blood tests for drugs. 'Threshold concentrations' of drugs (above which driving can be assumed to be impaired to a level similar to the legal limit for alcohol and driving) are being developed.

There is a need to increase testing for drugs in fatal crashes so that:
- trends can be monitored over time
- drug testing procedures across nations can be standardized
- the effects of drug-driving and drinking-driving laws can be better evaluated
- the proportions of people killed in drug-driving crashes other than the drug-using driver can be identified
- imputation models can be developed that predict which crashes involve drugs when drug test results are not available.

Penalties for driving when drugs are detected

- Ketamine, when confirmed by medical and laboratory evaluation, will lead to licence refusal or revocation in the UK until abstinent for 6 months.
- Persistent use of, or dependence on, heroin, morphine, methadone, cocaine, and methamphetamine confirmed by medical and laboratory evaluation, will lead to licence refusal or revocation until a minimum 1 year period free of such use has been attained.

Guidance for clinicians

- Clinicians should inform patients who are using drugs, whether illicit or prescribed that their driving may be impaired and that they should self-refer to the licensing authorities.
- Failing this, the clinician should consider the risk of the patient continuing to drive compared with risk of the individual leaving treatment. If the risk to the individual or the public is undeniably high, the clinician should inform the licensing authorities.
- Particular attention should be paid to older drivers, polydrug users, and those using benzodiazepines, or any drugs with alcohol.
- MDMA is not safe to consume if intending to drive; combining it with alcohol is contraindicated for safe driving.
- The clinician should check what requirements exist for patients prescribed methadone to self-report or be reported to the appropriate licensing authorities.

Further reading

Driver and Vehicle Licensing Agency (May 2014). *At a Glance Guide to the Current Medical Standards of Fitness to Drive*. Issued by Drivers Medical Group. www.gov.uk

Wolff K, Brimblecombe R, Forfar JC, et al. (2013). *Driving Under the Influence of Illicit Drugs*. Report from the Expert Panel on Drug Driving. London: Department for Transport. Available at: https://www.gov.uk/government/uploads/system/uploads/attachment_data/file/167971/drug-driving-expert-panel-report.pdf

Seizures and driving

Overview

The occurrence of a seizure while driving increases the risk of motor vehicle accidents, and may lead to catastrophic injuries and loss of life.

- Alcohol and/or sedative-hypnotic withdrawal seizures contribute substantially to morbidity and mortality because they may constitute up to 50% of seizures in some settings.
- As patients with a history of seizures are at risk of injury to themselves and/or to others, the clinician has a duty of care to advise the patient with a seizure not to drive for a proscribed seizure-free period of time.
- Following a single alcohol-related seizure an individual's licence will typically be revoked or refused. The length of time varies from country to country.
- Regulations governing restoration of licence with regard to seizure-free periods range from 3 to 36 months (between different countries and between different states in the same country).

Legislative requirements

- In several countries anyone who has experienced an alcohol-related (e.g. withdrawal) seizure is required to undergo medical assessment with blood analysis prior to having their licence restored. They should be free from alcohol misuse/dependence and seizure free for the appropriate period.
- To prevent non-compliance and under-reporting, and to preserve individual freedom, less stringent and shortened seizure-free periods are being advocated by some.
- Addiction specialists should be aware of relevant national and state legislation and medical guidelines regarding a person's fitness to drive after an alcohol- or substance-related seizure (see Box 26.2).
- People who have experienced a withdrawal seizure may be required to undergo an independent medical assessment with appropriate blood tests prior to having their licence restored.
- Referral to a neurologist for further investigation, including an EEG (to differentiate withdrawal seizures from epilepsy or to exclude concurrent epilepsy) should be considered.

Examples of national approaches

In Australia, following an acute symptomatic seizure, which includes seizures related to withdrawal from alcohol and other drugs, a conditional licence maybe considered by the driver's licensing authority subject to an annual review and a seizure free period of at least 6 months and EEG shows no epileptiform activity. For commercial vehicles (lorries,

---

Box 26.2 Seeking advice

Seek advice from local driving authorities and from legal and medical defence unions with regard to patient confidentiality and other issues.

buses), a conditional licence may be considered subject to annual review by a neurologist and there have been no further seizures for at least 12 months and an EEG shows no epileptiform activity.

In the UK, following a single alcohol-related seizure, an individual's licence will be revoked or refused for a minimum 6-month period from the date of the event (reduced from the previous 12 months). Medical enquiry to confirm an appropriate period free from alcohol misuse or dependence with blood analysis and consultant's report will normally be necessary. When more than one seizure has occurred, epilepsy regulations apply. For commercial vehicles (lorries, buses) following a solitary alcohol related seizure, the licence may be revoked or refused for a minimum 5-year period from the date of the event. Licence restoration requires no underlying cerebral structural abnormality, off-antiepileptic medication for at least 5 years, abstinence from alcohol (if previously dependent) and review by an addiction specialist or neurologist.

In the US, driving regulations do not distinguish between epilepsy and unprovoked first seizures and the proscribed seizure-free period varies between different states from 3 months to 36 months. Some states require physicians to immediately report in writing, persons diagnosed with epilepsy or unprovoked first seizures.

Further reading

Austroads and National Transport Commission (2012). *Assessing Fitness to Drive for Commercial and Private Vehicle Drivers: Medical Standards for Licensing and Clinical Management Guidelines March 2012.* Available at: http://www.onlinepublications.austroads.com.au/items/AP-G56

Driver and Vehicle Licensing Agency (2013). Alcohol related seizures. In *Current medical guidelines: DVLA guidance for professionals.* [Online] Available at: https://www.gov.uk/government/collections/current-medical-guidelines-dvla-guidance-for-professionals

Lingford-Hughes AR, Welch S, Nutt DJ. (2004). BAP consensus statement on the treatment of addiction. *J Psychopharmacol* 18:2933–5.

Winston GP, Jaiser SR. (2012). Western driving regulations for unprovoked first seizure and epilepsy. *Seizure* 21:371–6

Child protection

Introduction

Substance use and substance use disorders not only affect individuals but families too. Children's health, safety, and emotional well-being can be seriously impaired when their parents, guardians, or siblings have substance use problems. Substance use in the family can harm children from conception onwards and lead to problems that persist into adult life. The needs of these children have all too often been overlooked by treatment agencies commissioned to provide services for adults. Whilst it may be true that substance use does not always impair parenting, the effects when it does so can cause significant and lasting harm to children and young people. See Table 26.2.

Epidemiology

- More than half of adults in substance use treatment in England are parents or have children living with them.
- Data from child protection studies show that an increasing level of social work intervention is linked with an increasing rate of parental substance misuse.
- Data from Australia and the US suggest that parental substance abuse contributes to at least 50% of all child welfare cases.

Harms experienced by children

- Intrauterine exposure to substances ingested by the mother leading to growth impairment, premature birth, and in some cases specific fetal damage (e.g. alcohol)
- Vertical transmission of blood-borne viruses (which may be acquired by the mother through injecting or sexual behaviour)
- Diminished antenatal care through poor attendance and higher incidence of birth complications
- Neonatal abstinence syndrome
- Neglect due to parents being preoccupied with substance acquisition and use, or intoxicated or withdrawing from substances
- Poverty because of parents using money for drug use (many such families are in lower socioeconomic groups)

Table 26.2 The scale of the problem

Country	Children (under 16 years) living with parent(s) with substance use disorders
United Kingdom	Up to 3% (or 350,000) living with parents who are problem drug users. Up to 9% (or 1.3 million) living with parents who misuse alcohol
United States	9% of children (6 million) live with a parent who abuses alcohol or other drugs
Australia	Between 10% and 13% of children live with a parent who abuses alcohol or other drugs

- Poor nutritional status, poor medical and dental care, lack of immunizations
- Unpredictable adult behaviour (intoxication and withdrawal) and mood swings
- Separation from parents due to incarceration and hospitalization
- Bereavement: parents may die from overdose, complications of alcohol and drug use, and suicide
- Alternative care provision (grandparents, statutory accommodation)
- Accidental and non-accidental injury
- Exposure to dangerous substances including drugs and drug use paraphernalia, and passive smoking; children have died from ingestion of methadone prescribed to adults
- Domestic violence, well known to be associated with substance use, such as alcohol
- Poor school attendance and little support with educational endeavours such as homework and projects
- Separation from extended family
- Stigma from local community: e.g. parents known to be using substances, mentally unwell, or seen to be intoxicated, begging, or involved with criminal behaviours
- Children having to parent adults, other children, and themselves
- Inappropriate adults visiting home with attendant child protection risks
- Exposure to violence associated with drug acquisition and drug use
- Exposure to inappropriate adult behaviours such as sex for money or drugs, injecting behaviour
- Drug- or alcohol-impaired driving accidents.

Indicators of potential harm: assessing the parent(s)

- All adults presenting for treatment of a substance misuse problem should be assessed with regard to the likely impact of their substance misuse on their children.
- This should include professionals visiting the home and talking with the child, wherever possible.
- Children may be reluctant or afraid to discuss problems at home; staff need to be trained and skilled at interviewing children.
- Any concerns should be reported to the relevant child protection services so that full assessment of the children's needs can be undertaken.
- In all cases the needs of the children are paramount.

The following features suggest a risk of greater harm to children:
- Dependence on, or use in large amounts of, substance(s)
- Substantial time taken to fund, obtain, and use the substance(s)
- Injecting use
- Mood swings and unpredictability
- Significant withdrawal symptoms
- Use of multiple substances (including alcohol) with episodes of intoxication and withdrawal, and chaotic behaviour
- Methods of procuring funding for substances such as sex work and criminal activity

- Presence of co-morbid mental illness
- Financial problems, housing problems, legal problems
- No non-substance-using adults in household.
- Coexisting substance misuse, domestic violence, and comorbid mental health disorders (the 'toxic triad')

Impact of substance use on parenting ability and the experience of children

Substance misuse is one of many factors that can impact on parenting ability and there are many other factors that can mitigate or exacerbate any problems caused.

The following factors need to be considered:

- Severity of and type of parental drug and alcohol problems: little is known about the relative risks of different substance types in terms of impact on parenting; however, heavy and/or chaotic use of any substance with episodes of intoxication and withdrawal is likely to impact negatively on parenting skills.
- One or both parents receiving effective treatment and achieving abstinence or stability is likely to be associated with better outcomes for the children.
- Co-morbid mental illness: parental mental illness has associated child protection risks in addition to those associated with substance misuse.
- School experience: positive school experiences have been shown to be associated with better outcomes for childhood adversity.
- Age of the child and child's needs: e.g. younger children are more vulnerable to physical neglect.
- Presence of at least one supportive parent or parental figure is associated with better outcome.
- Level of social support to family: strong social support networks are associated with better outcomes for childhood adversity as is the presence of a committed mentor or other person outside the family.
- Financial status of family: a stable home with adequate financial resources is likely to be associated with better outcomes.
- Parents' ability to prioritize children's needs and general parenting skills (parents may have poor baseline parenting skills).
- Family routines: families report that routines are often difficult to establish where there are substance misuse problems; better outcome for children when routines and activities are preserved.

Adverse consequences for children from parental substance misuse

The potential effects of parental problem drug use on children are serious and can cause potentially life-long difficulties.

They include the following:

- Poor physical and dental health during childhood
- Incomplete immunizations
- Acquisition of blood-borne viruses
- Poor educational attainment and difficulty in relationships with peers

- Emotional and behavioural disorders, such as antisocial acts, truanting, impulsivity, hyperactivity, inattention, aggression, conduct disorders, depression, and anxiety
- Early initiation of smoking, alcohol, and drug use
- Increased risk of problem alcohol and drug use
- Increased risk of offending and criminality
- Increased risk of teenage pregnancy and STIs.

Interventions

A prerequisite for intervention is the identification of children living with adults with substance misuse problems by the relevant agencies. The needs of the children must be paramount and referrals to children's safeguarding services instituted when risks are identified.

For children

- Individual specific support for children—depends on age and needs—nursery, after school, counselling, peer support groups, educational support.
- Work with children to prevent early initiation of drug and alcohol use.
- Suitable alternative accommodation for children if necessary—where parents are in hospital/prison/unable to provide adequate care.

For parents

- Rapid entry to effective substance misuse treatment for parents. If medications such as methadone are prescribed to parents, the agencies must ensure that the risks to children from ingestion of such medication are minimized. This must include a risk assessment, parental education about the dangers to children, supervised administration of medication, or safe storage facilities (such as lockable medication cabinets) in the family home.
- Access to high-quality sexual health clinics for adults. Incentivizing contraception/sterilization for substance misusing women has been a controversial suggestion but nonetheless it is important for women to have access to contraceptive services to prevent unwanted pregnancies.

For families as a whole

- Specific programmes for families with substance misusing parents— research has shown that it is possible to recruit and retain high-risk families with substance misuse into structured programmes addressing parenting skills and deficits as well as substance misuse. Such interventions address many aspects of families' lives, including parental emotional and mental health, rather than focusing on a single issue.
- Social support for families including housing, financial, legal, and social support.
- Support should be given to alternative carers such as grandparents.

- Long-term residential care outside the family may be indicated if risks cannot be reduced by other interventions. Such decisions are complex and account needs to be taken of the timescales suitable for children and the timescales needed for the recovery of the adults.
- The use of Family Drug and Alcohol Courts, a multidisciplinary team working within a legal framework that appears to have better outcomes for families than conventional legal proceedings in cases of child protection.

Further reading

Adfam (2014). *Medications in Drug Treatment: Tackling the Risks to Children*. [Online] Available at: http://www.adfam.org.uk/cms/docs/adfam_ost_fullreport_web.pdf

Advisory Council on the Misuse of Drugs (2003). *Hidden Harm. Responding to the Needs of Children of Problem Drug Users*. London: Home Office.

Barnard M. (2007). *Drug Addiction and Families*. London: Jessica Kingsley Publishers.

Barnard MA, McKeganey NP. (2004). The impact of parental drug problem use on children: what is the problem and what can be done to help? *Addiction* 99:552–9.

Cleaver H, Unell I, Aldgate J. (1999). *Children's Needs—Parenting Capacity. The Impact of Parental Mental Illness, Problem Alcohol and Drug Use, and Domestic Violence on Children's Development*. London: Department of Health.

Dawe S, Frye S, Best D, et al. (2007). *Drug Use in the Family: Impacts and Implications for Children*. Canberra: Australian National Council on Drugs.

Harwin J, Alrouh B, Ryan M, et al. (2014). *Changing Lifestyles, Keeping Children Safe: An Evaluation of the first Family Drug and Alcohol Court (FDAC) in Care Proceedings*. London: Brunel University.

Prime Minister's Strategy Unit (2004). *Alcohol Harm Reduction Strategy for England*. London: Cabinet Office.

Interpersonal violence

Domestic violence is any actual or threatened behaviour by one partner in a relationship to cause psychological, physical, or sexual harm and gain power and control over another person's life. The most common example of domestic violence is the use of force by men to maintain control over their partners. One in four women is likely to be subjected to domestic violence. The WHO estimates that, worldwide, 35% of women report domestic violence, and that 40–75% of female murder victims are killed by their intimate partners in the context of an abusive relationship.

Some forms of domestic violence
- *Physical violence:* intentional use of physical force such as punching, hitting, kicking, pushing, slapping, biting, burning, choking, or the use of restraints or weapons.
- *Sexual violence:* being forced to have sex (rape), sexual abuse, indecent assault, being forced to look at pornography.
- *Psychological or emotional violence:* threats or verbal abuse of physical or sexual violence, injury or death, or abuse or actions which threaten, degrade, humiliate, or insult a person and cause fear; it may involve being stopped from seeing family or friends.
- *Economic abuse:* being denied access to, or having no control over money or other resources, and/or being forced to live without money.

Interpersonal violence is often related to use of alcohol and other drugs, in particular psychostimulants, by the perpetrator. The perpetrator may also have underlying psychological/psychiatric problems. Domestic violence is a crime in most Western countries. Acts of domestic violence and the subsequent outcomes are deemed the sole responsibility of the perpetrator.

Risk factors

Risk factors (in the victim):
- Female (especially younger age, pregnancy/postpartum)
- At risk of alcohol or other substance use
- High-risk sexual behaviour
- Childhood history of witnessing or experiencing violence
- Mental health problems (depression)
- Less educated
- Unemployed or being below the poverty line.

Risk factors (in the perpetrator):
- Alcohol and other substance use disorders (in particular psychostimulants)
- Psychological/psychiatric disorders (PTSD)
- Parental history of abuse.
- Recent job loss, or instability
- Exposure to childhood violence.

Outcomes of domestic and intimate partner violence

There is increasing risk to the victim of psychological and/or physical harm due to *worsening* of abuse and assaults over time.

Physical harm
- Varies from minor scratches, bruises to more serious injuries, knife wounds, broken bones, signs of strangulation
- Medical complaints—including headache, pain (back, chest, musculoskeletal), gynaecological disorders, STIs, HIV/AIDS, urinary tract infections, pregnancy complications, postpartum depression.

Psychological harm
- Fear, low self-esteem, and loss of self-confidence by victims
- Mental health problems (anxiety, dissociative disorders, PTSD; depression; suicide attempts; sleep disorders; eating disorders)
- Alcohol and other substance use disorders
- Relationship/family break-up.

Other outcomes of domestic violence
- Assault, homicide, suicide
- Criminal charges, imprisonment.
- Psychological and/or physical harm to children and young people who witness the domestic violence

Clinical assessment

Domestic/intimate partner violence is often undiagnosed as the victims are afraid or ashamed of their abuse. It is therefore important to look for clues, as indicated here:

History
- Psychological/psychiatric problems: inappropriate affect, evasive or hostile behaviour, fear, anxiety, panic attacks, depression, overdose, suicide attempts
- Repeated presentations with a vague, variable, or bizarre history of injury, which is inconsistent with the physical findings
- Social isolation
- Delay in seeking treatment, non-compliance, missed appointments
- Alcohol and other substance use problems.

Physical examination
A victim of domestic violence may be reluctant to undress or have a genital or rectal examination. Signs to look for include:
- poor health, bruising, lacerations, welts, bites, scratch marks, burns, scalds over the face, neck, head, or other parts of the body
- multiple injuries or bruises, trauma, fractures, head injuries
- bruising, injuries, tears, or bleeding from the genitalia or anus; genital warts or evidence of STIs/HIV/AIDS.

Signs in the perpetrator
A perpetrator of domestic violence may:
- appear overly concerned about the victim
- speak for partner or children
- show some signs, e.g. facial scratches and injuries, by the victim fighting back.

Intervention and management

In serious cases, medical care for injuries may be needed. It is important to document signs of injury found on clinical examination (a photographic record may be valuable for any later legal action).

Assess for safety

Safety is paramount to prevent harm or death.

Support

Offer support in a non-judgemental and empathetic way. Validate the victim. Ensure that the victim knows that acts of domestic violence and the subsequent outcomes are due to the perpetrator's behaviour and the sole responsibility of the perpetrator.

Assistance

Offer help and assistance. The clinician can encourage a victim to report an incident to the police; however, it is important to respect the patient's right to decide whether she or he wishes to take this action. In some cases, the victim is rightly afraid of the consequences to themselves should they speak to the police. Let the victim know of the range of legal actions open to them including placing criminal charges or (in many regions) seeking a court order designed to protect them. Such a court order may restrain the perpetrator from approaching them (often known as a restraining order or apprehended violence order). In other cases, a magistrate may order the partner not to drink or use substances in the home.

- Subsidized legal aid may be available
- Domestic violence help lines are available in many regions. The patient can call for ongoing advice and support
- Family support services may be able to offer support to children in the family.

Where there are children in the family who are placed at risk from domestic violence, the clinician is legally obliged to report domestic violence to the government department responsible for child protection in many countries. Reporting must occur when children and young persons under the age of 18 years are at risk of physical, psychological, or emotional harm as a result of what is done (physical, sexual, or psychological abuse) or not done (neglect) by another person responsible for their care.

The victim may use alcohol or other psychoactive substances to cope with the after effects of domestic violence. Psychotherapy can also target developing more productive responses. In some cases, the victim's own substance use, or disinhibited behaviour as a result of substance use, may be a trigger for domestic violence. While this never excuses the violence, the patient's safety may be enhanced by increasing awareness of the triggers to violence and how to avoid these, and/or other self-protective action that may be effective.

Further reading

World Health Organization (2014). Violence by intimate partners. In *World Report on Violence and Health*. Geneva: WHO. Available at: http://www.who.int/violence-injury-prevention/violence/global-campaign/en/chapter4.pdf

Workplace safety and interventions

There has been increasing focus in recent years on the issue of use of alcohol and other drugs in the workplace. The concern has arisen from four separate considerations:

- Concern about the negative impact on productivity of employees (at various levels) who are impaired as a result of substance use
- Concern about the legal and ethical implications of employees affected by psychoactive substances particularly in transportation and other industries where public safety is paramount
- Increasing expectation that employees will have a safe workplace, as enshrined by the development of health and safety legislation
- Acknowledgement that the workplace potentially offers a setting in which people with substance use disorders can seek advice and treatment through self-referral or employer-initiated mechanisms.

Effects of substance use on work

- Absenteeism due to illness or disciplinary suspension
- Reduced performance and productivity
- Inappropriate behaviour towards other workers, including those reporting to the individual
- Theft and other crime
- Work accidents
- Poor relationships between workers
- Increased turnover of staff
- Low morale in the workforce.

Work accidents

It is estimated that 20–25% of all workplace accidents involve alcohol in some way. Alcohol consumption impairs concentration, judgement, and coordination, and accidents can affect the drinker and those around them. Employers have legal responsibilities regarding the safety of employees and, where relevant, the general public. Drinking even small amounts of alcohol before or while carrying out work that is 'safety sensitive' will increase the risk of an accident.

Surveys of many industries have shown a high prevalence of alcohol and other drug use in workforces. In part, this reflects community patterns of substance use. However, other key influences are the sociodemographic make-up of the workforce, and also the nature of the product or service provided. Certain workforces have a particularly high prevalence of substance use. For example, workers in hospitality and catering industries, and in particular those involved in the production or sale of alcohol, have a high rate of alcohol misuse. Workgroups who have ready access to prescribed medications, such as healthcare professionals, have higher rates of dependence on prescribed sedative hypnotics and opioids. In the financial industry there is reportedly a high prevalence of psychostimulant use; whether this involves methamphetamine or cocaine depends on the geographical area.

In the music industry and other creative arts there is a high prevalence of multiple substance use, including cannabis, alcohol, heroin, and psychostimulants. In some industries (e.g. trucking), stimulants are sometimes used to increase wakefulness or stamina but pose major safety hazards. Stimulant use has also been associated with the modelling industry, where weight loss is often a desired outcome.

Workplace alcohol and drug policies

Substance use and related disorders in the workplace should be considered from a health as well as a legislative perspective. Policy should be linked to one or more of an organization's procedures on managing health and safety, as well as personnel and/or general management issues.

An alcohol and drug policy will be more successful if supported by a programme of training that raises alcohol awareness and supports managers in its application. Employers may have parallel or combined policy on alcohol and drug use.

Current approaches to the prevention of substance misuse in the workplace include the following:

- A policy covering the use of alcohol or other drugs prior to or during the working day, which is agreed through negotiation with employee groups, unions, and management representatives
- Provision through an employee assistance scheme of assessment and referral on a confidential basis of employees who are affected by psychoactive substances. Typically, this would include an employer-initiated process where impairment of work performance or the detection of psychoactive substances has occurred. Secondly, self-initiated referral also occurs where an employee recognizes that their alcohol or drug use is causing problems
- Routine and random testing for alcohol and other drugs has been introduced progressively in recent years into many industries particularly those where there are safety critical working conditions, e.g. using machinery or where there is a responsibility for public safety, as in the transportation industries. Such policies may require employees to provide a urine or saliva sample, which will be tested for drugs or a breath or urine sample for testing for alcohol. The consequences of a positive test will depend on the organization's policy, but may include a warning, a requirement to participate in an employee assistance programme, or, particularly with repeated infractions, loss of employment.
- Sometimes the workplace can offer supervision of medication, such as disulfiram to increase adherence to treatment regimens.

Testing

Testing employees or potential employees for alcohol use or related problems remains controversial, raising both industrial relations and civil liberty issues. In many countries, employers have a responsibility to 'take reasonable care' to prevent an accident if an employee's ability to work safely is impaired. This need to prevent alcohol- or drug-related accidents has led companies in the transport sector to introduce testing to prevent employees' substance use in the workplace.

Methods of testing

Alcohol testing indicates whether an individual is under the influence at that time. Drug testing differs, sometimes showing traces of drugs used in the past, but not confirming impairment at the time of testing. Alcohol use can be determined by breath or blood testing. Breath tests are convenient and inexpensive. Blood testing is the most accurate measure of alcohol in the body, but is more invasive than a breath test and not routinely carried out, except in safety critical jobs, e.g. after a positive breath test is returned.

Screening can be undertaken in several ways:

- *Recruitment screening* usually involves testing as part of assessing the health of potential employees during the recruitment process.
- *Routine testing* is done at specified times and gives a clear message that it is not acceptable to be affected by alcohol when working. It might be used in situations where employees are in 'safety critical' posts, such as operating public transport or machinery.
- *Random testing* is used as a deterrent to identify previously undetected alcohol misuse. Again, this is more likely to be used in safety critical settings.
- *'With cause' and post-incident testing* might be used if a manager has reason to believe that an employee has been drinking, by their behaviour or is smelling of alcohol, for instance. After an incident at work, such as an accident, it can be a part of the post-incident investigation.

Getting specialist help

Workforce programmes and interventions tend to be offered by specific organizations which specialize in this area. On occasion an employee may be referred to a public sector or private facility to undergo treatment. In such circumstances it is vital for the clinician to understand the nature of the referral request and any reporting requirements. This is essential to ensure the integrity of the treatment is maintained and that there is a clear understanding by all parties on whether the treatment and response is subject to usual medical confidentiality provisions or whether the clinician or agency is required to provide periodic reports on progress. This is especially important where a person's professional registration or business operating licence is at threat if adherence to treatment is inadequate.

Some larger employers will have an occupational health department or employee assistance programme that may include an in-house counselling service with expertise in alcohol problems. Alternatively, individuals might be encouraged to approach their GP, seek to be referred to a community alcohol service, or attend Alcoholics Anonymous. In-patient detoxification and residential treatment facilities may sometimes also be available, although normally these would be through referral following a full assessment.

Further reading

Drug Policy Forum (2007). *Tackling Drugs and Alcohol in the Workplace*. Available at: www.cityoflondon.gov.uk/ldpf

Involuntary treatment and diversion programmes

Involuntary drug and alcohol treatment

This refers to coerced detention and treatment which is legally sanctioned and the individual has no choice about entry into treatment
- Includes court-mandated diversion programmes where referral to treatment is required by the police or the criminal justice system.
- Includes compulsory prison-based drug treatment which is seen as contentious as it is often abstinence based, lacks rigorous evidence for effectiveness, and evidence-based treatments such as opioid maintenance may be excluded.
- 'Civil commitment' involves compulsory treatment for individuals who are outside the criminal justice system (non-offenders) but whose substance dependence is high risk or life-threatening.
- Clinicians are often reluctant to use involuntary treatment, viewing it as a violation of basic human rights including personal liberty and patient autonomy. Treatment is often seen as only likely to be effective if the patient is motivated for change.
- The evidence base for involuntary treatment is limited but expanding. Case reports indicate some individuals clearly benefit from short-term involuntary treatment with restoration of capacity to make decisions about substance use and personal well-being, leading to reduced substance use, improved health, and psychosocial function.
- Where involuntary treatment occurs, it is essential that the loss of liberty be balanced by access to a choice of appropriate treatments.

Coercive treatment and diversion

This occurs when an individual is given the choice of complying with treatment for substance misuse or receiving 'alternative consequences' as prescribed by the enforcement of the law, policy, or agency.
- 'Alternative consequences' may include prison or probation, loss of child custody, or loss of employment or benefits.
- May involve court diversion into treatment (including drug courts) for persons found guilty of a drug-related offence. Diversion into treatment is offered as an alternative to other penalties such as imprisonment.
- Diversion into treatment may also occur when the person is apprehended by the police and is referred to an education session or a short-term intervention instead of being arrested. This typically involves possession of cannabis in amounts considered for personal use only.
- Research on coercive treatment demonstrates mostly efficacy and cost benefits, including reduced substance use and criminality, improved health and employment.
- Those participating in community treatment under 'legal pressure' do as well as those entering treatment without legal coercion, with reductions in substance use and criminal behaviour.

Persons with substance use disorders may fall within the scope of a country's mental health legislation and provision (See Box 26.3).

Box 26.3 Mental Health Acts (MHAs)

Individuals with substance misuse may fall within the scope of the MHA if they have a coexisting mental illness and are a significant risk of harm to themselves and/or others because of the mental illness

The definition of 'mental illness' depends on the provisions of the MHA in the local jurisdiction.

Some jurisdictions also allow for the short-term detention and treatment of 'mentally disordered' persons under the MHA if the person's behaviour is so irrational that temporary care, treatment, or control is necessary to protect the person or others from serious harm

Guardianship and financial management

Provisions for guardianship and financial management are available in many national and international jurisdictions, and the local legislature should always be consulted.

Guardianship

- A guardian is a substitute decision-maker who has the authority to make lifestyle or personal decisions for someone who is incapable of making these decisions for themselves. This may include where someone lives, what medical treatment they receive, and what services they need.
- Guardianship orders are generally not applicable to a person who lacks the capacity to make decisions because of substance dependence alone, unless there is also evidence of a disability such as acquired brain injury, dementia, or mental illness which renders them incapable of making decisions about care and treatment.

Financial management

- An application for a financial management order may be required if the person is not capable of managing their financial and legal affairs and they need a substitute decision-maker (in the form of a financial manager) to manage their affairs.
- Financial affairs refers to things such as operating bank accounts, paying bills, investing money, selling or buying property, and includes legal affairs such as instructing a solicitor to act in legal proceedings.

Further reading

Broadstock M, Brinson D, Weston A. (2008). *The Effectiveness of Compulsory, Residential Treatment of Chronic Alcohol or Drug Addiction in Non-Offenders. Health Services Assessment Collaboration Report*. Christchurch: University of Canterbury.

Hall W, Lucke J. (2010). Legally coerced treatment for drug using offenders: ethical and policy issues. *Crime Justice Bull* 144:1–12.

Resources

Diagnosis and classification *590*
  ICD 10 diagnostic terms *590*
  DSM-IV-TR and DSM 5 diagnostic terms *597*
  ASAM diagnostic terms *599*
Screening instruments and questionnaires *600*
  Alcohol: AUDIT, AUDIT-C, and FAST *600*
  Nicotine: Fagerström Test *603*
  Drugs: DrugCheck *603*
  Internet Addiction Test (IAT) *604*
Withdrawal monitoring scales *606*
  Alcohol Withdrawal Scale (AWS) *606*
  Clinical Institute Withdrawal Assessment for Alcohol—
  Revised (CIWA-AR) *608*
  Clinical institute Withdrawal Assessment for Benzodiazepines
  (CIWA-B) *612*
  Subjective Opioid Withdrawal Scale (SOWS) *614*
  Objective Opioid Withdrawal Scale (OOWS) *615*
  Cannabis *616*
Cognitive function tests *617*
  Addenbrooke's Cognitive Examination (ACE-III) *617*
Risk assessment *625*
  Suicide screen *625*
Miscellaneous *627*
  The 12 steps of Alcoholics Anonymous *627*
  Useful websites *628*

Diagnosis and classification

ICD 10 diagnostic terms

ICD 10 Clinical Descriptions and Diagnostic Guidelines cover all physical and mental complications of alcohol and substance use.

They are subdivided into diagnostic entities and substance groups. The following substances are covered:

- Alcohol
- Opioids
- Cannabinoids
- Sedative hypnotics
- Cocaine
- Other stimulants, including caffeine
- Hallucinogens
- Tobacco
- Volatile solvents
- Multiple drug use and use of other psychoactive substances.

F1x.0. Acute intoxication

A transient condition following the administration of alcohol or other psychoactive substance, resulting in disturbances in level of consciousness, cognition, perception, affect or behaviour, or other psychophysiological functions and responses. This should be a main diagnosis only in cases where intoxication occurs without more persistent alcohol- or drug-related problems being concomitantly present. Where there are such problems, precedence should be given to diagnoses of harmful use (F1x.1), dependence syndrome (F1x.2), or psychotic disorder (F1x.5).

Acute intoxication is usually closely related to dose levels (see ICD 10). Exceptions to this may occur in individuals with certain underlying organic conditions (e.g. renal or hepatic insufficiency) in whom small doses of a substance may produce a disproportionately severe intoxicating effect. Disinhibition due to social context should also be taken into account (e.g. behavioural disinhibition at parties or carnivals). Acute intoxication is a transient phenomenon. Intensity of intoxication lessens with time and effects eventually disappear in the absence of further use of the substance. Recovery is therefore complete except where tissue damage or another complication has arisen.

Symptoms of intoxication need not always reflect primary actions of the substance. For instance, depressant drugs may lead to symptoms of agitation or hyperactivity, and stimulant drugs may lead to socially withdrawn and introverted behaviour. Effects of substances, such as cannabis and hallucinogens, may be particularly unpredictable.

Moreover, many psychoactive substances are capable of producing different types of effect at different levels. For example, alcohol may have apparently stimulant effects on behaviour at lower dose levels, lead to agitation and aggression with increasing dose levels, and produce clear sedation at very high levels.

F1x.1. Harmful use

A pattern of psychoactive substance use that is causing damage to health. The damage may be physical (as in cases of hepatitis from the self-administration of injected drugs) or mental (e.g. episodes of depressive disorder secondary to heavy consumption of alcohol).

Diagnostic guidelines

The diagnosis requires that actual damage should have been caused to the mental or physical health of the user.

Harmful patterns of use are often criticized by others and frequently associated with adverse social consequences of various kinds. The fact that a pattern of use or a particular substance is disapproved of by another person or by the culture, or may have led to socially negative consequences such as arrest or marital arguments is not in itself evidence of harmful use.

Acute intoxication (see F1x.0), or 'hangover' is not itself sufficient evidence of the damage to health required for coding harmful use.

Harmful use should not be diagnosed if dependence syndrome (F1x.2), a psychotic disorder (F1x.5), or another specific form of drug- or alcohol-related disorder is present.

F1x.2. Dependence syndrome

A cluster of physiological, behavioural, and cognitive phenomena in which the use of a substance or a class of substances takes on a much higher priority for a given individual than other behaviours that once had greater value. A central descriptive characteristic of the dependence syndrome is the desire (often strong, sometimes overpowering) to take psychoactive drugs (which may or may not have been medically prescribed), alcohol, or tobacco. There may be evidence that return to substance use after a period of abstinence leads to a more rapid reappearance of other features of the syndrome than occurs with nondependent individuals.

Diagnostic guidelines

A definite diagnosis of dependence should usually be made only if three or more of the following have been present together at some time during the previous year:

- A strong desire or sense of compulsion to take the substance
- Difficulties in controlling substance-taking behaviour in terms of its onset, termination, or levels of use
- A physiological withdrawal state (see F1x.3 and F1x.4) when substance use has ceased or been reduced, as evidenced by: the characteristic withdrawal syndrome for the substance; or use of the same (or a closely related) substance with the intention of relieving or avoiding withdrawal symptoms
- Evidence of tolerance, such that increased doses of the psychoactive substances are required in order to achieve effects originally produced by lower doses (clear examples of this are found in alcohol- and opiate-dependent individuals who may take daily doses sufficient to incapacitate or kill non-tolerant users)
- Progressive neglect of alternative pleasures or interests because of psychoactive substance use, increased amount of time necessary to obtain or take the substance or to recover from its effects

- Persisting with substance use despite clear evidence of overtly harmful consequences, such as harm to the liver through excessive drinking, depressive mood states consequent to periods of heavy substance use, or drug-related impairment of cognitive functioning; efforts should be made to determine that the user was actually, or could be expected to be, aware of the nature and extent of the harm.

See Table 27.1 for a comparison of these diagnostic findings with DSM IV substance definitions and DSM-5 substance use disorders.

F1x.3. Withdrawal state

A group of symptoms of variable clustering and severity occurring on absolute or relative withdrawal of a substance after repeated, and usually prolonged and/or high dose, use of that substance. Onset and course of the withdrawal state are time-limited and are related to the type of substance and the dose being used immediately before abstinence. The withdrawal state may be complicated by convulsions.

Diagnostic guidelines

Withdrawal state is one of the indicators of dependence syndrome (see F1x.2) and this latter diagnosis should also be considered. Withdrawal state should be coded as the main diagnosis if it is the reason for referral and sufficiently severe to require medical attention in its own right.

Physical symptoms vary according to the substance being used. Psychological disturbances (e.g. anxiety, depression, and sleep disorders) are also common features of withdrawal. Typically, the patient is likely to report that withdrawal symptoms are relieved by further substance use. It should be remembered that withdrawal symptoms can be induced by conditioned/learned stimuli in the absence of immediately preceding substance use. In such cases a diagnosis of withdrawal state should be made only if it is warranted in terms of severity.

F1x.4. Withdrawal state with delirium

A condition in which the withdrawal state (see F1x.3) is complicated by delirium.

F1x.5. Psychotic disorder

A cluster of psychotic phenomena that occur during or immediately after psychoactive substance use and are characterized by vivid hallucinations (typically auditory, but often in more than one sensory modality), misidentifications, delusions and/or ideas of reference (often of a paranoid or persecutory nature), psychomotor disturbances (excitement of stupor), and an abnormal affect, which may range from intense fear to ecstasy. The sensorium is usually clear, but some degree of clouding of consciousness, though not severe confusion, may be present. The disorder typically resolves at least partially within 1 month and fully within 6 months.

Diagnostic guidelines

A psychotic disorder occurring during or immediately after drug use (usually within 48 hours) should be recorded here provided that it is not a manifestation of drug withdrawal state with delirium (see F1x.4) or of late onset. Late-onset psychotic disorders (with onset more than 2 weeks after substance use) may occur, but should be coded as F1x.75.

Psychoactive substance-induced psychotic disorders may present with varying patterns of symptoms. These variations will be influenced by the type of substance involved and the personality of the user. For stimulant drugs such as cocaine and amphetamines, drug-induced psychotic disorders are generally closely related to high dose levels and/or prolonged use of the substance.

A diagnosis of psychotic disorder should not be made merely on the basis of perceptual distortions or hallucinatory experiences when substances having primary hallucinogenic effects (e.g. lysergic acid (LSD), mescaline, cannabis at high doses) have been taken. In such cases and also for confusional states, a possible diagnosis of acute intoxication (F1x.0) should be considered.

F1x.6. Amnesic syndrome

A syndrome associated with chronic prominent impairment of recent memory; remote memory is sometimes impaired, while immediate recall is preserved. Disturbances of time sense and ordering of events are usually evident, as are difficulties in learning new material. Confabulation may be marked but is not invariably present. Other cognitive functions are usually relatively well preserved and amnesic defects are out of proportion to other disturbances.

Diagnostic guidelines

Amnesic syndrome induced by alcohol or other psychoactive substances coded here should meet the general criteria for organic amnesic syndrome (see F04). The primary requirements for this diagnosis are:

- Memory impairment as shown in impairment of recent memory (learning of new material); disturbances of time sense (rearrangements of chronological sequence, telescoping of repeated events into one, etc.)
- Absence of defect in immediate recall, impairment of consciousness, and of generalized cognitive impairment
- History or objective evidence of chronic (and particularly high-dose) use of alcohol or drugs.

Personality changes, often with apparent apathy and loss of initiative, and a tendency towards self-neglect may also be present, but should not be regarded as necessary conditions for diagnosis.

Although confabulation may be marked it should not be regarded as a necessary prerequisite for diagnosis.

F1x.7. Residual and late-onset psychotic disorder

A disorder in which alcohol- or psychoactive substance-induced changes of cognition, affect, personality, or behaviour persist beyond the period during which a direct psychoactive substance-related effect might reasonably be assumed to be operating.

Diagnostic guidelines

Onset of the disorder should be directly related to the use of alcohol or a psychoactive substance. Cases in which initial onset occurs later than an episode(s) of substance use should be coded here only where clear and strong evidence is available to attribute the state to the residual effect of

Table 27.1 Diagnostic criteria for ICD 10 dependence, DSM-IV substance abuse and substance dependence and DSM-5 substance use disorders

	ICD 10 Alcohol Dependence/Substance Dependence	DSM-IV Alcohol Dependence/Substance Dependence	DSM-5 Alcohol Use Disorder/Substance Use Disorder
Stem	When three or more of the following criteria have been present together at some time during the previous 12-month period:	A maladaptive pattern of alcohol (or other substance) use, leading to clinically significant impairment or distress, as manifested by three or more of the following occurring at any time in the same 12-month period:	A problematic pattern of alcohol (or other substance) use, leading to clinically significant impairment or distress, as manifested by at least two of the following occurring within a 12-month period:
1 New in DSM-5	A strong desire or sense of compulsion to take alcohol or other psychoactive substance (*craving or compulsion*).	No equivalent criterion—mentioned in text.	Craving or a strong desire or urge to use alcohol (or other substance).
2	No equivalent criterion but text states that the subjective awareness of compulsion is most commonly seen during attempts to stop or control alcohol (or other substance) use.	There is persistent desire or unsuccessful attempts to cut down or control alcohol (or other substance use).	There is persistent desire or unsuccessful efforts to cut down or control alcohol (or other substance) use.
3	Difficulties in controlling alcohol or other substance-taking behaviour in terms of its onset, termination, or levels of use *(loss of control)*.	Alcohol (or other substance) is often taken in larger amounts or over a longer period of time than was intended.	Alcohol (or other substance) is often taken in larger amounts or over a longer period than was intended.
4	Progressive neglect of alternative pleasures because of psychoactive substance use, or increased amount of time necessary to obtain or take the substance or to recover from its effects.	Important social, occupational or recreational activities are given up or reduced because of drinking or psychoactive substance use.	Recurrent alcohol (or other substance) use resulting in a failure to fulfil major role obligations at work, school, or home.

5	Subsumed in above criterion.	A great deal of time is spent in activities necessary to obtain, or use, alcohol (or other substance), or recover from its effects.	A great deal of time is spent in activities necessary to obtain alcohol (or other substance), use alcohol (or other substance), or recover from its effects.
6.	Tolerance: such that increased doses of the psychoactive substances are required in order to achieve effects originally produced by lower doses.	Tolerance: as defined by either (a) a need for markedly increased amounts of alcohol (or other substance) to achieve the desired effects or (b) markedly diminished effect with continued use of the same amount of the substance.	Tolerance is defined by either of the following: (a) a need for markedly increased amounts of alcohol (or other substance) to achieve intoxication or desired effect or (b) a markedly diminished effect with continued use of the same amount of alcohol (or other substance).
7.	A physiological withdrawal state when substance use has ceased or been reduced, as evidenced by the characteristic withdrawal syndrome for the substance; or use of the same (or a closely related substance) with the intention of relieving or avoiding withdrawal symptoms.	Withdrawal as manifested by either (a) the characteristic withdrawal syndrome for alcohol (or other substance) or (b) the same (or a closely related) substance is taken to relieve or avoid withdrawal symptoms.	Withdrawal is manifested by either of the following: (a)the characteristic withdrawal syndrome for alcohol (or other substance) or (b) alcohol (or a closely related substance such as a benzodiazepine) (or other substance) is taken to relieve, or avoid withdrawal symptoms.
8.	Persisting with substance use despite clear evidence of overtly harmful consequences.	Alcohol (or other substance) use is continued despite knowledge of having a persistent or recurrent physical or psychological problem that is likely to have been caused or exacerbated by the substance.	Continued alcohol (or other substance) use despite having persistent or recurrent social or interpersonal problems caused or exacerbated by the effects of alcohol (or other substance).

Table 27.1 (Contd.)

	ICD 10 Alcohol Dependence/Substance Dependence	DSM-IV Alcohol Dependence/Substance Dependence	DSM-5 Alcohol Use Disorder/Substance Use Disorder
9.	Former DSM-IV abuse (presence of one criteria)	Continued alcohol (or other substance) use despite having persistent or recurrent social or interpersonal problems caused or exacerbated by the effects of alcohol (or other substance), e.g. arguments with spouse about consequences of intoxication, physical fights).	Alcohol (or other substance) use is continued despite knowledge of having a persistent or recurrent physical or psychological problem that is likely to have been caused or exacerbated by alcohol (or other substance).
10.	Former DSM-IV abuse	Recurrent alcohol (or other substance use) in situations in which it is typically hazardous (e.g. drink driving).	Recurrent use in situations in which it is physically hazardous.
11.	Former DSM-IV abuse	Recurrent alcohol (or other substance) use which results in failure to fulfil major obligations at work, school or home.	Important social, occupational or recreational activities are given up or reduced because of alcohol (or other substance) use.
	Omitted	Recurrent substance-related legal problems (e.g. driving an automobile or operating a machine when impaired by substance use).	

Note: in DSM-5 the diagnosis of alcohol (or substance) use disorder is further classified according to severity: mild: presence of 2 to 3 symptoms; moderate: presence of 4 to 5 symptoms; severe: presence of 6 or more symptoms.

the substance. The disorder should represent a change from or marked exaggeration of prior and normal state of functioning.

The disorder should persist beyond any period of time during which direct effects of the psychoactive substance might be assumed to be operative (see F1x.0, acute intoxication). Alcohol- or psychoactive substance-induced dementia is not always irreversible; after an extended period of total abstinence, intellectual functions and memory may improve.

The disorder should be carefully distinguished from withdrawal-related conditions (see F1x.3 and F1x.4). It should be remembered that, under certain conditions and for certain substances, withdrawal state phenomena may be present for a period of many days or weeks after discontinuation of the substance.

DSM-IV-TR and DSM-5 diagnostic terms

DSM-IV-TR is the text revision of the Fourth Edition of the *Diagnostic and Statistical Manual of Mental and Behavioral Disorders*, published by the American Psychiatric Association in 2000. DSM-5 is the Fifth Edition of the manual and was published in 2013.

DSM-IV-TR

1. *Alcohol abuse/Substance abuse* is defined as a mainly social disorder resulting from repetitive use causing personal or social problems.
2. *Alcohol dependence/Substance dependence* is defined as a pattern of repetitive use leading to significant impairment or distress which includes any three of the following criteria:
   - tolerance
   - withdrawal
   - persistent desire or unsuccessful attempts to cut down or control use
   - use in larger amounts or over a longer period than was intended
   - excessive time spent in obtaining the substance, using the substance or getting over its effects; important social, occupational or recreational activities are given up
   - continued use despite persistent or recurring psychical or psychological problems.

DSM-5

1. Alcohol Use Disorder/Substance Use Disorder

In DSM-5 alcohol abuse/substance abuse and alcohol dependence/substance dependence are subsumed under the broad term 'Alcohol use disorder' or 'Substance use disorder'. A diagnosis of alcohol use disorder or substance use disorder is made when two or more of the 11 criteria occur within a 12-month period. The severity of the disorder is further classified on the number of criteria met viz. mild: 2 or more; moderate: 4–5; severe: 6 or more.

Nine substances are covered: alcohol, caffeine, cannabis, hallucinogens, inhalants, opioids, sedative/hypnotic/anxiolytics, stimulants and tobacco. In addition, a section on gambling addiction has been also introduced.

Table 27.1 compares the diagnostic criteria for ICD 10 dependence, DSM-IV substance abuse and substance dependence, and DSM-5 substance use disorders.

2. Alcohol-Induced Disorder/Substance-Induced Disorder

2.1 Alcohol/substance intoxication and withdrawal

DSM-5 diagnostic criteria for alcohol intoxication/substance intoxication:

A: Recent ingestion of alcohol or substance (reversible and substance specific)

B: Clinically significant problematic behavioural or psychological changes that develop during or shortly after ingestion of alcohol /substance

C: Symptoms are attributable to physiological effects of alcohol or the substance

D: The signs and symptoms are not attributable to another medical condition and are not better explained by another mental disorder or intoxication with another substance.

DSM-5 diagnostic criteria for alcohol withdrawal/substance withdrawal:

A: Cessation or reduction of heavy prolonged heavy, repetitive use of alcohol or other substance

B: Two or more signs/symptoms (specific to alcohol or other substance), developing within hours to days after cessation or reduction in use

C: The signs and symptoms of withdrawal cause clinically significant distress or impairment in social, occupational or other areas of functioning

2.2 DSM-5 Substance/medication-induced mental disorders

The alcohol/substance is capable of producing the mental disorder and the symptoms of the mental disorder develop during or soon after alcohol/substance intoxication or withdrawal. This includes:

a. Substance/medication-induced psychotic disorder

b. Substance/medication-induced depressive disorder

c. Substance-induced anxiety disorder

d. Substance/medication induced neurocognitive disorders (referred to in DSM-IV-TR as dementia, delirium, amnestic and other cognitive disorders).

DSM-5 criteria for substance/medication-induced mental disorder:

A. The disorder represents a clinically significant symptomatic presentation of a relevant mental disorder

B. There is evidence from history, clinical examination or laboratory results that:

    a. The mental disorder developed during or within 1 month of substance intoxication or withdrawal

    b. The involved substance is capable of producing the disorder

C. The disorder is not better explained by an independent mental disorder evidenced by the following:

    a. The mental disorder preceded the onset of intoxication, withdrawal or exposure to medication

    b. The mental disorder persists for a substantial period of time (e.g. at least 1 month) after cessation of severe intoxication or acute withdrawal (does not apply to persisting substance induced

neurocognitive disorders or hallucinogen induced perception
disorder)

D. The disorder does not occur exclusively during the course of a delirium

E. The disorder causes clinically significant distress or impairment in social,
occupational or other important areas of functioning.

American Society of Addiction Medicine (ASAM) definition of addiction

Addiction is a primary, chronic disease of brain reward, motivation, memory, and related circuitry. Dysfunction in these circuits leads to characteristic
biological, psychological, social, and spiritual manifestations. This is reflected
in an individual pathologically pursuing reward and/or relief by substance
use and other behaviours.

Addiction is characterized by inability to consistently abstain, impairment in behavioural control, craving, diminished recognition of significant
problems with one's behaviours and interpersonal relationships, and a dysfunctional emotional response. Like other chronic diseases, addiction often
involves cycles of relapse and remission. Without treatment or engagement
in recovery activities, addiction is progressive and can result in disability or
premature death.

Further reading

American Psychiatric Association (2000). *The Diagnostic and Statistical Manual of Mental Disorders*
(4th ed, text rev). Washington DC: American Psychiatric Association.

American Psychiatric Association (2013). *Diagnostic and Statistical Manual of Mental Disorders* (5th
ed). Washington DC: American Psychiatric Association.

Latt N, Conigrave KM, Saunders JB, *et al*. (2009). *Addiction Medicine* (1st ed). Oxford: Oxford
University Press.

Saunders JB, Latt NC (2015). Diagnostic definitions, criteria and classification of substance use disorders. In El-Guebaly N, Carra G, Galanter M (eds) *Textbook of Addiction Treatment: International
Perspectives* (Vol. 1), pp. 167–89. New York: Springer Reference.

World Health Organization (1992). *The ICD 10 Classification of Mental and Behavioural Disorders:
Clinical Descriptions and Diagnostic Guidelines*. World Health Organization, Geneva.

Screening instruments and questionnaires

Alcohol: AUDIT

Fig. 27.1 shows the Alcohol Use Disorders Identification Test (AUDIT).

1. How often do you have a drink containing alcohol?				
Never	Monthly or less	2–4 times a month	2–3 times a week	4 or more times a week
2. How many standard drinks containing alcohol do you have on a typical day when you are drinking?				
1 or 2	3 or 4	5 or 6	7–9	10 or more
3. How often do you have six or more drinks on one occasion?				
Never	Less than monthly	Monthly	Weekly	Daily or almost daily
4. During the past year, how often have you found that you were not able to stop drinking once you had started?				
Never	Less than monthly	Monthly	Weekly	Daily or almost daily
5. During the past year, how often have you failed to do what was normally expected of you because of drinking?				
Never	Less than monthly	Monthly	Weekly	Daily or almost daily
6. During the past year, how often have you needed a drink in the morning to get yourself going after a heavy drinking session?				
Never	Less than monthly	Monthly	Weekly	Daily or almost daily
7. During the past year, how often have you had a feeling of guilt or remorse after drinking?				
Never	Less than monthly	Monthly	Weekly	Daily or almost daily
8. During the past year, have you been unable to remember what happened the night before because you had been drinking?				
Never	Less than monthly	Monthly	Weekly	Daily or almost daily
9. Have you or someone else been injured as a result of your drinking?				
No		Yes, but not in the past year		Yes, during the past year
10. Has a relative or friend, doctor or other health worker been concerned about your drinking or suggested you cut down?				
No		Yes, but not in the past year		Yes, during the past year

Scoring the AUDIT: Scores for each question range from 0 to 4, for questions 1–8 the first response for each question (e.g. never) scoring 0, the second (e.g. less than monthly) scoring 1, the third (e.g. monthly) scoring 2, the fourth (e.g. weekly) scoring 3, and the last response (e.g. daily or almost daily) scoring 4.

For questions 9 and 10, which only have three responses, the scoring is 0, 2 and 4 (from left to right).

A score of 8 or more is associated with harmful or hazardous drinking, a score of 13 or more is likely to indicate alcohol dependence.

Further reading

Babor TF, Higgins-Biddle JC, Saunders JB, et al. (2001).AUDIT. The Alcohol Use Disorders Identification Test—Guidelines for Use in Primary Care (2nd ed). Geneva: WHO, Department of Mental Health and Substance Dependence 2001. Available at: http://whqlibdoc.who.int/hq/2001/WHO_MSD_MSB_01.6a.pdf

Saunders JB, Aasland OG, Babor TF, et al. (1993). Development of the Alcohol Use Disorders Identification Test (AUDIT): WHO Collaborative Project on Early Detection of Persons with Harmful Alcohol Consumption—II. Addiction 88:791–804.

Alcohol: AUDIT-C

Consists of the first 3 questions of AUDIT and is scored in the same fashion. Cut-off scores are usually 3 for women and 4 for men, although for expediency in large-scale screening programmes, sometimes a cut-off of 4 is used for both.

1. How often did you have a drink containing alcohol in the past year?

Never	(0 points)
Monthly or less	(1 point)
Two to four times a month	(2 points)
Two to three times per week	(3 points)
Four or more times a week	(4 points)

2. How many drinks containing alcohol did you have on a typical day when you were drinking in the past year?

0 drinks	(0 points)
1 or 2	(0 points)
3 or 4	(1 point)
5 or 6	(2 points)
7 to 9	(3 points)
10 or more	(4 points)

3. How often did you have six or more drinks on one occasion in the past year?

Never	(0 points)
Less than monthly	(1 point)
Monthly	(2 points)
Weekly	(3 points)
Daily or almost daily	(4 points)

Scoring varies according to standard drink size and local needs:

- In the US, a total score of 4+ for a man or 3+ for a woman is used to indicate unhealthy use.
- In the UK, if a patient scores 5+ then they are then asked to complete the remaining seven questions of the AUDIT
- Note that a US standard drink is 14 g and a UK standard unit is 8 g

Alcohol: FAST

For the following questions please circle the answer which best applies.
Note: 1 drink = ½ pint of beer or 1 small glass of wine or 1 single measure of spirits/aperitifs or 1 small glass of sherry

1. MEN: How often do you have EIGHT or more drinks on one occasion?

   WOMEN: How often do you have SIX or more drinks on one occasion?

   Never   Less than Monthly   Monthly   Weekly   Daily or almost daily

2. Only answer the following questions if the answer above is Never, Less than Monthly or Monthly. Stop here if the answer is Weekly or Daily.

   How often during the last year have you been unable to remember what happened the night before because you had been drinking?

   Never   Less than Monthly   Monthly   Weekly   Daily or almost daily

3. How often during the last year have you failed to do what was normally expected of you because of your drinking?

   Never   Less than Monthly   Monthly   Weekly   Daily or almost daily

4. In the last year has a relative or friend, or a doctor or other health worker been concerned about your drinking or suggested you cut down?

   No   Yes, but not in the last year   Yes, during the last year

Scoring

Questions 1 to 3: Never = 0, Less than Monthly = 1, Monthly = 2, Weekly = 3, Daily or almost daily = 4

Question 4: No = 0, Yes, but not in the last year = 2, Yes, during the last year = 3

If score is 0, 1 or 2 on the first question, continue with the next three questions. If score is 3 or 4 on the first question, stop. A score ≥3 indicates probable hazardous drinking.

Further reading

Hodgson R, Alwyn T, John B, *et al.* (2002). The FAST alcohol screening test. *Alcohol Alcohol* 37(1):61–6.

Nicotine: Fagerström Test

Fig. 27.2 shows the Fagerström Test for Nicotine Dependence.

PLEASE TICK (✓) ONE BOX FOR EACH QUESTION		
How soon after waking do you smoke your first cigarette?	Within 5 minutes	☐ 3
	5–30 minutes	☐ 2
	31–60 minutes	☐ 1
Do you find it difficult to refrain from smoking in places where it is forbidden? e.g. Church, Library, etc.	Yes	☐ 1
	No	☐ 0
Which cigarette would you hate to give up?	The first in the morning	☐ 1
	Any other	☐ 0
How many cigarettes a day do you smoke?	10 or less	☐ 0
	11–20	☐ 1
	21–30	☐ 2
	31 or more	☐ 3
Do you smoke more frequently in the morning?	Yes	☐ 1
	No	☐ 0
Do you smoke even if your are sick in bed most of the day?	Yes	☐ 1
	No	☐ 0
	Total Score	
SCORE	1–2 = low dependence 5–7= moderate dependence	
	3–4 = low to mod dependence 8 + = high dependence	

Fig. 27.2 Fagerström Test for Nicotine Dependence.

Add up scores from the questionnaire.

Reproduced from *Br J Addict.*, 86(9), Heatherton TF et al., The Fagerström test for nicotine dependence: a revision of the Fagerström Tolerance Questionnaire, pp. 1119–27, Copyright (2006), with permission from John Wiley and Sons

Drugs: DrugCheck

Questions

In the last 3 months:

1. Did (substance) cause any money problems for you?
2. Did (substance) make you have problems at work, or at school (College/University/training courses)?
3. Did you having housing problems because of (substance)?
4. Were there problems at home or with your family because of (substance)?
5. Did you have any arguments or fights because of (substance)?
6. Has (substance) caused any trouble with the law, or the police?
7. Has (substance) caused any health problems or injuries?
8. Have you done anything 'risky' or 'outrageous' after using (substance)? (e.g. driving under the influence; unprotected sex; sharing needles)?

Further reading

Kavanagh DJ, Trembath M, Shockley N, et al. (2011). The DrugCheck Problem List: A new screen for substance use disorders in people with psychosis. *Addictive Behaviors* 36:927–32.

Internet Addiction Test

Young's Internet Addiction Test (IAT) (Fig. 27.3) is useful as a measurement. The IAT identifies and evaluates the severity of Internet addiction. Since most of Internet Addiction is Internet gaming, the IAT could be used for gaming addiction. The IAT is a five-point scale test.

---

0 = Not Applicable. 1 = Rarely. 2 = Occasionally.

3 = Frequently. 4 = Often. 5 = Always.

1. How often do you find that you stay online longer than you intended?

2. How often do you neglect household chores to spend more time online?

3. How often do you prefer the excitement of the Internet to intimacy with your partner?

4. How often do you form new relationships with fellow online users?

5. How often do others in your life complain to you about the amount of time you spend online?

6. How often do your grades or school work suffer because of the amount of time you spend online?

7. How often do you check your e-mail before something else that you need to do?

8. How often does your job performance or productivity suffer because of the Internet?

9. How often do you become defensive or secretive when anyone asks you what you do online?

10. How often do you block out disturbing thoughts about your life with soothing thoughts of the Internet?

11. How often do you find yourself anticipating when you will go online again?

12. How often do you fear that life without the Internet would be boring, empty, and joyless?

13. How often do you snap, yell, or act annoyed if someone bothers you while you are online?

14. How often do you lose sleep due to late-night log-ins?

15. How often do you feel preoccupied with the Internet when off-line, or fantasise about being online?

16. How often do you find yourself saying "just a few more minutes" when online?

17. How often do you try to cut down the amount of time you spend online and fail?

18. How often do you try to hide how long you've been online?

19. How often do you choose to spend more time online over going out with others?

20. How often do you feel depressed, moody, or nervous when you are off-line, which goes away once you are back online?

Fig. 27.3 (*Contd.*)

> **Score (sum of responses)**
>
> **20–39 points:** You are average on-line user. You may surf the Web a bit too long at times, but you have control over your usage.
>
> **40–69 points:** You are experiencing frequent problems because of the Internet. You should consider their full impact on your life.
>
> **70–100 points:** Your Internet usage is causing significant problems in your life. You should evaluate the impact of the Internet on your life and address the problems directly caused by your Internet usage.

Fig. 27.3 Internet Addiction Test (IAT).

Reproduced from *CyberPsychology and Behavior*, 1(3), Young KS, Internet addiction: the emergence of a new clinical disorder, pp. 237–244, Copyright (1998), with permission from Mary Ann Liebert, Inc.

Further reading

Young KS. (1998). Internet addiction: the emergence of a new clinical disorder. *CyberPsychol Behav* 1:237–44.

Withdrawal monitoring scales

Alcohol Withdrawal Scale (AWS)

(The following Fig. 27.4 describes the AWS.)

Scoring
- Perspiration   (0–4)
- Tremor   (0–3)
- Anxiety   (0–4)
- Agitation   (0–4)
- Axilla temperature   (0–4)
- Hallucinations   (0–4)
- Orientation   (0–4)

Total (maximum possible is 27).

Perspiration

0 No abnormal sweating

1 Moist skin

2 Localized beads of sweat, e.g. on face, chest

3 Whole body wet from perspiration

4 Profuse maximal sweating—clothes, linen are wet.

Tremor

0 No tremor

1 Slight tremor

2 Constant slight tremor of upper extremities

3 Constant marked tremor of extremities.

Anxiety

0 No apprehension or anxiety

1 Slight apprehension

2 Apprehension or understandable fear, e.g. of withdrawal symptoms

3 Anxiety occasionally accentuated to a state of panic

4 Constant panic-like anxiety.

Agitation

0 Rests normally during day, no signs of agitation

1 Slight restlessness, cannot sit or lie still. Awake when others asleep

2 Moves constantly, looks tense. Wants to get out of bed but obeys requests to stay in bed

3 Constantly restless. Gets out of bed for no obvious reason

4 Maximally restless, aggressive. Ignores requests to stay in bed.

Fig. 27.4 (*Contd.*)

Axilla temperature

0 Temperature of 37.0°C

1 Temperature of 37.1°C

2 Temperature of 37.6–38.0°C

3 Temperature of 38.1–38.5°C

4 Temperature above 38.5°C.

Hallucinations (sight, sound, taste or touch)

0 No evidence of hallucinations

1 Distortions of real objects, aware that these are not real if this is pointed out

2 Appearance of totally new objects or perceptions, aware that these are not real if this is pointed out

3 Believes the hallucinations are real, but still orientated in place and person

4 Believes him/herself to be in a totally non-existent environment, preoccupied and cannot be diverted or reassured.

Orientation

0 The patient is fully orientated in time, place, and person

1 The patient is fully orientated in person, but is not sure where s/he is or what time it is

2 Orientated in person, but disorientated in time and place

3 Doubtful personal orientation, disorientated in time and place; there may be short periods of lucidity

4 Disorientated in time, place, and person. No meaningful contact can be obtained.

Withdrawal severity

1–4   Mild

5–9   Mild to moderate

10–14 Moderate to severe

15+   Severe

Fig. 27.4 Alcohol Withdrawal Scale (AWS).

Reproduced from New South Wales Drug & Alcohol Withdrawal Clinical Practice Guidelines, Copyright (2007), with permission from NSW Health Department

Further reading

Mental Health and Drug & Alcohol Office, NSW Department of Health (2007). *NSW Drug & Alcohol Withdrawal Clinical Practice Guidelines*. Sydney: NSW Department of Health.

Clinical Institute Withdrawal Assessment for Alcohol—Revised (CIWA-AR)

(The following Fig. 27.5 shows the CIWA-AR.)

Patient .... Date .... Time ....

Pulse or heart rate, taken for one minute: ....

Blood pressure: .... / ....Rater's initials ....

Key to scoring

- Nausea and vomiting (0–7)
- Tremor (0–7)
- Paroxysmal sweats (0–7)
- Anxiety (0–7)
- Agitation (0–7)
- Tactile disturbances (0–7)
- Auditory disturbances (0–7)
- Visual disturbances (0–7)
- Headaches, fullness in head (0–7)
- Orientation and clouding of sensorium (0–4)

Total (maximum possible is 67).

Nausea and vomiting

Ask "Do you feel sick to your stomach? Have you vomited?" and observe.

Score

0 No nausea and no vomiting

1 Mild nausea with no vomiting

2

3

4 Intermittent nausea with dry heaves

5

6

7 Constant nausea, frequent dry heaves and vomiting

Tremor

Observe patient's arms extended and fingers spread apart.

Score

0 No tremor

1 Not visible, but can be felt fingertip to fingertip

2

3

4 Moderate, with patient's arms extended

5

6

7 Severe, even with arms not extended

Fig. 27.5 (*Contd.*)

Paroxysmal sweats

Score

0 No sweat visible

1 Barely perceptible sweating, palms moist

2

3

4 Beads of sweat obvious on forehead

5

6

7 Drenching sweats

Anxiety

Observe, and ask "Do you feel nervous?"

Score

0 No anxiety, at ease

1 Mildly anxious

2

3

4 Moderately anxious, or guarded, so anxiety is inferred

5

6

7 Equivalent to acute panic states as seen in severe delirium or acute schizophrenic reactions

Agitation

Score

0 Normal activity

1 Somewhat more than normal activity

2

3

4 Moderately fidgety and restless

5

6

7 Paces back and forth during most of the interview, or constantly thrashes about

Fig. 27.5 (*Contd.*)

Tactile disturbances

Ask "Have you any itching, pins and needles sensations, any burning, any numbness or do you feel bugs crawling on or under your skin?"

Score

0 None

1 Very mild itching, pins and needles, burning or numbness

2 Mild itching, pins and needles, burning or numbness

3 Moderate itching, pins and needles, burning or numbness

4 Moderately severe hallucinations

5 Severe hallucinations

6 Extremely severe hallucinations

7 Continuous hallucinations

Auditory disturbances

Ask "Are you more aware of sounds around you? Are they harsh? Do they frighten you? Are you hearing anything that is disturbing to you? Are you hearing things you know are not there?", and observe.

Score

0 Not present

1 Very mild harshness or ability to frighten

2 Mild harshness or ability to frighten

3 Moderate harshness or ability to frighten

4 Moderately severe hallucinations

5 Severe hallucinations

6 Extremely severe hallucinations

7 Continuous hallucinations

Visual disturbances

Ask "Does the light appear to be too bright? Is its colour different? Does it hurt your eyes? Are you seeing anything that is disturbing to you? Are you seeing things you know are not there?", and observe.

Score

0 Not present

1 Very mild sensitivity

2 Mild sensitivity

3 Moderate sensitivity

4 Moderately severe hallucinations

5 Severe hallucinations

6 Extremely severe hallucinations

7 Continuous hallucinations

Fig. 27.5 (*Contd.*)

Headaches, fullness in head

Ask "Does your head feel different? Does it feel like there is a band around your head?"

Do not rate for dizziness or lightheadedness. Otherwise, rate severity.

Score

0 Not present

1 Very mild

2 Mild

3 Moderate

4 Moderately severe

5 Severe

6 Very severe

7 Extremely severe

Orientation and clouding of sensorium

Ask "What day is this? Where are you? Who am 1?"

Score

0 Orientated and can do serial additions

1 Cannot do serial additions or is uncertain about date

2 Disorientated for date by no more than 2 calendar days

3 Disorientated for date by more than 2 calendar days

4 Disorientated for place and/or person

Withdrawal severity

Mild withdrawal: Score < 10

Moderate withdrawal: Score 10–20

Severe withdrawal: Score > 20

Fig. 27.5 Clinical Institute Withdrawal Assessment for Alcohol—Revised (CIWA-AR).

Reproduced from *Br J Addict*, 84(11), Sullivan J *et al.*, Assessment of alcohol withdrawal: the revised clinical Institute withdrawal for alcohol scale (CIWA–AR), pp. 1353–1357, Copyright (1989), with permission from John Wiley and Sons.

Further reading

Sullivan J, Sykora M, Schneiderman J, *et al.* (1989). Assessment of alcohol withdrawal: the revised. Clinical Institute withdrawal for alcohol scale (CIWA–AR). *Br J Addict* 84:1353–7.

Clinical Institute Withdrawal Assessment for Benzodiazepines (CIWA-B)

(The following Fig. 27.6 shows the CIWA-B.)

Clinician observation For each of the following items, please circle the number which best describes the severity of each symptom or sign. *Patient self-report* For each of the following items, ask the patient to circle the number which best describes how he/she feels.					
1. Observe behaviour for restlessness and agitation	0 Home, normal activity	1	2 Restless	3	4 Paces back and forth, unable to sit still
2. Ask patient to extend arms with fingers apart, observe tremor	0 No tremor	1 Not visible, can be felt in fingers	2 Visible but mild	3 Moderate with areas extended	4 Severe, with arms not extended
3. Observe for sweating, feel palms	0 No sweating visible	1 Barely perceptible, palms moist	2 Palms and forehead moist, reports armpits sweating	3 Beads of sweat on forehead	4 Severe drenching sweats
4. Do you feel irritable?	0 Not at all	1	2	3	4 Very much
5. Do you feel fatigued?	0 Not at all	1	2	3	4 Severely
6. Do you feel tense?	0 Not at all	1	2	3	4 Very much
7. Do you have difficulties concentrating?	0 No difficulty	1	2	3	4 Can't concentrate
8. Do you have any loss of appetite?	0 No loss	1	2	3	4 No appetite
9. Have you any numbness or burning sensation on your face, hands or feet?	0 No	1	2	3	4 Severe
10. Do you feel your heart racing?	0 No	1	2	3	4 Constantly

Fig. 27.6 (*Contd.*)

11. Does your head feel full or achy?	0 No	1	2	3	4 Severe
12. Do you feel muscle aches or stiffness?	0 Not at all	1	2	3	4 Severe
13. Do you feel anxious, nervous or jittery?	0 Not at all	1	2	3	4 Very much so
14. Do you feel upset?	0 Not at all	1	2	3	4 Very much so
15. How restful was your sleep last night?	0 Very restful	1	2	3	4 Not at all
16. Do you feel weak?	0 Not at all	1	2	3	4 Very much so
17. Do you think you didn't have enough sleep last night?	0 No	1	2	3	4 Not nearly enough
18. Do you have any visual disturbances? (sensitivity to light, blurred vision)	0 Not at all	1	2	3	4 Yes, extreme
19. Are you fearful?	0 Not at all	1	2	3	4 Very much so
20. Have you been worrying about possible misfortunes lately?	0 Not at all	1	2	3	4 Very much so

Total score (Total of Items 1 to 20) ....
Rater's initials ....

1–20 = mild withdrawal
21–40 = moderate withdrawal
41–60 = severe withdrawal
61–80 = very severe withdrawal

Fig. 27.6 Clinical institute Withdrawal Assessment for Benzodiazepines (CIWA-B).

Reproduced from *Journal of Clinical Psychopharmacology*, 9(6), Busto UE *et al.*, A clinical scale to assess benzodiazepine withdrawal, pp. 412–416, Copyright (1989), with permission from Wolters Kluwer Health, Inc.

Further reading

Busto UE, Sykora K, Sellers EM, *et al.* (1989). A clinical scale to assess benzodiazepine withdrawal. *J Clin Psychopharmacol* 9:412–16.

The Subjective Opioid Withdrawal Scale (SOWS)

The following Fig. 27.7 shows the SOWS.

	Date .... Time					
		Please score each of the 16 items below according to how you feel now (circle one number)				
	Symptom	Not at all	A little	Moderately	Quite a bit	Extremely
1	I feel anxious	0	1	2	3	4
2	I feel like yawning	0	1	2	3	4
3	I am perspiring	0	1	2	3	4
4	My eyes are teary	0	1	2	3	4
5	My nose is running	0	1	2	3	4
6	I have goosebumps	0	1	2	3	4
7	I am shaking	0	1	2	3	4
8	I have hot flushes	0	1	2	3	4
9	I have cold flushes	0	1	2	3	4
10	My bones and muscles ache	0	1	2	3	4
11	I feel restless	0	1	2	3	4
12	I feel nauseous	0	1	2	3	4
13	I feel like vomiting	0	1	2	3	4
14	My muscles twitch	0	1	2	3	4
15	I have stomach cramps	0	1	2	3	4
16	I feel like using now	0	1	2	3	4

Range 0–64.

Fig. 27.7 The Subjective Opioid Withdrawal Scale (SOWS).

Reproduced from *American Journal of Drug and Alcohol Abuse*, 13(3), Handelsman, L et al., Two New Rating Scales for Opiate Withdrawal, pp. 93–308, Copyright (1987), with permission from Taylor & Francis.

Objective Opioid Withdrawal Scale (OOWS)

The following >Fig. 27.8 shows the OOWS.

Date .... Time			
Observe the patient during a 5 minute observation period Then indicate a score for each of the opioid withdrawal signs listed below (items 1–13). Add the scores for each item to obtain the total score			
	Sign	Measures	Score
1	Yawning	0 = no yawns	1 = ≥ 1 yawn
2	Rhinorrhoea	0 = < 3 sniffs	1 = ≥ 3 sniffs
3	Piloerection (observe arm)	0 = absent	1 = present
4	Perspiration	0 = absent	1 = present
5	Lacrimation	0 = absent	1 = present
6	Tremor (hands)	0 = absent	1 = present
7	Mydriasis	0 = absent	1 = ≥ 3 mm
8	Hot and cold flushes	0 = absent	1 = shivering/huddling for warmth
9	Restlessness	0 = absent	1 = frequent shifts of position
10	Vomiting	0 = absent	1 = present
11	Muscle twitches	0 = absent	1 = present
12	Abdominal cramps	0 = absent	1 = Holding stomach
13	Anxiety	0 = absent	1 = mild–severe

Range 0–13

Fig. 27.8 Objective Opioid Withdrawal Scale (OOWS).

Cannabis

Fig. 27.9 shows the Cannabis Withdrawal Scale.

Please indicate whether or not you have experienced these symptoms over the past 12 hours and rate their severity:	None	Mild	Moderate	Severe
1 Craving to smoke cannabis	0	1	2	3
2 Headaches	0	1	2	3
3 Decreased appetite	0	1	2	3
4 Nausea/vomiting	0	1	2	3
5 Nervousness/anxiety	0	1	2	3
6 Increased anger	0	1	2	3
7 Increased aggression	0	1	2	3
8 Mood swings	0	1	2	3
9 Irritabilitiy	0	1	2	3
10 Restlessness	0	1	2	3
11 Stomach pains	0	1	2	3
12 Vivid/unusal dreams	0	1	2	3
13 Sweating	0	1	2	3
14 Sleep difficulty	0	1	2	3
15 Shakiness/tremulousness	0	1	2	3
Other symptoms: (Please record)				
TOTAL				

Patients with cannabis dependence should be asked about the aboce symptoms twice daily The scale should be administered for the first two weeks after admission or after last known use of cannabis (marijuana).

Fig. 27.9 Cannabis Withdrawal Scale.

Reproduced from *Archives of General Psychiatry*, 58(10), Budney A. et al., Marijuana Abstinence Effects in Marijuana Smokers Maintained in Their Home Environment, pp. 917–924, Copyright (2001), with permission from the American Medical Association.

Cognitive function tests

Addenbrooke's Cognitive Examination (ACE-III)

The ACE-III is a brief cognitive test that assesses five cognitive domains: attention, memory, verbal fluency, language, and visuospatial abilities. The total score is 100 with higher scores indicating better cognitive functioning. Administration of the ACE-III takes, on average, 15 minutes and scoring takes about 5 minutes.

ADDENBROOKE'S COGNITIVE EXAMINATION – ACE-III UK Version A (2012)						
Name: Date of Birth: Hospital No. or Address:		Date of testing: _____/_____/_____ Tester's name: _____/_____/_____ Age at leaving full-time education: _____/_____/ Occupation: _____/_____/ Handedness:				
ATTENTION *(Sum together only the items in BOLD for the M-ACE score)						
➤ Ask: what is the	**Day**	**Date**	**Month**	**Year**	Season	**Attention** [Score 0-5] * ▢▢
➤ Ask: Which	No./Floor	Street/Hospital	Town	County	Country	Attention [Score 0-5] ▢
ATTENTION						
➤ Tell: "I'm going to give you three words and I'd like you to repeat them after me: lemon, key and ball." After subject repeats, say "Try to remember them because I'm going to ask you later". ➤ Score only the first trial (repeat 3 times if necessary). ➤ Register number of trials: _____						**Attention** [Score 0-3] ▢
ATTENTION						
➤ Ask the subject: "Could you take 7 away from 100? I'd like you to keep taking 7 away from each new number until I tell you to stop." ➤ If subject makes a mistake, do not stop them. Let the subject carry on and check subsequent answers (e.g., 93, 84, 77, 70, 63 – score 4). ➤ Stop after five subtractions (93, 86, 79, 72, 65): _____ _____ _____ _____ _____						**Attention** [Score 0-5] ▢
MEMORY						
➤ Ask: 'Which 3 words did I ask you to repeat and remember?' _____ _____ _____						**Memory** [Score 0-3] ▢

Fig. 27.10 *(Contd.)*

FLUENCY

➤ Letters		
Say: "I'm going to give you a letter of the alphabet and I'd like you to generate as many words as you can beginning with that letter, but not names of people or places. For example, if I give you the letter "C", you could give me words like "cat, cry, clock" and so on. But, you can't give me words like Catherine or Canada. Do you understand? Are you ready? You have one minute. The letter I want you to use is the letter "P".	Fluency [Score 0 – 7]	

≥ 18	7
14–17	6
11–13	5
8–10	4
6–7	3
4–5	2
2–3	1
0–1	0
total	correct

➤ Animals		
Say; "Now can you name as many animals as possible. It can begin with any letter."	Fluency [Score 0 – 7]	

≥ 22	7
17–21	6
14–16	5
11–13	4
9–10	3
7–8	2
5–6	1
<5	0
total	correct

MEMORY

➤ Tell: "I'm going to give you a name and address and I'd like you to repeat the name and address after me. So you have a change to learn, we'll be doing that 3 times. I'll ask you the name and address later." Score only the third trail.				Memory [Score 0 – 4]

	1st Trial	2nd Trial	3rd Trial	
Harry Barnes 73 Orchard Close Kingsbridge Devon	—— —— —— ——	—— —— —— ——		

Fig. 27.10 (*Contd.*)

MEMORY	
➢ Name of the current Prime Minister ➢ Name of the woman who was Prime Minister ➢ Name of the USA president ➢ Name of the USA president who was assassinated in the 1960s	Memory [Score 0 – 4] ☐

LANGUAGE	
➢ Place a pencil and a piece of paper in front of the subject. As a practice trial, ask the subject to **"Pick up the pencil and then the paper."** If incorrect, score 0 and do not continue further. ➢ If the subject is correct on the practice trial, continue with the following three commands below. • Ask the subject to **"Place the paper on top of the pencil"** • Ask the subject to **"Pick up the pencil but not the paper"** • Ask the subject to **"Pass me the pencil after touching the paper"** Note: Place the pencil and paper in front of the subject before each command.	Language [Score 0-3] ☐

LANGUAGE	
➢ Say: "I want you to write two sentences. It can be about anything that you like. I want you to write in full sentences and avoid abbreviations." If the subject does not know what to write about, you could suggest a few topics. "For instance, you could write about a recent holiday, your hobbies, your family or childhood." If the subject writes only one sentence, then prompt for a second one. Sentences must contain a subject and a verb. Spelling and grammar are penalized. Sentences do not need to be about the same topic. See scoring guidelines for more information.	Language [Score 0-2] ☐

LANGUAGE	
➢ Ask the subject to repeat: 'caterpillar'; 'eccentricity'; 'unintelligible'; 'statistician' Score 2 if all are correct; score 1 if 3 are correct; and score 0 if 2 or less are correct.	Language [Score 0-2] ☐

LANGUAGE	
➢ Ask the subject to repeat: 'All that glitters is not gold'	Language [Score 0-1] ☐
➢ Ask the subject to repeat: 'A stitch in time saves nine'	Language [Score 0-1] ☐

Fig. 27.10 (Contd.)

LANGUAGE

> Ask the subject to name the following pictures:

Language
[Score 0-12]

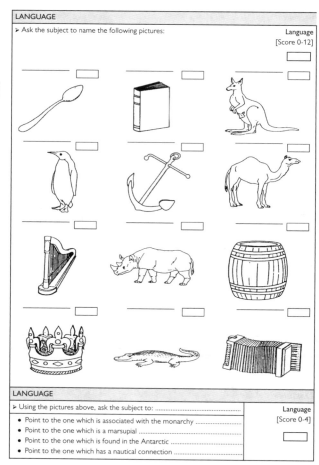

LANGUAGE

> Using the pictures above, ask the subject to: ....

• Point to the one which is associated with the monarchy ....
• Point to the one which is a marsupial ....
• Point to the one which is found in the Antarctic ....
• Point to the one which has a nautical connection ....

Language
[Score 0-4]

Fig. 27.10 (*Contd.*)

LANGUAGE

> Ask the subject to read the following words: (Score 1 only if all correct)

Language
[Score 0-1]

sew
pint
soot
dough
height

VISUOSPATIAL ABILITIES

> Infinity Diagram: Ask the subject to copy this diagram.

Visuospatial
[Score 0-1]

> Wire cube: Ask the subject to copy this drawing (for scoring, see instructions guide).

Visuospatial
[Score 0-2]

> Clock: Ask the subject to draw a clock face with numbers. Then, ask the subject to put the hands at ten past five. (For scoring see instruction guide: circle = 1, numbers = 2, hands = 2 if all correct).

Visuospatial
[Score 0-5]

Fig. 27.10 (Contd.)

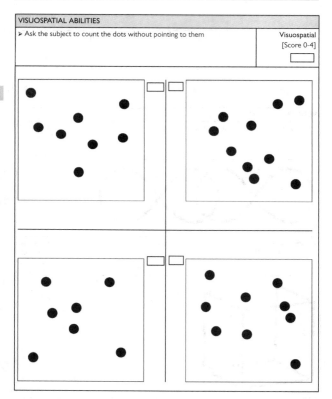

Fig. 27.10 (*Contd.*)

VISUOSPATIAL ABILITIES

> Ask the subject to identify the letters

Visuospatial
[Score 0-4]

MEMORY

> Ask "Now tell me what you remember about that name and address we were repeating at the beginning"

Harry Barnes	....	Memory
73 Orchard Close	....	[Score 0-7]
Kingsbridge	....	
Devon	....	

Fig. 27.10 (*Contd.*)

MEMORY						
▶ This test should be done if the subject failed to recall one or more items above. If all items were recalled, skip the test and score 5. If only part was recalled start by ticking items recalled in the shadowed column on the right hand side; and then test not recalled items by telling the subject "ok, I'll give you some hints: was the name X, Y or Z?" and so on. Each recognised item scores one point, which is added to the point gained by recalling.					Memory [Score 0-5]	

Jerry Barnes		Harry Barnes		Harry Bradford	recalled	
37		73		76	recalled	
Orchard Place		Oak Close		Orchard Close	recalled	
Oakhampton		Kingsbridge		Datington	recalled	
Devon		Dorset		Somerset	recalled	

SCORES	
TOTAL ACE-III SCORE	/100
TOTAL M-ACE SCORE	/30
Attention	/18
Memory	/26
Fluency	/14
Language	/26
Visuospatial	/16

Fig. 27.10 Addenbrooke's Cognitive Examination (ACE III).

Reproduced from Addenbrooke's Cognitive Examination-III (ACE-III).

Risk assessment

Suicide screen

Fig. 27.11 Suicide screen.

SUICIDE RISK ASSESSMENT AND RESPONSE		NSW✚HEALTH
A. CLIENT RISK ASSESSMENT		
SELF-HARM/SUICIDALITY: YES / NO		
Immediacy – Current thoughts? YES / NO		Comment:
Current plan: YES / NO		If YES, what is the plan
Current attempts? YES / NO		If YES, what happened:
Precipitating factors?		
Past attempts? YES / NO		If YES, where and when and what happened:
Precipitating factors?		
Family history of suicide? YES / NO		
Isolation risk? What social support does the client have?		
Is client talking/thinking about future?		
Current Overall Rating: HIGH MEDIUM	LOW	NONE

SUICIDE RISK RATING – Add 1 to the score if there has been a recent attempt		
0	NONE	No thoughts or intent of harm
1	LOW	Some current suicideal thoughts. No intent.
2	MODERATE	Suicidal preoccupation.
3	HIGH	Suicidal intent. Ill defined plan. History of attempt.
5	EMERGENCY	Clear plan and intent. Means at hand.

SUCIDE RISK ASSESSMENT SCORE = ☐

Fig. 27.11 (Contd.)

B. SERVICE RESPONSE	
Immediate response	Longer Term Response
• If a person's SUICIDE RISK ASSESSMENT SCORE is 2 or higher **you must consult** with the mental health service	• Ongoing monitoring of risk
• **Engage with client** – address the problem with the client & establish trust	• Identify triggers and safe responses
• **Identify supports** & contact if needed	• Establish protective factors
• **Develop management plan** to include health services and family supports	• Maintenance of supports for client & clinician
• **Specify follow up** contact times	• Develop coping strategies and action plan for client

Fig. 27.11 Suicide screen.

Reproduced from *Framework for Suicide Risk Assessment and Management for NSW Staff*, Copyright (2004), with permission from NSW Department of Health

Further reading

NSW Department of Health (2004). *Framework for Suicide Risk Assessment and Management for NSW Staff*. Sydney: NSW Department of Health.

Miscellaneous

The 12 steps of Alcoholics Anonymous

- We admitted we were powerless over alcohol and that our lives had become unmanageable
- We came to believe that a Power greater than ourselves could restore us to sanity
- We made a decision to turn our will and our lives over to the care of God, as we understand him
- We made a searching and fearless moral inventory of ourselves
- We admitted to God, to ourselves, and to another human being the exact nature of our wrongs
- We were entirely ready to have God remove all these defects of character
- We humbly asked Him to remove these shortcomings
- We made a list of all the persons we had harmed and became willing to make amends to them all
- We made direct amends to such people wherever possible, except when to do so would injure them or others
- We continued to take personal inventory and when we were wrong promptly admitted it
- We sought through prayer and meditation to improve our conscious contact with God as we understand him, praying only for knowledge of His will and the power to carry that out
- Having had a spiritual awakening as a result of these steps, we tried to carry this message to others, and to practice these principles in all our affairs.

(From Alcoholics Anonymous, USA.)

Useful websites

- http://www.asam.org
- http://www.bestpractice.bmj.com
- http://www.cochrane
- http://www.efnsguideline
- http://www.niaaa.nih.gov
- http://www.nhmrcgov.au/guidelines
- http://www:nice.org.uk/guidance
- http://www.samhsa.gov/about/csat.aspx
- http://www.sign.ac.uk/guidelines
- http://www.nida.nih.gov
- http://www.uptodate.com
- http://www.who.int/substance_abuse/terminology/icd_10/en/
- http://progressinmind.elsevierresource.com/
- http://www.mocatest.org/
- https://www.neura.edu.au/frontier/research/test-downloads/
- http://www.lkpz.nl/docs/lkpzpdf_1310485469.pdf

Index

A

abdominal pain 79
aboriginal, *see*
    indigenous people
acamprosate 202,
    205, 206–11
acceptance 60, 107, 275
ACE III 617
acetaldehyde 36,
    154–5, 157
acupuncture 148
acute care 85–101
acute withdrawal
    syndromes 90–3
Addenbrooke's Cognitive
    Examination (ACE
    III) 617
addiction 1–6
    ASAM definition 599
    schematic representation 6;
        see also dependence
Addiction Severity Index
    (ASI) 183
addictive disorders 1–6
addictive substances 2–3, 33
ADHD 446, 448, 481
adjustment disorder 468
adolescents 496–502
    harm reduction 501
    management 499–500
    polysubstance
        use 393–4, 498
    prevention 501
    risk factors and protective
        factors 497–9
    tips for parents 502
    warning sign of substance
        abuse 499
adrenergic toxidrome 398
adulterants 259, 418
advertising 4
affect 73
affective disorders 465
aftercare 62, 111,
    212–13, 291
age 8, 11
aggression 381, 453, 553–5
agitation 553–5
agoraphobia 466
AIDS 96
alanine transaminase 181
alcohol 151–233
    abuse 162, 597
    anxiety 229
    assessment 171

benefits of 153, 158
biomarkers 171, 179–82
birth defects 514
blood alcohol concentra-
    tion (BAC) 180, 190,
    564–6
brain damage 220, 226–7
breast milk 513
brief
    intervention 171–4,208
burden of disease 8
cardiomyopathy 223
cirrhosis 216, 222
cocaine and 334
core clinical
    syndromes 162–6
delirium 96
dental
    complications 485, 486
dependence, *see* alcohol
    dependence
depression 228
driving 564–9
drug interactions 232–3
epidemiology 8–11, 153
fetal alcohol spectrum
    disorders 228, 514–17
genetics 52–3
hallucinosis 228
harm reduction 64, 231
hazardous/harmful
    use 162
health impacts 10, 153
hepatitis 215–18, 221–2
hypertension 223
intoxication 162,
    184–5, 598
liver
    disease 215–18, 221–2
memory 226–7
metabolism 154–5
neurobiology 156
non-dependent
    disorders 162
opioids and 396, 402
paranoia 228
pathophysiology 156–7
pharmacology 34,
    36, 154–5
policy context 27
pregnancy 158, 509
prison inmates 539
safe levels of drinking 158
screening 169–71, 600–2
spectrum of use and
    misuse 158–61

standard drink 158–61
unhealthy use, *see*
    unhealthy alcohol use
units 158–61
withdrawal, *see* alcohol
    withdrawal
workplace policy 584
alcohol dehydroge-
    nase 36, 154–5
alcohol dependence 152,
    163, 164, 594, 597
continuing care 212–13
eliciting evidence of 176
in-patient treatment 211–13
mortality 168
neuroadaptation 156
ongoing treatment 200–13
overview of
    management 186
pharmacotherapy
    for relapse
    prevention 200–11
prognosis 167–8
psychosocial
    interventions 207
residential
    treatment 211–13
treatment options 152
withdrawal, *see* alcohol
    withdrawal
Alcohol-Related
    Problems (ARP)
    Questionnaire 183
alcohol use disorders 163,
    164, 597–9
    assessment 175–83
    diagnosis 182
    diagnostic
        schedules 182–3
    gambling and 434
    harm reduction 231
    history 175–9
    laboratory tests 179–82
    legal complications
        229–30
    natural history 167–8
    palliation 231
    physical
        examination 178–82
    psychosocial
        interventions 207–12
    social complications 229–30
Alcohol Use Disorders
    Identification Tests
    (AUDIT/AUDIT-C)
    169–71, 183, 600–1

alcohol withdrawal
  acute care 92
  blood alcohol
    concentration 190
  delirium tremens 96, 188,
    189, 193
  detox units 199
  diagnosis 187–91, 598
  differential diagnosis 189
  elective detoxification 197
  home/ambulatory
    detoxification 197–9
  in hospital 190–7
  investigations 189–90
  management 190–9
  monitoring 188, 190, 191
  rating scales 188,
    192, 606–11
  seizures 195–6
  syndrome 165–6
Alcohol Withdrawal Scale
  (AWS) 183, 188, 191,
    608
Alcoholics Anonymous
  (AA) 62, 110–11,
    113–15, 209–10, 627
alcoholism 163; see also
    alcohol dependence
aldehyde dehydroge-
    nase 36, 154–5
alertness 5–6
alprazolam 42, 310
ambulatory
    detoxification 197–9, 321
American Society of
    Addiction Medicine
    (ASAM) 599
amnesia, anterograde 314
amnesic episodes 214–15
amnesic syndrome 593
amotivational
    syndrome 242–3
amphetamine 12, 13
  driving 571
  epidemiology 12, 15,
    19, 329
  intoxication 337
  pharmacology 34, 43–4,
    332–3, 335
amphetamine-type
    stimulants (ATS)
  driving 571
  epidemiology 12, 328–31
  intoxication 337, 348
  natural history 22–4, 342
  pharmacology 43–4,
    332–3
  withdrawal 341
amyl nitrite 379
anabolic steroids 380–2
anaemia 223
ankle swelling 79

antihistamines 383–4, 386
antipsychotics 100, 194
antisocial personality
    disorder 434
anxiety 80, 229, 240, 242–3,
    248, 262, 290, 314–15,
    351, 360
anxiety disorders 434,
    465–8, 471, 477–8, 480
appearance 71, 73, 87–8,
    178, 344–6
applications (apps) 452
areca nut 367–8
Argyreia nervosa 356
arousal 490
ASAM diagnostic terms
    599
aspartate aminotrans-
    ferase 171, 181
Asperger's syndrome 446
  assessment 78
  alcohol 171
  alcohol intoxication 184
  alcohol use
    disorders 175–83
  benzodiazepine overdose/
    intoxications 317–18
  cannabis 245
  domestic violence 581
  elderly 519
  exercise addiction 456
  food addiction 457
  gambling 435–7
  gaming 447
  instruments 82, 183
  opioids 272–4
  psychiatric
    comorbidity 470–2
  psychosis, acute 98
  psychostimulants 344–7
  social networking
    addiction 451
  tobacco 132
  withdrawal, acute 90–2
at-risk youth 523
atrial fibrillation 88, 214
attention 74
attention deficit hyperac-
    tivity disorder 446,
    448, 481
AUDADIS 182–3
AUDIT/AUDIT-C 169–71,
    183, 600–1
autistic spectrum
    disorders 481–2
availability 4
ayahuasca 45, 46, 356

B

baclofen 204
  withdrawal 96

bacterial
    endocarditis 419, 423
bacterial infections 259–
    60, 419–20
barbiturates 96, 323
Barratt Impulsivity Scale 437
bath salts 525–6
behaviour 73
behaviour addictions
    and impulse control
    disorders 459
behavioural
    interventions 145–8
beliefs 527
benzodiazepine
    receptor 42–3
benzodiazepines
  abuse 311–12
  alcohol withdrawal 191,
    192, 193–4, 198, 199
  ambulatory
    detoxification 321
  anxiety 314–15
  clinical indications 308
  complications of
    use 314–15
  conversion table 310
  core clinical
    syndromes 311–12
  dependence 312, 319
  diazepam equivalents 310
  diazepam tapering
    regimen 321–2
  driving 571
  education 322
  epidemiology 24–5, 308
  good prescribing
    practices 116–18
  half-life 310
  harmful use 311
  injecting 314
  intoxication 311, 317–18
  misuse/hazardous use 311
  natural history 316
  neonatal withdrawal
    syndrome 511
  neuropsychiatric
    complications 314–15
  non-dependent
    misuse 311–12
  opioid maintenance
    and 284–5
  opportunistic
    intervention 316
  overdose 311, 317–18
  pharmacology 34,
    42–5, 309
  polysubstance use 396
  pregnancy 510
  prevention 325
  psychiatric
    comorbidity 315

psychological therapy 322
psychosis 315
resuscitation 87
screening 316
side effects 309
substance misuse with 478
tranquillization 100
withdrawal assessment scale (CIWA-B) 614
withdrawal delirium 96
withdrawal management 319–22
withdrawal syndrome 92, 312, 313
benzylpiperazine (BZP) 330–1, 335, 388–9
beta blockers 396, 478
beta-keto-N-methylbenzodioxolyl-propylamine 330–1
beta-ketonated amphetamines 388–9
betel 367–8
biomarkers
alcohol 171, 179–82
tobacco 134–5
bipolar disorder 480
bk-MBDB 330–1
blackouts 80, 214–15
blood alcohol concentration (BAC) 180, 190, 564–6
blood-borne infections 222, 260, 273–4, 289–90, 412–17, 506
blood pressure 87–9
body clock 490
body temperature 87–8
bradycardia 88
brain abscess 96
brain damage
alcohol-related 220, 226–7
hallucinogens 360
breastfeeding 140–1, 512–13
Brief Biosocial Gambling Screen 436
brief intervention
alcohol 171–4, 208
cannabis 246
opioids 263
psychostimulants 343
tobacco 131
bromazepam 42, 310
bruises 71
buprenorphine
equianalgesic doses 303
maintenance 278–85
and naloxone maintenance 281, 282

overdose 265
pharmacology 39–40, 41, 253, 254–5
polysubstance use 396, 402
tapering 268–71, 269
weaning off 285
withdrawal symptoms, onset and duration 267
bupropion 142–4, 353–4
buspirone 478
butylone 330–1
BZP 330–1, 335, 388–9

C

caffeine 34, 364–5, 366
calcium acetylhomotaurinate (acamprosate) 202, 205, 206–11
cancer 125, 130, 216
Candida albicans 260, 420
candidate genes 52–3
cannabidiol 37, 237–9
cannabinoid
analogues 236, 388–9
cannabis 13, 235–48
adolescents 500
assessment 245
breast milk 513
brief intervention 246
chemistry 237–9
core clinical syndromes 240–1
dental complications 485
dependence 239, 241, 247
detoxification 246
diagnosis 245
driving 570
epidemiology 12, 15, 21, 236
hashish (oil) 236, 237
hazardous/harmful use 241
history 245
intoxication 240, 246
laboratory tests 245
medical complications 242
medical marijuana 239, 244
natural history 22, 244
neuropsychiatric complications 242–3, 248
non-dependent use 241
pathophysiology 239
pharmacology 34, 37, 238–9
physical examination 245
policy 244
prevention 244
psychosis 243, 248
receptors 37, 238

schizophrenia 243
sinsemilla 237–9
skunk 37, 236, 237–9
social complications 243
therapeutic use 239
withdrawal 93, 241, 246
Cannabis indica 236
Cannabis sativa 236
Cannabis Withdrawal Scale 616
carbohydrate deficient transferrin (CDT) 171, 181
carbon monoxide 96, 134
cardiomyopathy 223
cardiovascular system 72, 79, 124, 130, 178, 223, 420
care coordination 208
care homes 521
care plan 89
caries 484
case management 208
Catha edulis 369
cathinones 330–1, 335, 388–9
CB₁ and CB₂ receptors 37, 238
CBT, see cognitive behavioural therapy
central nervous system, see CNS effects
central pontine myelinolysis 227
cerebellar degeneration 226–7
cerebral neoplasms 96
cerebrovascular accidents 96
chest pain 79
child pornography 453
child protection 575–9
children 3–4, 211, 494–5, 582
Chlamydia trachomatis genital infection 508
chlordiazepoxide 42, 192, 199, 310
chlorpheniramine 383, 386
cholesterol 181
CIDI 82, 182–3
circadian rhythm disorder 489
cirrhosis 216, 222
civil commitment 586
classical conditioning 5
classification 590–9
clinical assessment, see assessment
clinical examination 71–2

Clinical Institute Withdrawal Assessment for Alcohol – Revised (CIWA-AR) 183, 188, 191, 612
Clinical Institute Withdrawal Assessment for Benzodiazepines (CIWA-B) 614
clinicians
  harm reduction role 64–5
  responsibilities 116
clobazam 42, 310
clonazepam 42, 310
clonidine 144–8, 270
clorazepate 42, 310
CNS depressants 32
CNS effects 34, 88, 156, 226–7, 421
CNS stimulants 32
cocaine 13
  alcohol and 334
  crack 23, 45, 330, 512
  driving 570
  epidemiology 12, 15, 20, 330
  genetics 53
  intoxication 339, 348–9
  myocardial infarction 349
  natural history 22–4, 342
  pharmacology 34, 43, 45, 333–4, 335
  pregnancy 512
  synthetic 388–9
  withdrawal 341
codeine
  equianalgesic doses 303
  over-the-counter 385
  pharmacology 38, 252
coercive treatment 586–7
cognitive behavioural therapy (CBT) 209, 288–9, 352–4, 438, 448, 477
cognitive
  development 496, 503
cognitive function tests (ACE III) 617
cognitive impairment 81, 240, 242–3
cognitive state 74
cold and flu remedies 386
collateral information 78
colleagues, impaired 541–2
coma 81, 214, 555, 561
communication,
  cross-cultural 528, 531–2
community-controlled treatment 532
community
  reinforcement 209
comorbidity 109; see also psychiatric comorbidity

Composite International Diagnostic Interview (CIDI) 82, 182–3
compulsions 467
compulsive buying disorder 458
compulsory
  treatment 426, 586
computer games, see gaming
concentration 74
conditioning 5
confusion 80, 95–7, 185, 215, 240
conscious awareness 74
constipation 261
consultation-liaison service 559–60
consulting room practice 549–50
contaminants 259, 418
contingency management 209, 352–4
continuing care, see aftercare
coping skills training 209
corroborative information 78
cortical processing 50
cotinine 134, 135
couples therapy 210–11
crack cocaine 23, 45, 330, 512
crash 93
cravings 350–1
creatinine 181
crime 538–9
crystal methamphetamine 23
cue exposure treatment 209
cultural competence 531–2
cultural contexts 4, 525–8
cyanide 96
cycling 380
cyclizine 384, 386
cytisine 144
cytochrome P450 system 36, 155

D

DALYs 17
dance parties 561–2
Danshukai 115
DBT (dialectical behavioural therapy) 288–9
decongestants 386
decriminalization 27
delirium 80, 95–7, 240, 242–3, 315, 555–8
delirium tremens 96, 188, 189, 193

delta 9-tetrahydrocannabinol (THC) 37, 237–9
delta
  receptors 38–40, 251–5
delusional beliefs 73–4
demand reduction 56
denial 491–2
dental complications 71, 261, 344–5, 421, 484–8
dependence
  syndrome 48–51, 591–2
depression 80, 228, 242–3, 248, 262, 290, 315, 351, 381, 465, 470–1, 474–8, 480
designer stimulants, see synthetic stimulants
detox units 199
detoxification 60, 108
  alcohol 197–9
  benzodiazepines 321
  cannabis 246
  opioids 275
  rapid/ultra-rapid of opioids 268–71
development 494, 495, 496, 497, 503
dexamphetamine 12
dextromethorphan 383, 385
dextrose 144
diabetes 223
diagnosis 60, 67–83, 108
  alcohol use disorders 182
  alcohol withdrawal syndrome 187–91
  as basis of management 105
  cannabis 245
  DSM-IV-TR terms 594, 597
  DSM-5 terms 594, 597–9
  fetal alcohol spectrum disorders 514–15
  gambling 435–6
  ICD-10 terms 590–9
  polysubstance use 392
  psychostimulants 345–6
  sexual addictions 454
  tobacco 132
Diagnostic Interview Schedule (DIS) 82, 182–3
diagnostic
  schedules 82, 182–3
dialectical behavioural therapy (DBT) 288–9
diamorphine, see heroin
diarrhoea 79
diazepam 42, 310
  alcohol withdrawal 191, 192, 198–9
  tapering regimen 321–2

dihydrocodeine 385
dimenhydrinate 384, 386
dimethyltryptamine (DMT) 356
diphenhydramine 383, 386
DIS 82, 182–3
disorientation 215
dissociative drugs 356; see also hallucinogens, 45–6
dissociative toxidrome 399
disulfiram 203, 205, 207, 353–4
diversion 299, 586–7
doctor shopping 492, 549
domestic violence 580–2
dopamine agonists 439
dopamine system 6, 48–50, 156, 430, 444
driving
  drinking and 564–9
  drugs and 570–2
  seizures 573–4
drug dependence 15
drug-induced psychosis 97
drug interactions
  alcohol 232–3
  polysubstance use 402
drug intoxication delirium 96
drug use history 344
DrugCheck 603
DSM-IV-TR 594, 597
DSM-5 594, 597–9
dual diagnosis 462–3
dyspepsia 79
dysphoria 240
dystonia, acute 100

E
e-cigarettes 142
early intervention 57
eating disorders 481
Ecstasy, see MDMA
education 196–7, 266, 275, 322
elderly 518–21
elective detoxification
  alcohol 197
  benzodiazepines 321
electrolytes 96, 181
electronic cigarettes 142
emboli 420
emergency
  department 552–8
endocarditis 419, 423
endocrine disease 130, 179
endogenous
  cannabinoids 37, 238
endogenous opioids 156
energy drinks 364–5, 366

engagement 60, 107, 275
environment 4, 62, 112, 292, 353
ephedra 331, 335
ephedrine 384, 386
epidemiology 8–25
  alcohol 8–11, 153
  amphetamine 12, 15, 19, 329
  amphetamine-type stimulants 12, 328–31
  anabolic steroids 380
  areca nut 367
  benzodiazepines 24–5, 308
  blood-borne viral infections 412
  cannabis 12, 15, 21, 236
  child protection 575
  cocaine 12, 15, 20, 330
  elderly 518
  gambling 428–9
  gaming 442–3
  GBL 376
  GHB 376
  hallucinogens 356–7
  heroin 12
  illicit drug use 11–25
  immigrants 535
  MDMA 329–30
  mephedrone 330–1
  methamphetamine 329
  nitrites 379
  opioids 12, 15, 18, 250
  pharmaceutical opioids 299
  polysubstance use 392–4
  prison inmates 538–9
  psychiatric comorbidity 462–3
  psychostimulants 328–31
  sedative-hypnotics 308
  synthetic stimulants 330–1
  tobacco 10–11, 120–1
  volatile solvent misuse 25, 370–2
epileptogenic toxidrome 401
erythrocyte mean cell volume 171
eszopiclone 324
ethanol 157; see also alcohol
ethical issues, see legal and ethical issues
ethyl alcohol, see alcohol
ethyl glucuronide 171, 181
ethylene glycol 96
excoriations 75
executive function 74–5
exercise addiction 456

extrapyramidal side effects 100
eyes 71, 379

F
Fagerström Test for Nicotine Dependence 136, 604
family history 70, 178, 273, 344
family interventions 210–11, 477, 578–9
family support 61, 109–11, 291, 352–4
Fantasy, see GHB
FAST 602
fatty acid ethyl esters 181
fentanyl 303
fetal alcohol spectrum disorders 228, 514–17
fetal alcohol syndrome 509, 514
fetal development 505
financial management 587
5As approach 131
FLAGS 171, 246, 316, 343
flashbacks 359
flephedrone 330–1
fluid imbalance 96
flumazenil 265–6, 318
flunitrazepam 42, 310, 314
4-fluoromethcathinone 330–1
flurazepam 42, 310
fluvoxamine 39, 252
food addiction 457
forensic history 70, 178
formication 74
formulation 83, 345–6
Framework of Tobacco Control 150
free market 27
frontal cortex 50
frontal lobe syndrome 226–7
full blood count 180
functional imaging 220–1
fungal infections 260, 420

G
G, see GHB
GABA_A receptors 42–3, 309
gabapentin 204, 478
gait 72
Gamblers Anonymous 438
gambling 427–39
  antecedents 433
  assessment 435–7
  clinical syndromes 431–2
  diagnosis 432, 435–6

gambling (Contd.)
  disordered gambling
    428–9, 431–2
  epidemiology 428–9
  experience of 431
  management 438–9
  negative
    consequences 434
  pathophysiology 430
  pharmacotherapy 439
  prognosis 437
  psychiatric and social
    comorbidity 434
  psychological
    treatment 438
  remote types 429
  screening 436
gaming 441–8
  antecedents 446
  assessment 447
  clinical syndromes 445
  epidemiology 442–3
  On-Line Gamers
    Anonymous
    (OLGA) 448
  pathophysiology 444
  psychiatric
    comorbidity 446
  treatment 448
  types of games 442
gamma butyrolactone
  (GBL) 376–8
gamma-glutamyl transferase
  (GGT) 171, 180
gamma hydroxybutyrate
  (GHB) 34, 46, 376–8
gastrointestinal system 72,
  79, 88, 130, 178,
  214, 420
GBL 376–8
Gee's Linctus 385
gender differences 8, 10–11,
  15, 25, 36, 154–5
general appearance 71, 73,
  87–8, 178, 344–6
generalized anxiety
  disorder 466
genetic factors 3–4, 52–3
genital herpes 508
geographical variation
  8, 9, 11, 12, 15,
  16, 18
GHB 34, 46, 376–8
gingivitis 486
glucose 144
Grievous Bodily
  Harm, see GHB
growth 495
guarana 364
guardianship 587

H

haematological
  disorders 223
hallucinations 74, 81,
  228, 240
hallucinogenic
  toxidrome 399
hallucinogens 32
  acute
    intoxication 359, 361
  chemistry 358
  chronic use 359
  clinical syndromes 359–60
  dependence 359
  epidemiology 356–7
  pathophysiology 358
  pharmacology 34,
    45–6, 358
harm reduction 58, 63–5
  adolescents 501
  alcohol 64, 231
  dance parties 562
  injecting drug use 63–4
  opioids 293
  prison inmates 540
  tobacco 64, 150
harmful alcohol use 162
harmful drug use 15
harmful opioid use 257
harmful use 68, 591
hashish (oil) 236, 237
Hawaiian baby
  woodrose 356
hazardous alcohol use 162
hazardous use 68
head injury 96
Health of the Nation
  Outcome Scales
  (HoNOS) 82
health professionals 541–2
heart murmurs 72, 88
heartburn 79
hepatic encephalopathy 96
hepatitis, alcohol-
  induced 215–18, 221–2
hepatitis B 222, 260,
  274, 290, 412–13,
  415–16, 507
hepatitis 222, 260,
  274, 289–90, 412,
  414–16, 507
hepatitis D 222, 413, 416
hepatocellular carcinoma
  screening 416
hepatomegaly 72
herbal products 386
heritability 3–4, 52
heroin
  acute heroin reaction 259

contaminants and
  adulterants 259, 418
epidemiology 12
genetics 53
maintenance 285–6
neonatal abstinence
  syndrome 511
overdose 264–5
pharmacology 34, 38, 41,
  251, 255
pregnancy 510
quantification 272
withdrawal symptoms,
  onset and duration 267
withdrawal syndrome 92
hijacking the reward
  system 2–3
history-taking 69–70
  alcohol use
    disorders 175–9
  benzodiazepine
    dependence 319
  benzodiazepine overdose/
    intoxication 317
  cannabis 245
  domestic violence 581
  opioids 272–3
  psychostimulants 344
HIV 96, 260, 274, 290, 413,
  416, 507
'homebake' 385
homelessness 523
5HTOL:5HIAA 181
hypercalcaemia 96
hyperglycaemia 96
hypertension 72, 79,
  87–8, 223
hyperthermia 87–8, 561
hyperthyroidism 96
hyperventilation 88
hypnotherapy 148
hypocalcaemia 96
hypoglycaemia 96
hypokalaemia 97
hypomagnesaemia 96
hypomania 381
hyponatraemia 97, 561
hypotension 72, 88
hypothalamic–pituitary
  axis 156
hypothermia 87–8
hypothyroidism 96
hypoventilation 88
hypoxia 96

I

ibogaine 45–6
ICD-10 590–9
ICD admission 89

ichthyosis 374–5
illicit drug use,
    epidemiology 11–25
illusions 74, 240
immigrants 534–7
immunotherapy 354
impaired health
    professionals 541–2
impulse control
    disorders 459
income levels 8
indigenous
    people 526, 529–33
individual predisposing
    factors 3–4, 121
infections 96, 222, 259–60,
    273–4, 289, 412–17,
    419–20, 506
information 59, 107,
    275, 322
inhalants 25, 370–3
inheritance 3–4, 52
injecting drug use 407–26
    adulterants 259, 418
    benzodiazepines 314
    blood-borne viral infec-
        tions 260, 412–17, 506
    contaminants 259, 418
    dental
        complications 421, 486
    harm reduction 63–4
    hospitalized users 422–3
    laboratory tests 422
    lifestyle 419
    marginalized
        populations 524
    medical complica-
        tions 259–61, 418–23
    overdose and overdose
        deaths 408–11, 423
    physical examination 421
    pregnancy 506
    psychosocial
        complications 424–6
    unsafe injecting
        practices 418
insight 75, 240
insomnia 80, 489
insula 430
intensive day
    programmes 211
Internet Addiction Test 447,
    606
interpersonal therapy 477
interpersonal
    violence 580–2
intervention
    child protection 578–9
    domestic violence 582
    drink-driving 568–9

emergency
    department 557–8
    over-the-counter
        drugs 386–7
    scope of 56–8
    see also brief intervention
interview skills 69
intimate partner
    violence 580–2
intoxication
    acute 68, 86–9, 590
    alcohol 162, 184–5, 598
    amphetamine 337
    amphetamine-type
        stimulants 337, 348
    benzodiaz-
        epines 311, 317–18
    cannabis 240, 246
    cocaine 339, 348–9
    GHB/GBL 377
    hallucinogens 359, 361
    management of acute
        intoxication 86–9
    MDMA 338, 348
    mephedrone 340, 349
    methamphetamine 337
    psychostimulants
        337–40, 348–51
    synthetic
        stimulants 340, 349
    tobacco 126
investigations
    acute intoxication/
        overdose 88–9
    alcohol withdrawal
        syndrome 189–90
    benzodiazepine
        overdose/intoxication
        317
    psychostimulants 346–7
    tobacco 134–5
    unhealthy alcohol
        use 216, 218
    see also laboratory tests
involuntary
    treatment 426, 586

J

Japanese mutual help/
    Danshukai 115
jaundice 71, 79
judgement 75

K

kaolin and morphine 385
kappa
    receptors 38–40, 251–5
kava 374–5, 525–6

ketamine 34, 46–7, 356,
    357, 360, 571
ketamine derivatives 388–9
khat 34, 331, 335, 369
Korsakoff's
    syndrome 226–7
kratom 388–9, 525–6
krokodil 525–6

L

laboratory tests 77
    alcohol use
        disorders 179–82
    blood-borne viral
        infections 413–14
    cannabis 245
    injecting drug use 422
    lying patients 491–2
    opioids 273
    psychostimulants 346
    tobacco 134–5
    unhealthy alcohol use
        216
lactation, see breastfeeding
language 73
laxatives 384, 386
legal and ethical issues 4
    alcohol use
        disorders 229–30
    child protection 575–9
    coercive treatment 586–7
    diversion 586–7
    drinking and driving 564–9
    drugs and driving 570–2
    guardianship 587
    interpersonal
        violence 580–2
    involuntary treatment 586
    opioid maintenance
        treatment 275–8
    seizures and driving 573–4
    volatile solvent misuse
        373
    workplace safety 583–5
leucocytosis 223
leucopenia 223
licensing systems 26–8
Lie–Bet Questionnaire 436
lifestyle 62, 112, 292,
    353, 419
Liquid Ecstasy, see GHB
liver cell cancer 216
liver disease, alcohol-
    related 215–18, 221–2
liver tests 179–82
lofexidine 270
lorazepam 42, 310
lower GI bleeding 79
LSD 45–6, 356, 357

lung cancer 125
lying patients 491–2
lysergic acid diethylamide
(LSD) 45–6, 356, 357

M

macrocytic anaemia 223
magic mushrooms 45–6,
356, 357
magnesium 156
magnesium aspartate 194
major depression 465
malignancies 223
management, see treatment
mania 381
Marchiafava–Bignami
syndrome 226–7
marginalized
populations 522–4
MDMA (Ecstasy) 12
driving 571
epidemiology 329–30
intoxication 338, 348
pathophysiology 336
pharmacology 34, 43, 44,
333, 335
MDPV 330–1, 388–9
mean cell volume 171
mecamylamine 145
medical history 69, 177, 272
medical marijuana 239, 244
medical practice 26–8
medication history 70, 178
megaloblastic anaemia 223
memory 74, 314
meningitis 96
Mental Health Acts 573
mental health disorders, see
psychiatric comorbidity
mental state
examination 73–6
5-MeO-DALT 388–9
mephedrone 388–9
epidemiology 330–1
intoxication 340, 349
pharmacology 34, 335
mescaline 356
metabolic disease 130
meth mouth 344–5, 484
meth sores 344–5
methadone
equianalgesic doses 303
maintenance 276–9,
281–5
neonatal withdrawal
syndrome 511
overdose 265
pharmacology 38–40, 41,
252, 255

polysubstance
use 396, 402
tapering 268–71
weaning off 285
withdrawal symptoms,
onset and duration 267
methamphetamine 12
crystal meth 23
driving 571
epidemiology 329
genetics 53
intoxication 337
natural history 342
pharmacology 43,
332–3, 335
methanol 96
methedrone 330–1, 388–9
methoxetamine
derivatives 388–9
4-methoxymethcathinone
330–1
methylenedioxypyrovalerone
(MDPV) 330–1, 388–9
4-methylmethcathinone,
see mephedrone
α-methyltryptamine 388
microcytic anaemia 223
microsomal ethanol oxidizing
system 155
midazolam 42, 310
mirtazapine 353–4
*Mitragyna
speciosa* 388–9, 525–6
moclobemide 476–7
modafinil 353–4
monitoring 89, 92, 188,
190–1
monoamine oxidase
inhibitors 476
Montreal Cognitive
Assessment (MOCA)
75
mood 73
mood disorders 434, 465
morning glory 356
morphine 38, 252, 303
motivational enhancement
therapy 208–9, 288–9
mu receptors 38–40, 251–5
multidisciplinary
management 106
multiple disorders 105
muscle weakness 72
musculoskeletal system 72,
179, 421
mushrooms, see magic
mushrooms
mutual help, see self-help
fellowships
myoglobinuria 223

N

nabilone 239
nalmefene 201–2, 265, 439
naloxone
buprenorphine/naloxone
maintenance 281, 282
nasal spray 410–11
opioid overdose
264–5, 410–11
resuscitation 87
naltrexone
alcohol dependence
200–2, 205, 206
gambling 439
opioid dependence
268–71, 286–9
smoking cessation 145
stimulant use
disorder 353–4
Narcotics Anonymous
(NA) 113, 114, 291
NARS 150
natural history 104
alcohol use
disorders 167–8
amphetamine-type
stimulants 22–4, 342
benzodiazepines 316
cannabis 22, 244
cocaine 22–4, 342
illicit drug use 22–5
methamphetamine 342
opioids 23–4, 23–56
psychostimulants 22–4, 342
tobacco 128–9
volatile solvent misuse
371
NBOMes 356, 388–9
neck stiffness 88
neonatal benzodiaz-
epine withdrawal
syndrome 511
neonatal heroin abstinence
syndrome 511
neonatal methadone with-
drawal syndrome 511
neonatal stimulant with-
drawal syndrome 512
nerve pressure palsy 215
neuroadaptation 156
neurobehavioural dis-
order associated
with prenatal alcohol
exposure 514–15
neurobiology 5–6, 48–51,
156, 455
neurological system
see also CNS effects,
72, 179

neuroplasticity 6
neuropsychiatric complications 80–1, 224–7, 242–3, 248, 314–15, 351–4, 421
new psychoactive substances 388–9
nicotine
  dependence 123, 126, 132
  Fagerström Test 136, 604
  genetics 52, 53
  hair and nails 135
  learning and 123
  metabolism 121, 122
  pathophysiology 124–5
  pharmacology 34, 35
  pregnancy 508–9
  toxicity 141
  withdrawal 126–7
  see also tobacco
nicotine-assisted reduction to stop (NARS) 150
nicotine gum 138
nicotine inhaler 139
nicotine lozenges 139
nicotine nasal spray 139
nicotine patches 138
nicotine replacement therapies 138–41, 146, 150, 509
nicotinic acetylcholine receptors 122–3
nitrazepam 42, 310
nitrites 379
nitrous oxide 356
non-dependent alcohol use disorders 162
non-dependent substance use 68
noradrenaline and specific serotonergic agents 476
noradrenaline system 156
nortriptyline 145

O

Objective Opioid Withdrawal Scale (OOWS) 616
obsessive–compulsive disorder 467
occupational situations 543–4, 583–5
On-Line Gamers Anonymous (OLGA) 448
ondansetron 204–5
one-item screening tool 436
operant conditioning 5

opioid
  receptors 38–40, 251–5
opioid toxidrome 397
opioids 13, 249–93
  adolescents 500
  aftercare 291
  assessment 272–4
  breast milk 513
  brief intervention 263
  complications of use 259–62
  core clinical diagnoses 257–8
  dental complications 261, 485, 487
  dependence 256, 258, 275–92, 297, 300, 302–3
  detoxification 275
  driving 271
  endogenous 156
  environment 292
  epidemiology 12, 15, 18, 250
  equianalgesic doses 303
  family support 291
  harm reduction 293
  harmful use 257
  history 272–3
  hyperalgesia 297
  laboratory tests 273
  lifestyle 292
  maintenance treatment 275–86
  medical complications 259–61, 289–91
  natural history 23–4, 256
  Objective Opioid Withdrawal Scale (OOWS) 616
  opioid use disorder 257
  over-the-counter 383, 385
  overdose 259, 264–6, 408–11
  pain management 295–306
  palliation 293
  pathophysiology 256
  pharmacology 34, 38–41, 251–5
  pharmacotherapy 275–89
  physical examination 273
  polysubstance use 396, 402
  pregnancy 510
  prevention 293
  principles of prescribing 301

prison inmates 539–40
protracted abstinence syndrome 262, 291
psychiatric comorbidity 262, 290–1
psychological therapies 288–90
rapid detoxification 268–71
self-help organizations 291
social complications 262
social support 291
Subjective Opioid Withdrawal Scale (SOWS) 615
ultra-rapid detoxification 268–71
withdrawal management 267–71
withdrawal scales 615, 616
withdrawal syndrome 92, 258
opium 12
opportunistic healthcare 316, 501
oral complications 484–8
organic brain syndromes 360
orientation 74
outcome 104
outpatient services 551
outreach 501
over-the-counter drugs 383–7
overdose 68, 86–9
  barbiturates 323
  benzodiazepines 311, 317–18
  buprenorphine 265
  GHB/GBL 377
  heroin 264–5
  injecting drug use 408–11, 423
  methadone 265
  opioids 259, 264–6, 408–11
  psychostimulants 340, 348–51
oxazepam 42, 310
oxycodone 303

P

p-methoxymethamphetamine 330–1, 335
pain management 295–306
  acute 304
  assessment 300
  chronic 302–3

palliation 150, 231, 293
palpitations 79
pan masala 367–8
pancreatitis 220, 223
panic attacks 240, 242–3
panic disorder 466,
471, 477–8
paradoxical inhibition 315
paranoia 228, 240, 242–3
paranoid delusions 81
parents
   of adolescent substance
      users 500, 502
   as substance users 494,
      495, 576–9
partial fetal alcohol
   syndrome 514
partygoers 561–2
passive smoking 10–11, 120
Pathological Gambling
   Modification of the
   Yale-Brown Obsessive
   Compulsive Scale 437
pathophysiology
   alcohol 156–7
   anabolic steroids 380–2
   areca nut 367
   cannabis 239
   gambling 430
   gaming 444
   hallucinogens 358
   MDMA 336
   opioids 256
   psychostimulants 336
   tobacco 124–5
Paullinia cupana 364
Pavlovian conditioning 5
peer pressure 4
perception 74, 240
periodontal disease 486
peripheral neuropathy 227
pethidine 303
pharmacology 2–3, 32–47
   alcohol 34, 36, 154–5
   amphetamine 34, 43–4,
      332–3, 335
   amphetamine-type
      stimulants 43–4, 332–3
   anabolic steroids 380
   areca nut 367
   benzodiazepines 34,
      42–5, 309
   buprenorphine 39–40, 41,
      253, 254–5
   caffeine 34, 364
   cannabis 34, 37, 238–9
   cocaine 34, 43, 45,
      333–4, 335
   codeine 38, 252
   dissociative drugs 45–6
   ephedra 335
   GBL 376–7

GHB 34, 46, 376–7
hallucinogens 34,
   45–6, 358
heroin 34, 38, 41,
   251, 255
kava 374
ketamine 34, 46–7
khat 34, 335, 369
MDMA 34, 43, 44,
   333, 335
mephedrone 34, 335
methadone 38–40, 41,
   252, 255
methamphetamine 43,
   332–3, 335
morphine 38, 252
nicotine 34, 35
opioids 34, 38–41,
   251–5
psychostimulants 43–6,
   332–5
sedative-hypnotics 42–5
synthetic stimulants 335
tobacco 35, 122–3
volatile solvents 371–2
pharmacotherapy 60–1, 108
   alcohol depend-
      ence, relapse
      prevention 200–11
   elderly 520
   exercise addiction 456
   food addiction 457
   gambling 439
   gaming 448
   opioid
      dependence 275–89
   sexual addictions 455
   smoking cessation 138–48
   stimulant use
      disorder 352–4
   young adults 503
phencyclidine 356, 357
phencyclidine
   derivatives 388–9
phenylethylamine
   derivatives 388–9
phenylpiperazine
   derivatives 388–9
phenytoin 39, 252
phospatidylethanol 171, 181
physical disorders 4
physical examination 71
   alcohol use
      disorders 178–82
   cannabis 245
   domestic violence 581
   injecting drug use 421
   opioids 273
   psychostimulants 344–6
   tobacco 133
Piper methysticum 374–
   5, 525–6

piperazines 330–1
PMA/PMMA 330–1, 335
police 562
policy context 26–9, 244,
   536–7, 584
polysubstance use 391–405
   acute presentations 396
   adolescents 393–4, 498
   diagnosis 392
   drug interactions 402
   epidemiology 392–4
   management 403–5
   non-acute
      presentations 395
   pregnancy 512
   reasons for combining
      drugs 395
   specific combination
      effects 396
   toxidromes 397
poppers 379
pornography 453
post-incident testing 585
post-traumatic stress disorder 467–8, 471, 479
prazosin 204–5
predisposing
   factors 3–4, 121
pregabalin 204
pregnancy 505–13
   alcohol 158, 509
   benzodiazepines 510
   cocaine 512
   heroin/opioids 510
   injecting drug use 506
   multiple substance
      use 512
   nicotine 130, 508–9
   nicotine replacement
      therapies 140–1
   opioid
      maintenance 280, 284
   STIs 508
preoccupations 73–4
prescribed
   medications 70, 405
prescribing practices
   116–18
prescription only 26–8, 29
presentations 68, 79
prevention 56, 89
   adolescents 501
   benzodiazepines 325
   blood-borne viral
      infections 417
   cannabis 244
   dental complications 487
   fetal alcohol spectrum
      disorders 516–17
   heroin/opioid overdose
      deaths 410–11
   immigrants 536

opioids 293
oral complications 487
over-the-counter product abuse 387
policy context 26–9
prison inmates 539
tobacco 150
volatile solvent misuse 373
primary healthcare 117–18, 131, 173–4, 546–8
primary intervention 56
prison inmates 538–40
problematic use 14–15
prohibition 27, 28
protracted abstinence syndrome 262, 291
pseudoephedrine 384, 386
psilocybin (magic mushrooms) 45–6, 356, 357
psychedelic drugs, see hallucinogens
psychiatric comorbidity 4, 61, 105, 109, 461–82
adapting addiction treatment 473
alcohol use 228–30
assessment 470–2
benzodiazepines 315
epidemiology 462–3
gambling 434
gaming 446
opioids 262, 290–1
prison inmates 538, 540
psychiatric management 472–3, 474–9
sexual addictions 454
psychiatric disorders 465–8
psychiatric history 69, 177, 272, 344
psychodynamic psychotherapy 477
psychological mechanisms 5
psychological therapy 61, 108–9
benzodiazepines 322
depression 477
elderly 520–1
gambling 438
opioids 288–90
psychosis 479
PTSD 479
sexual addictions 455
stimulant use disorder 352–4
psychomotor impairment 240
psychosis 97, 98–101, 243, 248, 315, 351, 359–60, 381, 469, 471, 479, 481
psychosocial complications 424–6

psychosocial development 496, 503
psychosocial interventions 100, 207–12, 503
psychostimulants 327–54
assessment 344–7
breast milk 513
brief intervention 343
clinical syndromes 337–41
dental complications 485, 487
diagnosis 345–6
epidemiology 328–31
formulation 345–6
history 344
intoxication 337–40, 348–51
investigations 346–7
laboratory tests 346
natural history 22–4, 342
neuropsychiatric complications 351–4
overdose 340, 348–51
pathophysiology 336
pharmacology 43–6, 332–5
pharmacotherapy 353–4
physical examination 344–6
screening 343
stimulant use disorder 340–1, 344–7, 352–4
substitution therapy 353–4
withdrawal 93, 341, 349–52
psychotic disorder (ICD-10) 592
public venues 561–2
pulmonary system 130, 261, 420
pulpitis 486
pulse rate 87–9
pupils 71, 88
pyramiding 380

Q

qat, see khat

R

random testing 584, 585
rapid opioid detoxification 268–71
rapport 73
raves 561–2
reboxetine 476
recovery from substance abuse disorder 56–8, 60–3, 109–11, 112
alcohol 208, 209, 210
food addiction 457

gambling 434, 438
opioid dependence 285, 296
residential services 551
self-help groups 113, 114–15, 116
SMART Recovery® 209–10
stimulant use disorder 349–51
recruitment screening 585
reduced consciousness 554–5, 561
referral 117–18, 547
refugees 534–7
regulation 27, 28–9
renal disease 261, 421
residential services (rehab) 211–13, 551
residual and late-onset psychotic disorder 593
respiratory system 72, 88, 124, 178, 214
resuscitation 87
retirement facility living 521
reward system 2–3, 5–6, 156, 444
rhabdomyolysis 88–9, 223, 261, 561
rifampicin 39, 252
rimonabant 241
risk assessment 86, 625–6
risk factors
adolescents 497–9
domestic violence 580
immigrants 534
impaired health professionals 499
indigenous people 529
smoking 121
risky use 68
roid rage 381
routine testing 584, 585

S

SADQ 183
safety-critical occupations 543–4
Salvia divinorum 388–9
SAM 82
Saturday night palsy 215
Schedules for Clinical Assessment in Neuropsychiatry (SCAN) 82, 182–3
schizophrenia 97, 243

screening
alcohol 169–71, 600–2
benzodiazepines 316
gambling 436
hepatocellular
carcinoma 416
instruments and question-
naires 82, 600–5
psychostimulants 343
tobacco 131, 136, 604
second-hand
smoke 10–11, 120
secondary intervention 57
sedating antihistamines
383–4, 386
sedation 91, 191
sedative-hypnotics
epidemiology 308
pharmacology 42–5
polysubstance use 403
toxidrome 397
withdrawal 312, 323, 324
seizures 80, 88, 195–6,
561, 573–4
selective serotonin reuptake
inhibitors 204–5, 474
self-help fellowships 62,
110–11, 113–15, 209–10,
291, 353, 438, 448
sepsis encephalitis 96
serotonin 156
serotonin and noradrenaline
reuptake inhibitors 475
serotonin
syndrome 97, 351–4
Severity of Alcohol
Dependence
Questionnaire
(SADQ) 183
sex workers 523
sexual addictions 454–5
sexual identity 523–4
sexual risk-taking 214
sexually transmitted
infections 261, 508
shopping compulsion 458
shortness of breath 79
sildenafil 386
silver acetate 145
silver nitrate 145
sinsemilla cannabis 237–9
skin 71, 179, 344–5
skunk 37, 236, 237–9
sleep disorders 489–90
SMART Recovery® 209–10
smoking, see tobacco
smoking cessation 137–49
acupuncture 148
behavioural
interventions 145–8
benefits 129
cold turkey 137

follow-up 148
hypnotherapy 148
nicotine replacement
therapies 138–41,
146, 509
pharmacotherapy 138–48
weaning off nicotine 149
sniffer dogs 562
social anxiety
disorder 466–7
social attitudes 526
social complications 215,
229–30, 243, 262
social factors 4, 519
social history 70, 178, 273
social learning 5
social media 450–1
social network therapy 209
social networking
addiction 450–1
social norms 526
social phobia 466–7
social support 61, 109–11,
118, 291, 352–4, 439
sodium oxybate 204
solvents 25, 370–3
South Oaks Gambling
Screen 436
specialist
services 117–18, 551
speech 72, 73
Spice 236, 525–6
splenomegaly 72
sponsors 114
stacking 380
stigmatization 527
stimulant use disorder
340–1, 344–7, 352
street names 32
stroke 215
subculture 4
subdural
haematoma 96, 215
Subjective Opioid
Withdrawal Scale
(SOWS) 615
substance abuse 68, 597
Substance Abuse Module
(SAM) 82
substance dependence 594,
68, 597
schematic
representation 6
substance intoxication
598
substance/medication-
induced mental disorders
(DSM-5) 598–9
substance use
epidemiology 8–25
genetics 52–3
neurobiology 48–51

policy and
prevention 26–9
substance use
disorder 68, 597–9
substance withdrawal
delirium 96
substance withdrawal
syndrome 68, 598
sudden death sniffing
syndrome 372
suicide risk 75–6, 94, 100,
215, 371
suicide screen 625–6
supplements 92
supply reduction 56
support 89, 92, 495
supportive
psychotherapy 477
suspiciousness 240
sweating 71, 80
sympathomimetics 384, 386
synthetic
cannabinoids 236, 388–9
synthetic cocaine 388–9
synthetic stimulants 388–9
epidemiology 330–1
intoxication 340, 349
pharmacology 335
syphilis 508
systematic
examination 72, 87–9

T

Tabex® 144
taboo 527
tachyarrhythmias 72, 88
tachycardia 72
tachypnoea 88
teeth, see dental
complications
temazepam 42, 310
Temperament and Character
Inventory 437
tertiary intervention 57–8
tetraethylthiuram disulphide
(disulfiram) 203, 205,
207, 353–4
tetrahydrocannabinol
(THC) 37, 237–9
thiamine 87, 184–5, 194–5,
225, 227, 231
thought content 73–4
thought form 73
thrombocytopenia 223
tobacco 119–50
biomarkers 134–5
breast milk 513
brief intervention 131
burden 10–11
clinical assessment 132
clinical syndromes 126–7